D0259682

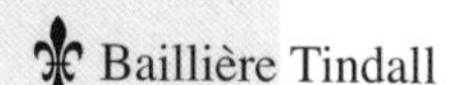
Baillière Tindall

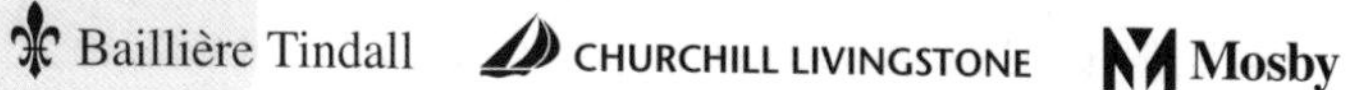
CHURCHILL LIVINGSTONE

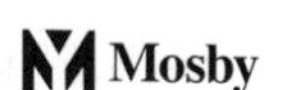
Mosby

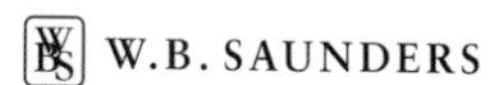
W.B. SAUNDERS

Clinical
PAEDIATRICS
and Child Health

For W. B. Saunders:

Commissioning Editor: Ellen Green
Project Development Manager: Sarah Keer-Keer
Project Manager: Frances Affleck
Designer: Sarah Russell

Clinical PAEDIATRICS and Child Health

David Candy MB BS MSc MD FRCPCH
Consultant Paediatric Gastroenterologist
St Richard's Hospital, The Royal West Sussex NHS Trust, Chichester, UK
Visiting Senior Lecturer, Department of Child Health, University of Southampton, UK

E. Graham Davies MA FRCP FRCPCH
Consultant Paediatrician and Immunologist
Great Ormond Street Hospital for Sick Children NHS Trust, London, UK

Euan Ross MD FRCP FRCPCH FFPHM DCH
Formerly Professor of Community Paediatrics
Department of Community Paediatrics, King's College, London, UK

With major contributions from:

Pamela Johnson MD MRCGP MRCOG
Senior Lecturer in Obstetrics and Gynaecology, Imperial College School of Medicine, London, UK

Michael Salman MB BS BSc MSc DCH MRCP
Division of Neurology, Hospital for Sick Children, Toronto, Canada

Susan Leech MA, MSc, MRCP, DCH
Consultant Paediatrician, King's College Hospital, London, UK

Illustrated by Paul Richardson

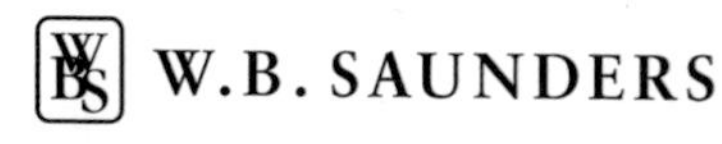

Edinburgh • London • New York • Philadelphia • St Louis • Sydney • Toronto 2001

W. B. SAUNDERS
An imprint of Harcourt Publishers Limited

First published 2001

ISBN 0 7020 1726 4

British Library Cataloguing in Publication Data
A catalogue record for this book is available from the British Library

Library of Congress Cataloging in Publication Data
A catalog record for this book is available from the Library of Congress

Medical knowledge is constantly changing. As new information becomes available, changes in treatment, procedures, equipment and the use of drugs become necessary. The editors and contributors, and the publishers have, as far as it is possible, taken care to ensure that the information given in this text is accurate and up to date. However, readers are strongly advised to confirm that the information, especially with regard to drug usage, complies with the latest legislation and standards of practice.

The publisher's policy is to use **paper manufactured from sustainable forests**

Printed in Spain

Contents

Acknowledgements

We would like to express our sincere thanks to our publishers who encouraged us to keep writing, re-writing and stay sane. Dr Pamela Johnson had a major input into the first chapter. We are very grateful to Drs Sue Leech and Michael Salman, clinical lecturers in Child Health at King's College Hospital, who did a great deal of editing work on early drafts, and to many consultant colleagues (listed below) who read through bits of the book when we needed further opinions, especially Dr Lesley Davidson in Oxford, and Dr Marion Crouchman and Dr Charles Buchanan at King's College Hospital. The philosophical thinking in this book was passed on to us by our own teachers; we hope that we have not misrepresented them too much. Finally, we are grateful to our wives and families for their forbearance.

D.C.
G.D.
E.R.

Chapter	Co-author	Affiliation
Accidents	**Lesley Davidson** Director, NPEU Honorary Consultant in Public Health Medicine	National Perinatal Epidemiology Unit Radcliffe Infirmary Oxford
Accidents	**Jonathan Sibert** Professor of Community Child Health	Department of Child Health University Hospital of Wales Cardiff
Cardiology	**Marion Crouchman** Consultant Neurorehabilitation Paediatrician	Paediatric Neurosciences King's College Hospital London
Cardiology	**Sandy Calvert** Consultant Neonatologist	St George's Hospital London
Child Abuse	**Aideen Naughton** Consultant Paediatrician (Community Child Health)	Newport, Wales
Endocrinology	**Charles Buchanan** Senior Lecturer in Paediatric Endocrinology	Variety Club Children's Hospital King's College Hospital London
Nephrology And Oncology	**Simon Meller** Consultant Paediatrician and Paediatric Oncologist	Royal Marsden Hospital Surrey
Respirology	**Gary Ruiz** Consultant Paediatrician	King's College Hospital London

Preface

The way paediatrics and child health is being taught is changing rapidly. This book has been written in an attempt to meet the challenge that such change poses. It is impossible to learn the whole subject in a few weeks as an undergraduate or in the early part of a hospital residency. The emphasis is now on knowing where to look rather than keeping vast stores of knowledge in one's head.

The book is divided into two sections. In Section 1 we go over general principles and how child health differs from the rest of medical practice. This book differs from its competitors because we have chosen to study the normal growing child in a chronological sequence and to deal with illnesses using a symptom-based approach. We have tried to avoid the repeated description of important disorders in succeeding chapters. We may mention important and common conditions, and we give the details in Section 2, which is essentially a brief encyclopaedia of childhood disorders. We spent much time agonizing over the conditions that should be listed or excluded.

We recommend that you read all of Section 1 of this book as soon as you start to study paediatrics. Before you start to see children, read up about their physical and psychological development. Know something about the pioneers of the subject, such as Dr Mary Sheridan on children's developmental progress, Noam Chomsky on the development of language, John Bowlby and Penelope Leach.

Where can you learn? In part this will be in paediatric wards and outpatient departments. Children encountered in these places are a selected group, especially in teaching hospitals, where rare disorders will be over-represented. Some exposure to unusual, often serious, acute and chronic conditions is important, particularly observation of the effects such illnesses have on the family. This could distort your understanding of the reality of present day child health, however. Contrasting experience from primary care, observing at first hand the work of family doctors and health visitors (who carry out most child health work in the UK) and from accident and emergency units will provide the necessary balance. Community child health services provide the organizational and specialist framework for out-of-hospital paediatrics, especially child protection, immunization and specialist care of children with disability. They work closely with acute paediatrics, child psychiatry, audiology, ophthalmology and public health services. They have close working links with local authority services, both social and educational.

We hope that you will wear this book out through hard use and supplement your reading from larger textbooks, journals and the Internet whenever you see a child with an unfamiliar condition. We would like to hear from you. If you find mistakes, feel disappointed that we have left out important conditions or want us to rewrite topics, please contact us.

D.C.
G.D.
E.R.

1

Paedriatric principles

a developmental approach

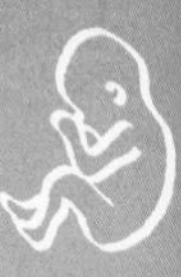

1 Birth and before birth

Introduction

Most pregnancies (about 90%) do not require medical intervention. Increasingly, midwives deal with normal pregnancies, often in the community setting. It is important that low risk pregnancies are distinguished from those at increased risk, in order to anticipate problems. Where these do occur, advances in medical care of the fetus have greatly improved the outlook. The fetus is no longer inaccessible, knowledge of fetal physiology and pathophysiology has increased dramatically in the past 20 years (Information box 1.1), and advances in ultrasound imaging have been crucial in this development.

For paediatricians, increasing knowledge of fetal life enhances their understanding of the problems faced by the neonate as well as greater understanding of how certain congenital problems develop. The events that occur in utero have long-lasting effects on the individual. A team approach permits optimal management of perinatal problems, with improved paediatric outcome.

Advances in diagnosis and therapeutics have created many ethical problems. These are of major concern to potential parents and those involved in care during pregnancy and the early life of the child.

Key issues

The main aim of those involved in fetal medicine is to optimize the outcome of pregnancy. Diagnostic procedures permit the gathering of information on

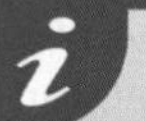

Information Box 1.1

The specialties of fetal and perinatal medicine embrace:

- Embryology
- Genetics
- Obstetrics
- Neonatology
- Paediatric surgery

which the parents, obstetricians and paediatricians can base their decisions. Options that need to be considered when presented with a fetus that is abnormal in any way include the termination of the pregnancy. Other management issues include the timing, mode and place of delivery. In rare cases, intrauterine surgery has been undertaken.

Definitions and statistics

Birth rate

In the UK, a population of 1000 people of all ages and both sexes produces 11–14 babies per year. This is the 'crude birth rate' and from this figure it is possible to estimate the expected local birth rate. Approximately 650 000 infants are born annually in the United Kingdom: an average of 2.1 children per family. The crude birth rate in developing countries is of the order of 50 babies per year.

The increase or decrease of the population of a country depends on the stillbirth rate, crude birth rate, infant and childhood mortality and adult mortality. These factors in turn are influenced globally by famine, war, and the incidence of infectious diseases, especially diarrhoea and pneumonia.

The birth rate in the UK and other high income nations is falling. As medical services improve and personal wealth increases, there is greater contraceptive usage and a gradual reduction in birth rate. The fall in birth rate is directly related to the increase in gross national product of a country.

Whilst the birth rate is higher in poorer countries, this is matched by higher maternal, perinatal and infant mortality rates. The level of deprivation in any particular region or country is accurately reflected in these figures.

Maternal mortality

A *maternal death* is defined as the death of a woman from any cause during pregnancy or within 6 weeks of delivery. The maternal mortality in England and Wales is currently 12.2 per 100 000 maternities. This compares favourably with the figure of 428 per 100 000 in 1928. In low income nations, however, the maternal mortality rate is still around 400 per 100 000, a risk of dying of 1 in 250.

Perinatal mortality

A *stillbirth* is defined as any baby born without signs of life after 24 weeks' gestation. Prior to 1992, a stillbirth was defined as a baby born dead after 28 weeks' gestation. It is a reflection of advances in neonatology that many babies born between 24 and 28 weeks now survive, and that this has necessitated a review of the definition of stillbirth (see Spontaneous miscarriage/therapeutic abortion, below).

The *perinatal mortality rate* is the number of stillbirths combined with the number of deaths within the first week of life, per 1000 still- and live births).

The perinatal mortality rate for England and Wales has more than halved in the past 20 years. Whilst there has been a decrease in these death rates, the rate of decline is now less than previously, and it may be that we are approaching the limit of avoidable deaths. Epidemiological data relating to perinatal mortality are given in Chapter 2 (p. 23).

The hazards of birth and the neonatal period are reflected in the fact that perinatal and neonatal mortality (death in the first 28 days of life) are greater than mortality at other ages. In any population these rates are influenced by a wide variety of factors, especially the rate of prematurity and therefore of low birthweight (LBW) and very low birthweight (VLBW) deliveries. Other factors include maternal nutrition and health (including smoking), socioeconomic status, and the incidence of genetic disorders (see Information box 1.2). Many of these factors influence intrauterine growth leading to the birth of infants who are small for gestational age (SGA).

Spontaneous miscarriage/ therapeutic abortion

A pregnancy loss before 24 weeks is defined as an abortion or miscarriage, and may be spontaneous or induced. Spontaneous miscarriage occurs most often during the first 12 weeks of pregnancy with up to 25% of conceptions being lost, many before the mother knows she is pregnant. There are numerous causes of

Information Box 1.2

Adverse maternal influences on perinatal mortality

- Pregnancy complications
- Smoking
- Low socioeconomic status
- Poor nutrition
- Very high parity
- Disease pre-dating the pregnancy
- Alcohol/drug abuse
- Age <16 or >35 years

spontaneous pregnancy loss, but it is well established that a proportion of pregnancies complicated by fetal chromosomal or structural abnormality will miscarry. This means that the true incidence of chromosomal abnormalities will be underestimated if account is not taken of chromosomally abnormal miscarriages.

The mechanism of attrition for fetuses with certain types of aneuploidy (having an abnormal number of a particular chromosome(s); p. 239) is poorly understood.

Induced abortion may be therapeutic or criminal, the latter being mercifully rare in the United Kingdom. The grounds on which a pregnancy may be terminated are covered by the Human Embryology Act, 1991, which permits termination up to 24 weeks of gestation on the grounds of potential physical or psychological harm to the mother. Where there is a substantial risk of the fetus having a very severe handicap, there is no gestational age limit. The proportion of terminations performed for fetal abnormality is around 1% (1752 out of 160 501 in 1992). Most of the others are performed for reasons involving maternal mental health. In some areas of the UK, the termination rate approaches that of the birth rate – a sobering statistic when one considers that contraception is freely available.

With advances in neonatology, there are now a number of babies born before 24 weeks' gestation who survive. Whilst the chances of this are small (<20%), it raises ethical problems for those staff who are faced with the problems of trying to save the lives of these babies whilst also being involved in termination of pregnancies at the same gestations. These ethical dilemmas are considered in Chapter 2 (p. 24).

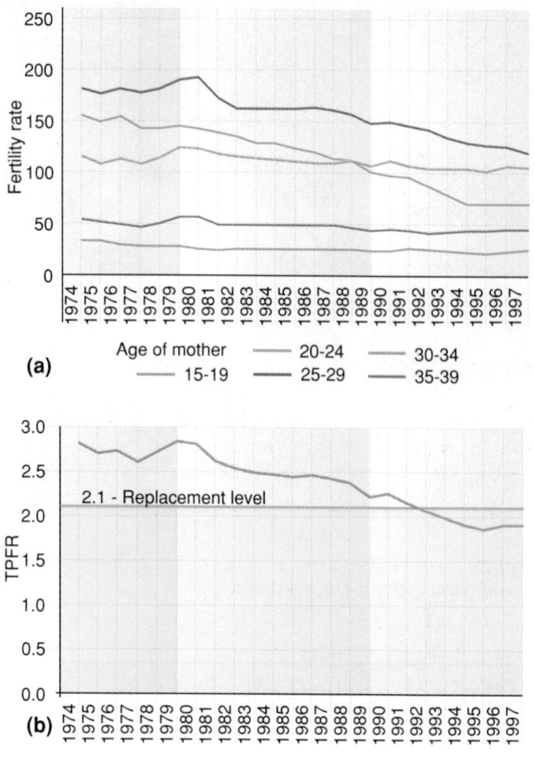

Fig 1.1
(a) Live births per 1000 women by age of mother, in Northern Ireland 1974–1997 (76th Annual Report of the Registrar-General, 1998).
(b) Total period fertility rate (TPFR) for 1974–1997 (same source). In western countries a TPFR of 2.1 is required to maintain long-term population levels, assuming no migration. Reproduced with permission of The General Register Office (Northern Ireland Statistics and Research Agency).

Fertility rates

The general fertility rate is expressed as the number of live births per 1000 women aged between 15 and 45 years. In the UK, the fertility rate has fallen in the last 20 years (Fig. 1.1). This fall in the fertility rate is partly due to the use of contraception and also due to the fact that, because fertility falls with increasing age, as women delay starting their families there are fewer pregnancies overall.

Multiple pregnancy

The majority of human pregnancies are singletons, but multiple pregnancies occur both naturally and as a result of assisted-conception techniques. In the UK, twin pregnancy occurs at a rate of approximately 1 in 80 births and naturally occurring triplets at 1 in 6400 (triplets have increased due to fertility treatment). One-third of twins are monozygotic (arising because of early division of the fertilized ovum) and two-thirds dizygotic (two ova are released and fertilized). There is often a family history of dizygotic twins. Monozygotic twin births occur at a relatively constant rate while dizygotic twinning varies in different races; the rate is highest in negro and lowest in mongolian races.

Twin and multiple pregnancies are more prone to obstetric complications. There is a greater likelihood of congenital anomaly, premature delivery and low birth-weight. Rarely, twins may be conjoined due to incomplete division of the zygote. The site and extent of conjoining varies and in the severest cases proves fatal for both twins, though successful surgical separation can sometimes be achieved. In monozygotic twins who share a placenta but have separate amniotic sacs (monochorionic, diamniotic) there is a risk of twin–twin transfusion, resulting in one twin (the donor) becoming anaemic and growth-restricted, with reduced amniotic fluid (oligohydramnios). The other twin becomes well grown, but polycythaemic with excessive liquor (polyhydramnios) (Fig. 1.2). Increased perinatal mortality and morbidity are associated with monochorionic twins.

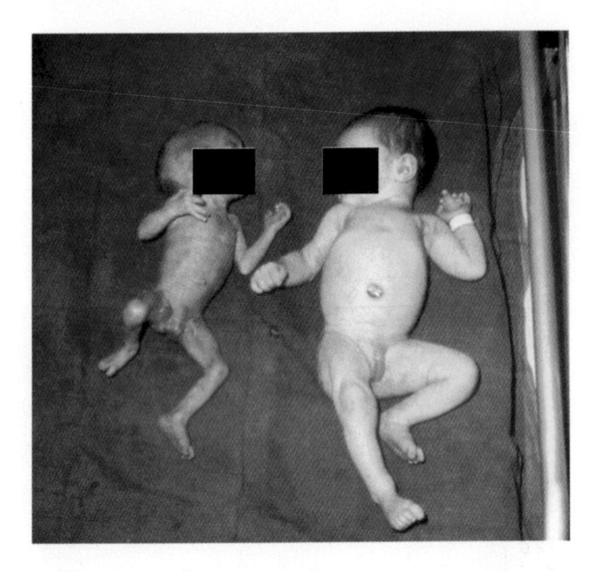

Fig 1.2
Severe example of twin–twin transfusion.

Clinical approach

Care before pregnancy and prevention of abnormality

The outcome of a pregnancy has the best prospect if the mother is healthy at the time of conception, and remains so during the pregnancy. Education and counselling before pregnancy are of definite value in encouraging women to stop smoking, reduce their alcohol intake and get fit. Women with preexisting medical problems, e.g. diabetes mellitus, benefit from high quality management before and during pregnancy. Control of such medical conditions gives the best fetal outcome if achieved preconceptually.

Couples with a history of fetal abnormality or loss need to be counselled before any subsequent pregnancy, with particular regard to the chances of recurrence and any preventative measures that may be available. The best example of the latter is the maternal administration of folic acid in all pregnancies, prior to conception and during the period of organogenesis, in the prevention of neural tube defects. Periconceptual folic acid supplementation of up to 4 mg per day has led to a 50–80% reduction of recurrence of neural tube defects.

Pre-pregnancy counselling also permits identification of risk factors for genetic disorders so that appropriate investigations may be performed as early as possible in the pregnancy, e.g. first-trimester chorionic villus sampling when both parents are carriers of the gene for cystic fibrosis.

Screening of immune status against certain infections can also be performed before pregnancy, the best example being checking the rubella antibody status of the mother (see p. 16). If a woman is not immune, the ideal time to offer immunization is before pregnancy. The need to avoid conception within 3 months of this immunization should be emphasized.

Antenatal care

Routine investigations performed during antenatal care are aimed at detecting maternal disease and complications of pregnancy, as well as the assessment of fetal wellbeing. When women book for antenatal care it is essential to identify any risk factors for complications as early as possible. These include smoking, alcohol intake, problems that have occurred in a previous pregnancy (e.g. intrauterine growth restriction) and preexisting medical conditions such as diabetes mellitus and systemic lupus erythematosus. It is essential that a full medical, surgical and obstetric history is taken from every woman and a complete examination performed.

It is well established that women who attend for antenatal care enjoy a better pregnancy outcome than those who do not. There are multiple reasons for this but it remains important to encourage women to attend their doctor or midwife during pregnancy. Antenatal visits provide an excellent opportunity for education of pregnant mothers and their partners about pregnancy, birth, breastfeeding and care of the newborn baby.

Assessment of fetal wellbeing and diagnosis of fetal abnormality

Noninvasive techniques

Until the advent of electronic fetal heart rate monitoring, the only methods of assessing fetal wellbeing were clinical assessment of growth, auscultation of the fetal heart rate and the mother's reports of fetal movements felt. These tests have now been augmented by electronic measurement of fetal heart and uterine contractions (cardiotocography), and ultrasound techniques including Doppler examination of fetal blood flow.

The aim of the assessment of fetal wellbeing is to deliver a healthy baby. At term, if there is evidence of fetal compromise, delivery can be expedited. However, if the fetus is premature, the level of compromise has to be balanced against the degree of prematurity. Good communication between obstetricians and neonatologists is essential in order to optimize the baby's chances of survival.

Noninvasive techniques, which do not pose any risk to the fetus, are increasingly used as screening tests of fetal wellbeing and for investigating potential problems. They include the following.

Cardiotocography (CTG). Electronic recording of the fetal heart rate provides information about fetal wellbeing. The fetal heart rate should be between 110 and 150 beats per minute at term, with a baseline variability of greater than 5 beats per minute. Accelerations in the fetal heart rate should occur in response to fetal movements or uterine activity and prior to labour there should be no decelerations. The risk of fetal demise within 24 hours of normal CTG findings is very low.

Ultrasound. A biophysical profile is based on an ultrasound examination that records liquor volume, fetal movements, fetal tone, heart rate and growth. Assessment of liquor volume is very important, particularly in the presence of growth retardation, a reduction in liquor indicating an element of fetal compromise as renal blood flow is reduced. Ultrasound examination also permits measurement of the fetus to assess fetal growth.

Doppler blood flow studies. Doppler studies of the umbilical artery can identify the presence of end-diastolic flow. In the absence of end-diastolic flow, there is a likelihood of fetal hypoxia. If there is actual reversal of end-diastolic flow, there is definite fetal hypoxia and delivery should be expedited (Fig. 1.3).

When a fetus is hypoxic, the brain is preferentially perfused at the expense of intra-abdominal organs. This redistribution can be demonstrated using Doppler blood flow studies of the middle cerebral artery and descending aorta. Reduced blood flow to the kidneys leads to oligohydramnios and the gut can become ischaemic as a result of reduced mesenteric supply. This may predispose to necrotizing enterocolitis (p. 56, 231) in the newborn baby. Thus, if a baby had abnormal umbilical artery blood flow antenatally, neonatal management might involve measures aimed at minimizing the risk of necrotizing enterocolitis, such as consideration of delaying enteral feeding, which should preferably be human milk.

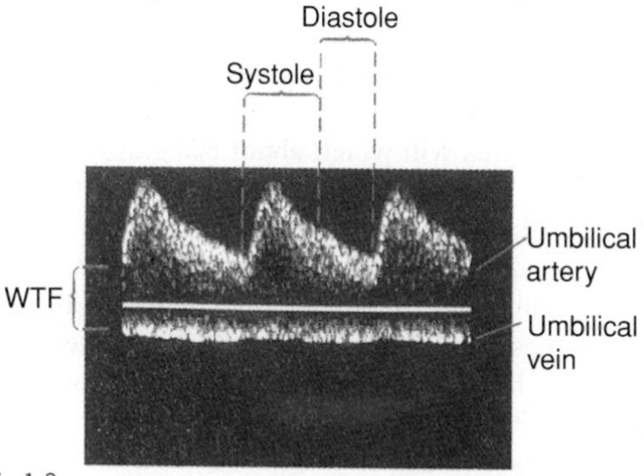

Fig 1.3
Doppler blood flow studies: normal umbilical artery waveform. Note continuous flow throughout cardiac cycle. Abnormal waveforms include absent or reversed flow at the end of the diastole.

Invasive procedures

Any invasive procedure carries a risk of fetal loss, and thus such tests are limited to cases where there is a high risk of an abnormal result. The loss rates after different procedures are presented in Table 1.1.

If the mother is Rhesus-negative, anti D must be administered after any invasive procedure to prevent sensitization to fetal Rhesus group antigens.

Amniocentesis. Amniotic fluid can be obtained by direct needling of the amniotic sac under continuous ultrasound guidance. The liquor obtained at amniocentesis is spun down and the fetal fibroblasts are isolated. These cells are then cultured using modern cytogenetic techniques, and when sufficient metaphase cells are available, the karyotype is examined. The duration of the culture is gradually being reduced and it is now possible to obtain a result within 2 weeks, although it may take longer. Application of techniques such as FISH (fluorescent in situ hybridization) may permit identification or exclusion of the major trisomies (p. 241) within 24 hours. The liquor can also be assessed for bilirubin level in the investigation of Rhesus isoimmunization (p. 19, 53).

With real-time ultrasound being used to guide the procedure, the incidence of failed or bloody taps (i.e. fluid contaminated with maternal blood) is low, and the risk of pregnancy loss after an amniocentesis is currently 0.5–1%. The procedure was originally performed between 15 and 16 weeks, but it is possible to karyotype a fetus by amniocentesis up to term. However, the main disadvantage of conventional amniocentesis is the late gestational age (well into the second trimester) at which the result becomes known. Termination of pregnancy at this stage is very stressful for the parents, their families and the staff involved in the provision of care. Further cytogenetic advances have led to the development of early amniocentesis, performed between 11 and 12 weeks, which permits the diagnosis of chromosome abnormalities during the first trimester. However, recent studies have indicated that there is an increased pregnancy loss rate after early amniocentesis.

Table 1.1
Risk of pregnancy loss after prenatal diagnostic procedure

Procedure	Risk of loss
Ultrasound	0
Amniocentesis	1:100
Chorion villus sampling	2:100
Fetal blood sampling	
Structurally normal fetus	1:100
Abnormal fetus	3:100
Hydropic fetus	25:100

Chorion villus sampling (CVS). This technique was first developed in China as a test for fetal sexing, where it was performed transcervically with no ultrasound guidance. It has subsequently been developed as an ultrasound-guided technique, using either a transcervical or transabdominal approach. Villi are aspirated or sampled with biopsy forceps. The advantage to the cytogeneticist is that the trophoblastic cells are rapidly dividing and are suitable for direct investigation of the chromosomes without the need to culture. The result may be available within 24–48 hours. It is also much easier to perform DNA studies on villi. CVS can be performed from 11 weeks until term. If performed earlier, there is a risk of limb reduction deformity in the fetus. The risk of pregnancy loss following CVS is not appreciably greater than that following amniocentesis (Table 1.1).

Fetal blood sampling. Amniocentesis and chorion villus sampling rely on the introduction of a needle into the uterus under continuous ultrasound guidance. These techniques have been adapted to obtain fetal blood from the umbilical cord, usually at the placental insertion, or the intrahepatic portion of the umbilical vein. The technique was developed in France for the investigation of pregnancies affected by toxoplasmosis but has a much wider application today. All tests that can be performed on postnatal blood can be performed on fetal blood, the main limitation being the volume available (maximum of 3 ml before 24 weeks, 6 ml thereafter). When used for karyotyping, the fetal lymphocytes are cultured and the result is available within 72 hours in the majority of cases. Fetal blood sampling, also known as cordocentesis, is generally performed from 20 weeks' gestation and carries a risk of pregnancy loss of approximately 1%, although if the fetus is very sick, the risk may be increased.

Breaking bad news

This is something in which all doctors need formal training. In perinatal medicine, there are the added problems of the expectation of normality and the life potential of the affected unborn individual. Many doctors and midwives are still poorly informed about many aspects of fetal health, and so have great difficulty in counselling parents. In any pregnancy, parents must be offered an opportunity to be fully informed about defects that have been detected so that they can be actively involved in working out a plan for the future. When parents are in a state of shock they may not be capable of listening fully, they may misunderstand what they are told and even deny that they have been told anything. The bearer of bad news can become a target for hostility. Sometimes the news is rejected or denied. Information may need to be repeated several times. It is vital that a consistent message is given. The involvement of other members of the perinatal team, that is neonatologists, paediatric surgeons, geneticists, etc., is essential at this stage.

Parents should always be given truthful and realistic explanations; they are extremely sensitive to any hint that their fetus might be in any way abnormal. Casual remarks by any member of the perinatal team, such as ultrasonographers and midwives, can readily be misunderstood. It is vital, where anomaly is suspected antenatally, that the parents understand the situation, and it is best to explain it to them straightaway rather than wait until the baby is born or later. It must be stressed that, in certain circumstances, the full diagnosis may not be apparent until after delivery. It is essential that these discussions are handled with skill and sensitivity. Often a written explanation and the loan of a video made by a parents' group may help. The use of 'before and after' photographs of surgically corrected abnormalities, such as cleft lip, is usually very helpful to the expectant parents.

Learning how to break bad news must be taught. It is good practice for clinical teachers to organize role-play exercises and take a student with them when they break bad news to parents, even though the student may find the experience quite distressing.

Growth, development and nutrition

Normal fetal growth

In a period of 280 days, the normal fetus grows from a single cell to an individual, capable of life outside the uterus, and weighing around 3 kg. The rate of growth is therefore rapid, and depends on an adequate supply of nutrients being carried across the placenta. Placental function depends on adequate trophoblast invasion of the uterine lining (decidua) and the maternal blood supply to the uterus.

A normal fetus will weigh about 500 g at 23 weeks, 1000 g at 27 weeks, 1500 g at 30 weeks, 2000 g at 33 weeks and 3000 g at 37 weeks. Fetal growth can be assessed by abdominal palpation of the mother and measurement of the pubic symphysis–fundal height. However, these clinical methods are insensitive even in experienced hands. Ultrasound biometry provides a more accurate assessment of fetal growth. Serial measurements of head circumference and abdominal circumference will demonstrate the pattern of growth, and these measurements are plotted on centile charts (see Fig. 1.4).

Abnormal fetal growth

Abnormal fetuses may be growth-restricted (intrauterine growth restriction, IUGR) or abnormally large (macrosomic; (Fig. 1.6) p. 10). Both growth abnormalities are associated with problems in fetal life, during labour and delivery and in the neonatal period. Abnormal fetal growth may be suspected because of maternal risk factors (previous IUGR, hypertension, diabetes), or clinically, when the uterus feels larger or smaller than expected. Serial ultrasound measurements will help identify those fetuses with an abnormal growth rate.

INTRAUTERINE GROWTH RESTRICTION (IUGR)

Babies who are born small for gestational age (i.e. with a birthweight less than the 3rd centile for gestational age) have an increased perinatal mortality and morbidity. Recent epidemiological work suggests that intrauterine growth restriction may also predispose an individual to cardiovascular disease and type 2 diabetes in adult life.

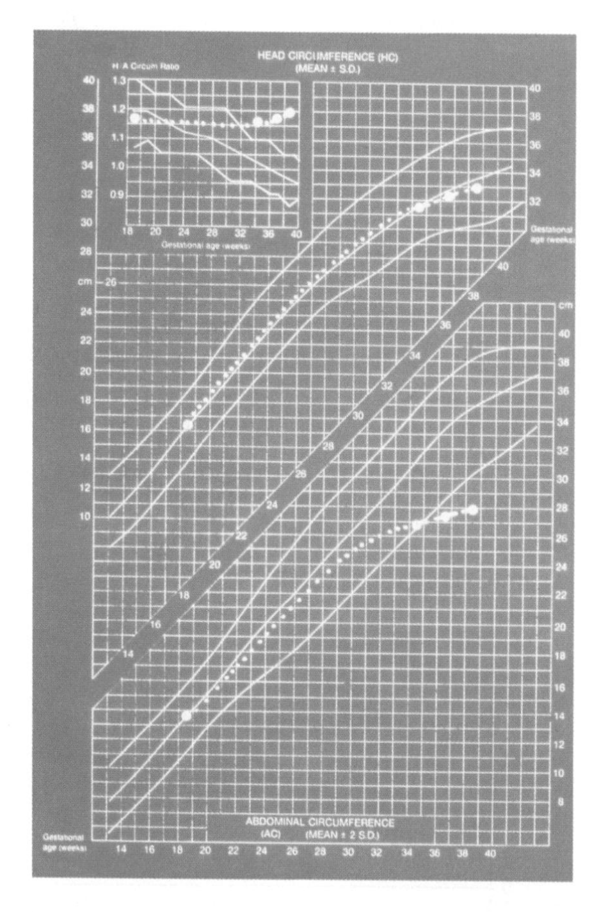

Fig 1.4
Chart of ultrasound measurement of fetal growth demonstrating a case of intrauterine growth restriction. Note that head growth is maintained while abdominal circumference falls off. Inset: shows ratio of the two.

The causes of IUGR can be divided into fetal and maternal (Information box 1.3). Fetal causes include structural and chromosomal anomaly and fetal infection, e.g. cytomegalovirus (p. 16). Maternal causes include abnormal placentation associated with hypertension, concurrent maternal disease, smoking, alcohol and drug abuse. Only in extremely severe conditions will maternal malnutrition affect fetal growth. A constitutionally small baby will grow at a normal rate and is not at increased risk.

The pattern of growth restriction may give a clue to the underlying cause. Poor placentation resulting in fetal malnutrition tends initially to spare head growth at the expense of abdominal growth (asymmetrical growth restriction; Figs 1.4 and 1.5). Inherent fetal problems such as chromosomal anomaly (p. 12) or congenital infection (p. 16) affect both head and abdominal growth (symmetrical growth restriction). IUGR caused by poor placental function is usually associated with reduced liquor volume.

The commonest cause of IUGR is placental insufficiency and this may lead to fetal hypoxia and eventually intrauterine death if no intervention occurs. If a fetus exhibits signs of intrauterine compromise, detected by cardiotocography or Doppler assessment, it is likely that labour will cause further compromise and the incidence of fetal distress is increased. In many situations, the baby may be delivered by elective caesarean section in order to minimize the risk of hypoxia.

In pregnancies in which IUGR is detected, careful monitoring of fetal wellbeing should be undertaken and investigation for underlying causes initiated. It is advisable to deliver a growth-restricted baby before 40 weeks of gestation.

Information Box 1.3

Causes and associations of intrauterine growth restriction (IUGR)

Maternal causes
Previous history of IUGR
Pregnancy-induced hypertension
Coexisting maternal disease
Poor socioeconomic status
Smoking
Alcohol and drug abuse
Extremes of childbearing age

Fetal
Fetal structural abnormality
Chromosomal abnormality
Fetal infection
Multiple pregnancy

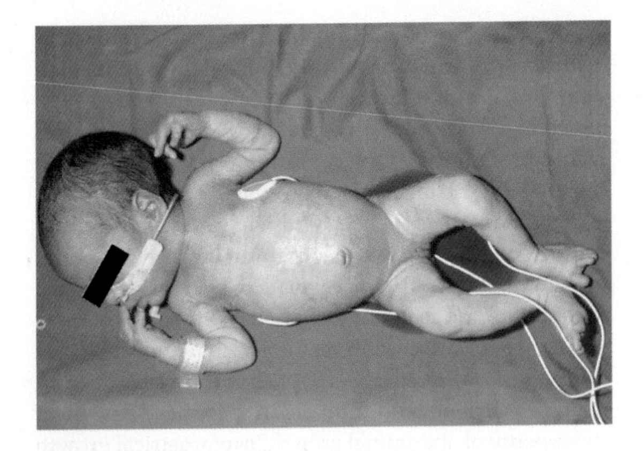

Fig 1.5
Asymmetric growth restriction. Normal head growth with poor abdominal growth.

MACROSOMIA

Macrosomic babies have a high birthweight due to increased body fat and enlarged viscera, puffy plethoric faces (Fig. 1.6). They are at risk of trauma and asphyxia during delivery, and often demonstrate metabolic abnormalities such as hypoglycaemia and hypocalcaemia in the neonatal period. The commonest association with fetal macrosomia is disturbed carbohydrate tolerance in the mother, particularly frank diabetes. There is an increased risk of unexplained intrauterine death towards the end of the third trimester in babies of diabetic mothers, as well as delayed fetal lung maturity which predisposes neonates to respiratory distress syndrome (p. 49).

PREMATURITY AND POSTMATURITY

The World Health Organization definition of prematurity is a baby delivered before 37 completed weeks of pregnancy measured from the first day of the last menstrual period. A baby of 2501 g or more at birth is regarded as normally grown. Babies weighing 1501–2500 g are described as low birthweight. Those weighing less than 1500 g are described as very low birthweight. The importance of these definitions is related to the differing perinatal mortality rates for the different groups (Figs 1.7 and 1.8).

Prematurity is the major cause of death in normally formed infants. There are many predisposing factors, both fetal and maternal, for prematurity. It is important to remember that premature delivery may be elective, for example in cases of IUGR with evidence of fetal hypoxia. In such cases, the risks of prematurity have to be balanced against the risks of further intrauterine compromise and possible intrauterine death.

Low birthweight may or may not be due to premature delivery; about 25% of babies who weigh under 2501 g at birth are of 37 or more weeks of gestation.

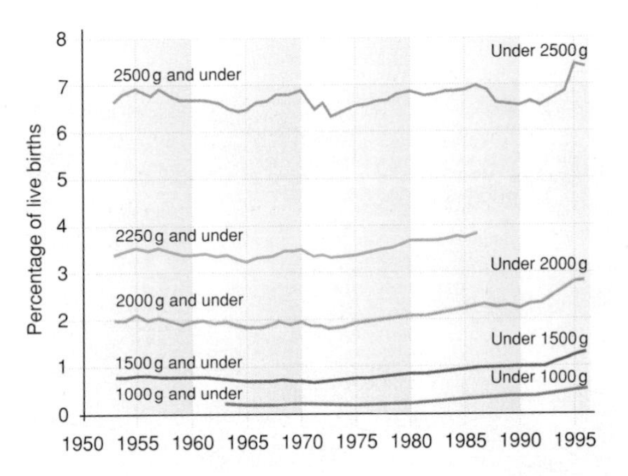

Fig 1.7
Incidence of low birthweight, England and Wales 1953–1996. (Sources: LHS 27/1 low birthweight returns for 1953–1986, and Office of National Statistics (ONS) Mortality Statistics, Series DH3, for 1983–1996 © Crown Copyright, reproduced with permission.)

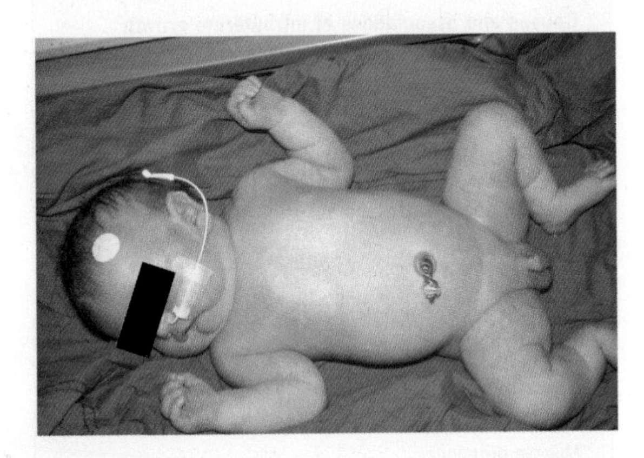

Fig 1.6
Macrosomic infant of a diabetic mother.

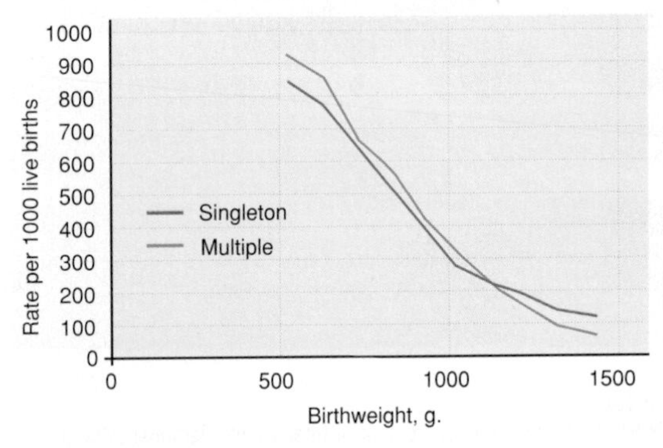

Fig 1.8
Infant mortality and birthweights under 1500 g, single and multiple births, England and Wales, 1983–1987 combined.

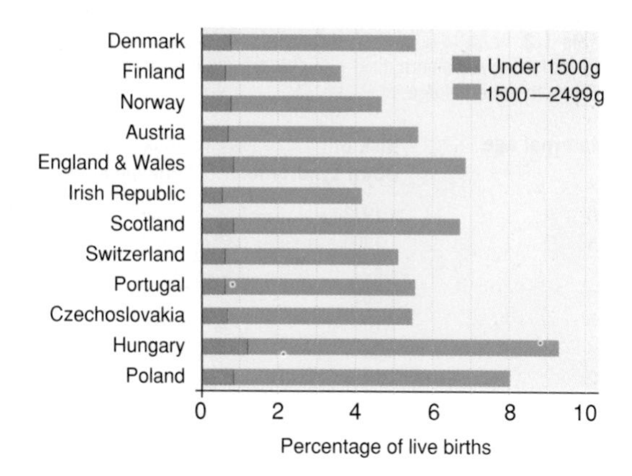

Fig 1.9
Low birthweight among live births in selected European countries, 1990 (from Masuy-Stroobant (1996) *Santé et Mortalité des Enfants en Europe*. Chair Quetelet, Academia-Bruylant, Louvain-la-Neuve).

The incidence of prematurity, and therefore low birthweight, has slowly increased in the last 15 years as a result of improvements in both obstetric care, allowing high risk pregnancies to reach the stage of viability, and also in neonatal care, permitting obstetricians to deliver earlier when pregnancy complications threaten the fetus. National low birthweight rates in high income countries range between 4% and 8% (Fig. 1.9).

The rate of low birthweight deliveries also varies with socioeconomic class, being 2–3 times higher in class V than in class I. The ethnic origin of the mother also has a major influence, low birthweight being most common in mothers of Asian origin.

Babies born after a prolonged pregnancy may be described as postmature. Normal pregnancy lasts from 37 to 42 weeks. As the pregnancy progresses beyond this, placental function is likely to fail. In such cases, the fetus can start to utilize its stores of glycogen and fat and thus apparently lose weight. The volume of liquor reduces and the fetal skin becomes dry and wrinkly. If delivery does not occur, there is an increased risk of intrauterine death in very prolonged pregnancies and therefore most obstetricians will intervene to induce labour at 42 weeks' gestation. If such intervention is against the mother's wishes, monitoring of fetal well-being is essential.

Screening

Ultrasound

The mainstay of prenatal diagnosis is the routine ultrasound scan (recommended for all pregnant women by the Royal Colleges of Obstetricians and Gynaecologists, and Radiologists) which is generally performed at 18–20 weeks of gestation. This scan permits accurate dating of the pregnancy (to within 10 days) and examination of fetal anatomy. The list of abnormalities detectable by ultrasound is very long (Information box 1.4). Gross structural abnormalities of all systems can be diagnosed with confidence, although subtle defects may be difficult to identify.

Routine anomaly scanning permits screening of the population for neural tube defects, cardiac anomalies and other potentially lethal defects. Accurate identification of defects which are associated with fetal or neonatal death, or severe handicap, offers the parents the option of termination of an affected pregnancy, resulting in less suffering for the affected individual, the family and society. For non-lethal conditions, accurate prenatal diagnosis permits optimization of management. For example, a baby with a diaphragmatic hernia (p. 213) can have a planned delivery at a unit with appropriate intensive care and surgical facilities. The parents can be prepared in advance for the problems that their unborn child is likely to face.

Information Box 1.4

Examples of abnormalities detected by prenatal ultrasound. (This list is not exhaustive but covers abnormalities commonly detected)

System	Abnormalities detected
Central nervous	Hydrocephalus Intracranial cysts Neural tube defects
Cardiovascular	Major congenital heart defects Heart failure
Gastrointestinal	Diaphragmatic hernia Meconium peritonitis (see cystic fibrosis) Gastroschisis Exomphalos Duodenal atresia
Urogenital	Hydronephrosis Renal agenesis Dysplastic kidneys Polycystic kidneys Bladder outflow obstruction
Skeletal	Osteogenesis imperfecta (severe) Talipes equinovarus Skeletal dysplasias: dwarfism Facial: cleft lip and palate

Alpha fetoprotein (αFP)

Maternal serum levels of αFP are elevated in conditions associated with open defects in the fetal body wall. The commonest type of defect is an open neural tube defect (p. 309), but other causes include exomphalos (p. 246) and gastrointestinal obstruction (p. 216). Traditionally, αFP is measured between 14 and 16 weeks as a screening test for neural tube defects. The range of αFP levels in normal pregnancies overlaps that of abnormal pregnancies, making interpretation of the results difficult. Before high-resolution ultrasound was available, an amniocentesis was carried out in women with elevated αFP. If the level of αFP in the liquor was also elevated, a diagnosis of neural tube defect was suspected. Ultrasound, however, provides a reliable diagnostic test and amniocentesis is no longer necessary in the diagnosis of neural tube defects. In areas of low prevalence, ultrasound has replaced αFP as a screening test. Low αFP levels may be found in conditions involving aneuploidy (see below).

Screening for Down syndrome and other chromosomal abnormalities

In addition to the detection of structural anomalies, ultrasound examination may suggest chromosomal and genetic abnormalities. However, for confirmation, invasive tests that carry a risk of pregnancy loss may be required. In order to maximize the value of invasive testing and minimize the loss of normal pregnancies, it is appropriate to consider screening the population to identify those individuals most at risk.

Until recently, screening for chromosomal abnormalities was based on maternal age: invasive testing was offered to women over the age of 35. Initially, following the introduction of amniocentesis for karyotyping, there was little reduction in the number of babies born with Down syndrome. However, with changes in the screening procedures, there has been a fall in the incidence of Down syndrome live births.

The incidence of chromosomal abnormality increases with maternal age (see Table 1.2); however, most babies with abnormalities are born to women below the age of 35 because these women have relatively more babies. Attempts have therefore been made to find a suitable screening test for Down syndrome and other trisomies. One such test, the triple test, is based on maternal serum biochemistry, using maternal serum αFP, human chorionic gonadotrophin and oestriol measurements in conjunction with gestational and maternal age, to obtain an estimate of the risk of a pregnancy being affected. Invasive tests are then offered to women with a risk factor above 1:250. In population studies, maternal serum screening identifies 60–70% of affected pregnancies. However, there is the problem that false-positive results engender much anxiety.

Table 1.2
Risk of having a live-born child with chromosomal abnormality, in relation to maternal age

Maternal age	Risk of Down syndrome	Risk of all aneuploidies
20	1:1923	1:526
25	1:1205	1:476
30	1:855	1:384
35	1:365	1:178
40	1:109	1:63
45	1:32	1:18
50	1:10	1:6

Ultrasound examination of the fetus in the late first trimester may demonstrate an echo-free area of oedema at the back of the fetal neck (Fig 1.10); this temporary phenomenon is called *nuchal translucency*. If the oedema measures greater than 3 mm, there is an increased risk of Down syndrome and all the other major trisomies. The risk increases with larger measurements, although the exact risk depends on the maternal age, gestational age of the fetus, nuchal translucency measurement and incidence of previous chromosomal abnormalities. A computer program is available which assesses the risk for any individual pregnancy. Initial studies of high risk populations suggested a possible 80% detection rate of aneuploidy, but general population studies suggest the test is slightly less effective. However, these methods do offer an alternative to purely invasive assessment and further studies are in progress.

Many structural abnormalities of the fetus are associated with aneuploidy, e.g. cardiac defects (p. 46, 240). If these are detected on routine ultrasound assessment, fetal karyotyping should be offered to the mother.

Infection screening

Maternal screening for rubella and syphilis is universal in the United Kingdom with routine screening for hepatitis B included recently.

The problem of screening for HIV infection is currently being addressed. Unlinked, anonymous screening of mothers has been in place for several years, with seropositive rates of up to 0.5% being found in some parts of inner London. In other areas

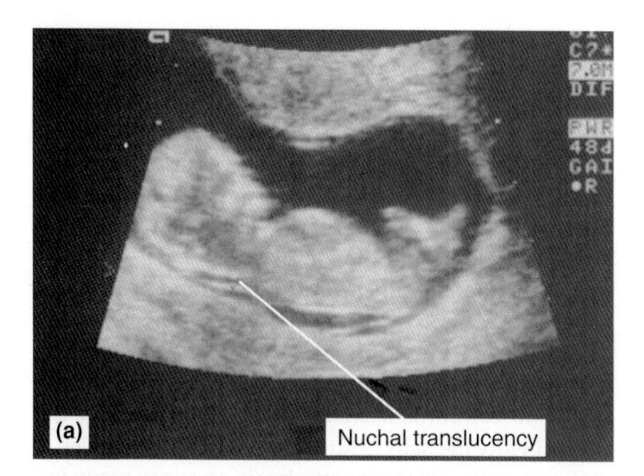

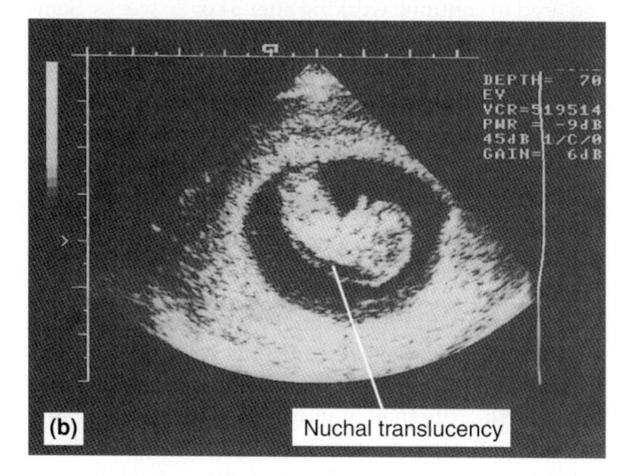

Fig 1.10
Ultrasound measurement of nuchal translucency: (a) normal fetus; (b) fetus showing increased translucency.

of the country the seroprevalence is extremely low (<0.01%). There is evidence that antiretroviral therapy, given to the mother antenatally and during labour and to the newborn infant for 6 weeks, greatly reduces transmission rates. The avoidance of breastfeeding also has a major impact in reducing transmission, and to a lesser extent delivery by caesarean section also reduces transmission. Many obstetric units are now routinely offering testing, allowing the identification of asymptomatic women who may then benefit themselves from treatment, as well as having a reduced likelihood of transmission of the virus to their children.

Criteria for the identification of mothers at high risk of group B streptococcal infection (in their infants) have been introduced in some units. This allows the selective use of intrapartum antibiotics to reduce the incidence of this serious infection in infants (p. 18).

Fetal problems

With advances in fetal medicine, the number of fetal problems which can be identified prenatally has grown enormously. Improvements in neonatal care have led to better survival and a reduction in perinatal mortality and morbidity. One problem associated with these advances is that we tend to have great expectations of modern technology. Healthcare professionals and parents alike may find it difficult to accept that in some cases, nothing can be done.

The abnormal fetus: genetic/inherited problems

A congenital problem is defined as a condition that started prenatally. Such disorders include those with a definite well established genetic basis, such as haemoglobinopathies (p. 251) and cystic fibrosis (p. 352). In other instances, genetic influences may be less well defined. The majority of structural abnormalities do not have a well established genetic background, although there is an increased risk of recurrence in some, for example congenital heart disease (p. 174). In the absence of chromosomal abnormality, a history of congenital heart disease in one of the parents, or in a sibling, increases the risk of recurrence by a factor of 10. In cases of structural abnormality associated with aneuploidy, e.g. duodenal atresia (p. 242) and Down syndrome, the risk of recurrence of the structural problem is the risk of recurrence of the chromosomal abnormality alone.

Chromosomal abnormality can take a number of forms:

- Gross abnormality of number, e.g. trisomy.
- Translocations (part of one chromosome displaced onto another), which may cause a number of genetic disorders. Translocations may be balanced, in which case the individual will usually be normal, or unbalanced, in which case the individual will have either too much or not enough genetic material. Severe neurodevelopmental delay is common in unbalanced translocations.
- Small deletions or duplications, only detectable through sophisticated karyotyping techniques using 'banding'. (This technique involves staining the chromosomes in characteristic bands, which helps highlight minor abnormalities of structure.)
- Single-gene defects where the DNA sequence for the suspected genetic problem is known, e.g. cystic fibrosis (p. 352).
- Genetic defects where the chromosomal localization is known, but the specific abnormality of the genetic code is unknown.

Methods of detection of genetic and chromosomal abnormalities are described in Chapter 12 (Genetics and dysmorphology).

Adverse influences on the fetus

Many diseases present at birth do not have a genetic origin but are acquired in utero. Some are believed to be due to environmental conditions present at the time of conception. The causes of many congenital abnormalities are still not understood. Despite advances in prenatal screening, some subtle structural and many functional problems may not be detected before birth.

Adverse socio-environmental factors are implicated in many fetal problems. They rarely exert their effect in isolation, making it difficult to establish a cause. For example, heavy cigarette smokers are more likely to have poor diets and to drink more alcohol than non-smokers. Families of low socio-economic status are also at increased risk of drug abuse. The fetus is potentially exposed to so many different influences during intrauterine life that it is often impossible to relate a problem directly to any single factor. However, there are some well characterized syndromes which are related to known risk factors.

A vast number of factors are known to influence intrauterine health. The health of the baby is intimately bound up with the health of the mother. The size of a baby is influenced by the mother's own birthweight. Small mothers, regardless of birthweight, tend to have small babies, even if the father is very large. This demonstrates that there are control factors concerned with fetal growth and development which pre-date maternal status during pregnancy.

Maternal factors which adversely affect fetal health

Maternal age and parity. Pregnancy at both extremes of a woman's reproductive life carries an increased risk of problems for the fetus. In many very young mothers poor education and poor socio-economic status lead to poor antenatal care with late detection of problems. IUGR (p. 9) and premature labour are more common in teenage pregnancies. At the other end of the childbearing age range, as the mother's age increases, there is an increased risk of chromosomal anomaly, IUGR, pregnancy-induced hypertension and multiple pregnancy. The perinatal mortality rate rises markedly in so-called 'grand multips', i.e. women with five or more children.

Socio-economic factors. Mothers who live in poor social conditions have repeatedly been shown to have an excessive perinatal mortality. This is largely associated with a low birthweight rate and an increased rate of premature delivery. It is harder to gauge the more nebulous effects of lack of rest, overwork and, in particular, 'stress'.

Single parenthood. Unmarried, unsupported mothers have increased risks, whatever their parity. The reasons for this are complex, but poverty leading to a poor diet is likely to be a major factor. Rates of single parenthood are continuing to rise.

Employment. Women who are in employment do not have an increased risk of fetal problems, even if they do a physical job. Providing that a pregnancy remains uncomplicated, women can continue to work for as long as they are comfortable. Many choose to finish work a few weeks before the baby is due. This time is often needed to make domestic arrangements, but in any case, many feel too tired to continue working after 34 or 36 weeks. Some occupations carry a potential risk to the fetus, including radiology and anaesthetics, and care is needed to minimize the risks. However, it is important to maintain a sense of perspective because it is very easy to incriminate any new environmental change as a possible cause of fetal abnormality. For example, in the 1980s there was a campaign to prevent pregnant women working with computers despite a lack of scientific evidence.

Maternal health. Preexisting medical conditions can have a profound influence on the course of a pregnancy and its outcome. Diabetes mellitus is associated with an increased incidence of fetal malformation, disorders of growth, pregnancy-induced hypertension and unexplained fetal death. Optimal control of diabetes helps to reduce the incidence of these problems, but does not completely prevent them. The secondary hyperinsulinism that occurs in the fetus of diabetic mothers leads to excessive fetal growth (p. 10), polycythaemia (p. 51) and a typical 'fleshy' appearance (Fig. 1.6). Tight control of blood glucose should ideally begin before conception and requires the collaboration of the mother, family, obstetrician, a physician specializing in diabetes and the family doctor.

Essential hypertension predisposes to IUGR and may be complicated by superimposed pregnancy-induced hypertension. Mothers with haemoglobinopathies, such as sickle cell disease, may be anaemic during the pregnancy, and may pass the disorder to the baby. Autoimmune disorders such as systemic lupus erythematosus carry an increased risk of miscarriage, IUGR and intrauterine death. In all cases of concurrent illness, a combined approach between an interested physician and an obstetrician is essential to minimize problems for the mother and fetus.

Drugs

Therapeutic drugs

Since the drug thalidomide was found to be causally associated with phocomelia (severe shortening of the limbs) in the early 1960s, there has been a major search for other teratogenic drugs and environmental factors. Whilst no other drug commonly used in pregnancy has been shown to have as predictable and devastating an effect as thalidomide, there has been a thorough review of existing medicines, and every new drug is extensively tested prior to introduction to human medicine. Some drugs exert a teratogenic effect in animal studies but not in humans. Licensing of drugs for use in pregnancy is extremely difficult, and many pharmaceutical companies do not license their products for use in pregnancy, to avoid the risk of litigation.

The exact role that drugs play in teratogenicity is often unclear. The list of known teratogenic drugs is quite long, and can easily be checked in the *British National Formulary*. Amongst existing drugs it was noted that phenytoin administered during the first trimester of pregnancy can be associated with cleft lip and palate (p. 215) and sodium valproate can be associated with spina bifida. In women with epilepsy, control of convulsions must be maintained during pregnancy and careful consideration (with expert help) of the options is required.

In order to exert a teratogenic effect, a drug or its metabolite must be able to cross the placental barrier. Women requiring anticoagulation during pregnancy pose a particular problem. Heparin is too large a molecule to cross the placenta, but has the disadvantage of requiring parenteral administration. Warfarin can be given orally, but if given in the first trimester it is associated with fetal abnormality, and if given near the time of delivery it can cause haemorrhage. For this reason heparin is given during organogenesis and just prior to delivery, while the woman is maintained on oral anticoagulant therapy in the middle and early third trimesters.

Drugs of abuse

There are no reports of fetal abnormality with maternal use of marijuana. However, so-called 'hard' drugs can have devastating effects on the fetus and newborn. Cocaine, barbiturates and opiates readily cross the placenta. Their use in pregnancy is particularly associated with problems of IUGR and neonatal difficulties. With drugs of addiction, the neonate is subjected to sudden withdrawal at birth and can develop jitteriness and seizures (p. 58). All babies born to mothers who have used addictive substances during pregnancy need to be closely monitored. During pregnancy, women who are addicted to opiates (usually heroin) are converted to regular and reducing doses of methadone. If the woman cooperates with this regime, the severity of withdrawal symptoms of the neonate is usually less. In addition, if women are willing to cooperate, they usually attend regularly for antenatal care with an improvement in perinatal outcome.

Women who abuse drugs are often at risk of other pregnancy complications by virtue of their tendency to have a poor diet, etc. There is an increased risk of prematurity, which can compound the problems of low birthweight due to IUGR. Such patients attend poorly for antenatal care.

Alcohol

Excessive consumption of alcohol during pregnancy is associated with IUGR. The 'safe' level of intake is not agreed but consumption exceeding 85 ml absolute alcohol per day (8 units) seems to be associated with fetal alcohol syndrome. In severe cases, the fetus has microcephaly, mental retardation and a characteristic face with short palpebral fissures, flat nasal bridge, micrognathia, hypoplastic maxilla and a thin upper lip. The Royal College of Midwives now recommends complete avoidance of alcohol in pregnancy.

Smoking

Cigarette smoking is associated with an average 180-g reduction in birthweight and a 10% increase in perinatal mortality. The mechanism by which this occurs has not been fully explained. Cessation of smoking in early pregnancy can reverse this effect. In smokers, there is an increase in the incidence of premature labour and placental abruption. However, there appears to be a lower incidence of pregnancy-induced hypertension. It is best that pregnant women stop smoking altogether, but a reduction in the number of cigarettes smoked each day still reduces the risk to the fetus. After birth, the infant of a mother who smoked during pregnancy is at increased risk of sudden infant death syndrome (p. 70) and respiratory problems, in particular asthma (p. 354).

Parental irradiation

Most evidence for the potential adverse effects of intrauterine irradiation derives from studies on survivors of Hiroshima and from studies of mothers treated with irradiation for cancer before they knew they were pregnant. There has been much controversy about the influence of radiation on fathers, particularly nuclear power station workers, and whether leukaemia in their children is more common than normal. The evidence is not conclusive. The wise student will follow the emerging debate with interest by reading papers in refereed scientific literature, as well as the media reports.

Congenital infections

These are infections acquired before or at birth. They include:

- Infections chronically carried by the mother and transmitted to the fetus in utero or to the infant around the time of birth, e.g. HIV, hepatitis B infections
- Primary infections acquired by the mother during pregnancy, e.g. rubella, parvovirus toxoplasma infections
- Reactivated latent infections developing during pregnancy, e.g. cytomegalovirus (CMV), herpes simplex infections.

As a rule viral infections acquired early in pregnancy and transmitted to the fetus are more likely to produce spontaneous abortion or embryopathy than those acquired later. Nevertheless, infections not associated with embryopathy may cause stillbirth or premature labour. Primary acquired infections at the very end of gestation and transmitted perinatally may lead to early symptomatic infection in the newborn which can be life-threatening. Examples include varicella zoster, primary genital herpes, enterovirus infections and listeriosis. Chronically carried infections transmitted perinatally may cause late disease, months or even years later, e.g. HIV, hepatitis B.

The important infections are caused by the following organisms.

Rubella

This is a markedly fetotoxic virus. Infection of the mother in the first trimester carries a high risk of embryopathy with the typical pattern of congenital cataracts, deafness and congenital heart disease. Infection later in pregnancy does not cause embryopathy but may still result in congenital infection (Fig. 1.11) with chronic viral excretion and risk of disease affecting the eyes (Fig. 1.12), cochlea or central nervous system. Prevention with vaccination (at 13–15 months of age) is the best approach. Women found to be seronegative should be vaccinated before pregnancy.

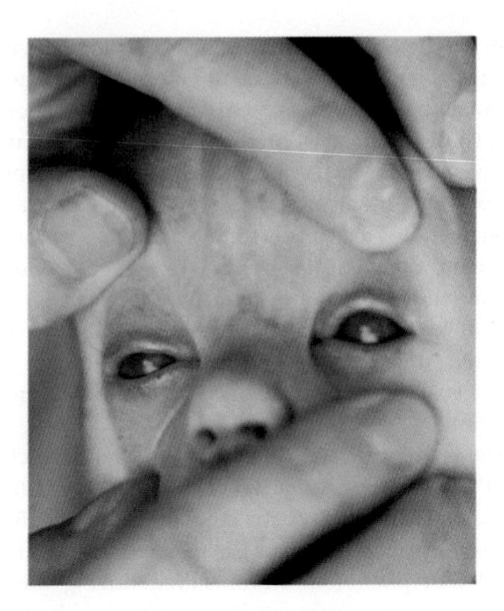

Fig 1.12
Cataracts due to congenital rubella (courtesy of Milupa).

The vaccine (live, attenuated) is contraindicated in women who may be pregnant.

Cytomegalovirus (CMV)

This is the commonest form of congenital infection affecting around 0.3% of infants in the UK. It is also the commonest cause of non-genetic deafness. Primary infection may occur in pregnancy or, as this is a herpes virus capable of latency, a seropositive mother can develop a reactivated infection during pregnancy. Around 90% of infants born with congenital cytomegalovirus infection do not develop permanent sequelae. Those that do may suffer IUGR, deafness, microcephaly, chorioretinitis and cerebral calcification (Fig. 1.13). Primary infection is more likely to produce serious problems though secondary disease has also been implicated. About 10% of seropositive mothers

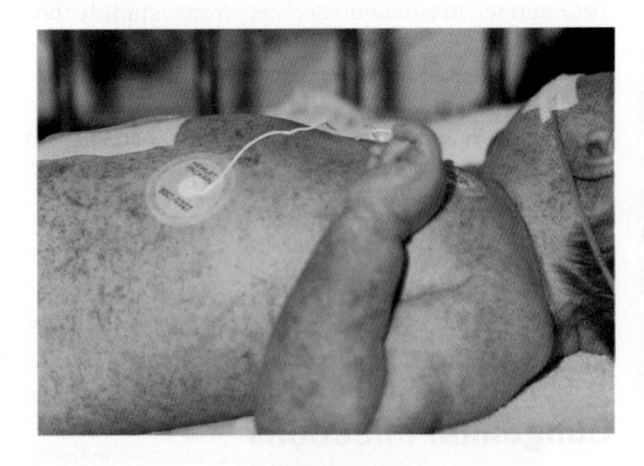

Fig 1.11
Congenital rubella (courtesy of Milupa).

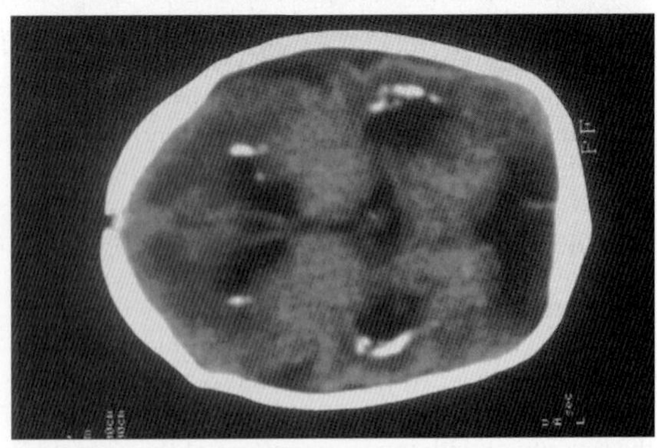

Fig 1.13
CT scan of an infant with congenital cytomegalovirus (CMV) infection, showing extensive periventricular cerebral calcification.

will reactivate CMV excretion at around the time of birth. The virus is excreted in breast milk and thus infects the baby. In healthy infants this causes no problems, but the possibility of acquisition of virus in this way may confuse attempts to confirm congenital infection in a baby with symptoms (see p. 18). Treatment of symptomatic congenital infection with the antiviral agent ganciclovir is controversial. It reduces viral excretion but its effects on long-term outcome are unknown.

Parvovirus

This virus is one of the causes of intrauterine heart failure, leading to hydrops fetalis (p. 20) as a result of fetal anaemia, and sometimes myocarditis. There are reports of successful in utero treatment of anaemia with intrauterine blood transfusions, resulting in intact survival.

Varicella zoster virus (VZV)

Infection with this virus during the first trimester can result in spontaneous miscarriage. Infection at all stages of pregnancy carries a 3% risk of fetal damage such as eye problems, mononeuropathy and severe scarring of the skin (Fig. 1.14). Maternal infection around the time of confinement is extremely dangerous for the neonate, as neonatal infection with this virus carries a high mortality. Infants at risk (those whose mothers developed chickenpox within 1 week before to 1 week after delivery) should be given varicella zoster immune globulin, observed closely and treated with aciclovir at the first sign of disease.

Syphilis (*Treponema pallidum*)

This is perhaps one of the oldest known causes of congenital infection. Fetuses with intrauterine infections with *Treponema pallidum* exhibit a classical syndrome of visceromegaly, thrombocytopenia (p. 20), osteochondritis (p. 348) and a degree of mental retardation. Asymptomatically infected babies can develop late-onset eye problems (interstitial keratitis), which after many years may result in blindness. Infection in pregnancy should be treated with a course of parenteral penicillin therapy, and postnatally all babies suspected of having this infection should also be treated.

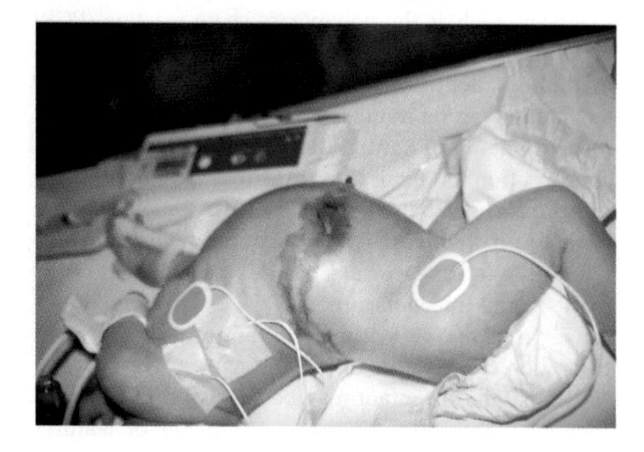

Fig 1.14
Cicatricial scarring as a result of intrauterine varicella zoster virus (VZV) infection.

Toxoplasma gondii

This can be acquired from cat faeces and raw meat. Infection during pregnancy carries a relatively low risk of fetal infection, and of those fetuses infected only a small proportion develop sequelae, which include IUGR, retinitis, hydrocephalus and mental retardation. The risk of fetal infection falls with increasing gestational length. Only in areas of high prevalence, such as France, is screening of the pregnant population appropriate. Proven infection during pregnancy can be treated with antimicrobials, which may reduce the risk of fetal infection, though the evidence for this is not strong. Treatment of the infant is not easy, requiring a prolonged course of antimicrobials. It is given to try to limit the damage in symptomatic disease or, in asymptomatic infants, to prevent the chance of development of retinal disease in later life.

Human immunodeficiency virus (HIV)

Transplacental passage of the virus can occur, but the greatest risk to the fetus occurs at the time of labour and delivery and during breastfeeding. If a mother with HIV is identified during pregnancy steps can be taken to minimize the risks to the baby (p. 12–13). Only women who have full-blown AIDS appear to be at risk of pregnancy complications such as IUGR.

Hepatitis B virus

Although in rare cases the virus can cross the placenta from a chronic carrier mother, most transmission occurs at the time of delivery. Even in the most highly infectious mothers, who are e-antibody-negative, this transmission can be interrupted by the administration of hepatitis B immunoglobulin and neonatal vaccination. In infants born to e-antibody-positive but surface antigen-positive mothers, administration of vaccine alone is sufficient. Three doses of vaccine are required altogether (p. 68).

Hepatitis C virus

Carrier mothers may transmit this virus, probably at the time of birth. The transmission rate is high in women with accompanying HIV infection (up to 50%). In otherwise healthy women, particularly those without detectable circulating viral DNA, the transmission rate is low (<5%). As yet there are no interventions available to reduce transmission.

Herpes simplex virus

This virus causes maternal genital infection. Infection may be primary or reactivated. Passage of the virus across the placenta to the fetus in early pregnancy is rare but results in fetal death or severe embryopathy. More commonly, the virus infects the infant at the time of birth, when the amniotic membranes have ruptured, and may lead to severe neonatal disease.

Papillomavirus

Mothers with a history of genital warts may transmit the virus to their newborn infants during birth. The virus has a long incubation period (2–3 years) and it may cause laryngeal or perianal papillomatosis in the infant (Fig. 1.15).

Enteroviruses

This group of small RNA viruses include ECHO and Coxsackie viruses which are common causes of mild illness. When mothers contract one of these illnesses at around the time of confinement, the infant may become infected and develop severe illness with hepatitis, myocarditis and encephalitis.

Listeria monocytogenes

This bacterium may be found in unpasteurized milk, soft cheeses, chicken and cooked cold meats. It is extremely fetopathic and acute infection often leads to sudden fetal demise. The mother is often systemically unwell and there is a risk of premature labour. The newborn infant may suffer septicaemia, pneumonia or meningitis.

Group B Streptococcus

This bacterium is part of the normal gut flora and colonizes the vagina up to 20% of women. Invasion of this organism across intact fetal membranes can result in premature labour. The infant acquiring the organism during birth may be born with congenital pneumonia and/or septicaemia (early-onset neonatal sepsis) with a high mortality rate. The incidence of this problem is around 1–2 per 1000 live births. Risk factors include premature labour, maternal fever, prolonged rupture of membranes and previous maternal history of a baby with Group B streptococcal disease. Intrapartum antibiotic prophylaxis, when given in high risk situations, is effective in reducing the rate of neonatal disease.

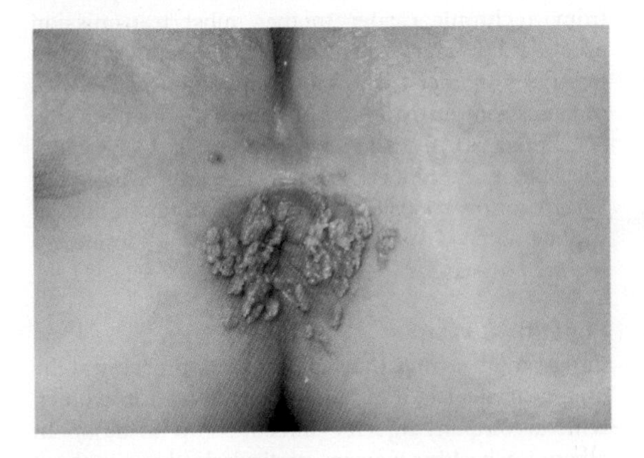

Fig 1.15
Perianal warts in a toddler due to vertical transmission of papillomavirus. The differential diagnosis should include child sexual abuse.

Neisseria gonorrhoea

Infection contracted during passage through the birth canal may cause severe conjuctivitis (ophthalmia neonatorum) with or without systemic sepsis (p. 60).

Ureaplasmas and *Mycoplasma hominis*

Infection of the genital tract with these organisms may induce premature labour.

DIAGNOSING INFECTION

The confirmation of maternal infection during pregnancy can be straightforward with the demonstration of rising titres of IgM and IgG. Most maternal infections lead to the passage of IgG but not IgM antibodies across the placenta. However the virus itself often does not cross. The detection of IgG antibodies in the fetus or infant is therefore not a useful test for congenital infection. The diagnosis of fetal infection can be very difficult. In cases of suspected rubella infection, isolation of viral DNA obtained by chorionic villus sampling (CVS) confirms transplacental passage of the virus, but not necessarily fetal infection. Investigation of pregnancies at risk involves liaison with microbiologists and careful counselling. Invasive procedures such as amniocentesis, CVS and fetal blood sampling may aid diagnosis. The presence of specific IgM in fetal blood confirms fetal infection, but IgG may be of maternal origin. Newer techniques in microbial diagnosis such as the polymerase chain reaction (PCR) for amplifying specific pieces of nucleic acid, can facilitate identification of the microbe. These techniques can be more sensitive and specific than the measurement of antibodies. With many agents, confirmation of fetal infection does not necessarily mean that the baby will suffer adverse sequelae. Before proceeding to invasive investigations which carry a risk to the fetus, each case has to be considered on its merits. Fetal infection must always be considered as a cause in cases of symmetrical intrauterine growth restriction and fetal hydrops.

Postnatally, an infant may be suspected of having a congenital infection because of a number of features (Information box 1.5).

Confirming the diagnosis can be difficult. The presence of specific IgM is diagnostic but some

> **Information Box 1.5**
>
> **Reasons for suspecting possible congenital infection**
>
> - Mother is known carrier of infection
> - Characteristic pattern of congenital abnormalities, e.g. cataracts, deafness, cardiac abnormality in rubella syndrome
> - Unexplained microcephaly (or occasionally hydrocephaly), especially if cerebral calcification found on X-ray
> - Unexplained nerve deafness
> - Visual problems associated with retinitis or cataracts
> - Unexplained hepatosplenomegaly with or without thrombocytopenia
> - Unexplained intrauterine growth restriction – though there are many other causes

infections may not induce this class of antibody, e.g. toxoplasmosis. Persistence of IgG (beyond the time that maternal IgG would be expected to persist), can be helpful but may take many months (18 months in the case of HIV). Increasingly, the approach taken is isolation of the organism or demonstration of microbial nucleic acid in the baby. However, in late-presenting infants one may not be able to exclude postnatal acquisition. For example, a urine sample taken at more than 3 weeks of age which grows CMV may represent postnatal infection, most probably via breast milk from a virus-excreting mother.

ADVICE FOR MOTHERS ON AVOIDING INFECTION

Rubella is currently preventable by immunization, and women are advised to have their immunity checked before embarking on their first pregnancy. Pregnant women are advised to avoid contact with cat faeces and the eating of raw or undercooked meat, which may transmit toxoplasmosis. Avoidance of unpasteurized dairy products, including soft cheeses, reduces the risk of listeria infection. Whilst it may be impossible for a mother to avoid contact with some of the common childhood infections (such as viral upper respiratory tract infections) it is advisable that children with acute infections of any sort should be excluded from the antenatal clinic.

Abnormalities of liquor volume

These can occur in association with fetal abnormality but are often idiopathic or secondary to another complication, e.g. premature (preterm) rupture of membranes. However, whatever the cause of the problem, there may be direct effects on the fetus.

Polyhydramnios. Excessive liquor can occur for a variety of reasons including fetal abnormality (such as inability to swallow and absorb amniotic fluid, as in intestinal obstruction) although, in the majority of cases, no cause is found. If the problem is severe, there is an increased risk of premature rupture of membranes and premature labour.

Oligohydramnios. A reduction in liquor volume may be due to either a reduced production (most dramatic in renal agenesis but also occurring as a consequence of other renal problems associated with oliguria and with placental insufficiency) or a loss of liquor (e.g. caused by premature rupture of membranes). Adequate liquor volume during the middle trimester is essential for normal lung growth and, in severe cases, the baby is at risk of pulmonary hypoplasia which is usually fatal. In addition, the fetus may have fixed flexion limb deformities, which will usually respond to physiotherapy after birth.

Rhesus immunization

Fetal red blood cells can enter the mother's circulation at any time during pregnancy but particularly following episodes of bleeding, invasive procedures and delivery. If the mother is Rhesus-negative and the fetus Rhesus-positive, exposure to the fetal blood cells causes the mother to produce antibodies to destroy the fetal cells. The commonest antibody produced is anti D. Once the mother is sensitized, any subsequent pregnancy with a Rhesus-positive fetus may lead to an increase in the level of maternal anti D antibodies which, being IgG, will cross the placenta and destroy the fetal red cells. This leads to fetal anaemia, heart failure and ultimately fetal death.

Advances in fetal medicine have radically altered the outlook for such pregnancies. The first useful therapeutic procedure was intrauterine blood transfusion used in the treatment of severe Rhesus incompatibility. The injection of Rhesus-negative blood into the peritoneal cavity of the fetus, originally performed under X-ray control, saved many babies. With the newer ultrasound-guided procedures, the fetal circulation is accessible for both sampling and transfusion. Such intrauterine transfusions are now given directly into the umbilical vein or intrahepatic vein, although administration by direct cardiac puncture has also been used. Rhesus isoimmunization is suspected if a Rhesus-negative mother develops anti D in her blood during pregnancy, and the condition is confirmed if the levels of that antibody rise. All Rhesus-negative women must have their antibodies tested repeatedly during pregnancy.

Information Box 1.6

Common causes of hydrops fetalis

- Severe Rhesus isoimmunization
- Nonimmune causes of fetal anaemia such as:
  - Parvovirus infection
  - Haemoglobinopathy, such as α thalassaemia
- Fetal dysrhythmias, tachycardia (such as supraventricular tachycardias) and bradycardias (such as complete heart block, associated with maternal systemic lupus erythematosus (SLE))
- Idiopathic (15–20% of cases)

Thrombocytopenia

A reduction in the platelet count in the fetal blood can occur in cases of maternal alloimmune thrombocytopenia where the fetus carries a rare platelet antigen (usually Pla-1) not present in the mother. Platelet transfusions can be given, which reduce the risk of fetal haemorrhage.

Hydrops fetalis

This is a relatively common condition, occurring in 1 in 2500–3000 pregnancies (Information box 1.6). It is characterized by extravascular fluid collections in the fetus. It may be associated with polyhydramnios.

The majority of cases involve a degree of fetal cardiac failure. Improvements in diagnostic techniques have led to great improvements in making a precise diagnosis, with the result that many fetuses can be successfully treated. Intrauterine transfusion can be employed in the management of fetal anaemia (see above), and dysrhythmias may be treated by either transplacental (administration to the mother) or direct fetal administration of antiarrhythmic agents, such as digoxin. Fluid collections, for example pleural effusions, can be drained as an ultrasound-guided procedure. This can be very valuable before delivery as it helps with normal lung development and eases the problems of resuscitation.

Birth

The passage through the birth canal is probably the shortest yet most hazardous journey that an individual can make. Nevertheless, in the great majority of births, it is achieved without ill-effect. It is essential for paediatricians to consider the potential problems encountered during the birth process, as they may be highly relevant to a number of problems in the infant.

Place of delivery

The potential hazards of birth have led most obstetricians in the UK to advise that babies should be routinely delivered in hospital, yet this policy remains a controversial matter. In the Netherlands (where distances from home to hospital are short and the average female pelvic diameter is approximately 1 cm greater than in the UK) a high proportion of babies are delivered at home. When mothers of equivalent social background from the UK and the Netherlands are compared, it is found that there is no difference in incidence of birth asphyxia and perinatal mortality. In the 1992 Winterton report, the House of Commons Select Committee on Obstetric Services recommended the encouragement of home deliveries in low risk pregnancies. However, few would argue against hospital delivery in pregnancies at high risk of perinatal problems, e.g. involving maternal pre-eclampsia, elderly primigravidae, maternal short stature or a history of previous birth complications.

Timing of delivery

Most pregnancies result in spontaneous onset of labour at term. When the risk to the baby and/or the mother is too great to allow a pregnancy to run its natural course, labour can be induced with prostaglandins and/or artificial rupture of the membranes. Induction may be indicated in a number of circumstances, particularly maternal diabetes, in which condition after 38 weeks there is an increased risk of intrauterine death and maternal complications. If a pregnancy continues beyond 42 weeks, there is also an increased risk of fetal morbidity and mortality and thus many obstetricians will consider induction of labour at this time.

Premature labour

Labour that occurs before 37 weeks is defined as premature. Prematurity is the commonest cause of perinatal mortality and morbidity in normal infants. Intrapartum complications are common, and may lead to birth trauma and asphyxia. Furthermore, the physiological adaptations in preparation for postnatal life are not complete, which leads to problems for the baby. This commonly results in surfactant deficiency in preterm infants. If time allows, this can be ameliorated by treating the mother with a course of corticosteroids (usually dexamethasone two doses 12 hours apart, 24 hours before delivery) to promote fetal lung maturation.

Problems in labour likely to affect the fetus

Monitoring of the fetal heart rate in labour is directed towards early detection of problems such as interruption or reduction in the blood supply to the baby, mechanical problems impeding vaginal delivery, infection of mother and/or baby and maternal exhaustion.

Interruption or reduction in the blood supply to the baby

During labour, uterine contractions can lead to cord compression and also a reduction in uterine blood flow leading to intermittent reduction of oxygenation. In a well grown fetus at term, this is unlikely to lead to any problems, but if the fetus is compromised, for example by growth-restriction or fetal hypoxia, distress may result. Signs of fetal distress in labour include abnormalities of the heart rate (reduction of baseline variability, decelerations, bradycardias and tachycardias) and the passage of meconium (opening of the bowels resulting in green/brown staining of the liquor). Decelerations of the fetal heart rate in conjunction with uterine contractions (early decelerations) are normal, but if the onset or recovery of the deceleration is delayed, the deceleration is described as late and it may indicate fetal compromise (Fig. 1.16). When signs that may indicate fetal compromise are detected, fetal state can be investigated by taking a sample of blood from the fetal scalp and measuring the blood gases and pH. If the pH is 7.25 or greater, there is no indication of fetal hypoxia at the time of the sampling. If the pH is below 7.2, delivery should be expedited by either caesarean section or instrumental delivery as appropriate.

Continuous fetal heart rate monitoring during labour is indicated in high risk pregnancies such as those with evidence of intrauterine growth restriction or pre-eclampsia in the mother. However, fetal distress can also occur unexpectedly in a previously normal pregnancy. It is thus important to regularly record the fetal heart rate through a fetal stethoscope (intermittent monitoring). The best time for detecting fetal distress is immediately following a uterine contraction.

Mechanical problems impeding vaginal delivery

Difficulty in achieving a vaginal delivery can be caused by problems relating to the passage (maternal anatomical problems, such as pelvic shape and size, pelvic masses, etc.) or problems of the passenger (fetal abnormalities, such as hydrocephalus). With good antenatal care, many of these problems can be anticipated before onset of labour.

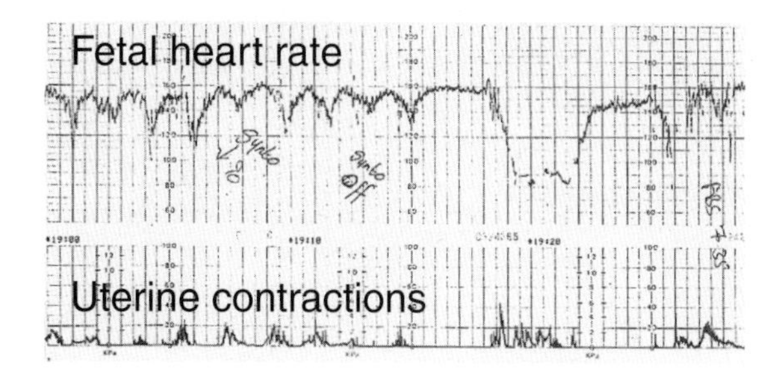

Fig 1.16
Fetal heart rate during contractions, showing shallow, late and variable decelerations. In this case the fetal pH was 7.35, which is normal.

Infection of mother and/or of baby

Both the mother and fetus are at risk of infection, usually by organisms normally present in the vagina. Infection may be the cause of spontaneous premature labour or may supervene during labour, the risk of the latter increasing the longer the amniotic membranes have been broken. Obvious signs of infection may not be apparent, but if present they include maternal fever, lower abdominal/pelvic tenderness, offensive vaginal discharge and fetal tachycardia. Infection is managed first by collecting blood and vaginal cultures followed by antibiotics given to the mother during labour and to the mother and the baby after birth. Delivery is expedited, particularly if there is evidence of fetal distress.

Maternal exhaustion

If the mother becomes dehydrated and/or exhausted during labour, fetal distress may occur, particularly if the mother becomes ketotic. Administration of fluids and analgesia will often correct this, although delivery may need to be expedited.

Abnormal delivery

Instrumental and operative deliveries carry an increased risk of maternal and neonatal morbidity. However, intervention is indicated when there is a risk of damage if the labour continues.

Instrumental delivery (forceps and vacuum)

Delivery may be expedited using forceps or the Ventouse vacuum extractor if the cervix is fully dilated and the head fully engaged in the pelvis. If the position of the fetal head is other than occipito-anterior, rotation can be effected manually with Ventouse or rotational forceps (Keillands). Instrumental deliveries almost always require an episiotomy.

Caesarean section

If vaginal delivery is deemed inappropriate, caesarean section may be performed either as an elective or emergency procedure. Elective caesarean sections are performed between 38 and 39 weeks in order to try to avoid problems of prematurity. However, a baby delivered by section does not have the normal period of physiological adaptation that occurs during labour. They may be affected by delayed clearance of lung fluid leading to usually mild respiratory distress. Emergency caesarean section is required when unexpected complications during labour necessitate a rapid delivery.

Abnormal presentations

If a fetus presents as a breech at the time of labour, there is an increased risk of fetal trauma and hypoxia. However, providing that the labour is managed well and the baby is estimated to weigh less than 3.5 kg with an adequate maternal pelvis, a trial of vaginal delivery with low threshold for caesarean section is reasonable. If the lie of the fetus is anything other than longitudinal (i.e. the longitudinal axis of the fetus parallel to the longitudinal axis of the uterus) delivery must be by caesarean section.

Fetal rights and ethics

There is no universal agreement concerning the rights of the fetus. Currently, investigation and treatment relies on maternal consent alone. However, there have been cases where the fetus has been made a ward of court and procedures performed on the mother without her consent. These have always related to operative delivery where the courts have felt the risk to the baby is so great that it will die if not delivered. Such cases are very rare, and deservedly so. Philosophers may help us in our quest for clarification of this type of problem. The question of whether the fetus feels pain has been addressed, and studies continue. As our knowledge of fetal physiology, health and disease continues to expand, the ethical dilemmas we face will also grow. However, by working as members of a team involving those from obstetric and paediatric disciplines we should be able to deal both effectively and ethically with the majority of problems we face.

New horizons

A small number of surgical procedures have now been carried out on the unborn child. The majority of these are ultrasound-guided, although an extrauterine approach has been used. The role of fetal surgery is limited, but this is an area of potential growth and development as we learn more about the natural history of some congenital conditions.

One application of these techniques is in the management of obstructive uropathies (p. 297), which can lead to renal damage. The drainage of hydronephrotic kidneys (Fig 17.1) has not been very successful, but insertion of a pigtail shunt into the bladder in cases of posterior urethral valves (p. 302) does appear to protect the kidneys from further damage and permit normalization of amniotic fluid volume and thus prevent pulmonary hypoplasia. Such interventions have probably improved the outcome in carefully selected cases. Other drainage procedures include the chronic drainage of pleural effusions, which if left may cause pulmonary hypoplasia. Fetal ascites may be drained prior to delivery and thus make resuscitation of the newborn easier. Hydrocephalus can be shunted in utero, but with a very low success rate, and it is rarely done today. There have been two successful cases of intrauterine balloon dilatation of stenotic aortic valves (p. 176), where a needle is inserted directly into the fetal left ventricle and a balloon passed across the aortic valve. This type of procedure has limited application.

One team in the United States has performed a number of extrauterine repairs of congenital diaphragmatic hernias. Such an approach involves performing a hysterotomy and carries significant morbidity for mother and fetus. The results have been disappointing, and this approach is unlikely to have many further applications.

FURTHER READING

Chamberlain GVP (ed) (1995) *Obstetrics by Ten Teachers.* London: Arnold.

Human Embryology Act 1991. London: HMSO.

Reed GB, Claireaux AE, Cockburn F (eds) (1995) *Diseases of the Fetus and Newborn.* London: Chapman and Hall.

Rodeck CH (ed) (1993) Prenatal diagnosis. In: *Trends in Childbirth Statistics.* Edinburgh: Churchill Livingstone.

2 The first month of life

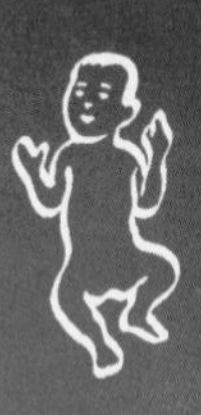

Introduction and epidemiology

The neonatal period (see Table 2.1 for definitions) is a period of great change for the infant and medical infant problems are relatively common. The newborn infant needs to adapt rapidly to postnatal independent life and failure to achieve such changes can result in disease, particularly in premature infants. In addition, major congenital malformations and genetic disorders will usually manifest at this age.

During labour, the physiological adaptation in the mature fetus which began towards the later stages of pregnancy accelerates in preparation for adaptation to extrauterine life. Examples of this adaptation during labour include:

- Absorption of lung fluid in preparation for the first breath
- A rise in neutrophil count (Fig. 2.1) to assist the change from a sterile to a bacteriologically contaminated environment.

The advancing sophistication of neonatal intensive care means that increasingly premature and sick infants have a chance of surviving (Fig. 2.2 and Table 2.2). Most neonatal intensive care units will report an upward trend in survival rates for those infants born from 24 weeks' gestation onwards and for those weighing upwards of 500 g, and even, sometimes, below these limits. Outcome studies in survivors of extreme

Table 2.1
Standard definitions in neonatology

Neonatal period	First 28 days of life
Premature birth	Birth before 37 weeks' gestation
Postmature birth	Birth after 42 weeks
Low birthweight (LBW)	<2500 g at birth
Very low birthweight (VLBW)	<1500 g at birth
Small for gestational age (SGA) infants	Infants born with weights <10th centile for gestation
Perinatal mortality	Stillbirths and early neonatal deaths
Neonatal mortality	Deaths in the first 28 days
Early neonatal mortality	Deaths at 0–6 days
Late neonatal mortality	Deaths at 7–27 days
Infant mortality	All deaths in the first year

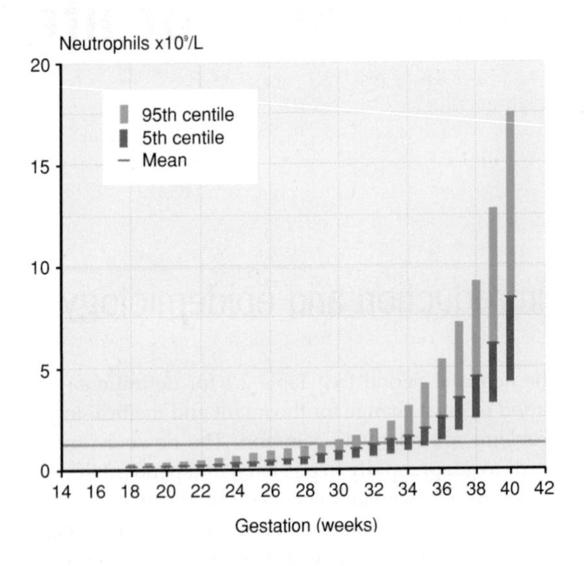

Fig 2.1
Neutrophil count at different gestations.

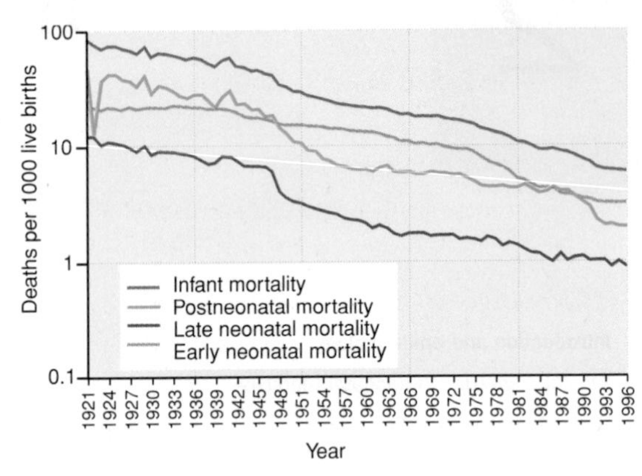

Fig 2.2
Neonatal mortality in England and Wales 1921–96. (From Platt MJ, *Archives of Disease in Childhood* 1998; 79: 523–7.)

Table 2.2
Improving rates of neonatal mortality (deaths per 1000 live births) at different gestational ages, in Scotland between 1984 and 1995. (Taken from Rennie and Roberton (1999) *Textbook of Neonatology*. Edinburgh: Harcourt Brace.)

	Gestational age, weeks							Total
	Less than 26	26–27	28–31	32–36	37–41	42 or more	Not known	
1984	793.1	472.4	165.6	20.0	2.0	2.2	16.0	6.4
1985	897.1	471.1	133.3	19.0	1.8	1.5	9.3	5.5
1986	763.2	454.5	128.9	15.5	1.7	2.3	9.9	5.2
1987	852.9	392.9	144.7	16.3	1.3	1.3	6.1	4.7
1988	700.0	384.6	89.6	13.9	1.6	1.0	13.4	4.5
1989	910.3	360.4	119.9	12.0	1.4	1.4	19.9	4.7
1990	802.3	283.2	102.3	11.7	1.5	0.8	7.5	4.4
1991	756.1	298.0	92.0	11.4	1.5	0.8	12.3	4.4
1992	666.7	382.8	60.2	14.4	1.7	0.9	4.5	4.6
1993	666.7	243.0	74.9	15.2	1.5	0.3	5.9	4.0
1994	710.5	292.0	59.7	9.1	1.1	3.1	2.7	4.0
1995*	823.5	355.6	63.8	10.5	1.3	0.7	0.0	3.9

*Provisional
(Source: Scottish Stillbirth and Neonatal Death Reports, 1988, 1989, 1994 and ISD unpublished data)

prematurity suggest that most of them do not suffer major handicap. However, as advances in treatment occur there is continued monitoring to ensure that the potential for a normal outcome in survivors is maintained.

Morbidity in this age group is as important as mortality. The most important causes of morbidity are those associated with neurological damage and long-term handicap such as cerebral palsy. Perinatal events leading to birth asphyxia certainly contribute to these and are important because they are potentially preventable. However in infants born at term, prenatal and genetic influences are more likely to be the cause of any neurological impairment. Cerebral palsy and other neurological problems are found more frequently in low birthweight infants. The rate is highest in the smallest infants, reflecting the greater severity of the perinatal problems that they are likely to suffer.

Areas of paramount importance to those involved in the care of newborn infants are summarized in Information box 2.1.

Ethical dilemmas in neonatal medicine

Neonatal medicine is subject to the usual ethical issues which occur throughout medical practice. Some of these

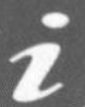

Information Box 2.1

Key issues in neonatal medicine

1. **The reduction of perinatal and infant mortality**. Though both have fallen in recent years (Table 2.3) this trend can easily be affected by changes in clinical practice in obstetrics or paediatrics. The new specialty of fetal medicine has an important role in this area.
2. **The prevention of handicap**. This is as important as the reduction in mortality. The quality of life of survivors of neonatal intensive care needs continued monitoring.
3. **Optimizing nutrition**. Paediatricians play an important role in facilitating the best start to the newborn infant's life at a critical stage in growth and development. Optimal nutrition may be of lasting benefit.

relate to the provision of care to very premature infants within the limited health care resources available. There are two specific issues which often present the clinician with a dilemma:

- Resuscitation at birth
- Withdrawal of supportive therapy.

Resuscitation at birth

As neonatal intensive care units treat ever smaller and more immature infants, the line between a viable infant (who should be resuscitated and given full intensive care treatment) and one who is non-viable becomes blurred. It is not possible to give a precise gestation or weight at which this distinction should be made; the merits of each case need to be assessed individually.

When it is clear that a mother with a pregnancy at the limits of neonatal viability is going to deliver, the paediatric staff should be involved prenatally and should meet the parents and discuss the issue of resuscitation and intensive care. This discussion will be guided by obstetric information about fetal size and wellbeing but often the decision as to whether to attempt resuscitation needs to be taken immediately after birth once the infant has been carefully assessed. This should be performed by a senior paediatrician. The parents' wishes must be taken into account. For infants with major congenital malformations at any stage in gestation, the same assessment will be applied.

Withdrawal of supportive therapy

In a newborn receiving intensive care support it may become clear that there is no chance of survival or that survival would only be possible with severe handicap. The situation may arise as a result of extreme prematurity with complications (such as extensive intracranial haemorrhage), or following severe birth asphyxia/injury or major congenital abnormality. It may become appropriate to withdraw life support treatments, resulting in the death of the infant (which would have occurred earlier had it not been for medical intervention). The decision to withdraw treatment must only be taken after full discussion with the family and members of staff. It should never be hurried.

Once the decision is taken, sensitive handling of the situation is essential (see p. 41). The staff on the unit, particularly those who are less experienced, will also need support at this time. Normal care (nursing as opposed to medical) should continue and this includes changing, dressing, feeding (if tolerated), keeping warm and providing comfort to infant and family. Steps should be taken to relieve pain and distress in the infant and in all concerned.

Clinical approach

Birth

The mechanics of birth are discussed in textbooks of obstetrics. Those issues relevant to fetal and neonatal medicine are discussed in Chapter 1.

The baby needing resuscitation

Infants may require cardiopulmonary resuscitation immediately after birth for a number of reasons (Information box 2.2).

Asphyxia is the most important cause. Asphyxia means lack of oxygen. In its medical usage, this carries the implication of possible hypoxia and ischaemia in the tissues and acidaemia.

Many of these problems are predictable before birth and a paediatrician experienced in resuscitation should attend the delivery (Information box 2.3).

Occasionally babies without any obvious risk factors have trouble establishing regular respiration after birth. Therefore it is essential that whoever attends a delivery, either in hospital or in the community, should be trained in neonatal resuscitation.

ASSESSMENT OF THE CONDITION AT BIRTH

Where it is obvious that a baby does not require resuscitation, or needs only minimal attention, a check for obvious congenital abnormalities should be made and if none are apparent he/she should be returned as quickly as possible to the mother to allow bonding to begin.

Infants who are apnoeic at birth need rapid assessment for the severity of asphyxia, if present, and

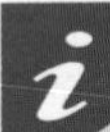

Information Box 2.2

Some of the reasons why a baby may need resuscitation at birth

- Acute intrapartum asphyxia
- Chronic intrauterine hypoxia
- Prematurity (immature respiratory drive, surfactant deficiency)
- Depressant maternal drugs (e.g. opiates)
- Severe birth trauma
- Hydrops
- Overwhelming sepsis
- Congenital disorder affecting:
  - Central nervous system
  - Neuromuscular system
  - Lungs (including hypoplasia)
  - Upper airway (obstruction)
  - Heart
  - Abdomen (causing massive distension)

for obvious major congenital abnormalities. At this stage there is no scoring system which reliably predicts the degree of asphyxia and hence the subsequent outcome. The one most widely used is the Apgar score (named after the late Dr Virginia Apgar, an anaesthetist from the USA) shown in Emergency box 2.1. Scores totalling 5 or under usually indicate the need for active resuscitation. Some infants with higher scores may need intubation because of apnoea while infants initially with very low scores may pick up following stimulation and face mask oxygen. The main problem with the Apgar scoring system is that it gives equal weight to all the parameters ignoring the fact that heart rate and respiration are the most vital; thus it is important to record a description of the infant's condition as well as the Apgar score.

Emergency Box 2.1

The basis of the AGPAR score

	Score		
	0	**1**	**2**
Response to stimulation	None	Grimace	Cry
Colour (of trunk)	White	Blue	Pink
Tone	Flaccid	Poor but present	Good
Heart rate	Absent	<100	>100
Respiration	None	Gasps	Regular

Information Box 2.3

Reasons for having a paediatrician present at delivery

- Forceps and Ventouse (vacuum) delivery
- Caesarean sections
- Breech delivery
- Multiple births
- Pre-37-week premature deliveries
- Where fetal distress has been detected or suspected
- Meconium-stained liquor
- Infants of diabetic mothers
- Hydropic infants
- Congenital abnormalities

As resuscitation proceeds it is essential to reassess the infant's condition on a regular timed basis. In cases of birth asphyxia, the results of the Apgar score measured 20 minutes after birth correlate better with subsequent neurological prognosis than do earlier scores. Another prognostic indicator in the asphyxiated newborn is the acid–base balance, which is best estimated by measuring the base deficit in an arterial blood sample.

Details of the baby's condition and the resuscitation procedures should be recorded accurately in writing, because where subsequent handicap is attributed to birth asphyxia, litigation may follow. Vital pieces of evidence such as fetal heart rate traces can easily be mislaid and must be kept safely.

THE PRINCIPLES OF RESUSCITATION

Published guidelines for neonatal resuscitation are available (see Further Reading), and paediatric units should have their own written procedure including any local modifications.

Resuscitation must be performed by an experienced individual capable of endotracheal intubation and rapidly establishing intravenous access through either peripheral or umbilical veins. A fully equipped resuscitation trolley (Practical box 2.1; Fig. 2.3) must be available and should be regularly checked and serviced.

It is important to ensure that the parents who are often anxiously watching events are kept informed of progress. Endotracheal intubation is the most important procedure, and in an apnoeic and bradycardic infant it should be undertaken as soon as possible. In an apnoeic infant with a good heart rate it is reasonable to delay intubation for a few minutes while inflating the lungs with oxygen via a bag and mask (Fig. 2.4).

When intubation is necessary, intermittent positive

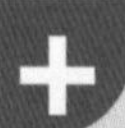

Practical Box 2.1

Essential equipment and drugs for the resuscitation trolley

- Flat surface for infant with slight head-down tilt
- Overhead heater
- Blanket or other wrap, foil
- Oxygen supply connected via water manometer
- Mucus extraction system connected to vacuum pump
- Stethoscope
- Laryngoscope
- Endotracheal tubes and appropriate connectors
- Butterfly needles for intravenous cannulation
- Umbilical vein catheters
- Drugs: adrenalin, naloxone, calcium chloride, atropine, sodium bicarbonate
- Surfactant
- Albumin 4.5% solution

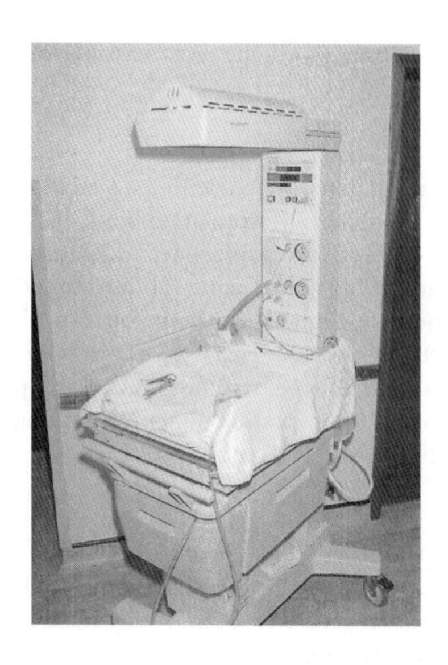

Fig 2.3
Typical resuscitation trolley.

pressure ventilation is commenced immediately (except in cases of meconium aspiration, see below). Often this results in rapid improvement in the infant's condition and extubation can rapidly follow.

If the infant fails to improve, the position of the tube must be checked, and intrathoracic problems (such as pneumothorax or diaphragmatic hernia), lung problems (such as hypoplasia), persistent fetal circulation (neonatal pulmonary hypertension) or major congenital heart defect should be considered. Correction of any hypoglycaemia, especially likely in low birthweight infants, should be performed.

When the heart rate is persistently very low, or absent, external cardiac massage as well as adrenalin, initially via endotracheal tube and then intravenously or by cardiac puncture, is given alongside intravenous sodium bicarbonate to correct acidosis. Further help should be sought in the most severe cases and the infant should be transferred to the neonatal intensive care unit. Most infants who have undergone a prolonged and difficult resuscitation will develop late complications (p. 28).

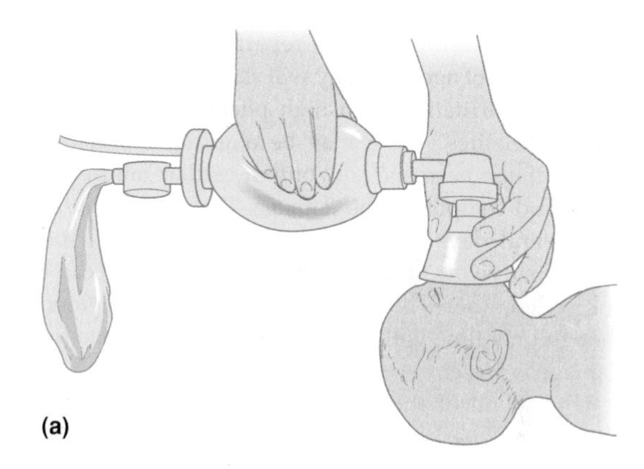

(a)

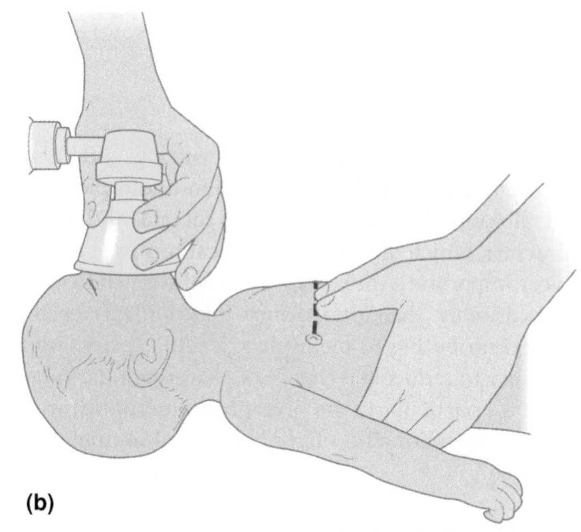

(b)

Fig 2.4
(a) Typical bag and mask used for neonatal resuscitation. (b) External cardiac massage of a newborn infant This can also be performed using two fingers of each hand, without holding the chest.

Common problems resulting from birth complications

BIRTH ASPHYXIA

Perinatal lack of oxygen leads to this condition in which the infant suffers from hypoxic ischaemic insult. Even though the neonate can withstand a lack of oxygen much better than older people, at least partly because of the presence of fetal haemoglobin, permanent damage can occur. Not surprisingly, the brain is the most susceptible organ and the least capable of repairing itself.

Causes

Several factors can interfere with the fetal blood supply, resulting in asphyxia (Information box 2.4).

When intrapartum asphyxia is diagnosed, prompt and efficient obstetric intervention together with paediatric resuscitation can limit the damage caused. With such intervention most babies born with moderate asphyxia will escape without long-term problems. Unfortunately, a proportion suffer lasting damage (see Information box 2.5).

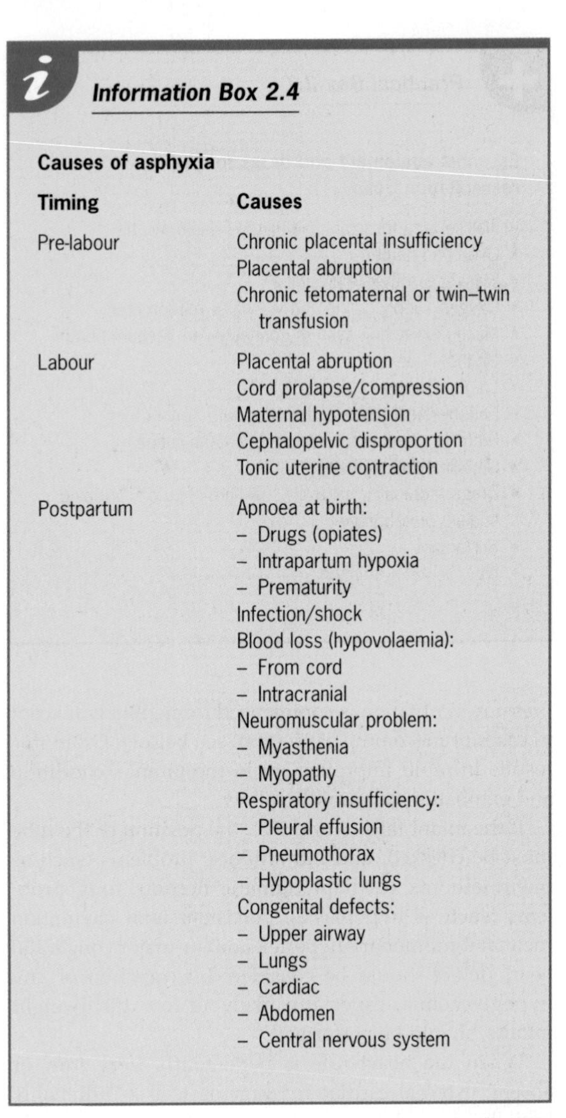

Information Box 2.4

Causes of asphyxia

Timing	Causes
Pre-labour	Chronic placental insufficiency Placental abruption Chronic fetomaternal or twin–twin transfusion
Labour	Placental abruption Cord prolapse/compression Maternal hypotension Cephalopelvic disproportion Tonic uterine contraction
Postpartum	Apnoea at birth: – Drugs (opiates) – Intrapartum hypoxia – Prematurity Infection/shock Blood loss (hypovolaemia): – From cord – Intracranial Neuromuscular problem: – Myasthenia – Myopathy Respiratory insufficiency: – Pleural effusion – Pneumothorax – Hypoplastic lungs Congenital defects: – Upper airway – Lungs – Cardiac – Abdomen – Central nervous system

Clinical signs

Asphyxiated babies are initially quiet and pale in appearance. In severe cases they may need ventilatory and circulatory support from birth.

The natural course of events is for the baby's condition to deteriorate before it improves and this is thought to be due to ongoing tissue damage as blood supply is restored, i.e. reperfusion injury. By 12–24 hours of age, the baby will show increasing signs of cerebral irritation with high pitched cry, jitteriness and/or seizures. There may be oliguria/anuria from acute tubular necrosis. Low output cardiac failure may occur and compound the damage. This stage may last for several days and in severe cases death ensues. Among survivors and those with seizures which can be controlled, there is usually gradual improvement, though only time will tell what persisting neurological damage is present.

Ultrasound of the brain provides some prognostic clues: early marked cerebral oedema and later echo-dense areas progressing to leucomalacia (necrosis of cerebal tissue, shown by ultrasound or CT scan) are bad prognostic signs.

Clinical management

This is largely supportive. Ensuring adequate oxygenation and treating hypotension (inotropic drugs and albumin infusions), hypoglycaemia and hypocalcaemia, which are all are complications of asphyxia, is very important. Antibiotics are usually given to cover the possibility that intrapartum infection has been a factor contributing to the asphyxia. Fluid restriction is necessary to reduce the chance of exacerbating cerebral oedema, particularly as inappropriate antidiuretic hormone secretion and oliguric renal failure may both be present.

Information Box 2.5

Reasons for poor outcome in asphyxia

- The threshold for damage was lowered by prolonged intrauterine hypoxia (from placental insufficiency).
- Intrapartum events were sudden or devastating or were unrecognized (or unrecognizable), so that obstetric intervention did not help.
- Postnatal resuscitation was not possible or was inadequate.

MECONIUM ASPIRATION

Meconium aspiration at birth may cause respiratory distress. The premature passage of meconium is usually due to fetal distress and is more common in post-term deliveries. The problems of birth asphyxia may therefore be superimposed. Attendants at deliveries where meconium has been produced should try to clear the airway of meconium as rapidly as possible (even before the trunk has delivered). The paediatrician should visualize the vocal cords with a laryngoscope and, using a catheter, suck out any meconium before any positive pressure ventilation is given.

Despite these efforts there are occasions when meconium finds its way to the lower airway. Symptoms of respiratory distress occur, and radiography usually shows a mixture of patchy atelectasis and hyperinflation. Pneumothoraces are common.

Treatment involves supplemental oxygen and management of any accompanying birth asphyxia. Ventilation may be necessary but should be avoided if possible, since it increases the problem of unequal air distribution and the risk of pneumothorax. In the most severe cases, extra corporeal membrane oxygenation therapy has been used. The respiratory distress may persist for several days but eventually settles, usually without any long-term problems.

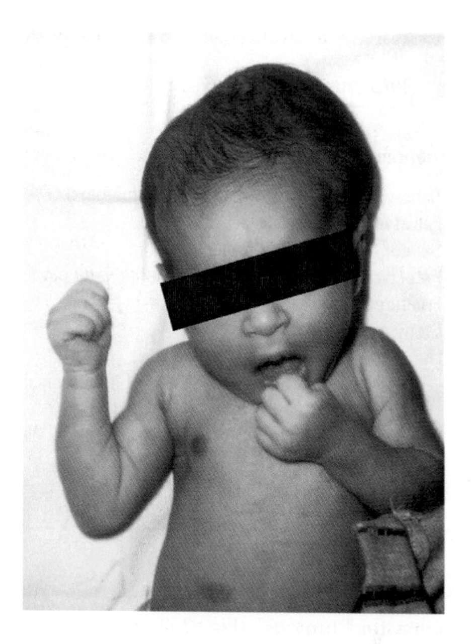

Fig 2.5
Cephalhaematoma.

BIRTH TRAUMA

Normal full-term newborn infants are fairly resilient. Most doctors and midwives can recall startling anecdotes of babies surviving mishaps unscathed, including being dropped on the floor or being born at home into lavatory bowls.

Physical injury to the infant may occur as a result of difficult vaginal delivery. This is more likely to occur with large babies (or those with congenital hydrocephalus), or with mechanical obstetric complications such as abnormal presentation of the fetus or small maternal pelvis. In these cases obstetricians often have to intervene and may be wrongly blamed for causing bruising with forceps, etc. Severe injury is relatively uncommon.

Physical injury mostly manifests as bruising or haematomas. Most commonly the haematoma is subperiosteal over one of the skull bones, most often the parietal bone (Fig. 2.5). Bruising should not be confused with mongolian blue spots (p. 31) which are common in highly pigmented races. Fracture of the clavicle may occur.

Nerve palsies, generally caused by stretching injury, are relatively common, mostly affecting the brachial plexus (Fig. 2.6). These usually improve spontaneously over time. Occasionally, serious injury such as fractured skull with or without intracranial haemorrhage, spinal cord injury or ruptured abdominal viscus, can occur, and these carry a risk of mortality and/or long-term morbidity. The situation is often complicated by accompanying birth asphyxia and this may be the important cause of any long-term problems.

The commoner minor birth injuries are listed in Information box 2.6.

In most cases no specific treatment is required but the parents will need reassurance because of the obvious disfigurement of their child. Heavily bruised infants may get more severe jaundice through absorption of broken-down blood. Infants with nerve palsies should be referred for physiotherapy. Some infants develop haemorrhage and swelling in a sternomastoid; this produces an area of hard swelling about the size of an acorn misleadingly known as a

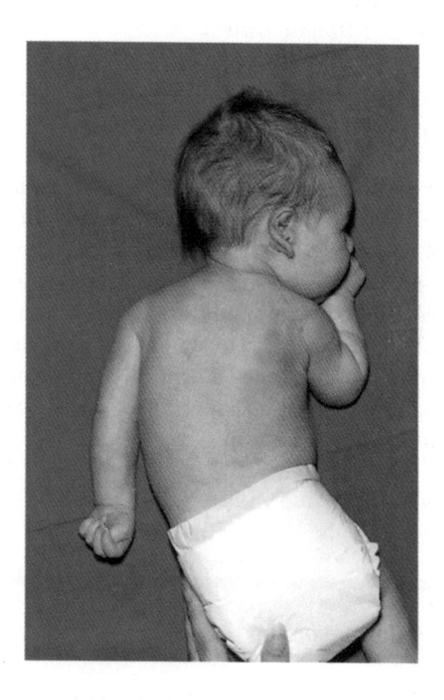

Fig 2.6
Infant with Erb palsy. Arm assumes the "waiter's tip" position.

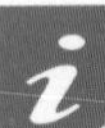

Information Box 2.6

Commoner (minor) birth injuries

- Subperiosteal haematoma (cephalhaematoma)
- Facial bruising/swelling
- Subconjunctival haemorrhages
- Petechial rash in distribution of superior vena cava
- Fractured clavicle
- Sternomastoid 'tumour'
- Nerve palsy
  - Erb; stretching of the upper roots of the brachial plexus
  - Klumpke; stretching of lower roots of brachial plexus
  - Facial nerve

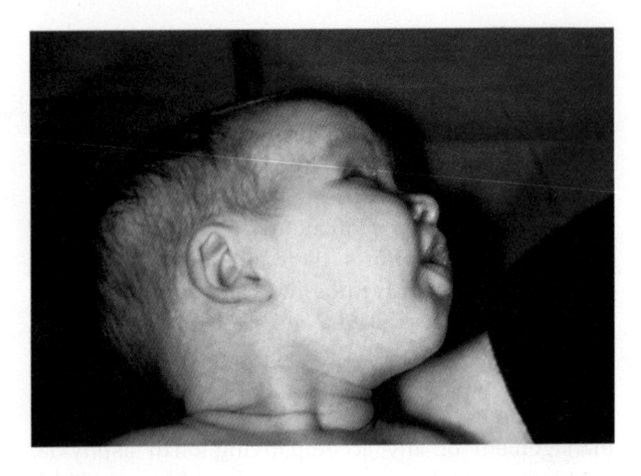

Fig 2.7
Sternomastoid tumour.

'sternomastoid tumour' (Fig. 2.7). Many such infants are referred to a physiotherapist though there is no evidence that this helps. In most cases the swelling resolves spontaneously.

The normal baby

At birth the normal full-term baby successfully adapts to extrauterine survival in a matter of seconds. In part the onset of respiration is a response to chemical influences such as prostaglandins and to physical factors including the lowering of pressure effects exerted by the uterus. The full process of physiological adaptation to extrauterine life continues during the following weeks (Information box 2.7). The control of this process remains poorly understood.

Information Box 2.7

Continuing adaptation to extrauterine life

- Production of surfactant
- Closure of the ductus venosus and ductus arteriosus
- Lowering the blood volume and haemoglobin content
- Production of digestive enzymes
- Coordination of swallowing and sucking through development of inborn reflexes
- Thickening of the skin
- Use of senses of vision, hearing and pain and an ability to adapt psychologically

Examination

Examination of the infant is required to detect congenital abnormalities, exclude disease processes and establish a baseline for future comparison, the latter being particularly important for neurodevelopmental assessment.

Examination must be carried out on a systematic basis, though it may need to be modified and repeated if the baby is restless or unwell. Ideally the infant should be in a quiet but wakeful state, and undressed apart from a nappy which must be removed during the examination so that the genitalia, anus, femoral pulses and hernial orifices can be examined.

The examination can be divided into physical and neurodevelopmental assessments.

PHYSICAL EXAMINATION

1. General external appearance of the baby

- **Central cyanosis** may indicate an underlying cardiorespiratory problem.
- **Jaundice**. This is relatively common between the 3rd and 5th days of life. Presence of jaundice, even mild, on the first day suggests haemolysis.
- **Pallor** suggests anaemia (possible feto-maternal haemorrhage or rarer bone marrow disorder).
- **Bruising** may be due to birth trauma but if extensive and associated with petechial skin haemorrhage warrants investigation for coagulation disorder or thrombocytopenia. NB: Mongolian blue spots (Fig. 2.8) commonly found over the buttocks and lower back but occasionally occurring elsewhere are common in black babies and can be confused with bruising; they gradually fade.

2. Examination of the skull

- **Swelling** may be due to 'caput' formation: oedema fluid resulting from the passage of the head through

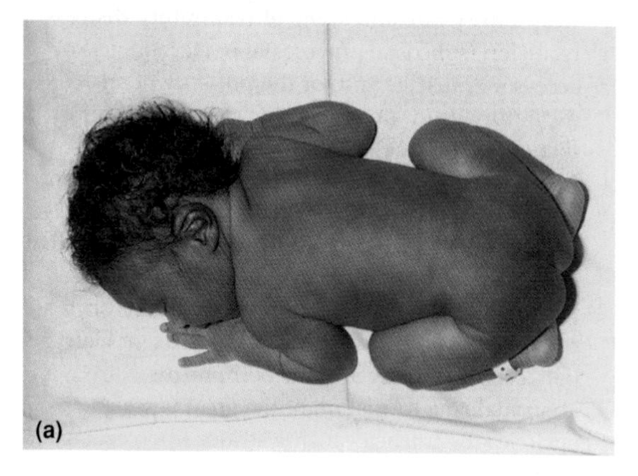
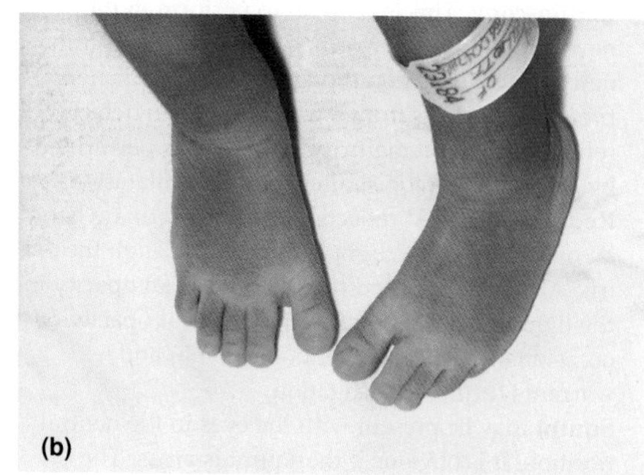

Fig 2.8 (a) & (b)
Mongolian blue spot.

the birth canal. This should not be confused with a *cephalhaematoma* (p. 29).

The swelling in the former crosses sutures whereas the latter is a subperiosteal haematoma limited to the area overlying one of the flat bones of the skull.

- **Size and tension of the fontanelles and sutures**. See Figure 2.9.
- **Occipitofrontal circumference**. Measure with a paper non-stretch measuring tape, taking the maximum circumference obtained on at least three different measurements. Measurements should be plotted on appropriate centile charts.

  Sequential measurements are more useful than single ones as they will give a trend. An abnormally small head size, or one falling off the growth chart centiles, implies that some insult has impaired brain growth. Megalencephaly (large head) is often of no significance, particularly if familial, but a head size crossing growth chart centiles upwards implies abnormal enlargement of the brain, most commonly due to developing hydrocephalus.
- **Asymmetry of the skull or face** may be the result of distortion following a difficult birth or, rarely, a developmental abnormality.

3. Examination of the face: general

- **Dysmorphic features** include the presence of epicanthic folds or disproportions in the facial measurements and the shape, structure and position of the ears. If in doubt measurements should be taken and compared with normative data (normal values in Smith's *Recognizable Patterns of Human Malformation*, see Further Reading). The opinion of a clinical geneticist may be helpful.

4. Examination of the eyes

- **Size and shape**. Normal ranges of measurements can be found in *Recognizable Patterns of Human Malformation* (see Further Reading).
- **Completeness of iris to exclude colobomata** (cleft of the iris).
- **Subconjunctival haemorrhages** may be present following passage through the birth canal and normally disappear shortly after birth.

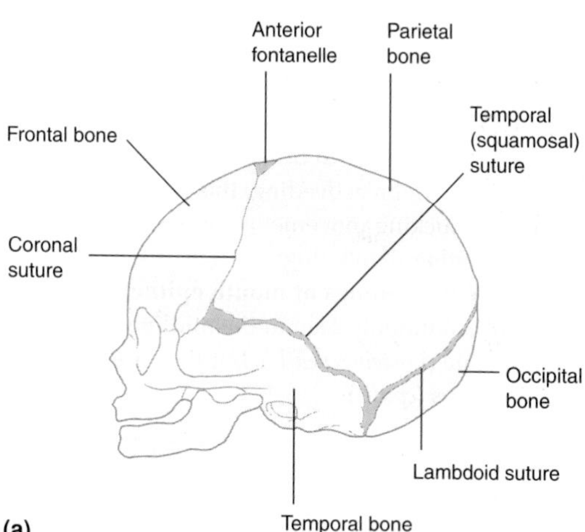

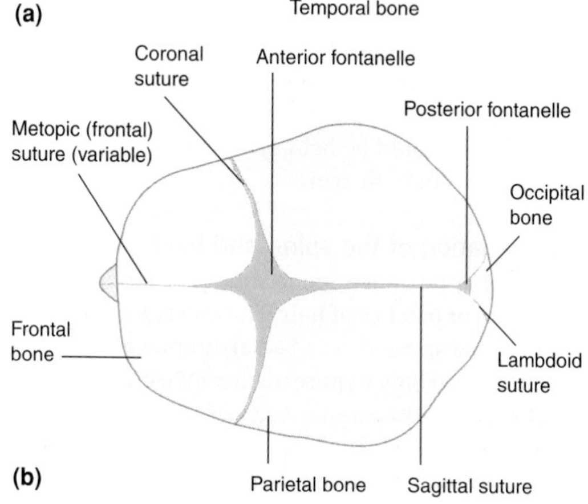

Fig 2.9 (a) & (b)
The fontanelles and sutures.

- **Retinoscopy**. This is difficult to perform in the newborn. It is not performed as part of the routine newborn examination though it is undertaken in premature infants from 6 weeks of age to detect retinopathy of prematurity. Usually it is performed by an ophthalmologist after pupillary dilatation.
- **Red reflex** is a red reflection from the retina when an ophthalmoscope light is directed through the iris. Absence of the red reflex suggests an opacity in the light path such as a cataract, corneal opacity or occasionally a tumour (retinoblastoma) and warrants further investigation.
- **Squint** may be present with the eyes in the neutral position. It is obvious if the squint is gross. The visual axes are not always parallel in newborns. An intermittent squint is common and rarely of importance in the newborn.

5. Examination of the mouth and lips

- **Cleft lip**.
- **Cleft palate**. The hard and soft palate should be examined for visible clefts, but the palate should also be felt with a finger to exclude submucosal clefts.
- **Appearance of the mouth**.
- **Size of the tongue and jaw**. An abnormally small jaw may suggest a number of syndromes such as Pierre Robin or Treacher Collins.
- **Teeth** are occasionally present from birth. Their presence either at birth or later rarely leads to problems with breastfeeding; this is done by powerful sucking movements involving the cheek muscle, rather than biting!
- **Cyst-like thickenings of mouth epithelium**. These are most commonly seen in the midline over the hard palate (*Epstein's pearls*), but they are also found on the gums (*epulis*).

6. Examination of the shoulders and neck

- **Integrity of the clavicles**. These should be palpated to exclude fractures acquired at the time of birth.
- **Range of neck movements**.
- **Presence of sternomastoid swelling.** Palpate sternomastoid muscles to exclude this.
- **Shoulders** should be held symmetrically with equal movements of both arms.

7. Examination of the spine and back

- **General appearance:** spine should be straight.
- **Dimples or patches of hair**. These may indicate an underlying spinal defect. Sacral dimples are very common and only require further investigation if the bottom of the pit cannot be seen when the skin is gently parted or if there is swelling or abnormal hair present. Sacral dimples should not be probed at the bedside.

8. Examination of the chest

- **Shape**.
- **Respiratory rate and signs of respiratory distress**: recession (subcostal, intercostal or sternal), use of accessory muscles and/or the presence of an expiratory grunt (a nonspecific sign of respiratory distress at this age).
- **Inspiratory noise**. This is most likely to be present with the baby lying supine. Inspiratory stridor usually with subcostal and intercostal recession may suggest a congenital laryngeal problem, such as laryngomalacia, or more serious conditions such as congenital web between the vocal cords, or cleft between the airway and the oesophagus. Rarely, an abnormal ring formation of the great vessels encircles the trachea causing stridor upon crying, feeding or neck flexion.

9. Examination of the cardiovascular system

- **Colour:** presence of central/peripheral cyanosis.
- **Pulse rate and character**.
- **Pulse in all four limbs**. Palpation of the femoral pulses requires patience and is best achieved in a baby who is not wriggling. If there is any suggestion of weakness of the femoral pulses, coarctation of the aorta needs to be excluded.
- **Measurement of blood pressure**. This procedure, straightforward in adults, can be difficult in infants and young children. The problems include getting a quiet relaxed child so that a meaningful measurement is obtained, and being able to hear the sounds with a stethoscope. The pressure cuff should cover two thirds of the upper arm. Doppler methods are available for measurement in infants and young children (p. 181). Normal blood pressures in newborn infants are shown in Tables 2.3 and 2.4.
- **The precordium.** This should be examined and palpated for position and character of the trachea, apex beat (should be in the 4th intercostal space), presence of any thrills, and a parasternal heave.
- **Auscultation** in the pulmonary, aortic, tricuspid and mitral areas and over the back. (Pulmonary murmurs and murmurs from patent ductus arteriosus (PDA) often radiate through to the back.) NB: the presence of a PDA murmur may be normal

Table 2.3
Normal blood pressure values on day 1 in healthy preterm infants (not receiving inotropes or intermittent positive pressure ventilation). Some infants in added inspired oxygen; some receiving continuous positive airway pressure. Some recordings were direct intra-arterial and some were oscillometric

Gestation (weeks)	Number	Systolic range (mmHg)	Diastolic range (mmHg)
<24	11	48–63	24–39
24–28	55	48–58	22–36
29–32	110	47–59	24–34
>32	68	48–60	24–34

From: Heggi, T. et al. J. Pediatrics, 1994; 124: 627–633.

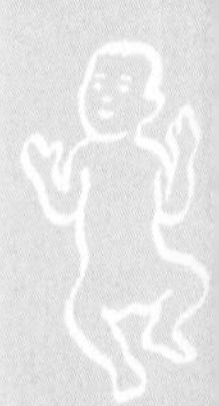

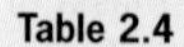

Table 2.4
Noninvasive (indirect) arm systolic blood pressures (mmHg) with pulse detected by Doppler probe. All infants 38 weeks' gestation or more

	Age, days					
	3	4	5	6	17	8–10
Awake						
Mean systolic BP (mmHg) ± SD	72 ± 6	74 ± 9	77 ± 10	77 ± 10	82 ± 9	88 ± 17
Numbers of infants	4	71	44	42	9	4
Asleep						
Mean systolic BP (mmHg) ± SD	68 ± 7	70 ± 8	72 ± 8	72 ± 9	72 ± 9	75 ± 9
Numbers of infants	72	681	426	322	47	18

(Derived from de Swiet M, Fayers P, Shinebourne EA (1980) Pediatrics 65: 1028–1035)

in the first 2–3 days of life while the duct is closing. When this is detected, the baby requires another check at a later stage to make sure that it has disappeared. Since right-sided heart pressures remain relatively high over the first few weeks of life, the presence of septal defects may not be detectable clinically as there is insufficient left-to-right shunting to produce a murmur.
- **Palpation of the abdomen** is part of the cardiovascular examination, looking for hepatomegaly, which is a sign of heart failure.

10. Examination of the abdomen
- **Appearance**: is there distension?
- **Palpation**: even the full abdomen should be soft and not tender.
- **Liver** is normally palpable up to 2 cm below the costal margin, but is often impalpable in infants with severe intrauterine growth restriction.
- **Spleen** should be impalpable.
- **Kidneys** are best palpated using a finger and thumb as shown in Figure 2.10 and should be barely palpable.
- **Anal size and position** should be noted.
- **Stool** at this stage is called *meconium*, a green/black viscous substance which should be passed within 24 hours of birth; failure to pass within 48 hours raises suspicions of rectal atresia, Hirschsprung disease, or meconium ileus, an early sign of cystic fibrosis.

11. Examination of the external genitalia: boys
- **Urethral orifice**. This should be at the tip of the penis. In *hypospadias* (Fig. 2.11) it is situated somewhere along the ventral surface of the penis: in mild forms, just at the ventral surface of the glans, and in severe forms, at the base of the penis.
- **Stream of urine**. A good stream largely excludes the problem of posterior urethral valves; a trickle demands repeat observation with a view to investigation.

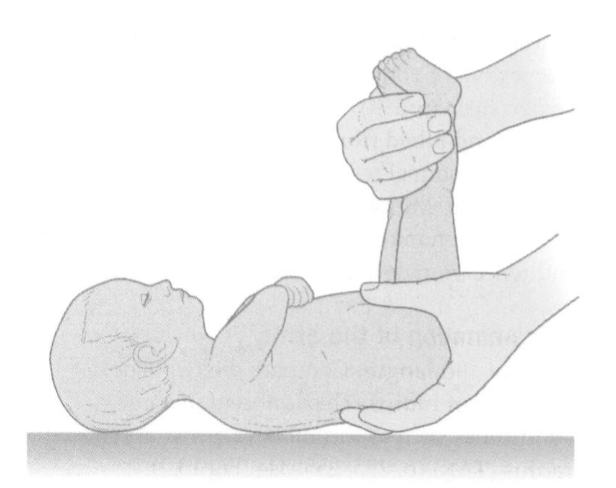

Fig 2.10
Single manual palpation of the kidneys.

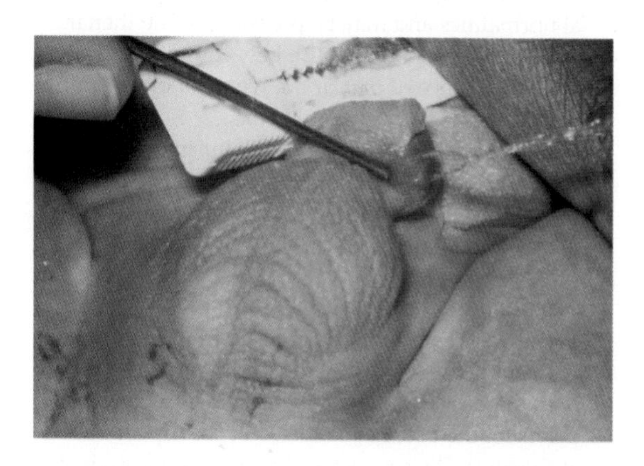

Fig 2.11
Hypospadias. (Courtesy of Ms. E. Gordon)

- **Prepuce (foreskin)**. This varies greatly in length. It is rarely retractile at birth; attempts should not be made to retract it at this age, and parents should be dissuaded if they request to have it removed (unless there are genuine religious reasons).
- **Penis**. If this is greatly oversized or pubic hair is present, consideration of possible congenital adrenal hyperplasia is warranted (p. 197).
- **Scrotum**. This should be palpated to check the descent of both testes. Hydrocele presents with a palpable fluid sac around the testis which sometimes extends up into the groin and communicates with the abdominal cavity through a patent processus vaginalis. The presence of abdominal contents in this sac constitutes a hernia. The scrotum shows increased pigmentation in congenital adrenal hyperplasia.

12. Examination of the external genitalia: girls
- **Fusion of the labia**.
- **Swellings in the labia majora** are possibly testes and if so are indicative of an intersex state.

- **Clitoral size (increased) and pigmentation** may be suggestive of conditions such as congenital adrenal hyperplasia (p. 197).
- **Mucus and blood from the vagina** at around 4 days of age is a normal response to maternal oestrogen withdrawal. Minor degrees of breast enlargement and lactation may occur in boys and girls under the influence of maternal oestrogen.

13. Examination of the arms

- **Posture** and **length.** Compare the two sides.
- **Presence of radius.** This is absent in some syndromes such as thrombocytopenia and absent radius (TAR) (p. 253, 255, 344, Fig 13.3).

14. Examination of the hands

- **Shape and structure**, especially of the **digits**. Accessory digits are relatively common minor abnormalities and may be preaxial (on the thenar side) or postaxial (Fig. 2.12). Less commonly there may be absence of part or the whole of one or more digits or webbing between them.
- **Palmar creases**. Abnormalities occur in certain conditions, most commonly in Down syndrome where there may be (but not always) a single crease in one or both hands.

15. Examination of the legs and hips

- **Posture** and **length** are compared, especially the length of the upper leg, measured by comparing the heights of both knees when the baby is held supine with the pelvis on the bed, flexed to 90° at the hip and at 90° at the knee. Discrepancy of length is suggestive of developmental dysplasia of the hip and is also seen in the rare Russell Silver syndrome (p. 205).
- **Hip examination** should be done gently; one hip at a time should be examined as this is less distressing to the baby. Forcible abduction of the hips is likely to upset the baby (and mother), and may damage the joint. Developmental dysplasia of the hip (DDH), formerly known as congenital dislocation of the hip, will be detected by Ortolani's procedure (Fig. 2.13). The thigh is abducted with the middle finger pressing the greater trochanter forward. It is confirmed if there is inability to fully abduct the hip, or the hip can be felt dislocating or a dislocated hip can be felt as it re-engages. The latter are felt as 'clunks'. 'Clicks' are more usually due to ligamentous laxity around the hip, rather than to true DDH. If there is uncertainty, a refinement of the test involves applying backward pressure with the thumb during abduction, to see whether the hip is unstable and can be dislocated backwards during the procedure. This is Barlow's test. Ultrasound scanning is a useful noninvasive test for infants where there is doubt about DDH.

16. Examination of the feet

- **Shape** and **structure** as for the hands. Rocker-bottom feet are found in trisomies 13 and 18.
- **Posture**. The normal foot is held neither everted nor inverted.
- **Dorsiflexion of the ankle** should allow the top of the foot to meet the lower leg just above the ankle. Occasionally babies may hold their foot inverted thus mimicking the position of *talipes equinovarus* (clubbed foot); a gentle effort should be made to return the foot to the normal position and if this can be achieved then true talipes is not present but rather a postural deformity probably related to the position of the foot in utero. The prognosis for this is excellent. In true talipes equinovarus the foot will not return to the normal position and will not dorsiflex fully; orthopaedic advice is needed.

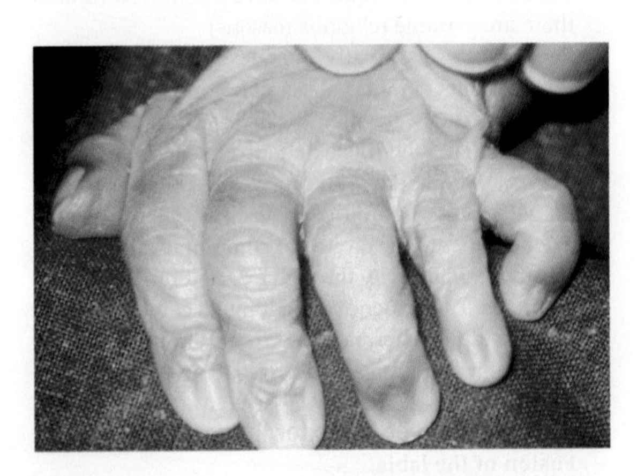

Fig 2.12
Postaxial polydactyly.

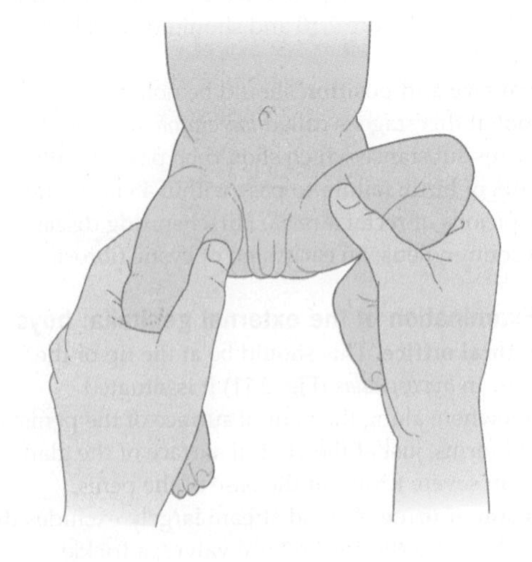

Fig 2.13
Detecting developmental dysplasia of the hip.

- **Puffy feet** suggest Turner syndrome and other chromosome disorders.
- **Digits**. Check for webbing, fusion or accessory digits.

17. Examination of the skin

- **Skin tags**. These may be present anywhere on the body but are found most commonly in the preauricular region. These should not be 'tied off' but referred to a plastic surgeon.
- **Dry peeling skin** is found in post-term infants.
- **Spots**. Tiny white pimples on the face, called *milia*, are present in a large proportion of infants. They represent blocked sebaceous glands and clear spontaneously. *Erythema toxicum* or *neonatal urticaria* is another common skin condition appearing at any stage from days 1 to 7. The lesions may be erythematous maculopapular, and in some places become vesicular. The aetiology is unclear but the condition is benign. The main problem is to distinguish them from staphylococcal septic spots (which require antibiotic treatment). Aspiration of the lesions of erythema toxicum reveals sterile fluid containing predominantly eosinophils.
- **Naevi**. Several types of haemangiomata may be present at birth or appear soon afterwards.
  Capillary haemangioma (*stork mark*) is often present around the head and neck particularly around the eyes and is of no consequence, usually disappearing over the first year (Fig. 9.5a).
  Cavernous haemangioma (*strawberry naevus*) is a florid, bright red, raised lesion which can appear anywhere on the body singly or multiply. Typically they are not present at birth but start to appear in the early weeks; they then gradually regress and fade leaving no scar by age 5–6 years. They can be a problem if situated over a site which can be readily traumatized resulting in bleeding and infection. Rarely, large lesions form around the eyes and interfere with visual fields or block tear ducts; in such instances corticosteroid treatment may help and, as a last resort, plastic surgery (Fig. 9.6).
  Capillary naevus (*port wine stain*) is potentially a more serious vascular malformation, which can occur anywhere but most commonly affects one side of the head and face in the distribution of the 5th cranial nerve. In this situation it is often associated with abnormal vascular malformation in the meninges covering the brain on the same side. This can interfere with brain development and function leading to convulsions and hemiplegia in severe cases (Sturge–Weber syndrome). The naevus is permanent (Fig. 9.5b).

NEUROLOGICAL EXAMINATION

The normal term baby adopts a flexed posture when placed prone (see Fig. 2.14). The posture should be symmetrical and all limbs should move equally. Asymmetry of posture may indicate a peripheral nerve palsy (most probably a result of birth trauma), a central nervous system abnormality or an orthopaedic problem such as congenital dislocation of the hip or talipes equinovarus. Abnormalities of tone may be apparent from the lack of this normal posture or may be detected when the baby is handled. The degree of head control can be assessed by pulling the baby up from the supine position, and trunk and limb tone by ventral suspension (Fig. 2.15).

So-called *primitive* or *neonatal reflexes* involve transitory neurological pathways and are of limited protective value to the infant. Generally they appear late in gestation and disappear over the early months of life. Eliciting these responses in infants is of some value: their absence in the neonatal period may occur after a severe neurological insult (such as severe birth asphyxia); asymmetry may indicate a unilateral neurological lesion, or persistence beyond 3–4 months of age may indicate a problem with motor development such as cerebral palsy.

Some of the more well known neonatal reflexes include:

- *Moro*: when the head is sharply extended there is startling outward movement of the arms, opening of the palms and extension of the legs. This is followed by a slow return to the flexed position.
- *Grasp*: flexion of the fingers or toes when the palmar or plantar surface is stimulated.
- *Stepping*: when the infant is held in a standing position and one foot placed on a surface, that leg extends and the other flexes as in a walking motion.
- *Rooting*: when a cheek is touched there is turning of the mouth and head towards the stimulus.
- *Asymmetric tonic neck reflex*: turning of the head to

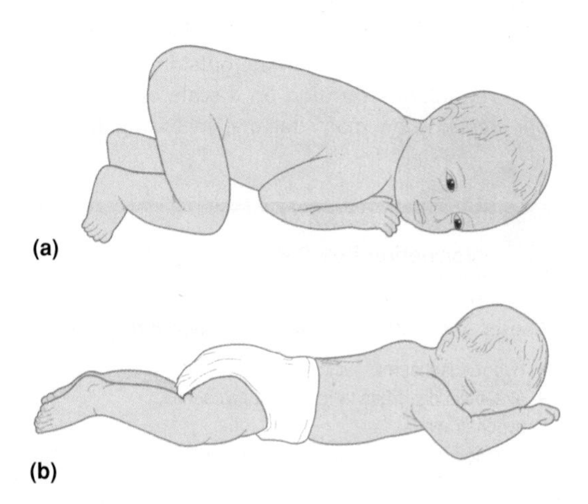

Fig 2.14
Normal posture: prone position. (a) Term baby. (b) 32-weeks' gestation baby.

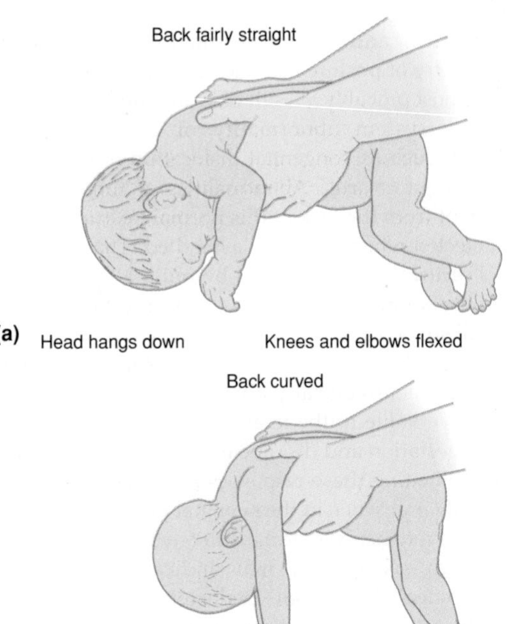

Fig 2.15
Ventral suspension in newborn infants. (a) Term baby. (b) Premature infant of 32 weeks' gestation.

one side results in flexion of the limbs on that side and extension of those on the opposite side.

The Moro reflex is most useful in assessing symmetry of movement.

The general alertness of the baby should be noted and the ability to fix and follow a brightly coloured object should be present from the first few days of life in a full-term baby. The neurological status of the baby is dependent on the gestational age; unlike most of the other body systems this is pre-programmed and continues at much the same rate outside the uterus as inside. The infant's position on a scale of irritability–torpor depends on many factors, including the time since the last feed or nappy change. It may be necessary to return and re-examine the infant before drawing definite conclusions about neurological status.

Possible causes of cerebral dysfunction in newborn infants are presented in Information box 2.8.

Encephalopathy in the newborn may produce either irritability or depression (see Information box 2.9).

Poor feeding is likely to be present with both sets of symptoms. Not uncommonly neurologically abnormal infants will fluctuate between the two extremes.

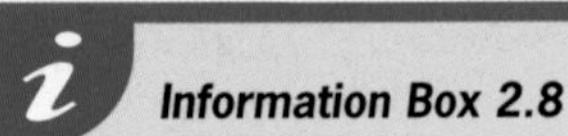

Information Box 2.8

Causes of cerebral dysfunction in a newborn infant

- Hypoxic ischaemic insult
- Metabolic disturbance (e.g. hypoglycaemia, hyponatraemia)
- Infection of the central nervous system
- Drug withdrawal (e.g. mother on drugs of abuse)
- Congenital abnormality of the central nervous system

Behaviour and bonding

Newborn babies respond to their mothers from birth. This relationship strengthens rapidly, the process being called bonding. Failure of this process is believed to be associated with long-term emotional difficulties between mother and child. It is therefore important that those caring for mothers and babies should take every opportunity to foster the development of this bonding process. This is particularly so when infants are sick and in need of medical treatment which may enforce separation of the pair for some of the time.

Initially it is difficult to observe infant responses to external stimuli. However, one can observe how an infant will 'still' in response to a loud noise and sometimes to tactile stimuli such as stroking. By the end of the first week a full-term baby will fix on large brightly coloured (especially red) objects and transiently follow such objects with the eyes. This process rapidly matures, with the following of a face and, by 3–5 weeks, smiling at the face. This social development reinforces the bonding process with the mother. Paternal bonding also occurs but more slowly and mainly beyond the neonatal period. In keeping with this social and visual development, hearing and early motor development can be seen with

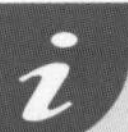

Information Box 2.9

Signs of cerebral irritation

- Hyperexcitability
- Irritability
- Jitteriness
- High-pitched cry
- Opisthotonus
- Seizures

Signs of cerebral depression

- Apathy
- Floppiness
- Somnolence

increasing responses to sound, in the form of eye, and later, head turning.

Physiological considerations in the care of the newborn infant

In the womb, many physiological processes are performed for the fetus by the mother via the placental and amniotic interfaces. The newborn infant must adapt rapidly after birth to establish these processes independently, and though the preliminaries to this adaptation will have occurred before birth, there may inevitably be some delays which may have consequences for the care and wellbeing of the infant. These consequences will be more marked in preterm infants. For most body systems, adaptation and development are triggered by exposure to the postnatal environment and so development of organ function in preterm infants can catch up with that in term infants. The exception is the nervous system in which development continues at the same pace both in and out of the womb.

These important physiological processes are discussed below.

TEMPERATURE REGULATION

The newborn has relatively immature mechanisms for controlling body temperature, and a high surface area-to-volume ratio which increases heat losses. This is even more evident in the preterm baby who additionally has thin, immature skin with increased evaporative heat loss. Preterm infants should be nursed in a thermally neutral environmental temperature range to minimize oxygen requirement (Fig. 2.16). When infants have to generate heat to maintain their body temperature, they metabolize brown fat which is very 'expensive' in terms of oxygen demand.

Babies who are small for gestational age have more difficulty maintaining body temperature partly because they have less subcutaneous and brown fat.

To prevent hypothermia, the newborn must be kept warm from the moment of birth. Babies needing resuscitation should be dried with a towel as soon as possible after birth and managed under an overhead heater. Low birthweight babies need to be nursed in especially warm environments (new staff need to adjust to the high temperatures in the neonatal unit). Infants weighing less than 1800 g need to be placed in a thermostatically controlled closed incubator or under an overhead heater. The head is a particularly important site of heat loss, and if ambient temperatures are low a hat is required.

FLUID BALANCE AND RENAL FUNCTION

The newborn has an excess of fluid which it excretes over the first few days of life, accounting for most of the early normal weight loss. Excessive fluid therapy in the labouring mother results in excess fluid in the infant followed by an apparent excess weight loss. If hypo-osmolar solutions are used the infant may become hyponatraemic, resulting in irritability, poor feeding and sometimes seizures. A relatively low fluid intake is therefore needed in the first few days (Table 2.5).

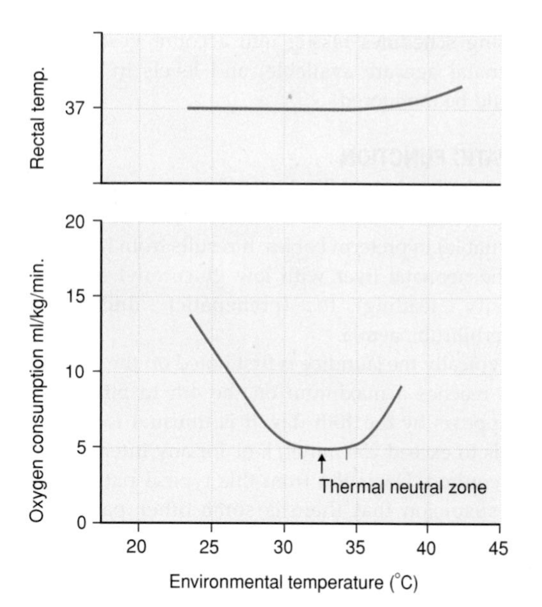

Fig 2.16
Oxygen demand of infants at different environmental thermal ranges. (Adapted from Klaus & Fanaroff (1993) *Care of the High-risk Neonate*, 4th edn. London: W.B. Saunders.)

Insensible fluid losses are greater in newborns because of the high surface area-to-volume ratio and the high permeability of the skin. This may pose problems for very immature preterm infants who will also suffer excess evaporative heat loss and should be nursed in an incubator with high humidity levels and given extra fluid. During the first week of life the skin becomes thicker and more impermeable.

Though infants pass urine in utero, renal function in newborns remains limited for several weeks. Excessive fluid or sodium is tolerated poorly by infants. Antibiotics excreted by the kidney, such as aminoglycosides, should be given in reduced dosage

Table 2.5
Neonatal fluid requirements

Day	ml/kg/day
1	60
2	90
3	120
4	150
5 (max)	180

(dosing schedules taking into account gestation and postnatal age are available) and levels in the blood should be monitored.

HEPATIC FUNCTION

Physiological hyperbilirubinaemia occurs in up to 50% of newborn babies. It is more common (but not inevitable) in preterm babies. It results from immaturity of the neonatal liver with low glucuronyl transferase activity leading to (prehepatic) unconjugated hyperbilirubinaemia.

Typically the jaundice is first noted on the 2nd to 3rd day, reaches a maximum on the 4th to 5th day and disappears by the 10th day. It is unusual for bilirubin levels to exceed 250 mmol/l. or for any intervention to be required. Deviation from this typical pattern raises the suspicion that there is some other pathological (rather than physiological) cause (see p. 53). Serum bilirubin measurements can be measured approximately and noninvasively using a portable icterometer or measured more accurately from a heel prick blood sample.

In the blood unconjugated bilirubin is carried bound to albumin. Drugs which compete for these binding sites, such as sulphonamides, should not be used in the neonatal period.

Other aspects of hepatic function are also immature, and drugs which are predominantly excreted in the biliary system, such as ceftriaxone, should not be used. Those drugs metabolized by the liver, such as opiates, should be used with care.

GASTROINTESTINAL FUNCTION

Sucking and swallowing are neurological activities, discussed below. Gut function in terms of peristaltic activity and digestion is stimulated by the ingestion of milk, particularly breast milk which is believed to contain soluble factors which promote these developments.

Enteral feeding also promotes gallbladder function, and hence infants who require prolonged total parenteral nutrition develop biliary sludging as well as cholestatic jaundice. When possible, small amounts of feed should be given enterally to these infants to prevent these problems.

Meconium is the name given to the viscid green/black stool which is present in the fetal bowel. First passage of meconium usually occurs within 24 hours of birth. Failure to do so by 48 hours should raise the possibility of some form of congenital intestinal obstruction (see p. 216).

After the first few meconium stools have been passed, the faeces change gradually in colour and consistency to normal infant stools. There is a wide range of normality from lemon yellow to dark green and from firm and pellet-like to loose (sometimes frothy) and unformed. Normal frequency varies greatly from 6 per day to 1 per 3 days. Breastfed babies tend to have looser, more frequent stools, but not invariably.

Vitamin K, either from the feed (though breast milk is a poor source), or from generation by gut bacteria is essential to the infant. Deficiency can lead to haemorrhagic disease of the newborn which can result in catastrophic brain haemorrhage. This is more common in breastfed infants, who should be given vitamin K. Following recent concerns (probably unfounded) that the injectable form might be associated with the later development of childhood malignant disease, most authorities recommended that it was given orally in a dose of 0.5 mg on three occasions (at birth, at 7–10 days and at 4–6 weeks). Subsequent studies failed to confirm this association. In preterm infants who are at greater risk, the first dose should be given by the intramuscular route.

RESPIRATORY FUNCTION

Immaturity of the neonatal respiratory centres results in a tendency for apnoea to develop, especially in premature infants where spontaneous apnoeas may occur in otherwise healthy infants. Immature responses to low partial pressure of oxygen in the circulation can paradoxically depress respiration, resulting in apnoea and bradycardia. This latter response can persist for several months after birth. Stimulant drugs such as theophylline or caffeine may be needed for premature infants who show this tendency. Care is required with depressant drugs, such as opiates or anti-epilepsy drugs, which may easily precipitate apnoea.

In the lungs, delayed clearance of lung fluid commonly causes relatively mild early respiratory distress. Any infant can be affected but it is more common after caesarean births. A chest radiograph typically shows streaky shadowing with fluid in the horizontal fissure (Fig. 2.17). It may be difficult to exclude infection. The symptoms normally resolve within a few hours of birth. If they persist for more than 24 hours another diagnosis is likely, such as surfactant deficiency. Apart from the occasional need for supplemental oxygen, treatment is not usually required.

The most significant immaturity in the lungs of newborns is surfactant deficiency; this occurs mainly in premature infants and causes hyaline membrane disease. Following birth the lungs may start making surfactant but by then it is often too late and lung disease (see p. 49) is established. If it is known that premature delivery is likely, a course of corticosteroids given to the mother will promote lung development and surfactant production in the infant.

In terms of oxygen transport, the newborn infant has mostly fetal haemoglobin which has a higher oxygen affinity than adult type. This partly explains the relative resistance of the newborn to the effects of hypoxia compared with older individuals. After birth, production switches to adult type but for the neonatal period fetal haemoglobin predominates.

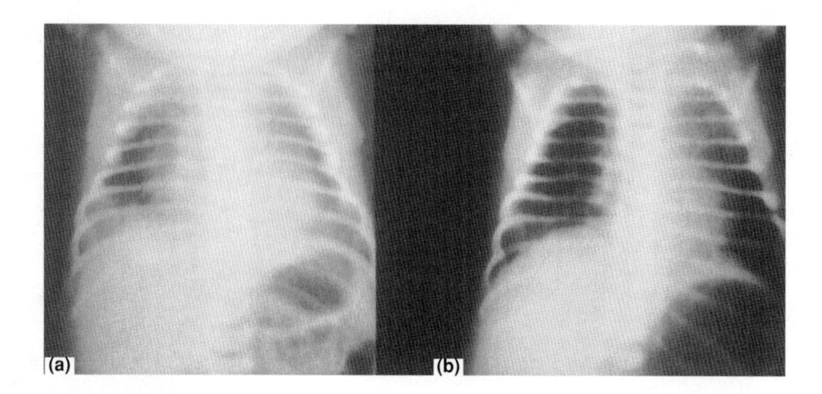

Fig 2.17
Chest radiograph showing delayed clearance of lung fluid: (a) 1st hour after birth; (b) 42 hours after birth (courtesy of Professor DV Walters).

STATUS OF THE CIRCULATION

Major changes in the circulation from fetal pattern to a transitional pattern (Fig. 2.18) must occur immediately after birth, and are triggered by lung inflation resulting in a sudden drop in pulmonary vascular resistance. The ductus arteriosus and oval foramen must close, increasing blood flow to the lungs. The placental circulation is no longer required, hence the umbilical arteries and vein close. Closure of the ductus venosus diverts portal blood, returning from the gut carrying nutrients, from the inferior vena cava to the liver. Failure to switch results in a condition of neonatal pulmonary hypertension in which the infant remains cyanosed in spite of oxygen therapy and assisted ventilation. The transitional pattern of circulation may last for several days and during this time physical signs may be difficult to interpret.

NEUROLOGICAL FUNCTION

In contrast to that of the other body systems, neurological development is preprogrammed and milestones occur at the same postconceptual age regardless of when the infant is born. Thus in preterm infants there is very little response to the extrauterine environment in the form of accelerated development.

The complex neurological coordination required for sucking and swallowing and the related airway-protective responses (such as cough) develop from around 32 weeks postconceptual age and are well established by 36 weeks. It is not possible to feed preterm infants orally before 33–34 weeks, and enteral feeds must be administered via a nasogastric tube, with great care during feeding to reduce the risk of aspiration.

IMMUNOLOGICAL FUNCTION

The fetus has little need of an active immune system. Indeed, it might be counterproductive to have one.

As soon as the amniotic membranes are ruptured, exposure to a variety of microbes occurs. The newborn baby is excessively susceptible to infection because immune responsiveness takes some time to develop. Within a few days adaptation begins and proceeds at similar rates in term and preterm infants.

However, preterm infants are at greater risk, partly due to lower (maternally transferred) immunoglobulin levels, and partly because under the stress of illness, such as hyaline membrane disease, immune function deteriorates. The neonate should therefore be regarded as an immunocompromised host and suspected or proven infection treated vigorously. Preventative measures include limiting the number of visitors, handwashing before handling the baby, breastfeeding, sterilization of feeding equipment if the baby is bottle-fed, and regular cleaning of the umbilical cord stump, which is a common portal of entry for bacterial infection.

Day-to-day care of the normal baby

Over the first few days of life, a pattern of sleeping and feeding gradually develops. Most babies sleep for long periods. Healthy full-term babies soon establish their own patterns of feeding and sleeping and demand appropriate amounts of feed, without the need for professional advice!

Sleeping. Babies should be put down to sleep in the supine position; this will establish a habit for later on. The supine position has been shown to be associated with a lower incidence of sudden infant death syndrome (SIDS). This position should not, however, be adopted in babies who have upper airway or laryngeal problems or in babies known to have marked gastrointestinal reflux, when side-lying with a degree of "head-up" to the mattress is advised.

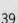

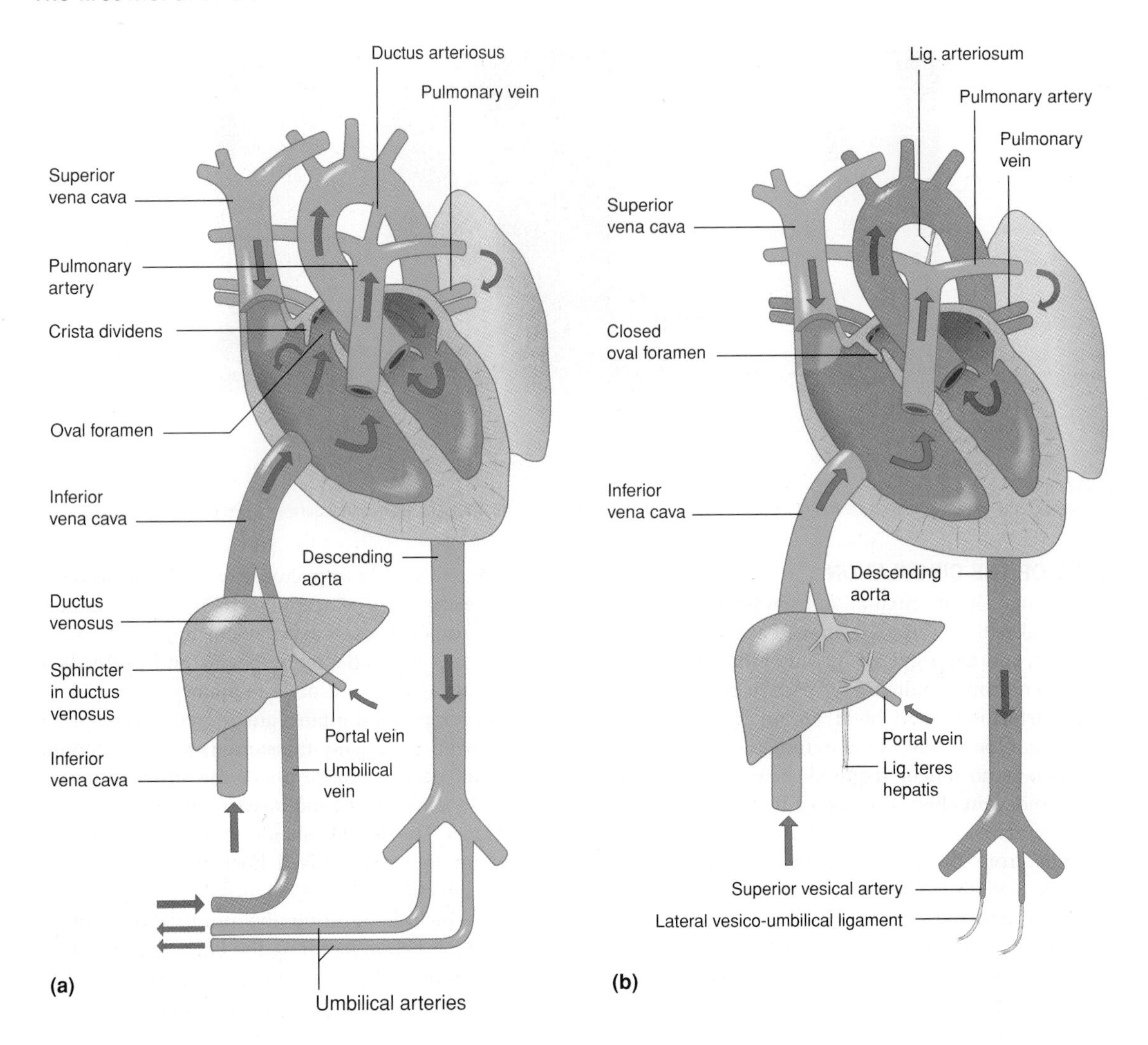

Fig 2.18
(a) Fetal pattern of circulation. Arrows indicate the direction of blood flow. (b) Circulation after birth.

Crying. This is a normal activity of newborn infants and often occurs for no apparent reason. It also occurs in response to discomfort including: pain, hunger, dirty nappy and bright lights. Persistent and inconsolable crying occurs in infants suffering from infant colic – a poorly understood condition in which the infant seems to suffer colicky abdominal pain. There is often an associated element of parental stress which apparently contributes to the symptoms as a vicious cycle. Fortunately the condition is usually transitory.

Bathing of a term or near-term newborn should not be advocated until the 4th or 5th day, to avoid the risk of hypothermia.

Dealing with clinical problems

Therapeutic considerations

Certain drugs are contraindicated in the neonatal period. Some displace bilirubin from albumin (e.g. sulphonamides); others may cause adverse reactions which are peculiar to this age group, e.g. chloramphenicol, which causes circulatory collapse ('grey baby syndrome'). Many drugs are excluded because of lack of clinical data concerning this age group.

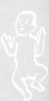

Dosages of drugs need precise calculation at this age (see Practical box 2.2).

Breaking bad news

In the neonatal period more than at any other time in childhood there is sometimes a need to transmit bad news to parents. This may be to tell them that their newborn baby has a serious congenital abnormality or genetic disorder, or that the baby has medical problems often as a result of birth problems or prematurity (p. 8).

Communicating bad news is never easy and it is difficult to teach the skills involved. A student learns more by quietly sitting in as the consultant talks to the parents than by reading books. Every doctor has to develop an individual style and approach for talking to patients and families. There is no right or wrong way, but some general principles are given in Information box 2.10.

Bereavement

Appropriate and sensitive handling of the family of the dying neonate is crucial to laying the foundation for a normal grieving process in that family. Badly handled situations can potentially lead to long-term emotional problems. When it is clear that a baby is dying, the most senior available member of the paediatric medical staff should talk to the parents and, with the parents' permission, to the relatives, about the treatment being given and the likely course of events. Precise predictions as to the time of death should be avoided as they invariably prove incorrect, but a general estimate should be given as this may have practical implications (for example for bringing grandparents along to see the baby before death). It is essential to be sensitive to the cultural and religious needs of the particular family. They should be encouraged, if they wish, to involve one of their own religious leaders.

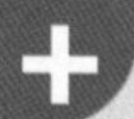

Practical Box 2.2

Considerations in determining drug dosages in newborn infants

- Body weight (surface area is not used partly because of the difficulty in measuring height accurately at this age)
- Gestation (reflecting the immaturity of systems especially the liver and kidneys)
- Postnatal age (reflecting the degree of maturation and adaptation since birth)

The family should be given as much time as possible with their dying infant and encouraged to touch and hold the baby. In most circumstances it is best that siblings in the family are fully involved in this process. They need to know what their baby brother/sister was

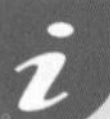

Information Box 2.10

Breaking bad news: general principles

1. Always set aside sufficient time for the meeting and try to prevent interruptions.
2. Try to see both parents together. In the case of single mothers it may be appropriate (with the mother's permission) to have another relative or a friend present. Fathers do need to be appraised of the situation, even if they are not living with the mother.
3. Always ensure that you are up to date with changes in the baby's condition, results of tests, etc.
4. It is often helpful to have a senior member of the nursing staff present. Parents often find it difficult to ask questions of the doctor at the time but can approach the nurse afterwards for clarification and further answers.
5. Always be completely truthful. However bad the news, the parents need to know. There is a temptation to understate the seriousness of a problem and to say what one thinks the parents would like to hear (and one would like to say!). Avoid this temptation.
6. One has to get to the point fairly quickly in the interview, but try to break the news gently and sensitively. Do not rush things but allow time for the information to sink in and for emotion to be expressed. Do not be afraid of prolonged silences during the interview.
7. Try not to overburden parents with too much factual detail. The amount you need to give will vary from family to family. It is good practice to arrange a second meeting shortly after the first to answer more detailed factual questions. It is very helpful for parents to be provided with written information about the condition and/or a contact telephone number/address of any appropriate support groups.
8. Whenever possible, try to leave the parent with at least some glimmer of realistic hope.
9. Parents often find it very stressful to transmit the bad news to their own relatives. One should, when possible, offer to do this on their behalf.
10. Finally, do not be afraid to sympathize with the family and say how sorry everyone is about the situation that the family is in. Even if the family later turn to a litigious frame of mind (which is still rare in the UK) saying sorry is not an admission of any error in management but simply the expression of a human feeling.

like and they need to be involved in the grieving process in the family. The family should be given as much privacy as possible during this period.

When the infant has died, the family should not be rushed and should be allowed to spend as much time as they wish with the baby, again in privacy. A senior member of the medical staff should talk to the parents explaining in simple terms what happened and why, and outlining the administrative process which will have to be undertaken. This will involve registering the death. Most often, the birth has not yet been registered so the family have to register both the birth and death at the same time. A death certificate can usually be completed immediately and handed to the parents with an explanation of the terms used. The question of autopsy will need to be addressed. In the newborn period it is rarely a legal necessity, but the benefits of performing such a study are:

- Providing information on the exact cause of death. This is particularly important if death was unexpected and the family are likely to benefit psychologically from more detailed knowledge of the problem. It also permits more accurate genetic counselling.
- Even if the cause of death is almost certain, detailed examination and studies may be undertaken to help increase knowledge about the underlying condition. This is not a direct benefit to the family but contributes to the general good.

Autopsy requires the family's written informed consent. If organs (e.g. brain or heart) are to be retained, specific permission is required. The reasons for the request and a sensitive account of what the autopsy involves should be given to the family. The best way to do this is to explain that the baby will undergo a series of 'operations' on different parts of the body to examine the internal organs. It should be made clear that small amounts of tissue may be retained for further studies. Not all families will agree to putting their dead child through what they see as further trauma. Important information can be obtained from limited studies such as skin biopsy for fibroblast culture to facilitate genetic studies or radiographic studies which can be undertaken quickly and with minimal trauma. In other cases there may be practical implications, such as delays in the funeral arrangements which go against cultural requirements. These may be overcome by close liaison with the pathologist. In any case it is important to talk to the pathologist who will perform the autopsy to give details of the precise questions being asked.

Before the family leave the hospital it is important to ensure that they have some continuing support. This may come from the general practitioner, the local religious community or specific counselling staff from the hospital or community services.

In all cases a follow-up appointment should be made, ideally with the doctor who saw the family at the time of death. At this appointment, further information available from autopsy, if performed, should be given, with a clear explanation of the implications. If these involve genetic risk in the family, referral to the clinical genetics department can be made.

Many families, at follow up, want to go through the perinatal events again in detail. An assessment of the emotional wellbeing of the family, including siblings, is needed and appropriate further help suggested. Finally, the family should be encouraged to come back for a further appointment should they feel that this is necessary. Often families take up this option many months later. They will also need extra care and counselling during future pregnancies.

Nutrition

Term babies are born with sufficient energy reserves (liver glycogen) to tide them over the first few days and have relatively little need for calories. This does *not* apply to premature and small-for-dates babies. The term baby also has a relative excess of fluid at birth so that immediate fluid requirements are low. The baby should be offered a feed within 2 to 3 hours of birth but most mothers will want to put the baby to their breast soon after delivery, and should be encouraged to do so.

In infants of less than 34 weeks' gestation, feeding needs to be given via a nasogastric tube (p. 39). Care is needed to ensure the correct siting of the tube and, if the infant has a tendency to regurgitate or vomit, there is a risk of milk aspiration. In such circumstances nasojejunal tubes may be passed or parenteral nutrition administered.

Infants with cleft palates have special problems; breastfeeding is difficult to establish though not impossible. Bottle-feeding is easier and maternal expressed milk can be given. Special cleft palate teats are available, but the benefit of using them has been questioned.

Approximate daily fluid (feed) requirements over the early days of life for a term infant are given in Table 2.5 (p. 37).

Breastfeeding (Fig. 2.19)

The relative merits of breast versus formula feeding remain a lively topic for debate. Most women can breastfeed if they wish, though some may need the help and support of a sympathetic midwife. Full-term healthy breastfed babies rarely need top-up feeds with formula and giving these is bad practice. Fluid

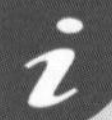

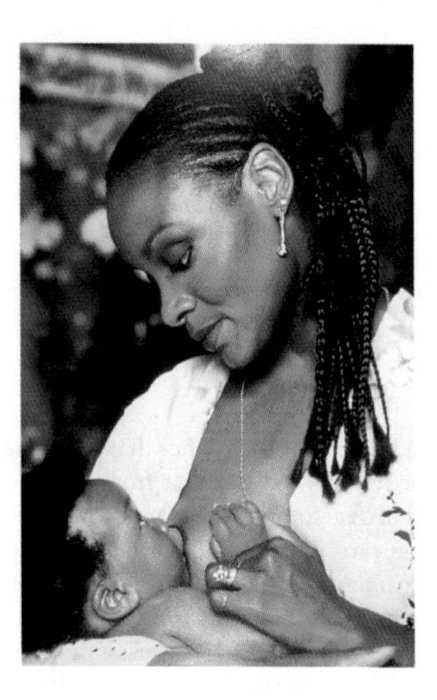

Fig 2.19
Breastfeeding. Note eye contact (Courtesy of Dr Angus Nicol).

Information Box 2.12

Contraindications to breastfeeding

1. Risks to infant: transfer of infection
   - HIV-positive mother
   - Active tuberculosis in mother
   - Breast abscess (avoid breastfeeding on that side)
2. Risks to infant: transfer of medications
   - Cytotoxics
   - Radio-isotopes
   - Chloramphenicol
   - Other medications (listed in the *British National Formulary*) are relative contraindications
3. Metabolic disorders in infant
   - Galactosaemia
   - Phenylketonuria
4. Maternal chronic ill health
   - Severe cardiac, respiratory or renal disease

requirements in the first few days are relatively small, so administering top-up formula feeds tends to give the baby excessive fluid and calories as well as reducing the stimulus for breast milk production. The advantages of breastfeeding over formula feeding are listed in Information box 2.11.

For full-term healthy babies in the UK, where living standards are generally high, the advantages of breastfeeding are less dramatic than in low income countries and mainly relate to a reduction in allergic disease; recent research suggests that there may be long-term benefit to brain formation in preterm infants who receive breast milk. In low income countries, however, the advantages of breast milk are much greater, particularly where pure water cannot be guaranteed and poverty reigns. For preterm babies and those with intestinal problems, it has recently been shown in the UK that the use of breast milk is associated with a reduced incidence of infection and necrotizing enterocolitis; however, it also produces a lower rate of growth, the significance of which is uncertain.

Information Box 2.11

Advantages of breastfeeding

- Provides a natural balance of nutrients
- Hygiene
- Cheapness
- Provides passive immunity through IgA*
- Important part of infant–mother bonding
- Associated in the child with reduced incidence of:
  - Obesity
  - SIDS
  - Cow's milk allergy
  - Eczema
- Associated in the mother with:
  - Reduced incidence of breast cancer
  - Some contraceptive value*

* These are particularly important in developing countries

Disadvantages of breastfeeding are few. Vitamin K deficiency is more common but with oral supplementation (see Physiological considerations in the care of the newborn infant, p. 37–38) the risks can be greatly reduced. Breastfeeding may exacerbate physiological jaundice, and in a small number of infants it causes prolonged (3–4 weeks) unconjugated hyperbilirubinaemia, due to hormonal interference with conjugation. The main consequence of this is the need to exclude other treatable causes of prolonged jaundice. There are a few other unavoidable problems in selected individuals which constitute contraindications to breastfeeding (Information box 2.12).

Artificial feeding (any non-breast milk feeding)

For those mothers who choose not to breastfeed or cannot breastfeed, a variety of formula feeds are available. The manufacturers are continually striving to approximate the formulation to mimic breast milk as

Table 2.6
Approximate composition of breast milk, cow's milk, cow's milk-based formula and preterm formula

Content (per 100ml)	Breast milk	Formula	Preterm formula	Cow's milk (doorstep)
Energy, kcal	74 (range 45–120)	63–70	74–80	70
Protein,[1] g	1.3	1.5–2.0	2.0	3.3
Fat,[2] g	4.1	3.4–3.8	3.6–4.4	3.8
Unsaturated fat, %	47	50–70	51–53	35
Carbohydrate,[3] g	7.2	7.2–8.4	8.3–8.6	4.7
Sodium, mmol	0.6	0.7–1.4	1.4	2.2
Calcium, mmol	0.9	1.1–2.1	1.5–1.9	3.0
Phosphate, mmol	0.5	0.9–1.8	1.3–1.5	3.1
Iron,[4] mmol	1.3	9–12.5	12.5	0.9

[1] Breast milk contains relatively more lactalbumin than casein; cow's milk has the reverse ratio. Formula milks may have a protein composition similar to breast or to cow's milk.
[2] Lipase in breast milk helps make fat more assimilable.
[3] Mainly lactose.
[4] Iron in breast milk is more bioavailable than that in formula milks.

closely as possible. Table 2.6 shows the composition of typical formula feeds compared with breast milk and natural cow's milk.

Several different brands of cow's milk formula are available with minor variations in composition. There is no logical reason for advocating one formula in preference to any other, nor for changing formulae in the belief that symptoms such as excessive regurgitation can be ameliorated. Natural cow's milk is unsuitable for infants because it contains too much protein, salt and phosphate. The formulae all contain reduced amounts of these constituents, which makes their composition closer to that of breast milk. Iron supplements are added to formulae but evidence suggests they are not as bioavailable as the much smaller amounts in breast milk. Preterm formulae have a higher protein content which produces a higher growth rate.

In low income countries the greatest risk of artificial feeding is infection from dirty water or utensils, combined with the absence of transferred IgA and other immunity factors found in breast milk. Formulae may be made up incorrectly. The poor and illiterate may grossly overdilute the feed. Overstrength feeds are also dangerous because they contain excessive sodium and cause greatly increased renal solute load.

Other formula feeds are designed for infants with specific problems; these include soya-based formulae and those based on hydrolyzed cow's milk protein which are used in cow's milk protein intolerance. They are rarely needed in the neonatal period. Soya protein itself may cause intolerance; the hydrolyzed preparations offer the advantage of containing peptides rather than whole protein molecules, thus reducing their antigenicity. In some cases of established eczema, avoidance of cow's milk may produce benefit and these alternative formulae

Table 2.7
Composition of a typical infant vitamin preparation (daily dosage)

Vitamin A	4000 IU
Vitamin D	400 IU
Thiamine (B1)	1 mg
Riboflavin (B2)	0.4 mg
Nicotinamide (B3)	5 mg
Pyridoxine	0.5 mg
Vitamin C	50 mg

can be used. There is no evidence that prophylactic usage of soya or hydrolyzed formula from birth reduces the likelihood of developing eczema or asthma.

In some rare metabolic disorders, such as galactosaemia or phenylketonuria, special milk formulations may be required.

Special milk preparations should not be used lightly and should be prescribed only by paediatricians with specialist knowledge supported by a paediatric dietician.

Micronutrients

It is standard practice to advise multivitamin supplements (Table 2.7) for all babies in the UK, though most full-term babies probably do not require any supplementation other than vitamin K to prevent haemorrhagic disease of the newborn (see Physiological considerations in the care of the newborn infant, p. 37).

Preterm infants definitely require vitamin supplementation, including vitamin D to prevent rickets of prematurity.

Preterm infants also require iron supplementation but this is only started at 1 month of age since iron may increase the risk of bacterial infections (being an essential growth factor for many bacteria). Those requiring regular 'top-up' blood transfusions do not need iron supplementation.

Growth and development

The normal newborn baby loses weight over the first few days of life. This loss is largely accounted for by fluid loss and should not exceed 10% of the body weight. It is normally complete by the 5th day and thereafter weight gain commences. Birthweight should be regained by the 10th day in a healthy term baby. This is unlikely to be achieved in a preterm infant especially one who is undergoing intensive care support.

Thereafter growth proceeds apace with a daily increment of 15–30 g over the first month. Brain growth is particularly rapid in this period and occipitofrontal circumference increases by up to 0.5 cm per week.

External sign	0	1	2	3	4
Oedema	Obvious oedema of hands and feet; pitting over tibia	No obvious oedema of hands and feet; pitting over tibia	No oedema		
Skin texture	Very thin gelatinous	Thin and smooth	Smooth; medium thickness. Rash or superficial peeling	Slight thickening. Superficial cracking and peeling especially of hands and feet	Thick and parchment-like; superficial or deep cracking
Skin colour	Dark red	Uniformly pink	Pale pink; variable over body	Pale; only pink over ears, lips, palms, or soles	
Skin opacity (trunk)	Numerous veins and venules clearly seen, especially over abdomen	Veins and tributaries seen	A few large vessels clearly seen over abdomen	A few large vessels seen indistinctly over abdomen	No blood vessels seen
Lanugo (over back)	No lanugo	Abundant; long and thick over whole back	Hair thinning especially over lower back	Small amount of lanugo and bald area	At least half of back devoid of lanugo
Plantar creases	No skin creases	Faint red marks over anterior half of sole	Definite red marks over >anterior 1/2; indentations over <anterior 1/3	Indentations over >anterior 1/3	Definite deep indentations over >anterior 1/3
Nipple formation	Nipple barely visible; no areola	Nipple well defined; areola smooth and flat, diameter <0.75cm	Areola stippled, edge not raised, diameter <0.75cm	Areola stippled, edge raised, diameter >0.75cm	
Breast size	No breast tissue palpable	Breast tissue on one or both sides, <0.5cm diameter	Breast tissue both sides; one or both 0.5–1.0cm	Breast tissue both sides; one or both >1cm	

(a)

Neurological sign	Score 0	1	2	3	4	5
Posture						
Square window	90°	60°	45°	30°	0°	
Ankle dorsiflexion	90°	75°	45°	20°	0°	
Arm recoil	180°	90°–180°	<90°			
Leg recoil	180°	90°–180°	<90°			
Popliteal angle	180°	160°	130°	110°	90°	<90°
Heel to ear						
Scarf sign						
Head lag						
Ventral suspension						

(b)

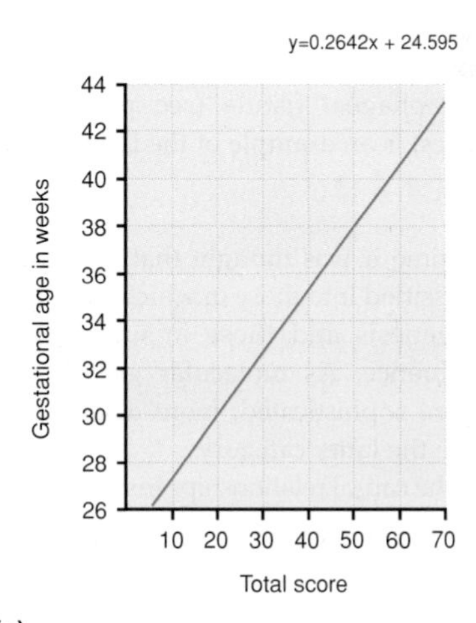

(c)

Fig 2.20
Assessment of gestational age of newborn infants. The Dubowitz system scores: (a) external appearance, and (b) neurological examination. (c) The gestational age (±2 weeks) of the infant is determined from the total scores using the conversion graph. (Adapted from Dubowitz LMS, Dubowitz V, Goldberg C (1970) Clinical assessment of gestational age in the newborn infant. *Journal of Paediatrics* 77: 1–10.)

Assessment of gestation

Antenatally there may be uncertainty as to the gestation of an infant (see p. 9). It is useful to know the gestation, particularly in premature infants, since this information may influence interpretation of clinical findings and calculation of drug doses.

Postmature infants show certain morphological changes, described in Chapter 1 (p. 10–11).

There are a number of scoring systems for assessing gestational age. The most widely used is the Dubowitz score. Two scores are derived, one for physical and the other for neurological signs of maturity (Fig. 2.20). To arrive at the neurological score, it is important to test the baby in a wakeful state for a valid result. If unexpected results are obtained the test should be repeated.

Congenital abnormalities and genetic disorders

See also Chapter 1, The abnormal fetus: genetic/inherited problems, page 13.

Significant congenital abnormalities (Figs 2.21–2.23) occur in up to 1.5% of all births. Nearly half are defects either wholly or partially involving the cardiovascular system. Often defects occur in association, producing recognized syndromes. There are over 2000 such syndromes and this number is increasing rapidly. Some of these, like Down syndrome (p. 241), have a recognized aetiology such as a chromosomal aberration (see Ch. 12); others do not and are simply recognized associations. The VATER association (vertebral, anal, tracheo-oesophageal fistula (see p. 214) and renal abnormalities) is an example of the latter.

CAUSES

For a long time it was thought that congenital defects could be classified into those in which mishaps occurred in embryogenesis and those in which there was a genetic influence. As molecular genetic techniques become more sophisticated, more disorders are being attributed to the latter category.

Some of the causal relationships involved in congenital abnormalities are presented in Information box 2.13.

DIAGNOSIS

Many abnormalities are easily detected after birth. Either the problem is detected on routine physical examination or the baby may exhibit symptoms. Dysmorphism is a common feature of many syndromes.

For the infant with multiple problems, and therefore a possibly recognized syndrome, it is important to involve the clinical genetics team at an early stage; they have access to databases of such syndromes.

Information Box 2.13

Some causal relationships in congenital abnormalities

1. *Maternal age*, e.g. Down syndrome (see p. 12).
2. *Maternal nutrition*, e.g. the association of neural tube defects with subclinical vitamin deficiency, probably of folic acid (see p. 6).
3. *Maternal illness*, e.g. the overall incidence of congenital disorders is increased at least twofold in diabetes mellitus.
4. *Maternal drug therapy*, e.g. the dramatic example of thalidomide. Steroid usage is associated with an increased rate of cleft lip and palate.
5. *Maternal drug abuse*, e.g. alcohol as the cause of fetal alcohol syndrome (see p. 15).
6. *Birth order*, e.g. neural tube defects are much commoner in first pregnancies.
7. *Congenital infection*; e.g. rubella contracted at a critical stage of organogenesis (see p. 16).

Commoner structural disorders

Some of the commoner abnormalities are listed in Table 2.8. Detailed descriptions of individual problems are given in Section 2.

Chromosomal disorders

These are described in detail in Chapter 12. They comprise trisomic disorders and those in which there has been deletion of part(s) of a chromosome. These are associated mostly with multiple abnormalities and there is a high probability of neurological development being affected.

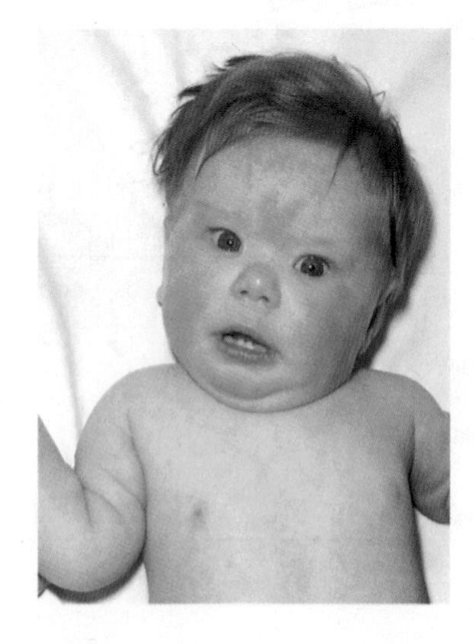

Fig 2.21
Congenital syndrome: Williams syndrome (p. 244) is associated with a chromosomal deletion.

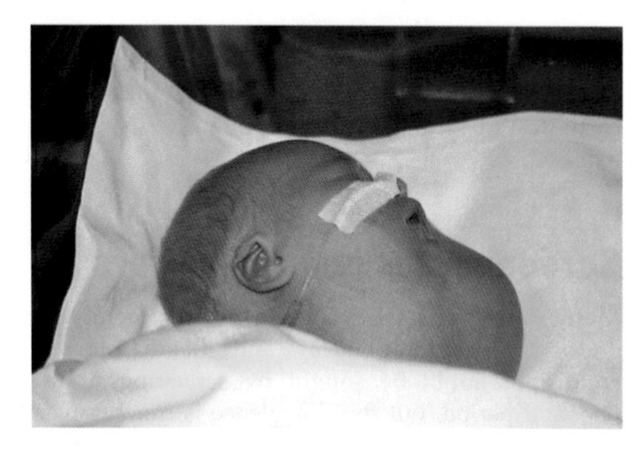

Fig 2.22
Cystic hygroma: this congenital lymphatic abnormality (p. 189) may present at birth or within 2 years. Courtesy of Mr K Holmes

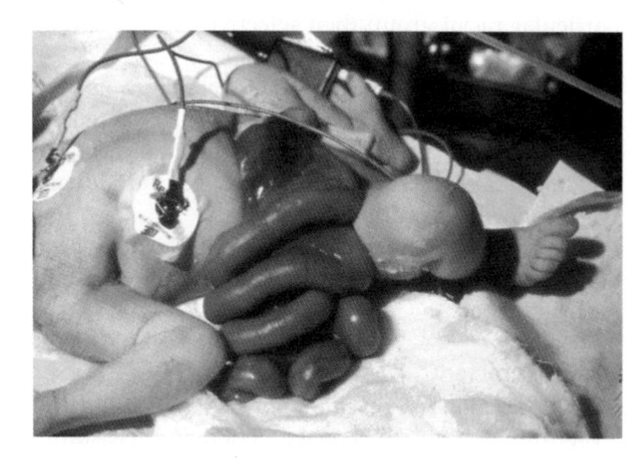

Fig 2.23
Gastroschisis. This anterior abdominal wall defect (p. 215) is not usually associated with other abnormalities. Courtesy of Mr K Holmes

Table 2.8
Congenital anomalies, England, 1987 and 1997*

Anomaly	Live births†		Stillbirths§	
	1987	1997¶	1987	1997¶
Babies born with anomalies				
Number	12650	4837	262	165
Rate	*196.6*	*79.2*	*4.1*	*2.7*
Central nervous system				
Number	401	148	80	38
Rate	*6.2*	*2.4*	*1.2*	*0.6*
Ear and eye				
Number	755	203	16	4
Rate	*11.7*	*3.3*	*0.2*	*0.1*
Cleft lip/cleft palate				
Number	780	527	17	7
Rate	*12.1*	*8.6*	*0.3*	*0.1*
Cardiovascular				
Number	829	412	24	16
Rate	*12.9*	*6.7*	*0.4*	*0.3*
Hypospadias/epispadias				
Number	1073	437	—	1
Rate	*16.7*	*7.2*	—	*0.0*
Reduction deformities of limbs				
Number	282	123	13	2
Rate	*4.4*	*2.0*	*0.2*	*0.0*
Talipes				
Number	2070	571	21	7
Rate	*32.2*	*9.3*	*0.3*	*0.1*
Chromosomal				
Number	544	321	21	19
Rate	*8.5*	*5.3*	*0.3*	*0.3*

Note: From January 1990 certain minor malformations are no longer notified, and have been excluded from the figures shown. For example, club foot of positional origin is now excluded from the category 'Talipes'. This change in notification practice largely accounts for the decrease in numbers of malformations reported in some categories.
* Provisional. † Rates per 10 000 live births.
§ Rates per 10 000 total births. ¶ Data as at 22 May 1998.
Source: Office for National Statistics (1998) *Congenital Anomaly Statistics Notifications*. London: The Stationery Office. © Crown copyright. With permission.

Single-gene disorders

These disorders, such as cystic fibrosis and sickle cell anaemia are also congenital abnormalities.

MANAGEMENT

In some cases the congenital abnormality will necessitate immediate intervention to save the infant's life. In others, there may be no immediate effects on wellbeing but potentially serious implications for the future. Once a syndrome or condition is suspected, it is important to proceed with any confirmatory tests as soon as practicable.

The parents must be carefully counselled and kept informed at all stages. It is likely to be very distressing for them to learn that their infant is not perfectly formed. They may be helped, for example, by seeing photographs of corrected disfiguring abnormalities such as cleft lip, by talking to other affected families (if available), or by being put in contact with the appropriate patient association/self-help group. Neonatal units should keep up-to-date information on such groups (the number of which is increasing) as well as information sheets about the commoner abnormalities.

Screening

The examination of the newborn baby is a useful screen for many congenital abnormalities. In addition screening tests can be justified on the basis of recognized criteria (Information box 2.14).

Phenylketonuria and hypothyroidism are screened for in all babies.

Information Box 2.14

Criteria for performing a screening test

1. The test is simple and non-invasive.
2. There is a high degree of sensitivity in detecting the condition.
3. Specificity is also relatively high but can be increased by further tests when necessary.
4. The condition being sought has a sufficient incidence and impact to justify the use of the resources involved.
5. There is some form of intervention which can be initiated to alter the natural course of the condition.

Phenylketonuria (PKU) (See also p. 288)

This has a relatively high incidence for a metabolic disorder (1 in 10 000). Screening is easily performed on a heel prick blood sample taken at 5 days of age (or after at least 72 hours of protein feeding). The highly sensitive test detects elevated circulating levels of phenylalanine. Mild to moderate elevation is usually due to transient hyperphenylalaninaemia which can be excluded by performing a further test. Babies affected by PKU develop mental retardation if not treated early. Screening allows early detection and the initiation of a low phenylalanine diet which prevents this complication from developing. The PKU screening programme undertaken on all babies in western countries thus meets all the criteria for a good screening test.

Hypothyroidism (See also p. 202)

Congenital hypothyroidism has an incidence in the UK of 1 in 3500 births. If left untreated beyond 2–3 months of age, it results in physical and mental changes (cretinism), the latter being irreversible. Screening of blood, on a Guthrie card blood spot, for thyroid stimulating hormone (TSH) allows detection of the great majority of cases. The circulating TSH level is grossly elevated.

In rare cases hypothyroidism has a central cause due to failure to produce TSH; these cases cannot be detected by the above test. To circumvent this problem, some screening programmes assay the circulating thyroxine (T_4) level. This test is far less specific involving a high number of false-positives necessitating further blood tests. Ideally both T_4 and TSH levels should be screened.

Given the narrow window of time in which treatment must be started to avert the risk of irreversible brain damage, a highly organized, efficient and audited system of collection of Guthrie cards, early testing and early distribution of results is required.

Screening for other disorders

Many other rare disorders including metabolic, endocrine, immunological and haematological conditions could be sought by screening in the neonatal period, but their incidence is much lower; this leads to arguments about cost efficiency. A good example is congenital adrenal hyperplasia due to 21-hydroxylase deficiency (see also p. 197). Where there is a positive family history of a disorder or a known local high incidence of a disease in a particular racial group then selective screening may be justified.

In a number of conditions, prenatal or antenatal screening of parents for carrier status or antenatal screening for an affected fetus may pre-empt neonatal screening or help direct it to selected individuals. Thalassaemia is a good example.

Two conditions in which extensive research has been done into the value of screening are cystic fibrosis and haemoglobinopathy.

Cystic fibrosis (CF)

In this condition, serum immunoreactive trypsin (IRT) levels are raised in the neonatal period and measuring these levels potentially allows early diagnosis. However, the test has relatively low specificity and to date has not been widely applied. Molecular genetic techniques to detect the ΔF508 mutation on chromosome 7 would detect the 70–80% of cases where this mutation is responsible. Techniques for identifying the mutations present in the other 20–30% of affected cases might make these techniques very useful screening tools. Certainly CF (with an incidence of 1 in 2000–2500 births and carrying the likelihood of early clinical problems (with chest infections and failure to thrive) would be a suitable condition for inclusion in a national neonatal screening programme. Screening would allow early treatment and genetic counselling.

Haemoglobinopathies

In high risk populations, sickle cell anaemia and β-thalassaemia major can usually be detected on umbilical cord or neonatal blood samples using high resolution haemoglobin electrophoresis. This cannot however be done on the Guthrie card blood sample and it is labour-intensive and costly. Molecular genetic techniques may supercede these tests. Ideally, parental carrier detection should enable the screening to be directed at specific families.

Screening as an epidemiological tool

Neonatal screening has been used to identify the prevalence of conditions in populations. A good example is the anonymous screening programme undertaken in many health regions for identifying the prevalence of HIV infection in pregnant mothers. This provides valuable information on the rate of heterosexual transmission of this virus in the community.

The sick baby

Symptoms in an unwell baby may be very nonspecific compared to symptoms of disease in older children. The younger the child, the less specific the symptoms. Furthermore an infant cannot help by giving a reliable history. When considering the diagnosis in an unwell baby numerous possibilities need to be considered.

The detection of abnormal signs was discussed under examination of the normal baby (p. 30). Some of the potential clinical problems are discussed here.

The baby with respiratory distress

CLINICAL SIGNS

These include tachypnoea, recession, grunting, central cyanosis and apnoea. Tachypnoea is a respiratory rate >60/minute. Recession occurs when the lungs are stiff. Grunting is the noise made by expiring against a partially closed glottis. This generates positive airway pressure which prevents lung collapse. The soft tissues of the intercostal spaces, base of neck and upper abdomen are drawn in as the baby breathes in (intercostal, suprasternal and subcostal recession). Apnoea is cessation of respiration >10 seconds.

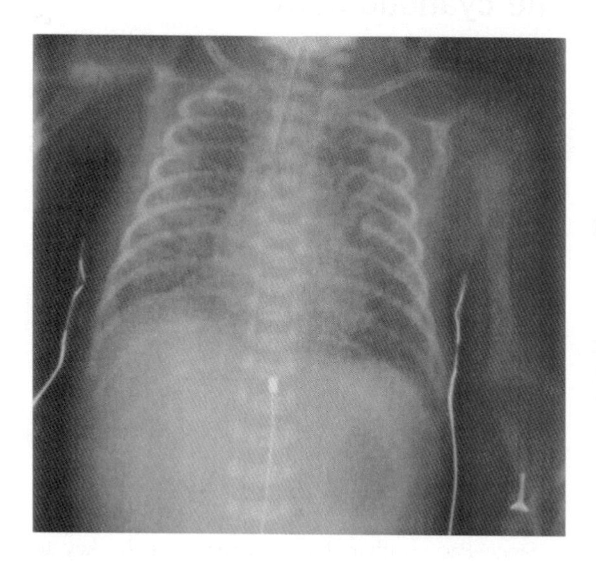

Fig 2.24
Chest radiograph in surfactant deficiency.

DIAGNOSIS

Surfactant deficiency

Surfactant deficiency (or idiopathic respiratory distress syndrome) leading to hyaline membrane disease is common in preterm infants but can occur in term babies. Chest radiographs (see Fig. 2.24) typically show a 'ground glass' appearance with an air bronchogram, but the appearances may vary and may not be distinguishable from those due to pneumonia (Fig 2.25) or retained lung fluid (Fig 2.17, p. 39).

Pneumonia

Congenital pneumonia is usually caused by bacteria derived from the mother's genital tract and is present at birth or develops shortly afterwards. The commonest cause is *Streptococcus agalactiae* (group B strep) but other agents include other streptococci, *Escherichia coli* and *Listeria monocytogenes*. Term and preterm infants are affected.

The symptoms and X-ray appearances (Fig. 2.25) may be undistinguishable from hyaline membrane disease. Features supporting a diagnosis of pneumonia include a history of maternal pyrexia, and/or prolonged rupture of the amniotic membranes and signs of septicaemia (e.g. circulatory failure, petechiae or other rash).

Later onset pneumonia (>48 hours of age) is more likely to occur in compromised babies, such as preterm infants, especially those on ventilatory support. The

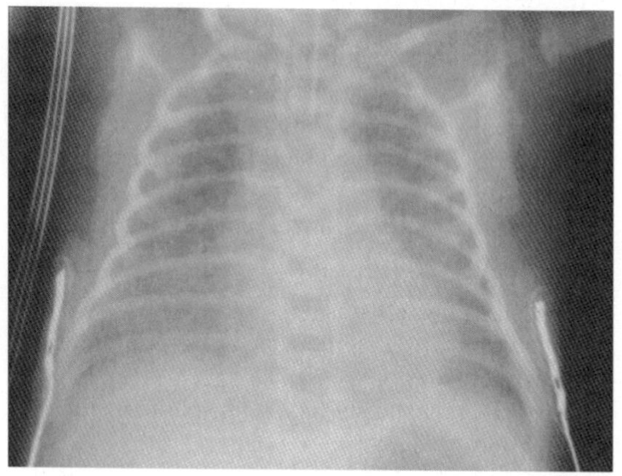

Fig 2.25
Chest X-ray in congenital pneumonia, in this case caused by *Listeria monocytogenes*.

range of organisms responsible is much wider and includes opportunistic environmentally acquired bacteria, including *Staphylococcus aureus*, *Klebsiella sp.* and *Pseudomonas aeruginosa*.

Atypical pneumonias include those caused by viruses, such as influenza, respiratory syncytial virus (RSV), ureaplasma/mycoplasma, and *Chlamydia trachomatis*. These usually start later in the neonatal period.

Delayed clearance of lung fluid

See Physiological adaptations, page 38, and Figure 2.17, p. 39.

Pneumothorax

Spontaneous pneumothorax at delivery occurs in up to 2% of births. It may be an incidental finding with no symptoms, or if tension develops it may cause severe respiratory difficulties. It may complicate meconium aspiration, hyaline membrane disease and positive pressure ventilation (for whatever reason). In the last of these situations there is almost always a need for drainage but in the asymptomatic term baby it may be left (with observation) to resolve spontaneously.

Meconium aspiration

See Birth complications, page 28.

Milk aspiration

Babies born before 34 weeks' gestation and those with neuromuscular or structural upper airway problems have poor airway protection and may aspirate milk. Careful nursing is required to minimize this. Those with respiratory distress and/or abdominal distension are also at risk and if the airway is not protected with an endotracheal tube it is often best not to feed enterally until symptoms improve. Massive milk aspiration can lead to 'collapse' or even death, and surviving babies will often require ventilatory support. Antibiotics are given because of the risk of secondary infection.

Congenital abnormalities

Conditions such as diaphragmatic hernia, lung cysts and tracheo-oesophageal fistula can cause respiratory distress. The chest radiograph is usually diagnostic.

Nonpulmonary causes of respiratory distress

These include:

- Congenital heart disease
- Metabolic disorders producing acidosis (and thus tachypnoea)
- Gross abdominal distension with splinting of the diaphragm.

MANAGEMENT

In idiopathic respiratory distress syndrome (due to surfactant deficiency) treatment involves supplementary inspired oxygen and, in more severe cases, ventilatory support. Recently the use of artificial or natural (porcine) surfactant has been shown to improve outcome when used either prophylactically or as an interventional treatment. Antibiotics are used for pneumonia and usually in other respiratory disorders because of the difficulty of excluding infection.

The baby with apnoea

See also Clinical approach, Physiological considerations in the care of the newborn infant, page 38.

CLINICAL SIGNS AND DIAGNOSIS

If an infant (term or preterm) is unwell the normal tendency to apnoea of prematurity increases; this may be an early sign of illness such as infection, anaemia, dehydration or metabolic upset. In infants with respiratory conditions, low partial pressure of oxygen in the circulation paradoxically depresses respiration resulting in apnoea and bradycardia (heart rate <120/minute). Likewise upper airway obstruction results in apnoea rather than the hyperpnoea characteristic of older age groups. This latter response persists for a number of months after birth.

MANAGEMENT

This involves identifying possible underlying causes and treating them where possible; respiratory stimulants and if these fail artificial ventilation may be needed.

The cyanotic baby

CLINICAL SIGNS

Peripheral cyanosis is common in the first hours of life and is usually of no consequence provided that the baby is well. Central cyanosis always indicates a problem and should be confirmed by demonstrating low oxygen saturation of haemoglobin. Cyanosis is dependent on the absolute amount of circulating reduced haemoglobin. In anaemic babies desaturation will be less apparent than in those with polycythaemia for any given partial pressure of oxygen ($Pa\text{O}_2$).

Confirmation of desaturation can be obtained by pulse oximetry which directly measures the proportion of reduced haemoglobin. Alternatively the $Pa\text{O}_2$ can be measured by arterial blood sampling with the advantage that the partial pressure of carbon dioxide ($Pa\text{CO}_2$) can also be measured as well as the acid–base status.

Since $Pa\text{O}_2$ (rather than saturation) is the key to oxygen delivery to the tissues it is measured in the first instance.

NB: Capillary blood samples give useful information on $P\text{CO}_2$ and acid–base status but are not helpful in assessing $P\text{O}_2$.

Transcutaneous oxygen and carbon dioxide electrodes are also useful for continuous monitoring of blood gas levels after an initial validating blood gas sample has been obtained.

DIAGNOSIS

When central cyanosis is accompanied by marked signs of respiratory distress the likely cause is one of the disorders discussed above. Cyanosis with only minimal signs of respiratory distress is likely to be due to a congenital heart disorder with a right-to-left shunt (see Information box 2.15) or neonatal pulmonary hypertension.

When accompanying lung disease results in pulmonary vascular constriction and therefore pulmonary (and right heart) hypertension, defects normally associated with a left-to-right shunt (such as ventricular septal defects) can show reversed flow (either consistently or intermittently) to produce cyanosis.

Neonatal pulmonary hypertension may be idiopathic or secondary to lung disease (see Information box 2.16). This was formerly called persistent fetal circulation. Right-to-left shunting may occur in affected babies in the absence of true congenital abnormalities, since the high right-sided pressures tend to reopen 'normal' communications (Information box 2.17) such as the ductus arteriosus or the foramen ovale (in the intra-atrial septum).

Information Box 2.15

Most common heart defects leading to early central cyanosis

- Truncus arteriosus
- Total anomalous pulmonary venous drainage (obstructed type)
- Transposition of the great vessels
- Tricuspid atresia

For details see Congenital heart disease, p. 174.

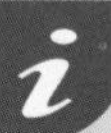

Information Box 2.16

Common causes of pulmonary hypertension

- Hyaline membrane disease
- Bacterial pneumonia
- Meconium aspiration
- Birth asphyxia

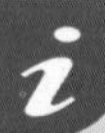

Information Box 2.17

Routes of paradoxical right-to-left shunt in babies

'Normal' – Foramen ovale
– Ductus arteriosus (early)
– Intrapulmonary shunting
Abnormal – Atrial septal defect (ASD): ostium primum
– AV canal
– Ventricular septal defect
– Ductus arteriosus (late)

Figure 2.18 (p. 40) shows the patterns of fetal and adult type circulation.

Diagnosing the cause of central cyanosis is not always easy. Chest radiography may show obvious pulmonary or cardiac abnormalities or may show the typical oligaemic lungs of neonatal pulmonary hypertension. ECG provides further information on cardiac conduction and high-definition echocardiography, available in major neonatal centres, provides extremely useful structural and haemodynamic information about the heart. Administering 100% inspired oxygen to the baby may help to distinguish pulmonary from shunting causes. The nitrogen washout test (as it is called) will reveal a significant rise in $P\text{O}_2$ where the cause is pulmonary but not in infants who are shunting.

MANAGEMENT

Management of the cyanosed baby depends on the primary cause. Pulmonary disorders are treated appropriately (see above). Severe congenital heart disease requires expert advice from a paediatric cardiologist who will be able to say whether or when palliative or corrective surgery should be undertaken. If pulmonary hypertension is a problem, vasodilators must only be used cautiously, as they reduce the systemic as well as the pulmonary blood pressure. Oxygen is the most potent and specific pulmonary vasodilator.

The plethoric baby

CLINICAL SIGNS

In babies plethora is due to excessive haemoglobin in the skin circulation. A ruddy complexion with the appearance of peripheral cyanosis is common.

The symptoms of polycythaemia include irritability – and sometimes convulsions, and poor feeding. There is often a relative bradycardia and sluggish capillary return in the skin when it is blanched. Hypoglycaemia is a common complication. Confirmation of polycythaemia is obtained by measuring the packed cell volume (PCV), ideally on an arterial blood sample. A PCV of above 65% is often associated with symptoms.

DIAGNOSIS

The most likely cause is polycythaemia (see Information box 2.18). Occasionally plethora may be due to congestive cardiac failure without polycythaemia. The signs of cardiac failure such as tachycardia, tachypnoea, hepatomegaly, oedema (not dependent) are usually present.

MANAGEMENT

Treatment involves a partial exchange transfusion with 20 ml/kg of human albumin (5% solution) or saline in the first instance to decrease haemoconcentration. Occasionally the packed cell volume will rise again after such a procedure necessitating a repeat exchange transfusion.

The pallid baby

CLINICAL SIGNS

Pallor is due to insufficient circulating haemoglobin in the blood vessels of the skin due to either anaemia or inadequate perfusion. Being cold or in pain also causes pallor.

DIAGNOSIS

Anaemia needs to be excluded. Causes are listed in Information box 2.19.

Not all pallid babies are anaemic. Other causes include inadequate circulation in the cutaneous vessels due to either frank hypotension or incipient hypotension with compensatory vasoconstriction (for example in dehydration).

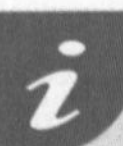

Information Box 2.18

Causes of polycythaemia in the newborn

- Intrauterine oxygen starvation, usually associated with intrauterine growth retardation
- Congenital cyanotic heart disease
- Placento-fetal or (in twins) feto-fetal transfusion
- Excess growth factors, e.g. in the infant of a diabetic mother or in macrosomic syndromes such as Beckwith–Wiedemann (p. 245)

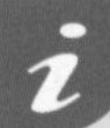

Information Box 2.19

Causes of anaemia in the newborn period

1. Blood loss – Feto-placental
   – Feto-maternal
   – Feto-fetal (twin–twin)
   – Cord clamp slippage
   – Intraventricular or cerebral
   – Pulmonary
   – Gastrointestinal
   – Result of prematurity
   – Acute haemorrhagic disease of newborn
2. Haemolytic – Rhesus or ABO incompatibility
   – Severe glucose 6-phosphatase deficiency (G6PD) (+ jaundice)
3. Bone marrow disorder – α-thalassaemia
   – Diamond–Blackfan anaemia

NB: Prenatal causes of fetal anaemia may result in fetal hydrops, fetal distress and intrauterine death (see Ch. 1).

MANAGEMENT (Practical box 2.3)

Treatment depends on the underlying cause.

The shocked baby

CLINICAL SIGNS

Severe circulatory decompensation predisposes to shock.

DIAGNOSIS (See Information box 2.20)

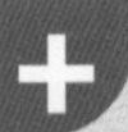

Practical Box 2.3

Assessment of the pallid baby

- Check the blood pressure.
- In severe cases measurement of the peripheral surface temperature in comparison to central temperature (a gap of more than 3°C indicates significant circulatory failure).
- Signs of dehydration should be sought (weighing the baby is helpful when assessing any fluid deficit).
- Full blood count, blood film, Coombs test and blood grouping.
- Urea and electrolyte analysis.

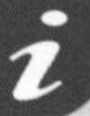

Information Box 2.20

Causes of shock in neonates

- Acute hypovolaemia, due to acute blood loss (e.g. feto-maternal or retroplacental bleeding or excessive blood loss from an inadequately clamped umbilical cord).
- Septicaemia. Overwhelming sepsis, due to a variety of possible causes, most commonly group B Streptococcus.
- Cardiogenic shock due to:
  (a) congenital heart disease, e.g. hypoplastic left heart syndrome
  (b) left ventricular dysfunction (myocardial failure) due to asphyxia, viral myocarditis or metabolic disorders.
- Salt and water loss, e.g. in the Addisonian crisis which can occur in babies born with congenital adrenal hyperplasia.

MANAGEMENT

A full account of the treatment of shock is beyond the scope of this book. Blood or fluid loss should be replaced as rapidly as necessary, but in the causes involving myocardial dysfunction inotropic drugs (e.g. dobutamine, adrenalin) are also necessary. There is nearly always accompanying acidosis and hypoxaemia which complicate the situation and these should be corrected as much as possible.

The acidotic baby

DIAGNOSIS

Respiratory acidosis occurs in many of the respiratory disorders of the newborn (see p. 49).

Persistent metabolic acidosis may be due to tissue hypoxia, sepsis or to inborn errors of metabolism. Very low birthweight babies, particularly those who are sick, requiring full intensive care, often persist in a hypercatabolic state for several days. Excessive protein given to babies at this stage will exacerbate the problem and they should be fed with an increased carbohydrate and relatively low protein intake until the acidosis resolves.

MANAGEMENT

Treatment of other causes of acidosis should be directed at the underlying cause. In an emergency, optimizing the circulating volume and cardiac output is of vital importance and to achieve this it may be necessary to administer alkali, usually in the form of 8.4% sodium bicarbonate. (NB: This is an extremely hyperosmolar agent and should be given very slowly and ideally diluted. Note that every mmol of bicarbonate administered is accompanied by another mmol of sodium; babies who receive excessive amounts of sodium bicarbonate may become hypernatraemic.)

The baby with thermal instability/fever

CLINICAL SIGNS

Excessive thermal instability may be a sign of illness in a newborn child. This may involve either hypothermia or hyperthermia which occurs despite attention to environmental temperature control.

DIAGNOSIS

Possible causes include sepsis (Fig. 2.26), dehydration or intracranial haemorrhage. The infant should be examined and investigated for signs of these problems.

Fever in this age group is relatively uncommon. Its absence does not indicate that infection is not present. When fever occurs it may signify infection, overheating (particularly in premature infants with poor temperature regulation) or intracranial (especially pontine) haemorrhage or a reaction to medications.

The baby with pathological jaundice

CLINICAL SIGNS

Physiological jaundice has already been discussed with reference to the normal baby. Pathological causes of jaundice are diagnosed when the pattern of hyperbilirubinaemia deviates from the typical normal

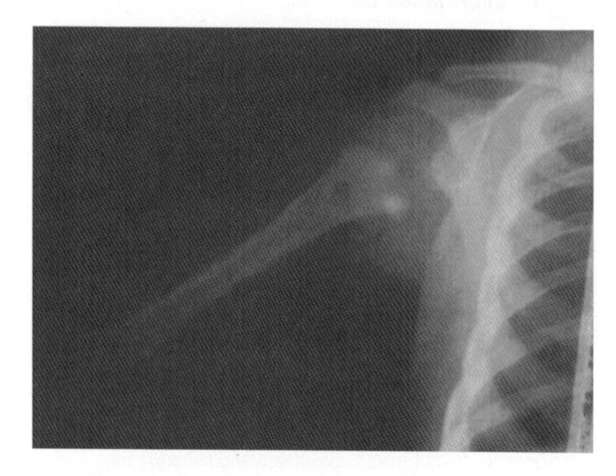

Fig 2.26
'Occult' sepsis: osteomyelitis of upper humeral metaphysis caused by group B Streptococcus.

pattern. This may involve the jaundice appearing early in the first 24 hours of life (jaundice detectable by the naked eye before 24 hours is usually abnormal); being of an excessive degree (it is unusual for the bilirubin to exceed 250 μmol/l in simple physiological jaundice), or persisting for an excessively long period (jaundice should have disappeared in the term baby by 10 days or in the preterm baby by 14 days).

DIAGNOSIS

Causes of early unconjugated hyperbilirubinaemia are listed in Information box 2.21, and those of prolonged jaundice in Information box 2.22.

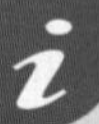

Information Box 2.21

Causes of 'pathological' early neonatal unconjugated hyperbilirubinaemia

1. Physiological, complicated by dehydration
2. Infection, urinary tract or septicaemia
3. Haemolysis
   - Immune (Rhesus or ABO incompatible)
   - Red cell abnormality, e.g. glucose-6-phosphatase deficiency (G6PD)
4. Excessive bruising with red cell breakdown (birth trauma)

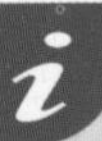

Information Box 2.22

Causes of prolonged jaundice

1. Liver disease
   - Inborn errors
   - Crigler–Najjar
   - Dubin–Johnson
   - Gilbert*
2. Infection
   - Bacterial especially urinary tract†
   - Viral, neonatal hepatitis type B, ? other
3. Hypothyroidism*
4. Galactosaemia*
5. Biliary atresia
6. Breast milk jaundice*

* unconjugated; † mixed conjugated and unconjugated; others are all conjugated

MANAGEMENT

The jaundiced baby requires investigation for possible underlying causes. Treatment is needed to prevent the serum unconjugated bilirubin from saturating the binding sites on albumin and eventually depositing in the tissues, particularly the brain, resulting in kernicterus. Preterm babies having lower serum albumin levels are liable to develop kernicterus at much lower serum bilirubin levels. These values are published in nomograms which suggest levels for commencing treatment at various gestational ages. Sick neonates, whether at term or preterm, may develop kernicterus at a lower bilirubin level than healthy babies, and so the threshold for commencing treatment should be lower in these infants. Acidosis is particularly associated with lowering of the thresholds.

Immediate treatment involves attention to fluid balance and acidosis, since abnormalities of these may exacerbate the problem. Specific treatments include phototherapy and exchange transfusion.

Phototherapy

Light of wavelength approximately 460 nanometres has the effect of converting bilirubin in the skin to water-soluble metabolites which can be excreted from the body without the need for conjugation. Babies nursed naked apart from a nappy and eye-protecting pads are bathed in light of the appropriate wavelength. Care is taken to ensure that the baby's temperature remains stable and that fluid depletion does not occur. An occasional side-effect is the development of loose stools which seems to be due to lactase deficiency which develops by unknown mechanisms. Phototherapy is usually initiated at a bilirubin level of 250 μmol/l in the healthy term baby but at much lower levels in preterm babies. In the majority of cases such treatment will avert the need for exchange transfusion.

Exchange transfusion

When the bilirubin level is not controllable by phototherapy, and particularly in haemolytic disorders where anaemia is likely to develop, the treatment required is an exchange transfusion performed through an umbilical arterial and/or venous cannula. The aim is to exchange usually in 5- to 20-ml aliquots (depending on the size of the baby), until two blood volumes have been exchanged.

The rationale is to:

- Reduce the bilirubin
- Correct the anaemia
- Reduce the ongoing haemolytic process.

In Rhesus disease the Rhesus-positive blood in the baby is exchanged for Rhesus-negative blood thus reducing future haemolysis. In addition, there is dilution of the causative antibodies, though this is a minor effect.

With the awareness of Rhesus haemolytic disease

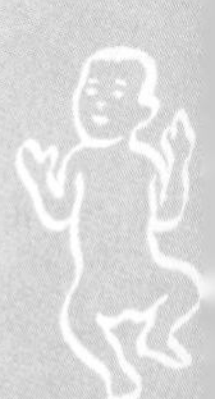

and the use of anti D as prophylaxis for this condition in Rhesus-negative women, the need for performing exchange transfusions has fallen considerably in recent years.

The baby with bruising/bleeding

CLINICAL SIGNS

Some bruising and petechiae, particularly around the head and face, can occur as part of the trauma of delivery, as can cephalhaematoma and subconjunctival haemorrhage. Mostly reassurance is all that is required but on reabsorption the blood may exacerbate neonatal jaundice.

DIAGNOSIS

More severe bruising and bleeding from orifices, umbilicus or venepuncture sites and appearance of new petechiae/purpura should cause concern and merit prompt investigation. The concern is that more severe (internal) bleeding will occur, such as cerebral, pulmonary or gastrointestinal haemorrhage. These are most likely to occur in premature babies undergoing intensive care. A family history may reveal coagulation disorder such as haemophilia or von Willebrand disease and a pregnancy history may reveal maternal thrombocytopenia. Examination of the infant may give clues; for example hepatosplenomegaly suggestive of congenital infection. Check the records to ensure that vitamin K has been given. Causes of bruising/bleeding in the newborn are shown in Information box 2.23.

MANAGEMENT

Investigation of bleeding/bruising requires a coagulation screen and a platelet count. The former requires a slickly taken (to avoid activation of clotting factors) sample of at least 1 ml (some laboratories require more), which is not always easy. Likewise difficult venesection may give spuriously low platelet counts, so again a slickly taken sample is required.

NB: The normal adult values for coagulation times are different for neonates and different again for premature infants.

Information Box 2.23

Causes of bleeding/bruising

Thrombocytopenia	Maternal autoimmune thrombocytopenia
	Isoimmune thrombocytopenia (anti pla-1 antibodies)
	Congenital infection (e.g. cytomegalovirus (CMV), rubella)
	Disseminated intravascular coagulation (DIC)
	Congenital deficiency (e.g. thrombocytopenia-absent radius (TAR) syndrome)
Coagulation disorder	Haemorrhagic disease of the newborn (vitamin K deficiency)
	Congenital clotting deficiency
	Haemophilia
	DIC*
	Drugs; heparin (overdose in intravenous lines)
	Extensive haemangiomata (consumption)

* DIC can have a number of causes; sepsis, asphyxia, necrotizing enterocolitis, twin death, amniotic fluid embolus. Treatment depends on the underlying cause.

The vomiting baby

CLINICAL SIGNS

Vomiting in the newborn may be a nonspecific sign of many medical problems ranging from meningitis to metabolic disorders. It may also of course be a symptom of gastrointestinal disease, either congenital (e.g. atresias) or acquired (e.g. necrotizing enterocolitis). It is important to distinguish between true vomiting, which is usually quite forceful and of relatively large volume, and relatively minor regurgitations. Regurgitation is extremely common in the newborn; it is usually of no consequence, though occasionally it may be more profound and of clinical significance.

DIAGNOSIS

Early vomiting within the first few days of life should raise the possibility of surgical disorders. **Bile-stained vomit is a particularly important sign and must be investigated to rule out small bowel obstruction.** Initially this will involve plain abdominal radiography but barium studies may be necessary and paediatric surgical opinion should be sought. Other conditions which can present with vomiting include infection, including that at distant sites, such as meningitis or pneumonia, or that involving the gastrointestinal tract, e.g. necrotizing enterocolitis or acute diarrhoea (see p. 221). Metabolic and some endocrine disorders presenting in early life may cause profuse vomiting which contributes to the biochemical disturbance.

MANAGEMENT

The infant with vomiting requires investigation and treatment for any underlying causes. At the same time it should be a priority to correct the inevitable fluid and electrolyte disturbance which involves replacement of sodium, chloride, potassium and water. Gastric juices are rich in sodium and it is usual practice to replace the lost fluid either with normal saline or half normal saline. If the intestinal losses are ongoing then it is usual to replace the fluid lost (ml for ml) with normal saline and added potassium. If vomiting persists after feeding has been stopped, i.e. the vomitus is being generated from intestinal secretions, then a nasogastric tube will drain the stomach and facilitate measurement of the losses, as well as reducing the risk of aspiration pneumonia.

The baby with diarrhoea

CLINICAL SIGNS AND CAUSES

Causes of diarrhoea are shown in Information box 2.24.

The presence of blood and/or mucus mixed with the stool suggests an inflammatory process, such as necrotizing enterocolitis (NEC) or infection. NEC follows ischaemic damage to the bowel wall. Gas producing organisms produce pneumatosis (gas in the bowel wall). Perforation of the bowel wall may occur. Fortunately, because of routine hygiene precautions, gastroenteritis is relatively rare in newborns. When it occurs the causes include the usual pathogens (see p. 221). The young infant may be unable to handle these organisms, so that bacterial infections such as salmonella may invade the body from the intestine to cause systemic disease, such as septicaemia, meningitis or osteomyelitis. By contrast, rotavirus causes a more benign or even asymptomatic infection in neonates, and colitis caused by *Clostridium difficile* rarely occurs at this age, even when the toxin-producing organisms can be found in the stool.

MANAGEMENT

Gastroenteritis in neonates is managed using the same principles as in other age groups. However there will be a lower threshold for commencing intravenous fluid therapy to prevent or correct the dehydration which can occur rapidly. Antibiotics are frequently used at this age for proven bacterial infections, particularly those due to salmonella species to prevent invasive disease. Cross-infection is a major hazard in neonatal intensive care and special care units, and the hospital infection control team may need to initiate special procedures to control an outbreak.

Information Box 2.24

Causes of loose/watery stools in the neonate

- Phototherapy
- Gastrointestinal infection
- Infection elsewhere (such as urinary tract)
- Necrotizing enterocolitis (NEC)
- Congenital disorders
  - Lactase deficiency
  - Chloride-losing
- Overfeeding
- Feeding with high osmolality feeds

The baby with constipation

CLINICAL SIGNS AND CAUSES

Failure of passage of meconium within the first 48 hours of life should raise the possibility of congenital intestinal obstruction, which may be mechanical (such as atresias) or functional (as in Hirschsprung disease, aganglionosis) (see p. 220). Usually there will be associated abdominal distension and vomiting. Hirschsprung disease is excluded by a suction rectal biopsy (to look for the presence of ganglia).

Constipation in the neonate is diagnosed if the stools are exceptionally hard and difficult to pass. Fissuring of the anal margin may occur resulting in streaking of the stool surface with bright red blood.

MANAGEMENT

The constipated infant requires attention to the diet to ensure sufficient fluid intake. Extra fluid will often cure the problem, and if calorie intake is sufficient it is best to use boiled water. Failure to respond to such measures should raise the possibility of the more serious disorders discussed above as well as hypothyroidism or hypercalcaemia. Laxatives are rarely used in the neonatal period.

The baby with abdominal distension

CLINICAL SIGNS AND CAUSES

Mild distension of the abdomen is common and may be seen after large feeds. More marked and persistent distension should always be taken seriously.

Gross distension of the abdomen present from birth is indicative of organomegaly due to tumour, such as neuroblastoma, or congenital malformation, such as hydronephrosis due to urinary tract obstruction.

Oedematous infants with hydrops fetalis (Fig. 2.27) will have distended abdomens.

More commonly distension develops hours or days after birth. This is the typical time for presentation of congenital intestinal anomalies such as atresias, which present as the intestine proximal to the obstruction fills up with air and fluid. There are usually accompanying symptoms of vomiting (bilious) and constipation. As a general rule, the lower the obstruction, the later these symptoms will develop. A relatively common cause of neonatal intestinal obstruction is meconium ileus which occurs in 15% of children with cystic fibrosis (see p. 352).

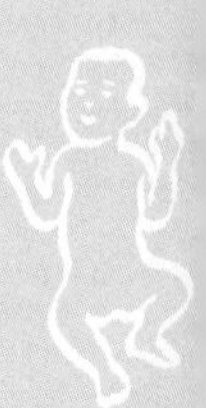

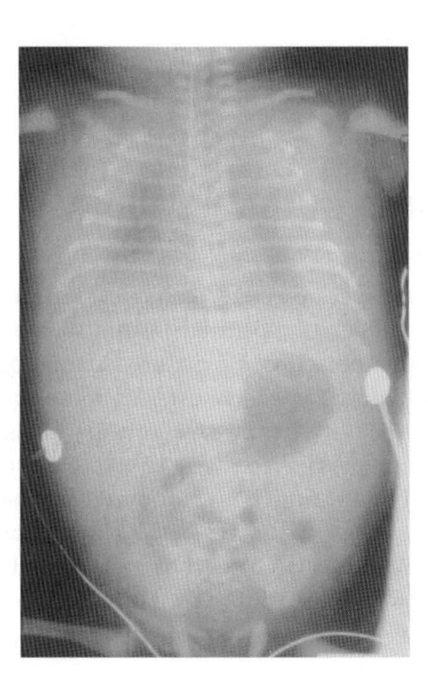

Fig 2.27
X-ray of a hydropic baby. Note bilateral pleural effusions, distended abdomen and thickened subcutaneous tissues due to oedema.

Partial obstructions due to intestinal stenoses often present later as feed volumes build up, while congenital gut malrotation can remain undetected for years before presenting with obstruction. Hirschsprung disease results in a functional intestinal obstruction presenting with constipation and abdominal distension; vomiting will be a late feature unless the complication of enterocolitis develops.

Abdominal distension may also occur in the absence of obstruction (Information box 2.25).

MANAGEMENT

This will be guided by the physical examination findings. A well infant with organomegaly requires less urgent intervention than an infant with a suspected surgical problem or sepsis. The sick infant requires an infection screen (lumbar puncture, urine and blood culture) followed by treatment with broad-spectrum antibiotics. Enteral feeding should be stopped, intravenous fluids given and a nasogastric tube passed. Plain abdominal radiographs should be obtained and unless there is an obvious nonsurgical cause specialist paediatric surgeons should be consulted at an early stage. Where the cause is obstructive, in most cases early surgery is required.

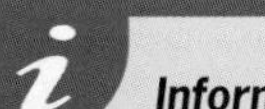

Information Box 2.25

Causes of nonobstructive acquired abdominal distension

- Ileus
  - Electrolyte imbalance, e.g. hypokalaemia
  - Other metabolic/endocrine disorder, e.g. hypercalcaemia, hypothyroidism
  - Sepsis
- Necrotizing enterocolitis
- Hirschsprung enterocolitis

The floppy baby

CLINICAL SIGNS

Relative hypotonia is a feature of prematurity and accounts for the different postures adopted by infants at varying degrees of prematurity (see Figs 2.14 p. 35, and 2.15, p. 36).

DIAGNOSIS

Acute illness in neonates and infants will often result in loss of muscle tone to produce nonspecific floppiness. Persistent and marked hypotonia should raise the possibility of neuromuscular disorder (see Information box 2.26).

MANAGEMENT

History and examination of the infant and mother may provide some clues. In central nervous system disease there may be other features such as irritability and seizures while deep tendon reflexes tend to be preserved.

Information Box 2.26

Causes of hypotonia in neonates

- Central nervous system damage or depression
  - Asphyxia
  - Haemorrhage
  - Infection
  - Metabolic disturbance
  - Drugs (e.g. opiates)
- Peripheral nervous system disease
  - Spinal cord damage at birth
  - Anterior horn cell disease (see p. 311)
  - Neonatal transient myasthenia gravis (in an infant born to an affected mother)
- Muscular disease
  - Inherited myopathy
  - Congenital muscular dystrophy (mother will also be affected)
  - Generalized metabolic disorder (e.g. glycogen storage disease)
  - Mitochondrial cytopathy

In peripheral disorders deep tendon reflexes are lost. Muscles should be examined for fasciculation and tests should include measurement of creatine kinase, electromyogram nerve conduction studies and, if necessary, muscle biopsy. If myasthenia is suspected a Tensilon test (administration of neostigmine) will confirm the diagnosis. More extensive metabolic tests will be required in some cases.

The baby with persistent crying

Crying in most instances is not associated with any underlying problem other than possibly the condition of infantile colic (see p. 39, Day-to-day care of the normal baby). However in some circumstances it may indicate a clinical problem. In the acute situation screaming attacks may suggest colicky pain indicating intestinal problems such as incarcerated inguinal hernia or an intra-abdominal problem. More persistent crying may be due to pain such as in osteomyelitis. High-pitched cry suggests cerebral irritation as in meningitis. The infant should be examined and if necessary investigated to exclude these diagnoses. Drug withdrawal should be considered as a cause of the symptoms. On most occasions nothing will be found and the symptoms settle spontaneously.

When chronic persistent crying presents, it is even less likely that a cause will be found. Neurological disorders should be considered, but once these are ruled out management should focus on the family since emotional factors are likely to have a major role in the problem. Practical help including close support from the health visitor and in extreme cases respite care may be beneficial.

The jittery baby

CLINICAL SIGNS

Jitteriness is a term that has been adopted by paediatricians to describe an infant who when stimulated is irritable and rather shaky. There is hypertonia and clonus can be elicited on examination. The cry may be high pitched.

DIAGNOSIS

Jitteriness has a variety of causes most of which cause excitation at neuromuscular junctions.

Common causes are shown in Information box 2.27.

MANAGEMENT

Occasionally jitteriness occurs in normal babies and remains unexplained, eventually settling down. Usually however it is a useful clue that all is not well and requires investigation.

Careful observation is required to detect whether the infant is likely to proceed to the next stage of irritation in which seizures may occur.

Seizures in the newborn

CLINICAL SIGNS

The neonatal period is the commonest time for seizures. A large number of potential insults to the brain can trigger these episodes. Premature infants, particularly those undergoing intensive care, are more susceptible.

Seizure activity in the newborn, particularly in the premature baby, may be very subtle. Deviation of the eyes, odd mouthing behaviour and apnoea can all indicate seizure activity. Full blown tonic–clonic convulsions can occur also. In ventilated and paralysed infants it is very difficult to spot seizures. An EEG may be helpful but is not routinely available in most neonatal units.

DIAGNOSIS

Causes of neonatal seizures are shown in Information box 2.28.

MANAGEMENT

Management of neonatal seizures involves identifying and remedying underlying causes such as hypoglycaemia or hypocalcaemia. Where this is not possible, anticonvulsant treatment should be commenced. Phenytoin is probably more useful than

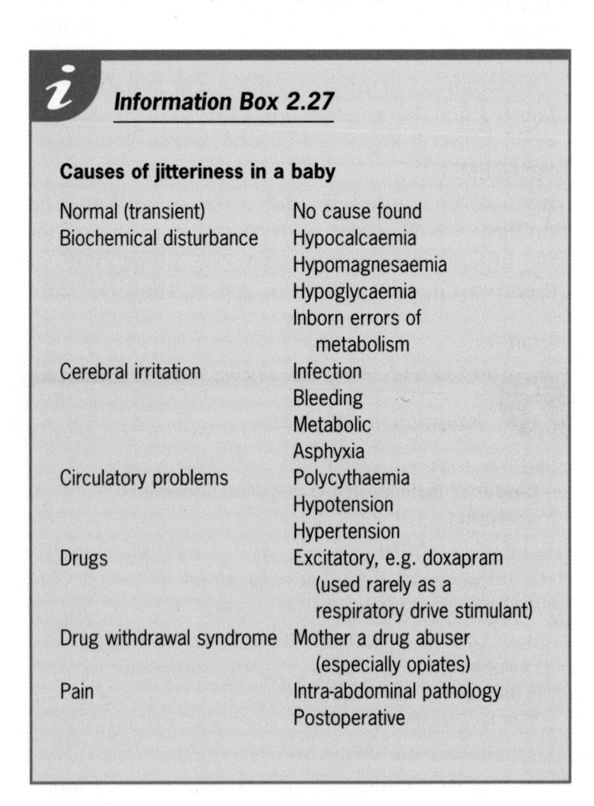

Information Box 2.27

Causes of jitteriness in a baby

Normal (transient)	No cause found
Biochemical disturbance	Hypocalcaemia Hypomagnesaemia Hypoglycaemia Inborn errors of metabolism
Cerebral irritation	Infection Bleeding Metabolic Asphyxia
Circulatory problems	Polycythaemia Hypotension Hypertension
Drugs	Excitatory, e.g. doxapram (used rarely as a respiratory drive stimulant)
Drug withdrawal syndrome	Mother a drug abuser (especially opiates)
Pain	Intra-abdominal pathology Postoperative

Information Box 2.28

Causes of neonatal seizures

Hypoxic ischaemic injury	Pre-birth: intrauterine problems At birth: birth asphyxia Postnatally: secondary to respiratory/cardiac disease
Birth injury	Haemorrhage – Subarachnoid – Subdural
Biochemical	Hypoglycaemia Hypocalcaemia Hypomagnesaemia
Drugs	Drug withdrawal
Metabolic	Inborn errors
Infective	Meningitis/encephalitis Septicaemia
Circulatory	Polycythaemia Hypotension Hypertension
CNS malformation	Sturge–Weber malformation (p. 325) Tuberose sclerosis (p. 325)

phenobarbitone. Benzodiazepines such as clonazepam are also useful.

The baby with superficial infection

CLINICAL SIGNS AND CAUSES

Infections causing rashes in the newborn include the following.

Candida

Oral candidiasis is common particularly in those who have received antibiotics (or whose mothers have received antibiotics). Oral candida manifests as white plaques which leave raw areas when scraped (as opposed to milk deposits). It should respond well to topical treatment such as nystatin, but inadequately sterilized dummies are a source of reinfection and in breastfeeding babies it is possible that maternal nipples will be a source of reinfection. Topical treatment for the mother will reduce this likelihood.

Napkin candidiasis is sometimes difficult to distinguish from simple nappy rash but there are some clues (see Fig. 3.27, p. 88). If there is doubt, infants should be treated with topical nystatin with added hydrocortisone if there is very marked inflammation.

In newborn infants receiving broad-spectrum antibiotics it is a good policy to prescribe a prophylactic nonabsorbable antifungal such as nystatin.

Rarely, candida may cause invasive disease (septicaemia) in very compromised infants undergoing intensive care and who usually have a history of prolonged antibiotic treatment and central venous feeding lines.

Superficial (staphylococcal) infection

Newborns are prone to superficial infection with *Staphylococcus aureus*. The organism may cause conjunctivitis, paronychias of fingers or toes (Fig. 2.28), septic spots and peri-umbilical sepsis. These need to be treated with systemic antibiotics (usually flucloxacillin) since the newborn is vulnerable to progressive and ultimately invasive infection with this organism.

Occasionally neonates may become infected with a toxin-producing staphylococcus which can produce the syndrome of toxic epidermal necrolysis or staphylococcal 'scalded skin' (Fig. 2.29 and p. 267). This is

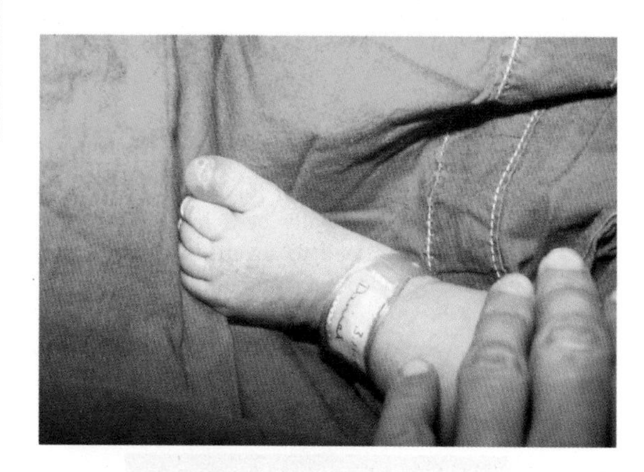

Fig 2.28
Paronychia.

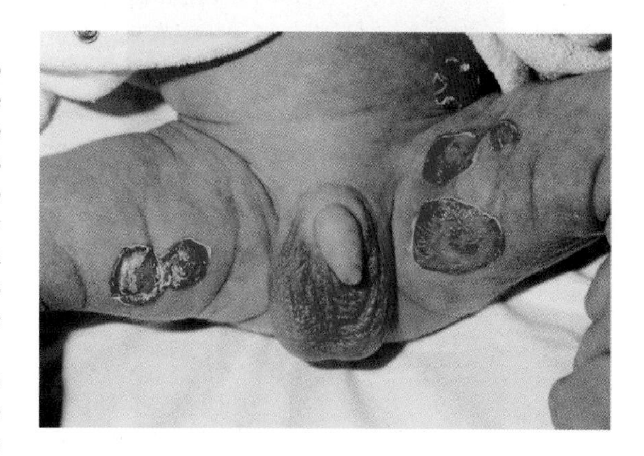

Fig 2.29
Staphylococcal 'scalded' skin.

potentially life-threatening and requires prompt treatment with parenteral antibodies.

Staphylococcal infection in postnatal wards and nurseries is not such a frequent problem as it was in the past thanks to hospital cross-infection policies and the use of chlorhexidine-containing soaps for staff in the relevant clinical areas.

Peri-umbilical sepsis

The umbilicus is a potential entry point for bacteria. Initially the cord itself may become sticky and purulent, but more worrying is the stage where peri-umbilical erythema and cellulitis starts to develop. Though it is often caused by *S. aureus* (see above), this is not always the case. A broad-spectrum combination of antibiotics such as flucloxacillin and gentamicin should be used.

MANAGEMENT

Topical nystatin is the treatment of choice for candidal infection. In bacterial infections, appropriate swabs and blood cultures should be taken.

Flucloxacillin (plus gentamicin in more serious cases including peri-umbilical sepsis) should be used for staphylococcal infection.

The baby with a discharging eye

A common problem (Fig. 2.30), this should be taken seriously as it can occasionally be a marker of more severe infection or can lead to severe local problems. The possibility of gonococcal ophthalmia neonatorum should always be considered, particularly when the problem begins within the first 3 days. Urgent swabs for microscopic examination should be taken. If positive, intensive treatment with local and systemic antibiotics (penicillin) should be given. Other less severe but common causes of bacterial conjunctivitis are *S. aureus* and *E. coli*. These can be treated with topical neomycin.

Conjunctivitis occurring from the beginning of the 2nd week onwards could be caused by *Chlamydia trachomatis* acquired from the mother's genital tract. If there is failure to respond to neomycin and particularly if bacterial swabs are negative, a swab scrape for this agent, diagnosed by a rapid immunofluorescence test (Fig. 2.31), should be taken. Chlamydial disease is treated with topical tetracycline and systemic erythromycin for 14 days; the latter is used to prevent the possible later development of chlamydial pneumonia (Fig. 2.32).

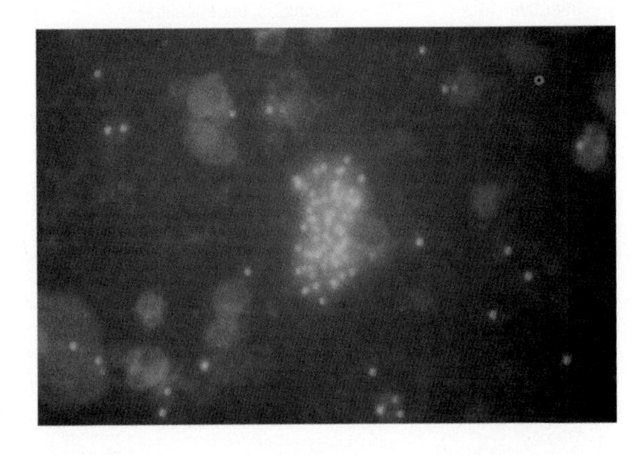

Fig 2.31
Immunofluorescence on conjunctival scraping showing elementary bodies of *Chlamydia trachomatis* (courtesy of Dr David Carrington).

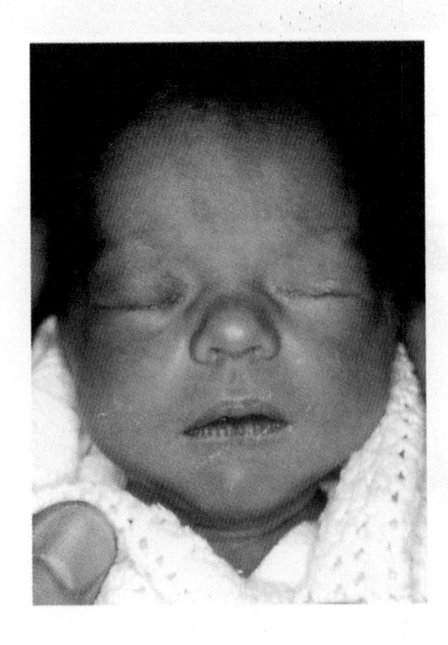

Fig 2.30
Neonatal conjunctivitis with cellulitis.

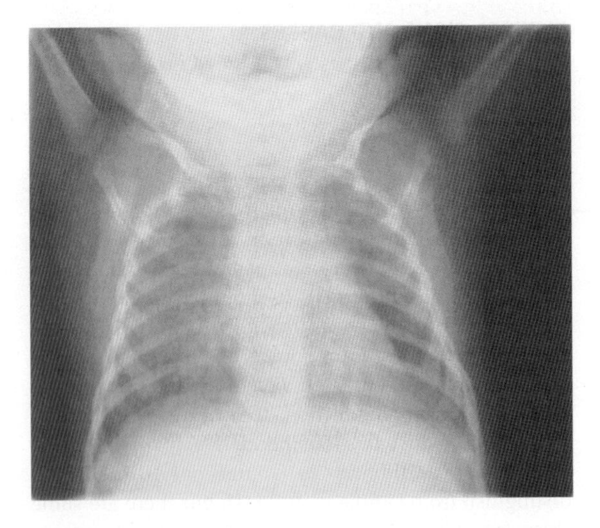

Fig 2.32
Chlamydial pneumonia presenting at 6 weeks of age. There was a previous history of neonatal conjunctivitis.

Chlamydia and gonococcus are sexually transmitted. If these are identified the mother and her partner(s) should be referred to a genitourinary medicine specialist.

Chloramphenicol, the most commonly used eye drop preparation, is inadvisable at this age as empirical treatment because it may partially treat chlamydial infection thus masking the signs. Such infants may present with chlamydial pneumonia at a later stage. Neomycin is preferable.

New horizons

Improvements in fetal and perinatal medicine

The continually improving care of the fetus and the early diagnosis of problems affecting either the fetus or the mother are likely to lead to a further reduction in birth complications. As a consequence we are likely to see further falls in neonatal morbidity and mortality. This may be offset by a continuing fall in the gestational age at which viability may be possible with modern intensive care support.

Managing lung disease of prematurity

The role of surfactant therapy is now established. Further refinement of the protocols for its use will maximize the benefits of this therapy. For those infants with severe lung disease not responding to conventional ventilation, newer strategies of ventilation such as oscillatory techniques are becoming established. The place of extracorporeal membrane oxygenation (ECMO) therapy has also now been established. Fluid phase ventilation is an exciting potential new method of ventilation aimed at reducing the incidence and severity of chronic lung problems in survivors of neonatal respiratory distress syndromes.

Reducing the incidence of neonatal sepsis

Several areas of research and development have the potential for reducing morbidity and mortality from infection in newborn infants. A conjugate vaccine against group B Streptococcus, currently under development, could if given to mothers reduce the incidence of sepsis and meningitis due to this organism. This is an increasingly important problem as other advances in neonatal care lead to survival of smaller, sicker and therefore more immunocompromised infants. Increasing understanding of the neonatal immune response may lead to strategies for immune modulation aimed at either preventing sepsis or enhancing its treatment. The use of immunoglobulin preparations or recombinant haemopoietic growth factors or other cytokines seems promising in this respect. The use of mother's breast milk and other strategies may help newborn infants who are undergoing intensive care to retain relatively normal colonizing bacterial flora, which are increasingly felt to be important in defence against infection.

All of these approaches will become increasingly important with what seems to be an inevitable rise in antibiotic-resistant pathogens, particularly in hospital settings.

Advanced surgical techniques

For those infants born with congenital abnormalities, advances in surgical techniques already offer advantages such as earlier repair of cleft lip and palate (thus reducing the associated feeding problems). Minimally invasive cardiac surgery such as the occlusion of patent ductus or ventricular septal defect by balloons and other devices inserted via arterial catheters is an area of rapid development, and will reduce the need for major invasive surgery in newborns. Minimally invasive techniques for abdominal surgery already utilized at other ages have a similar potential for application to newborns.

FURTHER READING

Rennie J, Roberton NRC (1999) *Textbook of Neonatology*. Edinburgh: Churchill Livingstone.

Jones KL (1997) *Smith's Recognizable Patterns of Human Malformation*. WB Saunders: London.

3 The infant from 1 month to 1 year

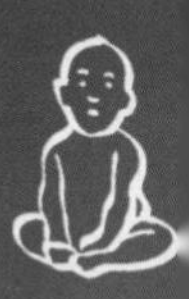

Introduction

The term infancy is used to cover the period in a child's life from birth to the first birthday. It therefore includes both the neonatal (first 28 days) and postneonatal periods. This phase of the child's life sees the maximum rate of development in physical, psychological and neurological terms. Overall growth and the growth of individual organs is at its maximal postnatal rate in the first year of life. The functional adaptation of organ systems to postnatal life continues.

Parental bonding is well established by the second half of the first year of life. Social development starts in this period. The infant's immune system, though developing rapidly, remains unable to handle some infections and this is a period where infection and infectious diseases are a major contributor to ill health. The rapidly developing organ systems are themselves particularly vulnerable to damage; examples include encephalopathic illnesses (usually due to infection or a metabolic cause) leading to profound brain damage; urinary tract infection causing renal scarring, and respiratory viral infections, such as bronchiolitis, which may result in long-lasting changes in the airways producing a persisting tendency to cough and wheeze.

First-time parents in particular need to undergo a continuous learning process during the first year. Even experienced parents may encounter uncertainty as second and subsequent children may have an entirely different behaviour pattern from earlier siblings. Twins produce more than twice the work of singletons. Several good books are available, but even the best of these tend to be rather dogmatic on some points and may fail to explain the great variability in behaviour amongst infants. Health visitors are the key professionals to help in supporting parents and provide advice and appropriate reassurance.

Epidemiology

Many illnesses of children are commonest in the first year particularly infections such as bacterial meningitis (Fig. 3.1). Respiratory tract infections comprise the greatest cause of acquired illness and include the syndrome of bronchiolitis which is confined exclusively to this age group.

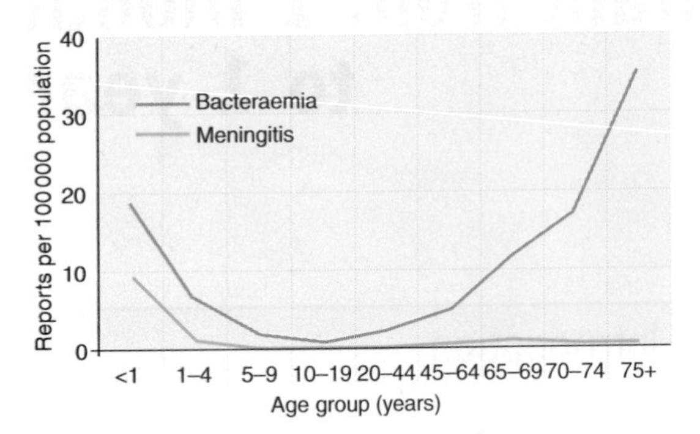

Fig 3.1
Mean annual age-specific incidence of laboratory reports for pneumococcal bacteraemia and meningitis, England and Wales, 1993–95 (From *Communicable Disease and Public Health Reports.* Vol. 1, 1998.) © Crown copyright 1998

Infant mortality is defined as deaths in the first year per 1000 live births, including neonatal and postneonatal mortality. It is inversely related to the affluence of a particular society, being lower in high income countries, and within those countries showing an inverse relationship with social class. Most western countries show falling infant mortality rates in recent years.

There has been a dramatic fall in infant mortality in the last 50 years (Fig. 3.2). The extent of the reduction varies with the cause. The highest fall is in infant mortality caused by infectious diseases (see Information box 3.1).

An example of a recent trend is the dramatic fall in sudden unexplained infant deaths (SIDS, see p. 70) or cot deaths, which followed the demonstration that the prone sleeping position was a risk factor (Fig. 3.3).

Social, cultural and environmental factors affecting child health

In infancy the child is completely dependent on his/her carers, and vulnerable to adverse influences stemming from background and circumstances. In their most extreme form these influences may result in child abuse.

Social factors

The developing infant needs a stable environment and caring parents. Unfortunately not all infants will automatically get these. Infants of young single mothers are particularly vulnerable. These families need close monitoring and support, provided primarily by the health visitor. Maternal instincts are not nearly as well developed in humans as in other animals. An inexperienced parent may not have sufficient instinct or knowledge to cope with the problems that may arise with feeding, weaning, sleeping, crying and bowel habits which are part of normal infant development. Grandmothers are usually helpful sources of support but can be counterproductive if they undermine the mother's own confidence. Add to these problems the fact that a sizeable proportion of babies are born into families with pre-existing social problems (financial, housing or marital) and it is not surprising that the incidence of child abuse is maximal in the infant age group.

Childcare facilities in the UK are sparse for this particular age group. The expertise and facilities required are expensive and neither the government nor individual employers have chosen to invest in these on a large scale. Mothers wishing to return to work in the first year are faced with difficult decisions (see Practical box 3.1).

Cultural factors

In the UK we live in a multicultural society. Childrearing holds an important place in many cultures and this should be borne in mind when seeing infants. Weaning practices vary considerably. For example in Asian cultures the progression from milk to solid feeds as the main source of nutrition is more protracted than in western cultures.

Although prolonged breastfeeding, if it delays the weaning process, may sometimes lead to suboptimal

Information Box 3.1

Factors contributing to the fall in infant mortality

- Improved standard of living
- Advent of antibiotics
- Introduction of vaccinations

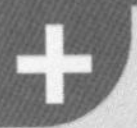

Practical Box 3.1

Problems faced by mothers returning to work in the first year after giving birth

- Emotional, with perhaps the necessity for prolonged periods of separation during the day
- Physical, tiredness
- Practical, such as the need to stop or reduce breast-feeding early
- Financial, in terms of employing a child carer

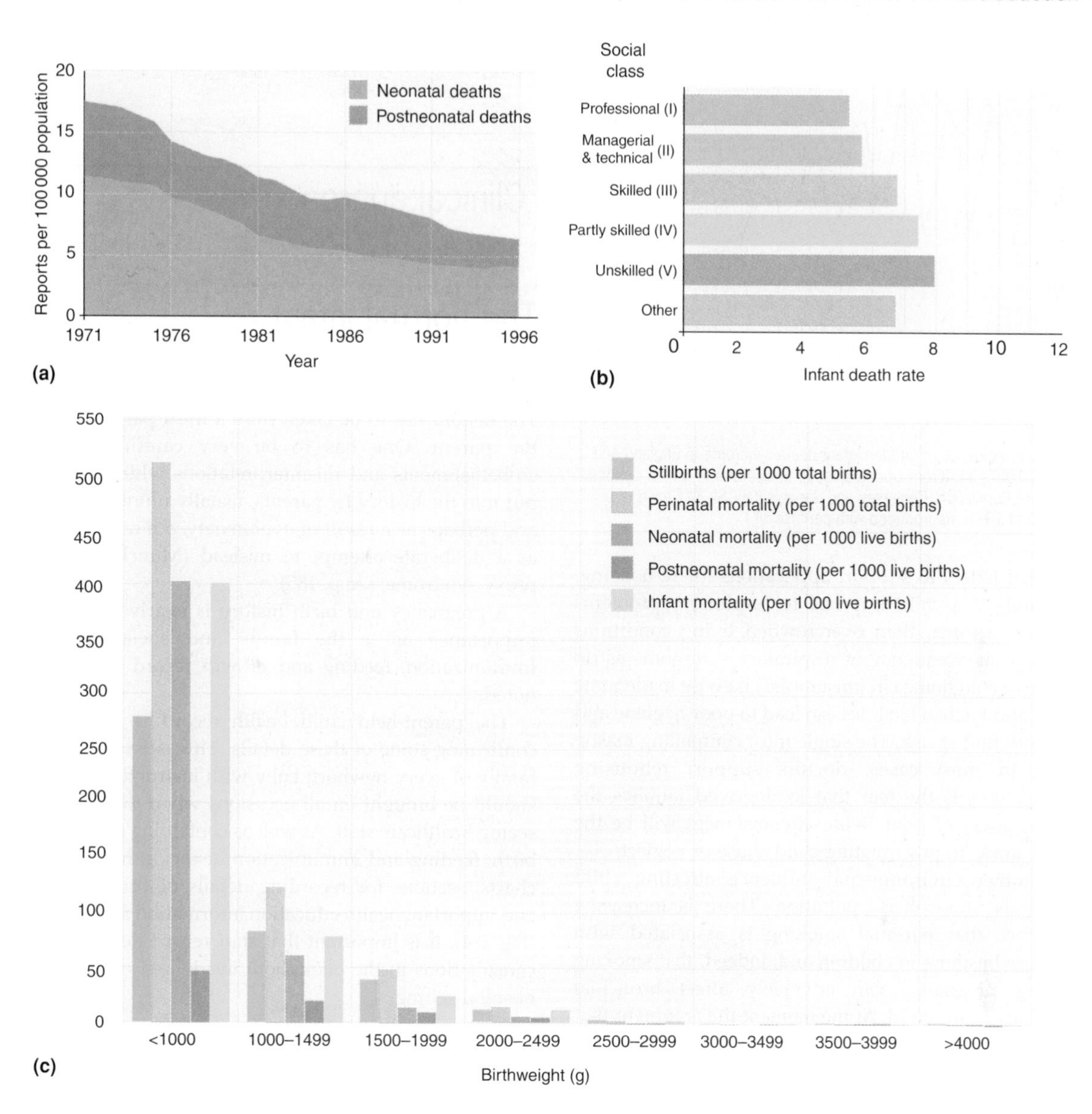

Fig 3.2
Infant mortality rates. (a) England and Wales, 1971–96. (b) In Northern Ireland, according to social class, 1991–95. (c) By birthweight, in England and Wales, 1996. (Sources: (a) and (c) from the Office for National Statistics (1998) *Mortality Statistics; Childhood, Infant and Perinatal, 1996*, Series DH3 no. 29, © Crown Copyright 1996. London: The Stationery Office; (b) from the *76th Annual Report of the Registrar-General, 1997*, Belfast: Northern Ireland Statistics and Research Agency, © The General Register Office (Reproduced with permission.)

calorie intake, in areas of great poverty it is useful as the best source of nutrition and protection against infection in the infant. It also has a partial effect as a contraceptive for the mother.

Developmental milestones can also vary; Negro children generally have advanced motor development compared with Caucasians and Asians.

The way one talks to parents needs to be adjusted in the light of cultural factors. In some cultures female emancipation lags behind that of western society. Some mothers don't speak English; beware of using the father or another male member of the family to interpret. They may decide to withhold certain key facts from the mother. Many areas now have trained 'link workers' who can not only act as language interpreters but help to explain relevant cultural nuances.

Even in continental Europe practices differ from those of the UK. In most European countries all children are seen regularly by family paediatricians whereas in the UK only those with problems will see specialist paediatricians. This difference needs to be explained to families from other European countries.

Environmental factors

Paediatricians and other doctors are continually asked by families, social workers and health visitors to write

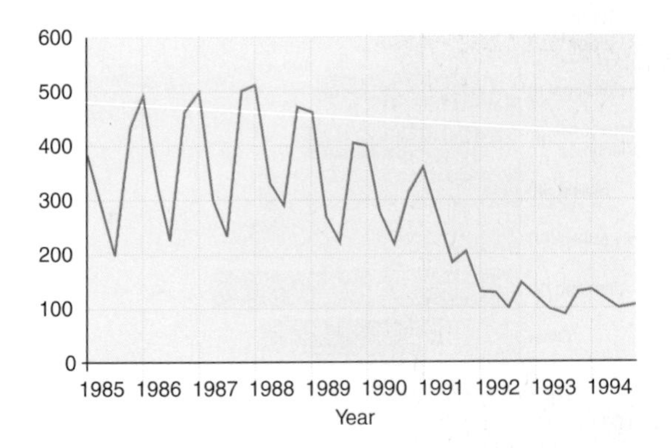

Fig 3.3
Trends in incidence of sudden infant death syndrome in England and Wales, 1985–94. (From *Updates*, issue 9, September 1995. London: Office of Population, Censuses and Surveys (OPCS). © Crown Copyright 1995. Reproduced with permission.)

medical letters to support applications for re-housing. Certainly if a child is prone to respiratory problems such as asthma, then overcrowded living conditions increase the frequency of respiratory symptoms as do damp or cold home circumstances. Likewise inadequate toilet and kitchen facilities can lead to poor hygiene and put the child at risk. The single most compelling reason why, in most cases, doctors support rehousing applications is the fear that in deprived families the added stress of poor living circumstances will be the 'final straw' in precipitating child abuse or neglect.

Another environmental influence affecting child health is atmospheric pollution. There is increasing evidence that parental smoking is associated with increased asthma in children and, indeed, that smoking during pregnancy can adversely affect bronchial reactivity in the child. At the moment the argument that industrial and car exhaust pollution contribute to childhood asthma problems is unproven. Similar rates of asthma are found in clean air places, such as Shetland, to urban areas in the UK.

Key issues

The three most important areas of concern to those caring for children in this age group are:

- Maintaining a high uptake of vaccines and promoting the development and introduction of new vaccines against infectious diseases which still produce significant mortality and morbidity (for example meningococcal disease).
- Continuing to develop appropriate infant screening programmes so that physical and neurodevelopmental disorders can be identified at the earliest opportunity.
- Encouraging further social change to promote greater availability of childcare support and to improve monitoring and support for deprived families.

Clinical approach

The normal infant

History taking

The history has to be taken from a third party, usually the parent. One has to be very careful to spot embellishments and misinterpretations which may be put into the history by parents, usually unintentionally and perhaps as a result of overanxiety, but occasionally as a deliberate attempt to mislead (Munchausen by proxy syndrome; see p. 185).

A pregnancy and birth history is nearly always of importance as is the family and social history. Immunization, feeding and growth record should be noted.

The parent-held child health record is useful for confirming some of these details. This is issued to the family of every newborn baby with instructions that it should be brought on all occasions when the infant is seeing healthcare staff. As well as containing a record of birth, feeding and immunization history it has growth charts, sections for recording details of consultations and important health education information for families (Fig. 3.4). It is important that staff record details of all consultations in the book, both inside and outside the hospital setting.

Physical examination

As at all ages this should be thorough and systematic. To keep the infant's cooperation it may be necessary to do things out of order; for example listening to the chest early before crying occurs, and deferring more unpleasant procedures (such as examining the throat) until the end.

In the last few months of infancy the child tends to become wary of strangers. The approach is therefore critical. During the time spent taking the history, exchange of eye contact and smiles may help reassure the wary infant, as well as providing important information about the child, the parent and their relationship. Whatever the reason for examining the child, the opportunity should be taken to screen for congenital or genetic disorders, which may have been missed or not presented during the neonatal period. Growth, development, emotional and family problems should also be identified.

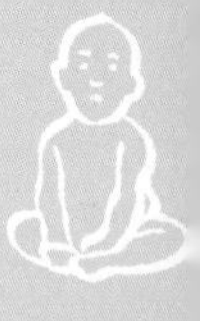

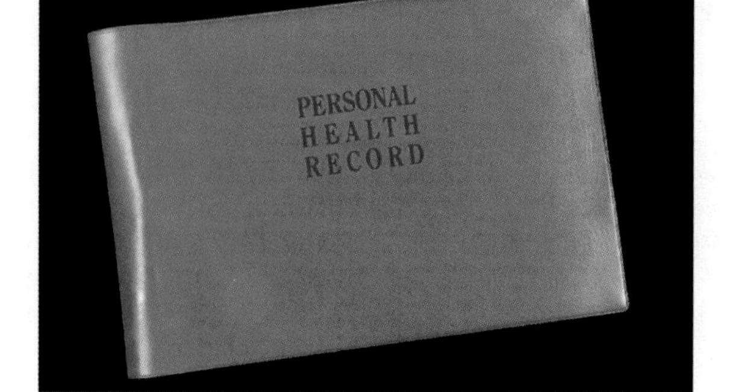

(a)

SUMMARY PAGE – For further details see main record

CLINIC CHECKS	
AGE DUE	DATE DONE
4–6 weeks	
7–8 months	
2–2½ years	
3½ years	

IMMUNISATIONS		
AGE DUE		DATE DONE
Diphtheria, Tetanus, Pertussis, Polio, Hib MenC	2 months	
	3 months	
	4 months	
M.M.R. 12–15 months		
Diphtheria, Tetanus, Polio MMR	3½ years	
B.C.G. 10–14 years		
Others		

TESTS	DATE	RESULT
P.K.U. (Guthrie)		
Thyroid		
Sickle Cell Status		
Others		

INCLUSION ON REGISTERS		
REGISTER	DATE ON	DATE OFF
Observation		
Special Needs		
Child Protection		

MAJOR HEALTH PROBLEMS – Allergies, Operations, Chronic Illness Etc.	DATE

(b)

Fig 3.4
(a) Child health record book; (b) summary page.

Neurodevelopmental assessment

See developmental screening, below.

Immunization

Infancy is a stage in life when the opportunity exists to protect a child against certain infections before he/she comes into contact with them. Factors determining the scheduling of immunization are listed in Information box 3.2.

Nearly every country has a different schedule, in some cases reflecting local circumstances (for example the need for earlier protection against measles in low income countries), in others reflecting a different approach to the same problem. The current UK schedule is presented in Table 3.1.

Contraindications to vaccination are few. In high income countries BCG is not given to HIV-positive children, though it is in Africa where the risk of TB is higher. Live vaccines should not be given to those who are (or are suspected of being) immunocompromised, with the exception of HIV-positive children where MMR vaccine can be given safely. An enhanced inactivated polio vaccine (eIPV), given by injection, is an

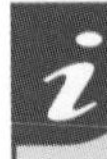

Information Box 3.2

Factors influencing the timing and nature of infant immunization

- The degree of maturity of the immune system.
- The amount of maternal placentally transferred antibody remaining in the infant which might interfere with the response of the child to live virus vaccines.
- The need to immunize before the child encounters the relevant infection.
- The need to keep the schedule simple and straightforward.

alternative to the live oral polio vaccine in immunocompromised patients and is equally efficacious. Household contacts of immunocompromised patients should also be given eIPV because of the risk of transmission of the live polio vaccine.

Any immunization is contraindicated during the acute febrile phase of a brief illness and in those in whom the particular vaccine has produced a severe generalized or local reaction previously (Fig. 3.5). In children with an evolving neurological problem (i.e. not a static problem such as cerebral palsy) the pertussis component of the triple vaccine should be deferred until the clinical picture becomes clearer. In children with diarrhoea the oral polio vaccine is best deferred for fear that it won't work. Many false contraindications have been used as excuses not to immunize in the past. The Department of Health now issues a *Green Book* to all doctors, clarifying the guidelines, and its introduction has helped to boost immunization rates in this country.

Since components of the measles, mumps and rubella (MMR) vaccine are produced on egg embryos there has been some worry about anaphylactic reactions in egg-sensitive children. Allergic reactions can occur very rarely, but there is no evidence to suggest that they are caused by egg proteins and they may be due to other constituents. If children are considered to be at high risk of type I (immediate) hypersensitivity reaction they can be observed for 2 hours after immunization with medical staff and appropriate facilities

Table 3.1
The current UK immunization schedule

Age*	Immunization	Comments
Birth	BCG (Bacillus Calmette–Guérin)	In some areas to all infants In others to high risk ethnic groups only In others only where there is recent family history of TB
Birth	Hepatitis B vaccine (Hep B)	Only to babies of carrier mothers
6 weeks	Hep B (second dose)	If mother is e antigen-positive a dose of Hep B immune globulin is also given
2 months	Diphtheria, tetanus pertussis, (DTP) (triple) + Oral polio vaccine (OPV) + Haemophilus influenzae B (Hib) vaccine + Meningococcal C conjugate vaccine (Men C)	
3 months	DTP OPV Hib	
4 months	DTP OP Hib Men C	
6 months	Hep B (third dose)	
12–14 months	Measles, mumps, rubella (MMR)	
4 years	Diphtheria, tetanus (DT) OPV MMR	Preschool booster
13–14 years	BCG	If Heaf test negative
15–16 years	dT† OPV	Booster

* Premature infants are commenced on triple vaccine at 2 months after birth rather than after the expected date of delivery
† dT is low-dose diphtheria vaccine (as opposed to standard-dose)

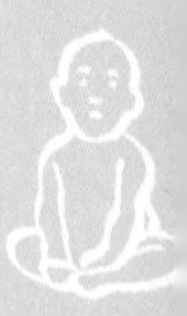

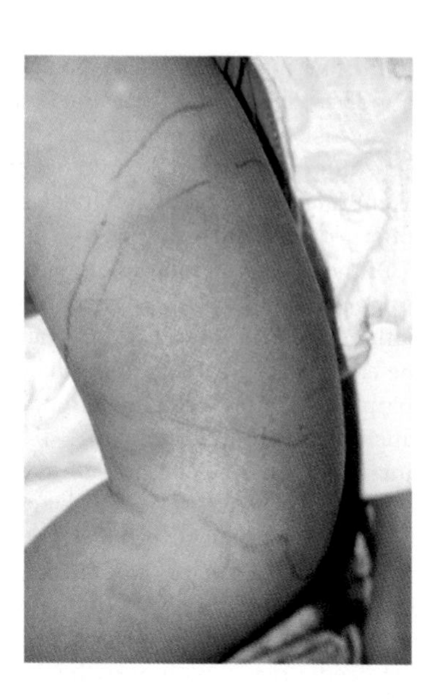

Fig 3.5
Severe local reaction to immunization (in this case pneumococcal vaccine).

available for emergency treatment if this becomes necessary.

Injectable vaccines are given by intramuscular injection (except in children with coagulation disorders who should receive them subcutaneously) either in the lateral compartment of the thigh or into the deltoid muscle. Some minor local irritation a few days later is common, but major reactions, producing redness and swelling over at least two-thirds of the upper arm (Fig. 3.5), are rare.

Minor general reactions may include low grade fever and irritability in the first 48 hours, and can be treated with paracetamol. Major generalised reactions are rare and result in high fever and often inconsolable crying. The oral polio vaccine does not produce any reactions.

Teething

At every medical examination the teeth should be studied, interest expressed in their condition, and co-operation with dentists urged.

Teeth that are occasionally found to be present at birth are usually precursors rather than true primary dentition and may soon be extruded. The primary dentition usually starts to erupt at around 5–7 months. There is a tendency to blame children's minor upsets too readily on 'teething'. Though a long-term temperature monitoring study showed a correlation between mild elevation of temperature and the eruption of teeth, ascribing fever to teething should be done very reluctantly and after exclusion of all other possibilities.

As soon as teeth erupt, daily wiping with moistened cotton wool and fluoride toothpaste should begin, and soft brushing commence at around 1 year. This early start establishes a pattern which is hard to introduce if commenced later. The family should discourage excessive consumption of sweets and sugary drinks.

Fluoride helps to reduce caries. If there is insufficient in local water, supplementation may be needed. The introduction of fluoride toothpaste has led to a dramatic improvement in children's dental health (Fig. 3.6). Gross dental decay is much less common than in the recent past. Its occurrence now suggests very poor care. Dentists are now paid to conserve rather than treat children's teeth and this should lead to a reduction of drilling; minor caries can be a self-healing condition.

Orthodontic advice is needed where there is gross crowding of teeth and malocclusion.

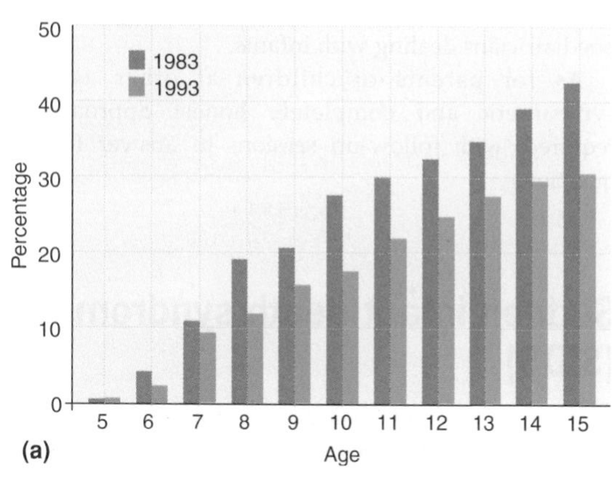

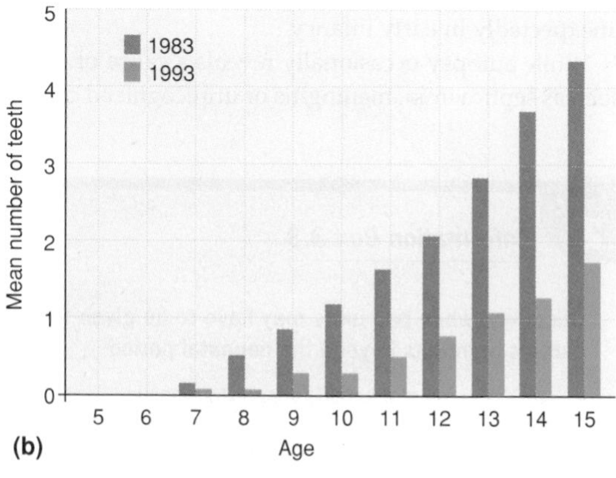

Fig 3.6
(a) Proportion of children with active decay in the permanent dentition, and (b) mean number of filled teeth; by age, United Kingdom, 1983 and 1993. (Source: OPCS ss 94/1, London: Office of Population, Censuses and Surveys. OPCS. © Crown Copyright. Reproduced with permission.)

Dealing with clinical problems

Therapeutic considerations

The ability of infants to metabolize and excrete drugs has matured markedly by the end of the neonatal period. Calculation of dosages must be performed with great care. By the latter part of infancy this is most accurately achieved using surface area (SA) calculated from a nomogram (see Appendix 1 on p. 367). In early infancy (<6 months) measurement and calculation of SA is not easily achieved and calculations are usually based on body weight.

The mobility and inquisitiveness acquired by the end of infancy make it mandatory that those caring for children should keep all medicines in childproof containers and in a cupboard (ideally lockable) out of the reach of determined children.

Breaking bad news

This is a not infrequent task (see Information box 3.3) for paediatricians dealing with infants.

As for parents of children at other ages, a sympathetic and completely honest approach is required, with follow-up sessions to answer further questions.

Sudden infant death syndrome (SIDS)

In recent years there has been a dramatic fall in the incidence of SIDS (see Fig. 3.3, p. 65). However, a number of previously healthy infants still die unexpectedly in early infancy.

While autopsy occasionally reveals a cause of death, such as septicaemia, meningitis or unrecognized cardiac abnormality, in the majority of cases no specific cause can be found. It is thought that these infants are particularly at risk because of immature patterns of control of breathing, and then some other factor such as intercurrent infection precipitates apnoea and death.

A number of risk factors for SIDS have been identified. Of these, sleeping in the prone position and overwrapping (and therefore overheating) are the stronger influences. The introduction of an education programme encouraging parents to put their infants to sleep in a supine position seems to be the main reason for the reduction in the SIDS rate.

When infants die of SIDS, because of its unexpected nature and the fact that the child was usually completely healthy previously, the impact on the family is often much greater than for other less unexpected child deaths. Careful and detailed bereavement counselling will be necessary. This is best undertaken by a consultant paediatrician, with or without the aid of a nurse counsellor who can keep in close contact with the family and conduct follow-up sessions.

Autopsy is mandatory in these cases and the results, together with the results of the screens for infection and metabolic disorders, should be made known to the family, with explanation. It is important that parents feel that they can return with further questions and that they receive extra support during and after future pregnancies.

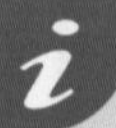

Information Box 3.3

Occasions when bad news may have to be given to parents of infants beyond the neonatal period

- Late diagnosis of a serious congenital/genetic problem.
- Recognition of neurodevelopmental problems which may only occur as the infant fails to achieve milestones.
- Serious acquired disorders which may be immediately life-threatening or may imply long-term disability.

Child abuse

When child abuse first became widely recognized it was known as the 'battered baby syndrome', reflecting the fact that physical abuse in infancy is perhaps the most overt form of abuse. Subsequently it was realized that more subtle and, in some ways, more cruel forms of abuse exist, including physical and emotional neglect, Munchausen by proxy syndrome and child sexual abuse. In infancy the common types of abuse are physical trauma and neglect or deprivation. These can occur in any family but certain risk factors can be identified (Information box 3.4).

For a general account of child abuse see page 183. This section will deal specifically with aspects of infant abuse.

Several patterns of physical injury are known to be associated with child abuse in the infant (see Information box 3.5).

In assessing injuries it is important to fully document all marks with drawings and measurements. Photographs are most helpful; for forensic use they must be taken by a police photographer in a standardized way. Radiographs of the full skeleton (skeletal survey) may show multiple old fractures which are not clinically obvious. A full coagulation screen is usually undertaken to rule out the (rare) possibility of clotting disorder if bruising is the presenting feature.

Neglect and deprivation abuse can also take different

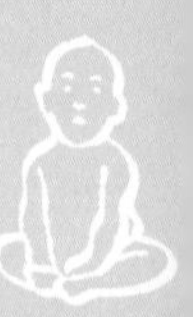

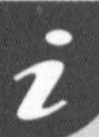

Information Box 3.4

Risk factors in infant abuse

- Low socioeconomic status
- Parental factors
  - Low ability
  - Low self-esteem
- Parents themselves abused as children
- Financial problems
- Poor housing
- Marital/relationship problems
- Child has handicap or medical problem

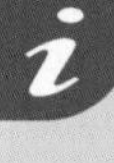

Information Box 3.5

Patterns of physical injury in infant abuse

Type of injury	Pattern of injury
Gripping injuries	Finger mark bruises Fractured ribs or limbs
Twisting injuries	Spiral fractures of long bones Avulsion fractures at metaphyses
Shaking injuries	Subdural haematoma Cerebral haemorrhage Retinal haemorrhages
Hitting injuries	Bruises especially around face and inside lips Torn frenulum of upper lip
Cigarette burns	Circular lesions
Scalding	Buttocks and legs; from over hot baths Mouth; from milk that is too hot
Bites	Usually on limbs

forms. Cases of gross neglect often make headlines in the newspapers but are fortunately rare. Such children may be starved and left alone for long periods. An example of more subtle neglect is the failure to change soiled napkins for long periods resulting in irritant napkin dermatitis.

It is sometimes difficult to distinguish between deliberate parental neglect and incompetence. The latter may occur with unsupported parents of limited ability, and often relates to feeding or emotional issues. Pure emotional deprivation is a form of neglect in which the child is cleaned and fed perfectly normally but not given any love or attention. Such infants often fail to thrive despite adequate calorie intake and are slow to achieve developmental milestones, especially the social ones. Older infants and toddlers may engage in self-stimulatory behaviour such as head banging, while younger infants often have a tell-tale bald patch over the occiput, on which they have lain for hours on end.

Munchausen by proxy syndrome (see page 185) can occur at any childhood age including the infant age group. It can take many forms, including imposed upper airway obstruction which is described in the section on Apnoea, on p. 85.

Child sexual abuse is uncommon in the infant age range, usually taking the form of inappropriate fingering of the genitalia.

Identifying cases of child abuse before serious damage or death occurs is clearly vitally important. Child health workers already have a low threshold for considering abuse, but it is important that GPs and staff in accident and emergency departments also consider this diagnosis when confronted by injured children or those with other unexplained problems.

MANAGEMENT

An experienced paediatrician and social worker should be involved at an early stage. The latter will take responsibility for planning the approach to the problem. The social worker will also inform the police child protection team at an early stage. The situation needs to be explained to the parents and if the child is considered to be at continuing risk while the investigation proceeds then he/she should be admitted to hospital, if appropriate, or taken into foster care, if necessary using an Emergency Care Order under the Children Act. A case conference (see Child Abuse, p. 70) will have to be convened to make long-term decisions regarding the protection of the child.

Accidents in infancy

A general discussion of accidents in childhood can be found in Chapter 6. Susceptibility to accidents develops in late infancy with the development of mobility.

Most accidents occur in the home (Fig. 3.7). Parents can't be expected to have 'eyes in the backs of their heads' and advice on sensible precautions should be provided (see Practical box 3.2).

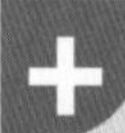

Practical Box 3.2

Accident prevention in infancy

- Fixing of guards on steps and stairs
- Fencing around swimming pools or other open water
- Avoidance of dangling electric flexes on kettles and irons
- Preventing access to small inhalable objects such as peanuts and tablets
- Preventing access to medicines, household cleaning reagents and garden chemicals

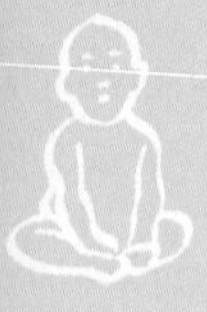

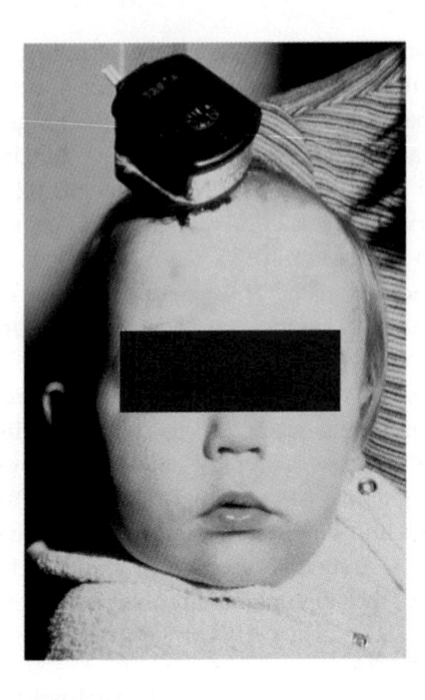

Fig 3.7
An unusual accident in the home. This child fell onto an upturned electric plug after being left unsupervised on a bed. He made a full recovery.

Adoption and fostering

These two processes are part of a continuum. Crises over care of children often arise. This may be a short-term matter, for instance an unsupported mother having a baby with no one to look after older children. Although such crises can usually be resolved by the family, this is not always the case and as a last resort social services may be called to 'look after' the child in terms of the Children Act 1989. Parenting may fail, most commonly due to child abuse, and children may have to be taken away from their parents. This process is regulated by the Children Act. In the past local authorities tended to place such children in residential homes, run either by themselves or by private agencies (such as Barnardos or National Children's Homes). Increasingly however, there has been a move towards placing children directly with approved registered foster parents. Provided the foster parents are satisfactory, this normally leads to a much superior quality of childcare. Children may bond closely with their foster parents and great problems can arise when the natural parents, who may be less devoted and less capable, have their children restored to them.

Foster children are thus vulnerable. One has to consider the original reasons why they needed fostering. Often children are psychologically disturbed and sometimes malnourished. Usually such children bloom with good parenting. In thinking about these children, one has to consider old injuries, shaking, fetal alcohol or narcotic damage. The local authority has a duty to support such children and pay their foster parents, and do whatever is feasible to keep them in touch with their birth parents. In some instances, it is clear that these children can never go back to their parents and long-term planning for the child's future is needed. Here the correct answer may well be an adoption.

Each social service department has an adoption and fostering service. They have the duty to review all children known to them where the possibility of adoption could arise. Such children are allocated to social workers, either in the local authority or working for an approved adoption agency, who have the duty to determine the child's social status. If attempts to help the natural parents to look after their own child fail, then a search is made for potential adoptive parents. This may be within the natural family, but the needs of the child rather than the wishes of the relatives are paramount, and it may be better to choose outsiders than aged grandparents or relatives who cannot give assurances that the child would receive an appropriate quality of care. Far more people wish to adopt children than there are children available. According to the Office of National Statistics, the number of adoptions in England and Wales fell from 21 299 in 1975 to 5962 in 1996.

Applicants for adoption are thoroughly studied. A shortage of available babies means that only those who are young, healthy and in regular lifestyles have much hope of being accepted as adoptive parents. An elaborate process is undertaken to ensure that the potential adopters are satisfactory. Information on both child and the adoptive parents are brought to an adoption panel and the casework for both the child and potential adopters is scrutinized. If it is agreed that adoption with such a family would be in the child's interests, the papers are taken before a judge in order to seek an Adoption Order. Once granted, an adoption is a permanent matter and the adoptive parents assume the full rights and duties of parents. New adoptive parents need a great deal of support. When adopted children reach 18 years old, they are now entitled to seek information about their original parents. Information is rigorously kept on the antecedents of adopted children and it is good practice to build up a life-story book for the child, though this does not include details of the birth parents.

The shortage of healthy babies for adoption means that potential adopters may go to great lengths to seek infants. There is much controversy over the question of inter-country adoptions and legislation has had to be adapted to cope with this growing trend. It is very important that no possibility of money changing hands is permitted. Although such adoptions are usually successful, problems can occur, particularly if an infant is brought in who subsequently proves to have a severe handicapping disorder and the potential adoptive parents change their minds.

Special efforts have been made to place children who were formerly regarded as 'unadoptable'. Organizations such as Parents for Children play a major role in bringing together potential parents and children with handicaps or severe disorders such as HIV infection.

Paediatricians play a major role in the adoption process. The child's future may depend on an accurate medical examination and an appropriate prognosis being given.

Nutrition

During infancy the diet changes from entirely milk to one of mixed solids and milk.

Most infants need to have solids introduced at somewhere between 3 and 4 months. Initially sloppy solids such as 'baby rice' or pureed fruit are used and gradually more complex and solid foods added. Eating habits start to form at this stage and it is important to establish reasonably fixed patterns for 'meal' times. Current practice is to recommend that gluten-containing solids are withheld until 6 months of age. There is no sound scientific basis for this, but the practice of later introduction of gluten does seem to have coincided with a reduction in the incidence of classical infantile gluten enteropathy (see Coeliac disease, p. 224).

By the end of infancy most children should be eating a mixed diet, which often consists of what the rest of the family is eating but cut into small pieces or pureed. There is usually still a significant milk intake but this has reduced as a proportion of calorie intake. Allowing too high a proportion of milk in the diet delays the development of the child's solid diet which can result in iron deficiency (see below).

A common question for parents to ask is when can they switch to ordinary (doorstep) cow's milk from formula feeds. In physiological terms the infant should be able to handle the higher protein, phosphate and sodium from about 6 months. However, current practice is to recommend continued use of formula feeds until 12 months, since these contain iron supplements while unmodified cow's milk has virtually no iron. Another question often asked is whether cow's milk should be boiled. For pasteurized milk there is no advantage in doing this.

Routine multivitamin supplementation is advocated for all babies under 2 years. A typical preparation contains vitamins A, B, C and D. These preparations do not however contain iron which will need to be given as a separate supplement in high-risk groups such as premature infants.

The method of feeding develops over the first year. Towards the end of this period infants will learn to feed from a trainer beaker and then a mug instead of a bottle with a teat. Older infants will be able to finger feed and have rudimentary abilities with a spoon (Fig. 3.8), though the natural tendency to turn the spoon over on the way to the mouth makes this a very messy experience!

Nutritional deficiencies

In many poorer parts of the world calorie deficiency, resulting in marasmus, or protein energy deficiency resulting in kwashiorkor (see pp 327–328) start to develop during infancy (Figs 3.9 and 3.10). These are very rare in the UK and are only seen in those families who abuse their children by making them conform to a very restrictive diet (e.g. a strict vegan diet).

Specific nutritional deficiencies do occur quite frequently in high income countries. Iron deficiency is the commonest (Information box 3.6).

Though breast milk contains very small amounts of iron, it is in a highly bioavailable form and therefore

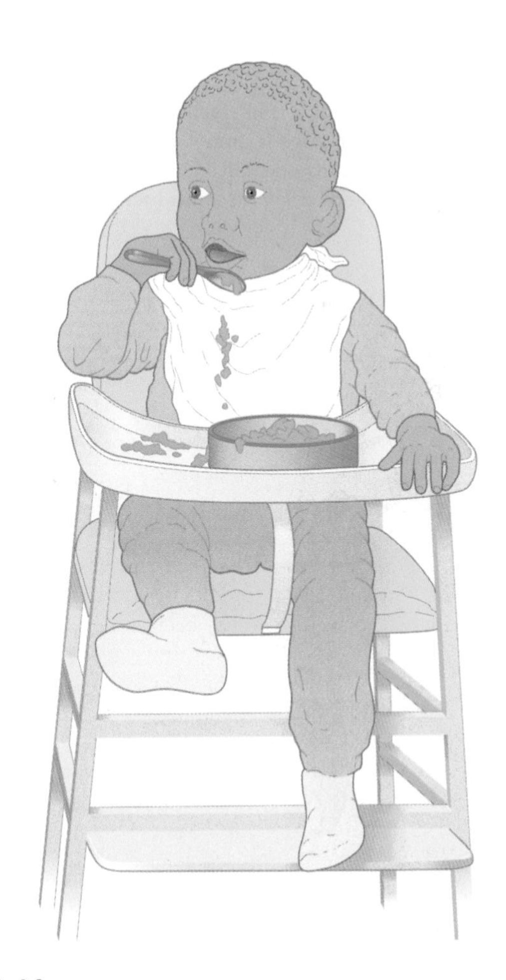

Fig 3.8
Early attempt to spoon feed. Learning to feed can be a messy business.

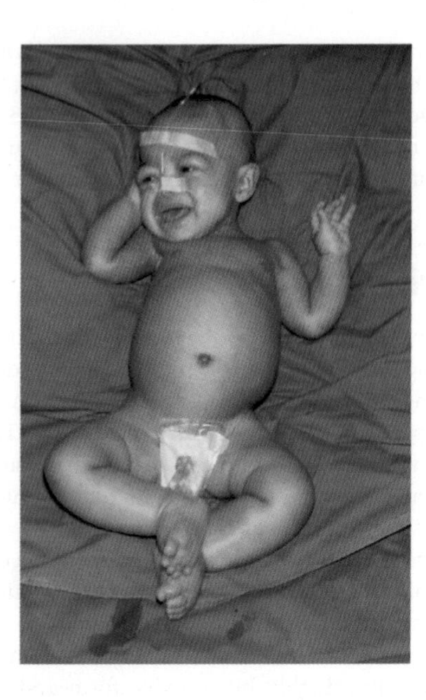

Fig 3.9
Infant with kwashiorkor. Note distended abdomen, peripheral oedema and pigmentary changes.

breastfeeding is not a risk factor in early infancy. However at a later stage it cannot provide the infant's requirements, and iron deficiency can then develop if there is associated delay in introduction of mixed feeding.

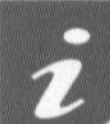

Information Box 3.6

Predisposing factors to nutritional iron deficiency

- Prematurity (less placental transfer).
- Delayed introduction of solids.
- Conversion too early from formula to unmodified cow's milk feeds.
- Over-emphasis on milk in the diet.
- Excess of iron-binding phytates in the diet. (Certain types of flour, used especially in Asian cooking, e.g. to make chapati, are rich in these.)

Policies for reducing the problem of iron deficiency are given in Practical box 3.3.

Vitamin D deficiency, which results in nutritional rickets (see p. 329), is now relatively rare. Certain groups are more susceptible than others, especially vegetarian Asian families where relatively low vitamin D levels may occur in the mothers and the diet, which is rich in phytates, may lead to reduced calcium and phosphate absorption. Well targeted health education programmes have helped reduce this problem in recent years. In addition the routine use of vitamin drops in infancy supplies most of the daily vitamin D requirement.

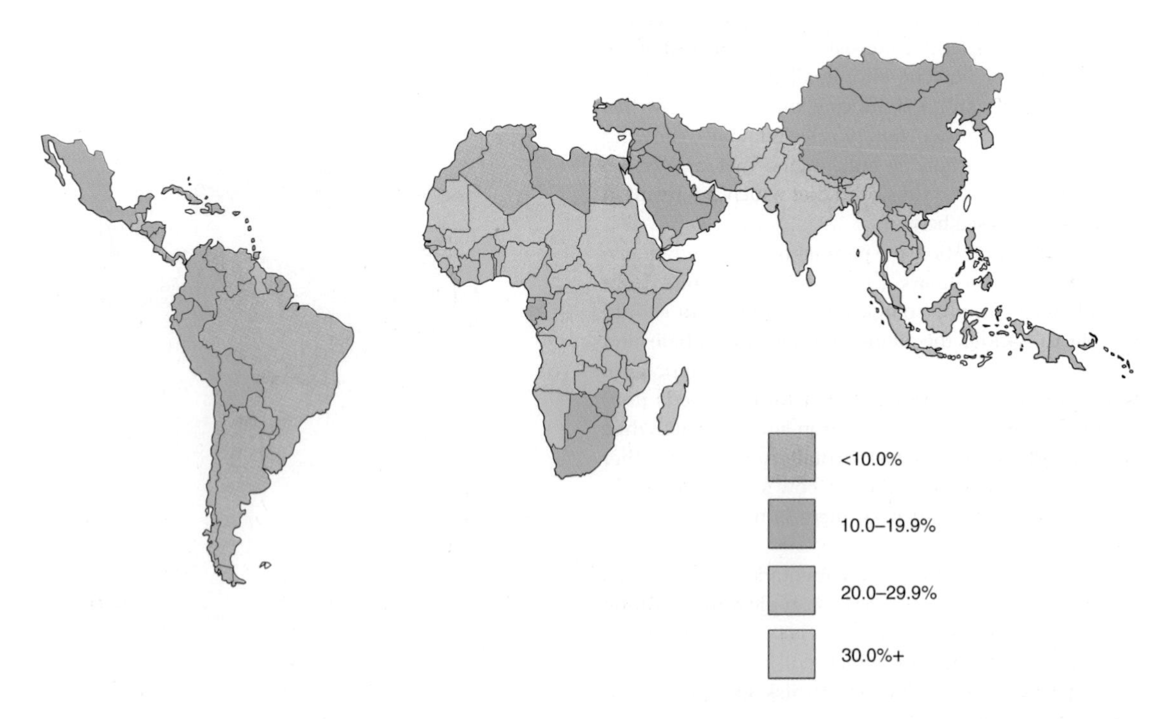

Fig 3.10
Proportion (%) of all children under 5 who were underweight in high income countries, as estimated for 1995. (Source: World Health Organization (WHO) global database on child growth and malnutrition, 1996. Geneva: WHO.)

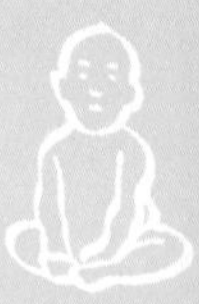

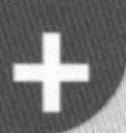

Practical Box 3.3

Reducing the problem of iron deficiency (UK policies)

- Iron supplementation from 1 month to 1 year in infants born prematurely
- Using supplemented formula feeds until 1 year in all infants
- Health educational advice directed specifically towards high risk groups such as Asian families

Other specific nutritional deficiencies are rare in the absence of intestinal disease.

Obesity and overfeeding

Obesity is relatively common in infancy. Bottle-fed babies are more susceptible than breastfed babies. Inexperienced parents should be advised that babies cry for a variety of reasons and crying does not always mean that they are hungry. Giving the baby a bottle to get some peace for the parents leads to excessive calorie intake, an exacerbation of any tendency to regurgitate or vomit (which itself causes parental anxiety) and a vicious cycle whereby some overfed babies demand more and more. Feeding at night when the baby cries is also to be avoided. By 6 months most healthy infants should be able to manage between 11 p.m. and 7 a.m. without feeding. Routinely offering feeds during these hours reinforces bad feeding and sleeping patterns.

Growth and development

Normal growth

Growth in all three major parameters, weight, height and head circumference, all occur at their maximal rates during the early part of the first year of life. For weight, the early rate is usually of the order of 30 g per day and the average baby has doubled his or her birthweight by 4 months of age and trebled it by 1 year of age. The average head circumference increases in the first year from around 35 cm at birth to around 47 cm by the first birthday reflecting the rapid brain growth that takes place at this time (Fig. 3.11).

It is important to record the baby's growth during infancy by regular plotting on centile charts which should highlight any deviation from normal at an early stage. In the first few months there may be some readjustment of centiles since intrauterine growth does not necessarily reflect postnatal growth, and a large baby may be genetically disposed to being small and therefore adjust downwards. Conversely, a baby with intrauterine growth retardation because of placental dysfunction may show catch-up growth over the first few months. Thereafter one expects a child to keep fairly closely to a given centile.

Normal development

At the same time as the child is physically growing there is rapid neurodevelopmental progress. This seems to be preprogrammed in that it occurs at a relatively fixed rate in relation to postconceptual age so that, on average, babies born prematurely achieve neurodevelopmental milestones at later postnatal ages than full-term infants. This contrasts with most other body systems; for example, in the gastrointestinal and immunological systems the maturation process is switched on by birth, irrespective of the degree of prematurity (hence the reason for not delaying immunization in premature infants).

Developmental milestones (see, for example, Figs 3.12 and 3.13) are for convenience divided into different categories: locomotor, social, vision and hearing. These are listed in Table 3.2, together with the average age of achievement. The normal age range for reaching these milestones is quite wide, and experience as well as more than one assessment is usually needed in judging when to diagnose a problem.

Table 3.2
Average age for reaching developmental milestones in infancy. NB: There is considerable normal variation

Age	Motor	Social
4 weeks	Head lag no longer complete	Smiles
8 weeks	Lifts head off couch when prone	Coos and gurgles
12 weeks	Holds, with crude grasp, objects placed in hand	Regards hands
16 weeks	Chest off floor in prone position	Laughs
20 weeks	Takes weight on feet when held upright	Smiles at own image in mirror
24 weeks	Anticipates with head when pulled to sitting Rolls prone to supine	Imitates sounds
32 weeks	Sits unsupported for several minutes	Looks for dropped toys
36 weeks	Uses thumb in opposition to fingers	Early suspicion of strangers
40 weeks	Crawls	Waves 'bye-bye'
48 weeks	Cruises (walks holding furniture)	Plays 'peek-a-boo'
52 weeks	Walks unsupported Mature pincer grip	Says 2–3 words

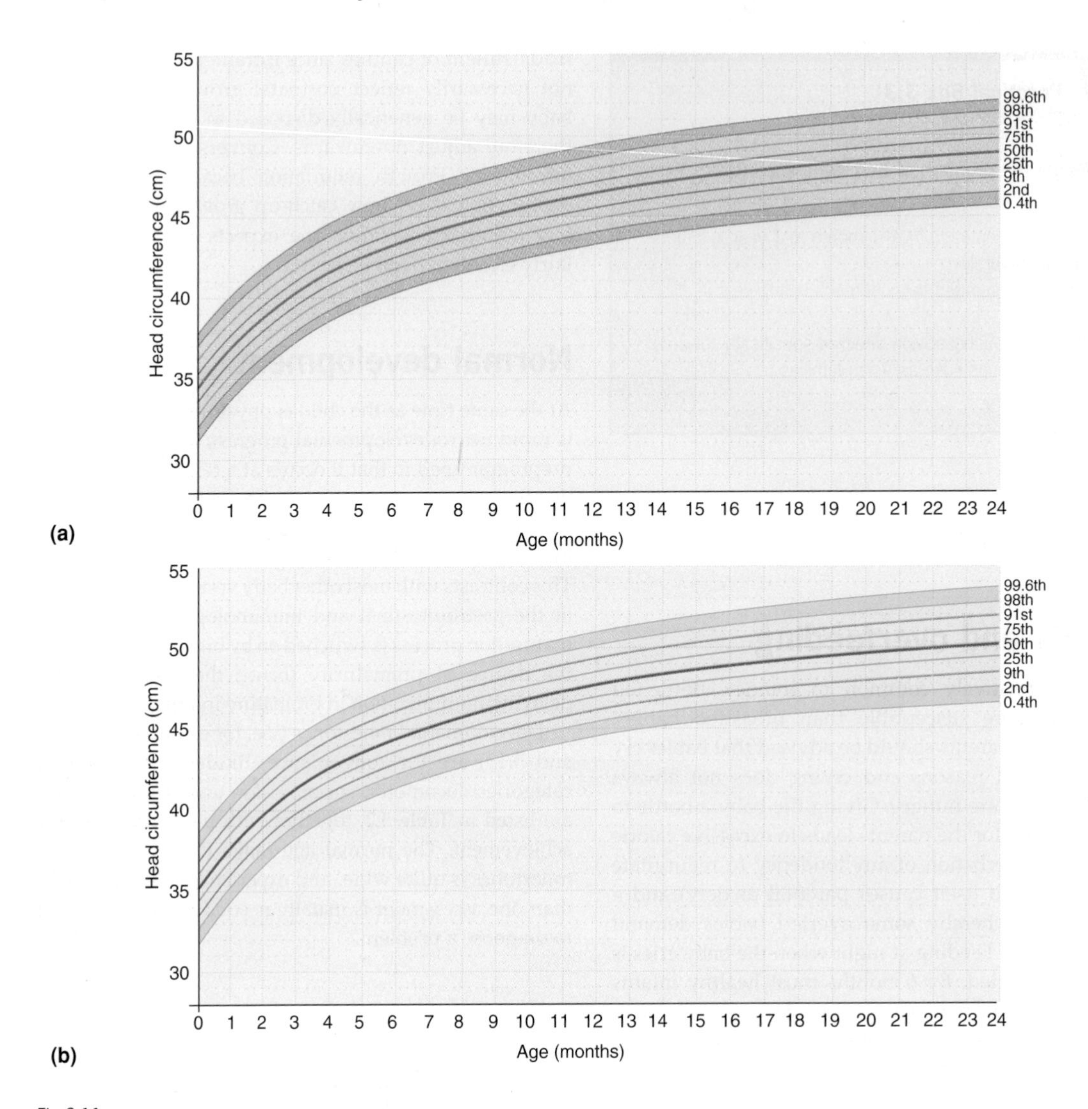

Fig 3.11
Head circumference chart, 0–24 months: (a) girls; (b) boys.

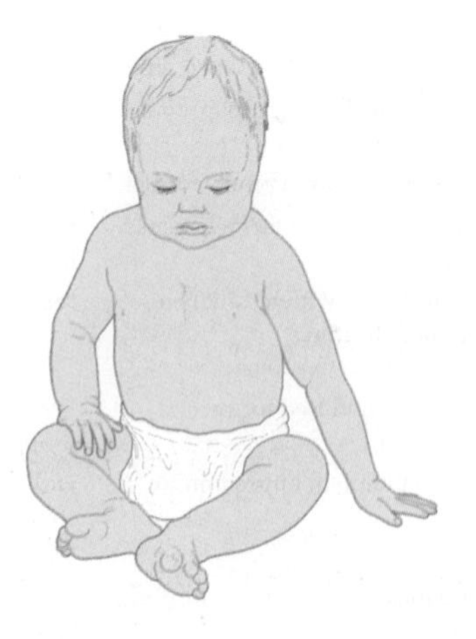

Fig 3.12
Sitting unsupported; note the hands being used for balance (24 weeks).

Abnormal growth

Failure to thrive

Infancy is the period when the most rapid growth and development of children occurs. Not surprisingly a great variety of factors can critically influence these processes. The failure of the child to grow at an adequate rate is termed 'failure to thrive'. Often, but not invariably, there is an accompanying failure of social development.

Recognition of the infant who is failing to grow can be difficult. Since there is considerable natural variation in the size of infants, single measurements, unless grossly outside the normal range, do not reveal that the child is failing to grow. Sequential measurements are much more useful and usually these can be obtained by consulting the parent-held child health book. Failure to thrive can then be diagnosed by showing that the

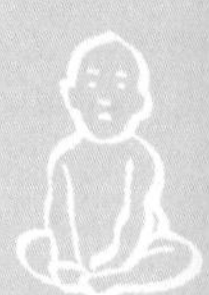

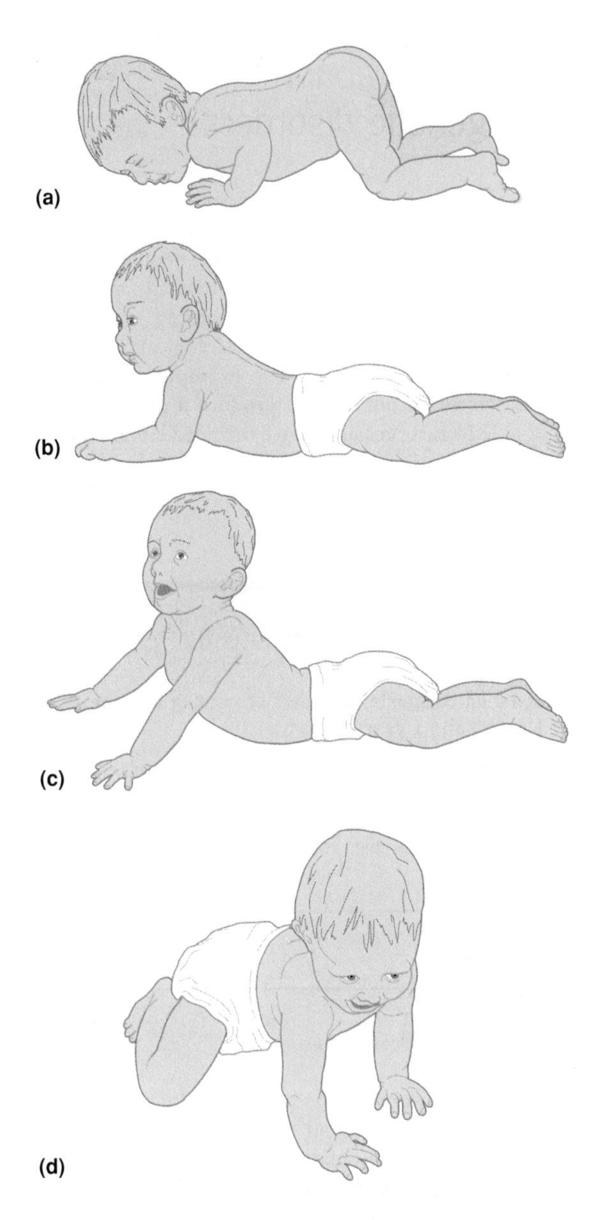

Fig 3.13
(a) Normal 4- to 6-week baby, prone position; (b) normal 12-week baby, prone position; (c) normal 24-week baby, prone position; (d) 40-week baby, vigorous at crawling.

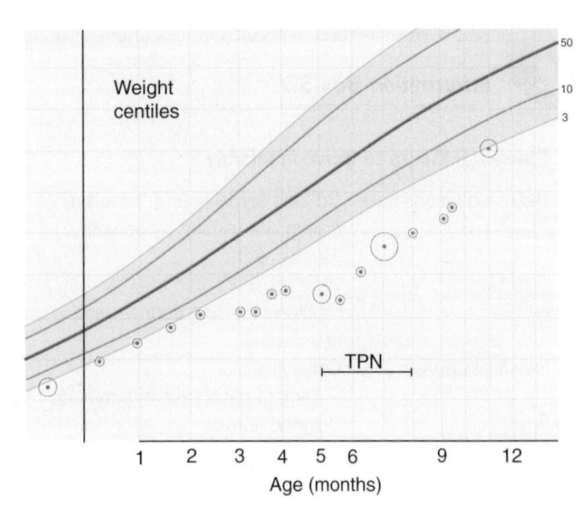

Fig 3.14
Growth chart of infant who is failing to thrive. TPN – total parenteral nutrition given.

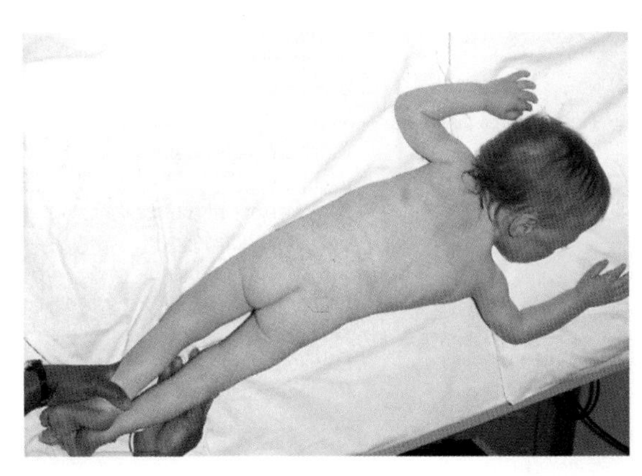

Fig 3.15
Infant who is failing to thrive. Note muscle wasting, especially of the buttocks.

child's growth has fallen across the centile charts over a period of time. There may be a certain amount of adjusting of centiles in the early months of life (see Normal growth, p. 75) but persistent crossing of centiles downwards is never normal. It is very unusual for babies to lose weight (unless they are acutely dehydrated) and what is observed is a slowing of the normal growth rate (Figs 3.14 and 3.15).

A common misdiagnosis is to label a child as failing to thrive whose height and/or weight are below the 3rd centile but are proceeding with time in a line parallel to the centiles. This is small stature which may be one extreme of normal or may indicate some underlying problem, but it is not failure to thrive.

Not surprisingly, growth may be critically affected in infancy by a variety of problems (Information box 3.7).

Abnormal development

Delay in achieving milestones should prompt a full physical examination, looking especially at the nervous system and for dysmorphic features. Different patterns of selective delay may emerge. If there is a global delay there may or may not be microcephaly, so head circumference should always be plotted on a chart.

Delayed motor development raises the possibility of a motor problem such as cerebral palsy (see p. 313). In this condition, relative hypotonia is often present early

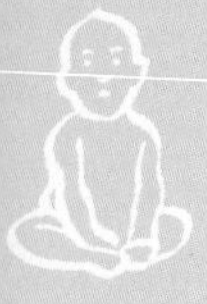

Information Box 3.7

Causes of failure to thrive in infancy

Decreased food intake	No food available (e.g. poverty) Inadequate feeding by parents 'Cranky' diets Child abuse Problems causing poor feeding (see below)
Intestinal disease	Congenital – Lack of pancreatic enzymes in cystic fibrosis Acquired – Coeliac disease – Infective enteropathy, e.g. giardiasis – Short-bowel syndrome, e.g. following neonatal resection for necrotizing enterocolitis – Post-gastroenteritis food intolerance – Vomiting
Nonintestinal disease	– Increased energy expenditure – Catabolic state, e.g. chronic infection – Inborn errors of metabolism – Endocrine deficiency – Neurological problems (especially affecting eating and swallowing)
Nonorganic causes	– Emotional deprivation – Primary behavioural disturbance

on but gradually hypertonia develops in certain muscle groups, leading to the characteristic features of the condition. Other neuromuscular conditions such as myotonic dystrophy and anterior horn cell disease (Werdnig–Hoffman) (see p. 311) will present in infancy. In children with delayed social development it is important to exclude visual and hearing impairment. If these are normal then the problem is one of intellectual delay or of emotional deprivation. See also Screening (below).

In infants with delayed vocalization, hearing defects and problems with palatal and tongue movements should be excluded. Specific investigation will depend on the findings. Asymmetrical neurological clinical signs should prompt a brain scan. The opinion of a clinical geneticist may be helpful if chromosomal disorders such as fragile X syndrome (see p. 240) or other neuro-dysmorphic syndromes are suspected.

Congenital abnormalities and genetic disorders

Many of these are discussed in Chapters 1, 2 and 12.

It should be noted that disorders may have a relatively late presentation, beyond the neonatal period (see Information box 3.8), or that if they are asymptomatic they can only be picked up during routine screening when certain physiological changes of maturation have occurred. For example, ventricular septal defects do not usually produce a murmur until right-sided heart pressures have dropped sufficiently to produce a significant left-to-right shunt (this may take several weeks).

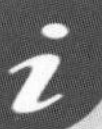

Information Box 3.8

Common congenital disorders presenting between 1 month and 1 year of age

- Congenital heart disorders with left-to-right shunt
- Cystic fibrosis without meconium ileus
- Central nervous system disorders resulting in seizures, hypotonia or developmental disorder

Screening

Screening programmes for anomalies in growth and development are designed to detect problems at an early stage when they may be corrected or minimized by intervention. All children born in the UK should be allocated a health visitor who will have a nursing background and particular training in child health and development. The health visitor works closely with the general practitioner and the community paediatric team. Amongst her responsibilities are monitoring growth and development and ensuring that the child is fully immunized.

Most health authorities will have set ages at which the child is screened for problems. Typically this might be at 8 weeks of age and again at 8 months. This screening is done by the health visitor and the general practitioner. Consultant community paediatricians have the responsibility for providing training and updating of GPs performing these functions. They will usually also be the specialists to whom the GP turns if a developmental problem is diagnosed or suspected.

Child health surveillance at 6–8 weeks of age

PHYSICAL EXAMINATION

The physical examination is important at this stage for detecting congenital abnormalities which were either missed or not detectable at the immediate postnatal examination. An example of the former might be developmental dysplasia of the hip. An example of the latter could be the presence of a ventricular septal defect which did not produce a murmur in the neonatal period because the right-sided heart pressures had not dropped sufficiently after birth for a significant shunt (and therefore murmur) to develop. Other problems such as prolonged neonatal jaundice may come to light at this stage and will require investigation (see Chps. 2 and 14). A complete physical examination along the lines of that performed on the newborn should be undertaken.

NEURODEVELOPMENTAL EXAMINATION

Motor

The child's general tone should have markedly increased from the newborn period. When drawing the baby up by the arms from a supine position, there should not be complete head lag (Fig. 3.16).

1. *Ventral suspension*. It should be possible to demonstrate some head and limb tone (Fig. 3.17).

The baby should be spontaneously moving all four limbs but cannot yet roll over and remains in the position in which he or she was placed.

2. *Primitive reflexes*. These are still largely present though stepping and palmar pressure reflexes are starting to fade. The Moro reflex is usually still present and should be symmetrical. If it is asymmetrical this may indicate a neurological problem such as cerebral palsy.

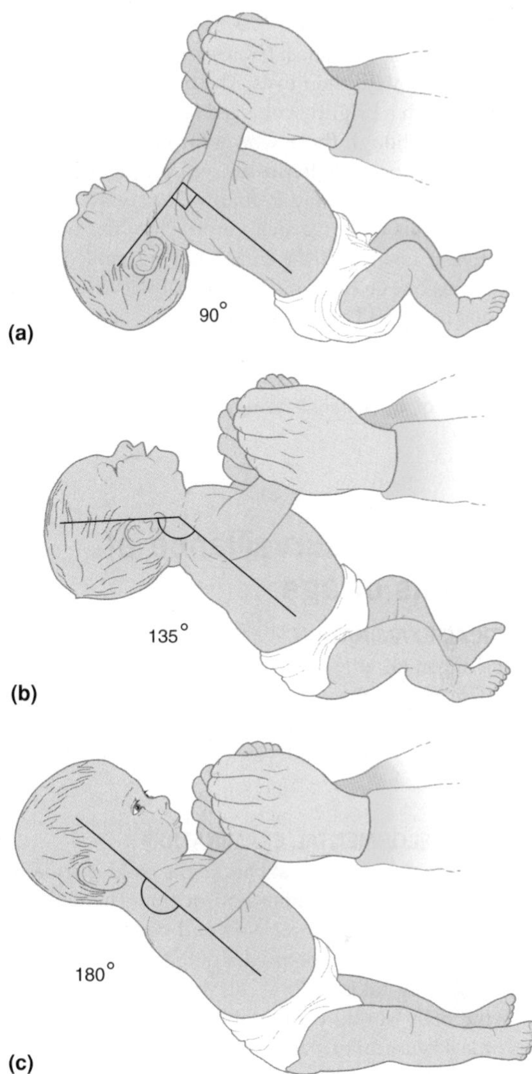
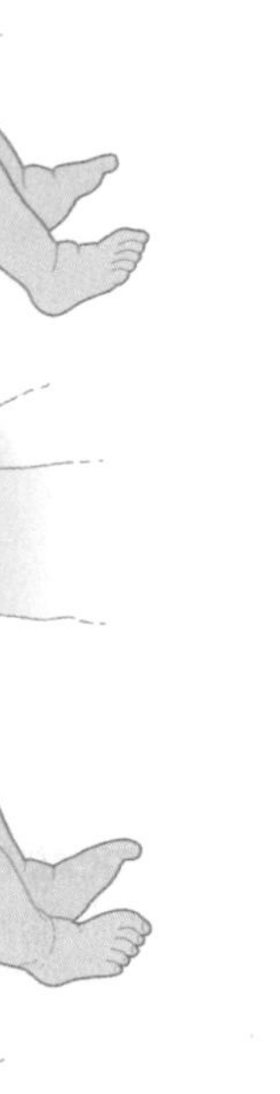

Fig 3.16
Head lag when pulled to sitting: (a) newborn, complete head lag; (b) normal 6-week infant; (c) 16-week infant, no head lag.

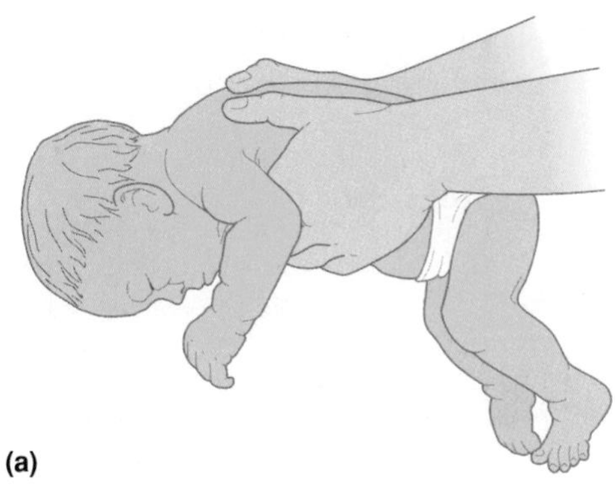

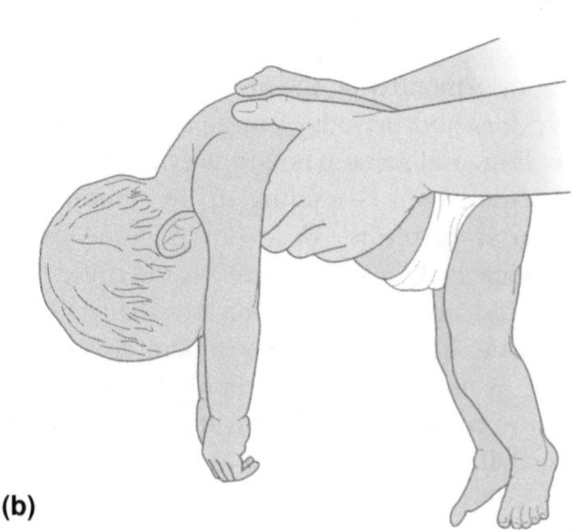

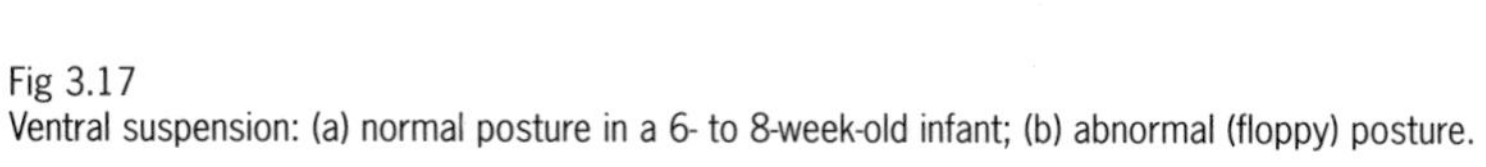

Fig 3.17
Ventral suspension: (a) normal posture in a 6- to 8-week-old infant; (b) abnormal (floppy) posture.

Social

By 8 weeks post-term most babies will have learned to fix and follow with their eyes. The best way of testing for this is with a brightly coloured large object such as a fluffy ball, though those who wear glasses find that the reflective spectacle lenses act as a bright and interesting object for the baby to follow. No sound should be made as this will give an auditory clue. The mother may give a history of the infant having smiled, and usually this can be confirmed (if the baby is awake and in a good mood and a comfortable position) by the examiner gently cooing and smiling at the baby. Failure of the baby to perform these activities should raise the possibility of a visual, hearing, motor or intellectual defect.

Child health surveillance at 8 months of age

PHYSICAL EXAMINATION

Most congenital physical abnormalities should have been detected by this stage. Nevertheless examination may pick up problems or may detect those such as hernias which have developed since the earlier examinations.

NEURODEVELOPMENTAL EXAMINATION

The 8-month developmental check on a child is usually a pleasure for infant, mother and doctor. The child at this age is usually very sociable and cooperative and has not yet learned to distrust strangers. The assessor should start by taking a brief history from the mother with the baby sitting comfortably on her lap. During this time it is useful to make some eye contact and smile at the infant to gain his or her confidence. The history will highlight any potential problems which can be addressed at the examination stage and will allow the mother to indicate any worries that she has.

Motor

Most babies by 8 months of age are capable of sitting unsupported for short periods. A large proportion will also be crawling, and some who are very advanced in motor terms may even be pulling up to standing or cruising around furniture, or even in some cases walking unsupported for a few steps. Bear in mind that there is a wide normal range for acquiring these abilities, and one should be at pains to point this out to the mother so as not to alarm her if her baby is average or even slightly below average. For testing gross motor skills it is usually necessary for the examiner and the mother to get down on the floor with the baby (a large rubber mat is useful).

Examination should include an assessment of muscle tone which by now should be very good. On pulling to sitting the head usually comes up in anticipation of the trunk. Muscle tone can also be assessed in a more conventional way by passive movement of the limbs.

Saving reflexes, such as putting out limbs in the appropriate direction so as to anticipate a fall, will have started to develop.

Fine motor

Infants of 8 months old will probably still use a grasp approach to picking up small objects but some more advanced children may already be starting to develop a pincer forefinger and thumb type approach.

Social

The 8-month-old will show great visual alertness. Smiles should be spontaneous and plentiful (Fig. 3.18) as well as chuckles and happy sounds such as cooing and babbling.

Hearing

At 8 months the baby's attention is largely unifocal. He or she will turn to the most dominant stimulus. Use of this is made in distraction testing whereby threshold-level noises are generated at ear-level to the side and slightly behind the baby and the baby's ability to hear the noises is seen by the head turning to the stimulus. One can only do this with the help of an assistant who sits in front of the baby and attracts his or her attention in the first place. This should be repeated on both sides. A degree of experience is required on the part of the distractor who should try to get the baby to lose interest in them at the instant the noise is to be made. Overconcentration on one stimulus may mean that the baby will choose to ignore the other. The sound sources should start at approximately 30 decibels (most people

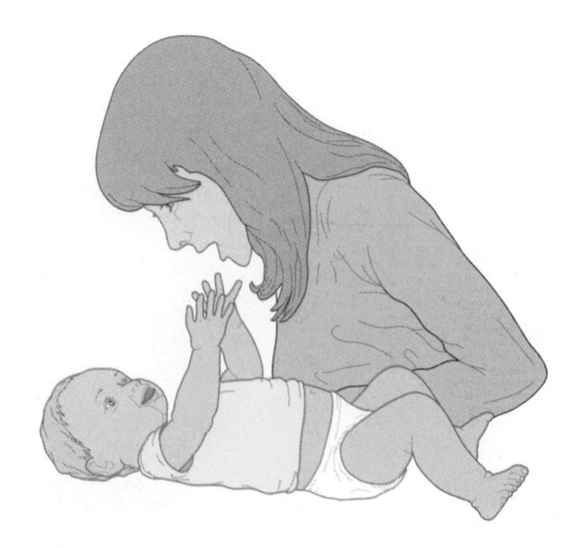

Fig 3.18
Social interaction between mother and baby at 6 to 8 months.

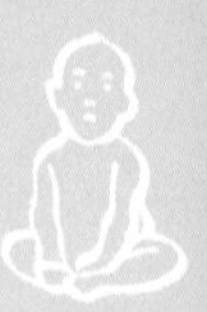

carrying out this test regularly practise making noises with a sound intensity measurer) and should be repeated with a high and low frequency sound source. Rattles of known frequency range (e.g. the Manchester rattle), or better, pure-tone generators should be used.

Hearing behaviour can also be tested by placing the source in a position 45° above a horizontal line from the baby's ear. Typically the baby should turn the head horizontally sideways and then upwards until the eyes fix the source. This tests not only hearing but also peripheral vision (as the head turns it is the peripheral vision that catches sight of the sound source and directs further movement of the head upwards), and is a measure of the ability to integrate hearing, vision and movement. Children with deficiency in any of these three areas will not be able to do this adequately. The ability to locate a sound directly above the head is usually not present in an 8-month-old. This does not develop until approximately 12 to 13 months of age. Previous history of middle ear problems, even though they may have resolved, will result in delayed acquisition of this hearing behaviour.

Vision

During the history taking the examiner should have noted whether or not there is any squint. While a physiological squint may have been apparent at the 8-week check-up this should have disappeared by 8 months. This should be tested formally, using the methods listed below, until the examiner is happy that a squint does not exist. If the mother reports that the baby is squinting, even if this cannot be demonstrated it is likely that she is correct. Latent squints may become manifest only intermittently, particularly when the child is tired.

Visual acuity for near and distant vision needs to be tested. For near vision, most examiners will use a variety of very small brightly coloured objects down to 1 mm in size which are deposited onto a green baize-covered table top, and it is usually quite easy to tell when the baby has seen and fixed on them. For distant vision (usually measured at 3 metres at this age) the ability to see small white balls projected from behind a screen can be used. The lens should be observed for cataracts. Fundoscopy may or may not be easily achieved in an 8-month-old, but if all the other vision tests appear normal it is not necessary.

The sick infant

Children at this age can become ill quickly and often without specific signs. The doctor will have to use his/her experience to judge whether the child has a serious problem or one of the numerous nonserious viral episodes that frequently develop in infants.

Although other disorders such as heart failure, metabolic disorders and seizures can occur, infections are the most common cause of illness at this age. During infancy the infant's immune system undergoes steady maturation. The neonatal susceptibility to overwhelming infection with pathogens such as *Herpes simplex* and group B Streptococcus passes, though the child remains excessively susceptible to other pathogens, especially the polysaccharide-encapsulated organisms: (pneumococcus, meningococcus and, until vaccinated, *Haemophilus influenzae* type b). Enteric pathogens such as salmonella species may cause invasive disease, and respiratory bacterial pathogens especially *Bordetella pertussis* may cause severe disease (Fig. 3.19).

Maternal antibody levels wane over the early months, and this manifests as a susceptibility to viral respiratory infections since the infant has not yet acquired a repertoire of immunological memory against the many agents in this group. The most notorious of these viruses is respiratory syncytial virus (RSV) which in the winter months is responsible for a large proportion of respiratory infections in this age group (Fig. 3.20). These viruses may cause a number of different clinical pictures from a simple cold to bronchiolitis and pneumonia (see p. 357, 359).

Various scoring systems have been devised in an attempt to increase the ability of clinicians and parents to spot seriously ill children, but none is perfect (see Information box 3.9).

The febrile infant

Individual infections are discussed in Chapter 15.

Assessing the child with presumed infection can be

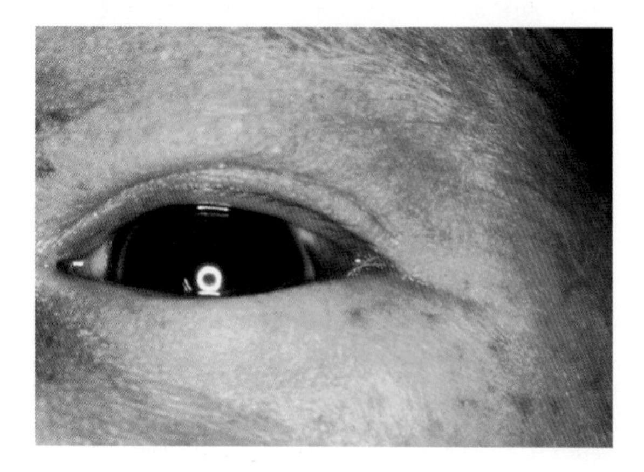

Fig 3.19
Pertussis: subconjunctival haemorrhage as a result of coughing paroxysms.

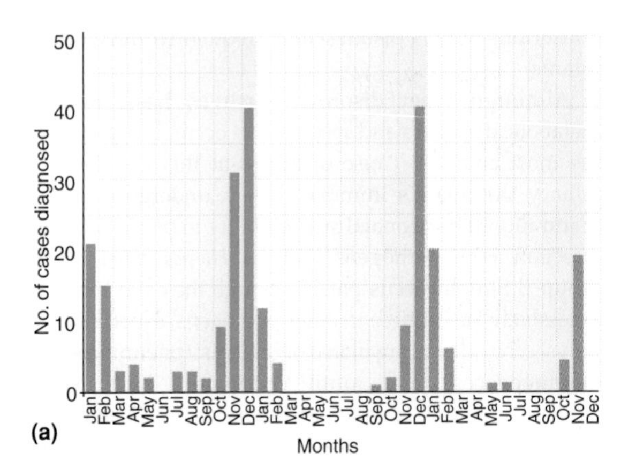

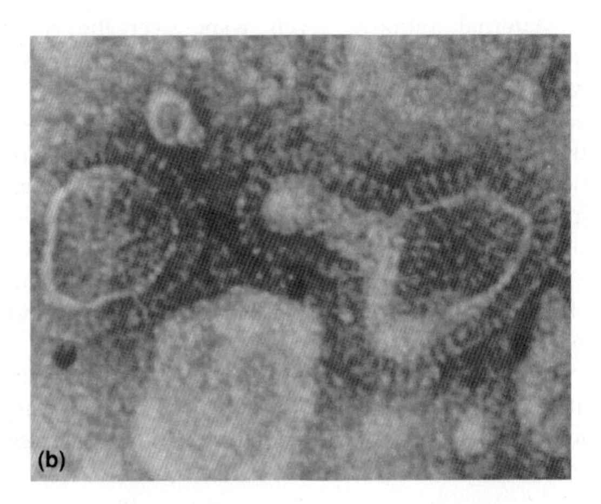

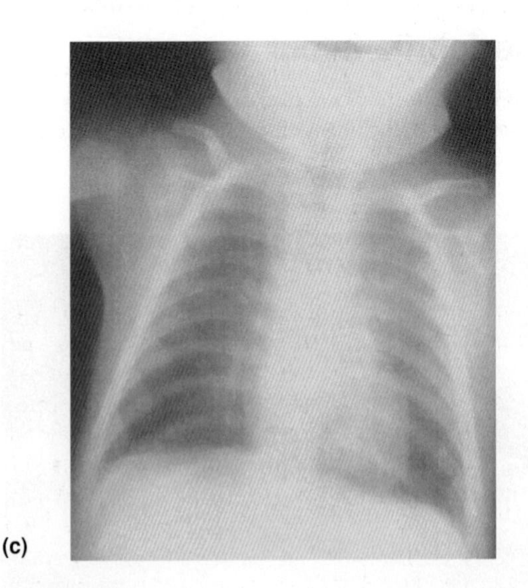

Fig 3.20
Respiratory syncytial virus (RSV). (a) Seasonality (data from St. George's Hospital, courtesy of the late Dr Jim Booth).
(b) Electronmicrograph of the virus. (c) Typical chest X-ray appearance. Note flattened and depressed diaphragms indicating hyperinflation of the lungs.

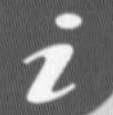

Information Box 3.9

Symptoms associated with serious illness in infants of less than 6 months

- Drowsiness
- Decreased activity
- Less than half normal feeds in 24 hours
- Fewer than four wet nappies in 24 hours
- Breathing difficulties
- Appears hot and pale

Positive predictive value of any one feature is >50%.
(From Hewson et al (1990) *Archives of Disease in Childhood* 65: (7): 750–6.Jul

difficult. Most will have mild self-limiting illnesses but one has to be alert for the more serious bacterial infections such as meningitis, septicaemia, pneumonia and urinary tract infection. The key point is that at this age few of these are likely to produce a specific clinical picture. The child is likely to be febrile and to look ill, but useful signs such as neck stiffness are unlikely to be present, even in established meningitis. The exception is the child with a purpuric rash which is highly suggestive of meningococcal infection.

Recognition of the sick child is helped by scoring systems and by experience, but one cannot always get it right. When in doubt one has to fall back on batteries of investigation ('septic screens', Information box 3.10) to rule out infection.

The infant with acute behavioural change

Nonspecific changes in behaviour in a previously well child are often the first signs of an acute illness, most commonly infective (Fig. 3.21) but occasionally due to

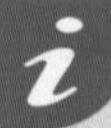

Information Box 3.10

'Septic screen' in infants

- Full blood picture
- Throat swab
- Blood cultures
- Lumbar puncture
- Urine microscopy and culture
- Chest radiograph

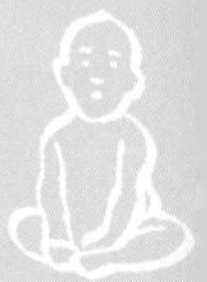

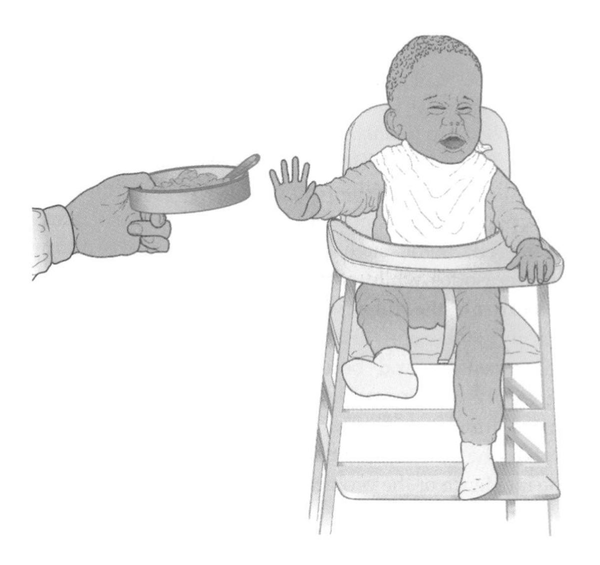

Fig 3.21
Early symptoms of infection, include nonspecific behavioural changes such as poor feeding and irritability.

other illness. These include poor feeding, drowsiness and irritability (Information box 3.9). The last two can occur together often in an alternating pattern. In the case of drowsiness the use of sedative medications (e.g. antihistamines or anticonvulsants) has to be excluded as a cause. The pathologically irritable infant may show signs of persistent, often inconsolable crying, high-pitched cry and jitteriness. These are all signs of cerebral irritation which may be due to infection, metabolic disturbance (for example hypoglycaemia), exposure to medications or toxins or congenital abnormality. Unexplained irritability should always be investigated thoroughly.

Infective causes of behavioural change can occur at any site, including the urinary tract and lungs, as well as the brain.

When these types of behaviour are more persistent they may indicate chronic disease or congenital abnormality.

The infant with persistent crying

Persistent crying may be due to pain, hunger, neurological disorder (cerebral irritation), emotional factors (neglect, abuse) or is sometimes completely unexplained. Common causes of pain include napkin dermatitis, earache and abdominal colic. More serious causes include occult fractures (child abuse), osteomyelitis and meningitis.

Earache

In older infants, in addition to crying, there may be rubbing of the ear or rubbing it against the pillow.

The most common cause (see Information box 3.11) will be otitis media. This may lead to perforation and

Information Box 3.11

Causes of earache

- Otitis media
- Otitis externa
- Blocked eustachian tube
  - Acute (during air travel)
  - Insidious (during upper respiratory tract infection)
- Wax impaction
- Foreign body (rare)
- Tonsillitis (referred pain)

discharge, the latter being apparent without an auroscope. Examination of the canal and drum with an auroscope is essential.

Treatment of otitis media should be with a broad-spectrum antibiotic such as amoxycillin. Though many episodes are viral and therefore self-limiting, there is no easy way of distinguishing the cause.

Infant colic

This is a very common and frustrating disorder in the first few months of life. Infants develop spasmodic bouts of crying inconsolably and appear to be in pain, presumed to be due to colonic spasm. Various dietary factors in the baby, or (if the infant is breastfed) in the mother, have been suggested as precipitants but there is no good evidence to incriminate these. Other theories postulate parental stress or tension, conveyed to the baby, as contributory factors. Fortunately, this phase usually passes by 3 months though it can occasionally persist for longer. The role of the doctor and health visitor is to provide reassurance. Infant colic remedies rarely make any difference and are best avoided.

The infant with a cough

Cough will usually indicate a respiratory problem. Viral infection is the most likely diagnosis and this may also trigger wheezing (see below). Some coughs will be characteristic such as the barking seal-like cough of acute laryngotracheobronchitis (croup) or the paroxysmal cough of pertussis. In young infants with pertussis the characteristic whoop at the end of a coughing paroxysm (see Practical box 3.4) is often absent and apnoea without a preceding cough may occur. Vomiting at the end of a bout of coughing is common at this age and is not diagnostically specific.

In examining the respiratory system one's eyes are more useful than the stethoscope in this age group. Count the respiratory rate (and know the approximate normal rates at different ages). Look for signs of

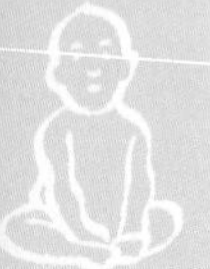

Practical Box 3.4

- In pertussis, a paroxysm of coughing occurs without any inspirations, i.e. it is one long expiratory effort.
- Partial closure of the larynx occurs to maintain some end-expiratory pressure. The sharp following inspiration with a partially closed larynx results in the characteristic whoop.
- In contrast, in other causes of bouts of coughing which are not true paroxysms (e.g. nocturnal coughing due to asthma), there is a series of short recurrent coughs with inspirations between.

respiratory distress: recession – intercostal, subcostal and supraclavicular. Look for accessory muscle usage and listen for added sounds: grunting or stridor. Only then listen to the chest. Wheeze or crackles may be heard, but at this age pneumonia may be present in the absence of any positive auscultatory findings (Fig. 3.22).

The wheezy infant

Recurrent wheezing in infancy is frequently encountered. It is nearly always triggered by viral respiratory infections and may not be atopic in nature. Most respiratory viruses can trigger these episodes but RSV is notorious. RSV can also cause true bronchiolitis, usually in children under 6 months of age who become acutely distressed with wheezing and tachypnoea.

Rapid viral diagnosis can be achieved by using immunofluorescent staining on naso-epithelial cells, obtained by naso-pharyngeal aspiration (NPA) via a catheter through the nose (Fig. 3.23). Once the catheter is positioned, a short sharp application of suction is required, to 'strip off' some epithelial cells, rather than only collecting mucus.

In the child with a virus-associated wheezing episode, the typical picture is of a wheezy child with a hyperinflated chest but who is not particularly distressed. Some such children only wheeze during viral episodes while others (often overweight infants) wheeze all the time without any apparent distress (happy wheezers) although they can unexpectedly decompensate and become ill. The response to β2 agonists is often poor though there may be a response to ipatropium bromide and to corticosteroids.

No one knows why children get this syndrome but the incidence of the problem does seem to be increasing. Most probably, an early viral infection alters the bronchial inflammatory/immunological response to subsequent viral challenges. Such altered bronchial responsiveness has been well documented after RSV bronchiolitis and some symptoms may last for many years. Most non-atopic wheezing infants do however 'grow out' of the majority of their symptoms by 2–3 years of age.

Wheeze may also be a feature of heart failure, in children with congenital heart disease. In older infants, beware the possibility of a foreign body (such as a peanut) lodged in the airway.

Other noisy breathing in infants

The acute onset of snuffly breathing usually indicates a viral upper respiratory tract infection. Mostly this is benign, though it can make feeding difficult. However, occasionally upper respiratory symptoms are associated with the onset of more serious infections such as

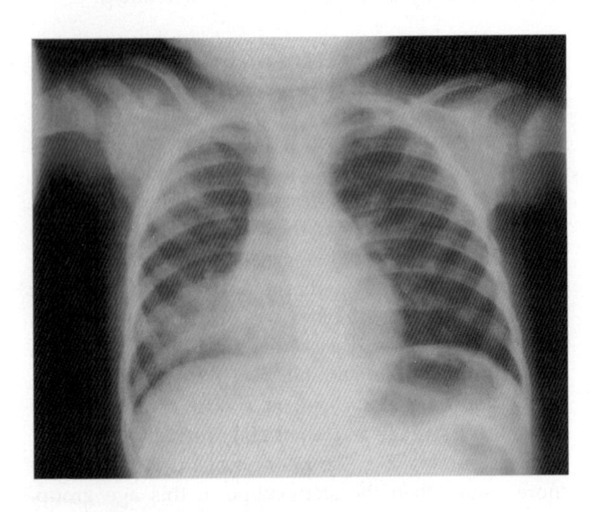

Fig 3.22
Right middle lobe pneumonia

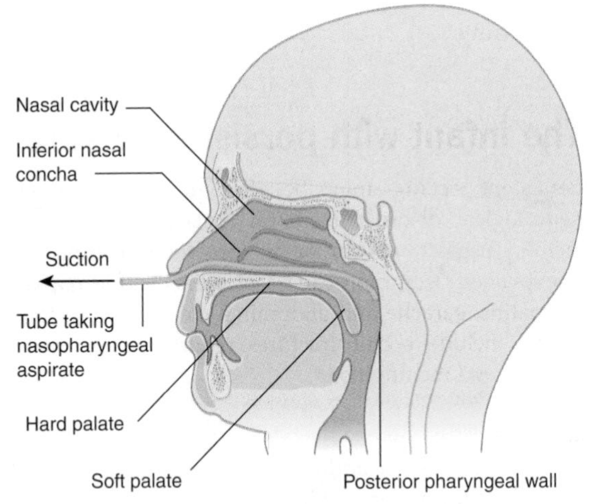

Fig 3.23
Collecting a nasopharyngeal aspirate.

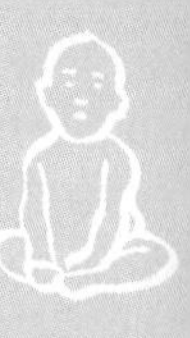

meningitis. These should be considered particularly in the child who has a continuing high fever and in the child who appears disproportionately unwell.

Persistent snuffly nasal breathing is not uncommon in young infants, and if they are feeding well it is likely to be of no consequence. If feeding is affected, congenital problems such as unilateral choanal atresia (the bilateral type would have presented earlier) or choanal stenosis should be considered. Children with motor problems such as cerebral palsy may pool secretions and generate pharyngeal rattling sounds during breathing. Some anticonvulsants such as clonazepam increase these secretions.

Stridor is an inspiratory noise produced by air passing through a narrowed larynx or trachea. As a general rule inspiratory stridor is caused by extrathoracic obstruction while intrathoracic problems produce expiratory wheeze, as in asthma. Obstructions in the trachea itself or main bronchii may produce biphasic stridor.

Persistent stridor in young infants is most probably due to a floppy larynx (congenital laryngeal stridor, see p. 353). If it is atypical or doesn't improve over the early months then other more serious problems (laryngeal webs or clefts) should be considered. Acute stridor is likely to be due to a viral laryngotracheobronchitis. Bacterial epiglottitis is a cause of stridor (see Emergency box 3.1). This is very rare since introduction of the Hib vaccination.

Emergency Box 3.1

Beware the child with stridor who looks grey and ill and can't swallow saliva: this is likely to be bacterial epiglottitis (Fig. 3.24) (see p. 358).

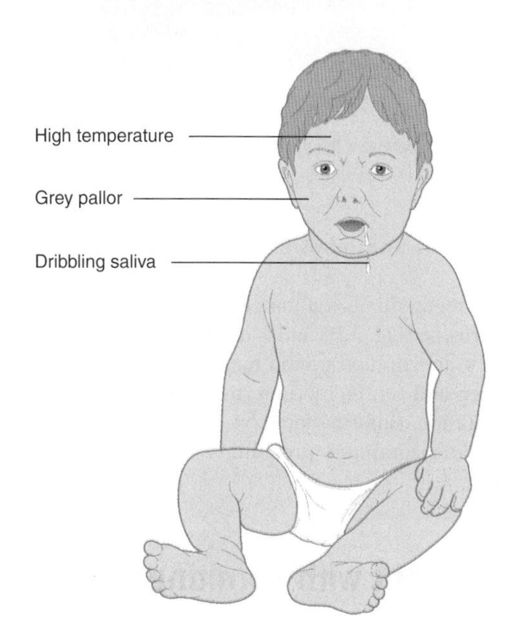

Fig 3.24
Acute epiglottitis.

Apnoea in infancy

An apnoeic episode in a young infant may be symptomatic of a number of underlying conditions. The commoner causes are listed in Information box 3.12.

In the history it is important to establish when the attack occurred in relation to feeding, who observed it, how long it lasted, and whether there were any convulsive movements. Seizures may both cause apnoea and be a consequence of it. What was the sequence of colour changes (usually pallor followed by cyanosis)?

Depending on the clues from the history and examination a number of investigations may be required (see Practical box 3.5).

When observed by covert video recording, a small proportion of the mothers of these infants have been found to be smothering their children: so-called imposed upper airway obstruction. This is a variety of Munchausen by proxy syndrome (see p. 185).

Information Box 3.12

Commoner causes of apnoea in infancy

Neurological	Seizures Raised intracranial pressure Central apnoea: immature breathing control
Cardiac	Arrhythmias Pulmonary hypertensive crisis (in congenital heart disease)
Respiratory	Obstruction to upper airway Aspiration (gastro-oesophageal reflux)
Metabolic	Hypoglycaemia Inborn errors
Infective	Pertussis Overwhelming infection: sepsis Meningitis/encephalitis
Drugs	Respiratory depressants Opiates/sedatives
Miscellaneous	Breath-holding attacks (usually toddler age group, see Ch. 4) Imposed upper airway obstruction (Munchausen by proxy)

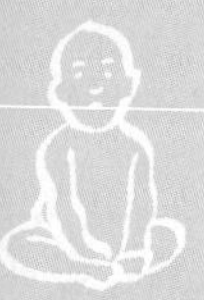

Practical Box 3.5

Investigation of apnoea

• Septic screen	If child acutely unwell
• Biochemical screen	Glucose, electrolytes, amino acids, ammonia, organic acids
• EEG	Including video recording
• ECG	12-lead and 24-hour tape
• Barium studies and/or oesophageal pH monitoring	

Information Box 3.13

Causes of floppiness in infants

- Cerebral palsy (preceding the spastic phase) (see Fig. 3.25)
- Congenital cerebellar malformation or hypoplasia
- Neuropathy, usually congenital, for example anterior horn cell disease (Werdnig–Hoffman)
- Myasthenia gravis (usually transient, occurring in infants born to affected mothers)
- Dystrophia myotonica
- Myopathies (see under specific myopathies in Chapter 18)
- Benign infantile hypotonia (a diagnosis of exclusion)

The infant suffering convulsions (seizures)

Convulsions and epilepsy are described in detail in Chapter 18. During infancy convulsions crop up as a relatively common problem. They may be symptomatic of underlying brain pathology, such as congenital malformations, inborn errors of metabolism or acquired problems such as meningitis or encephalitis. Alternatively they may be idiopathic and represent the onset of epilepsy. Febrile seizures are the commonest type in infancy occurring from 6 months onwards. A peculiar form of convulsion in infancy is caused by the disorder known as infantile spasms in which a characteristic hectic EEG pattern (hypsarrhythmia) is associated with repeated convulsive movements in which the arms are thrown outwards and the head flexed with adduction of the arms (salaam attacks).

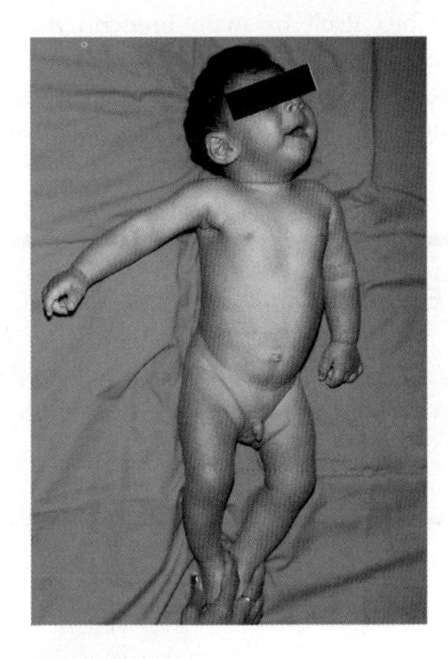

Fig 3.25
Cerebral palsy; note also the microcephaly.

The floppy infant

Infants may become acutely floppy in the context of an intercurrent illness. Of more concern is the persistent floppiness which signifies a possible neuromuscular disorder (Information box 3.13). These disorders are discussed in Chapters 2 and 18.

In mild form, the only effect may be of delayed motor milestones but in severe form there may be poor feeding, inability to feed or swallow at all, and respiratory compromise which is likely to be exacerbated by even mild respiratory infections.

The infant with diarrhoea

In infants acute diarrhoea is not always synonymous with gastroenteritis. As with vomiting it may be a nonspecific symptom in a febrile child with infection elsewhere (urinary tract infection, meningitis, otitis). It may also be a manifestation of food (e.g. cow's milk) allergy.

Gastroenteritis has a variety of different causes (e.g. rotavirus, see Fig. 3.26) and is discussed in Chapter 11. In infancy dehydration occurs more quickly than in older children and can be more devastating. Hypernatraemic dehydration (Information box 3.14) is a particularly dangerous condition predominantly affecting young infants.

The infant with vomiting

In all children but particularly in infants vomiting is a very nonspecific symptom. Just about any acute paediatric illness can cause vomiting.

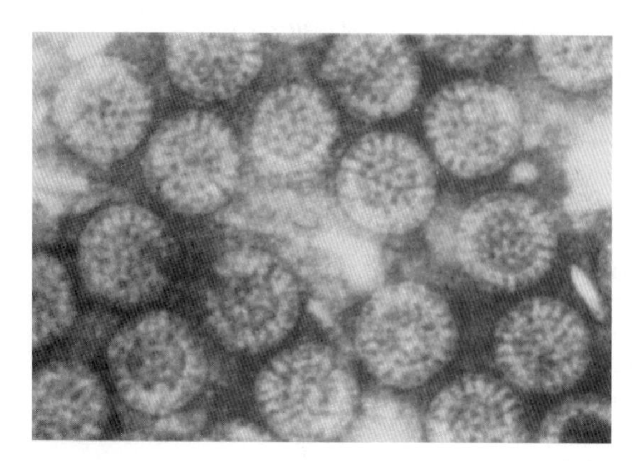

Fig 3.26
Electronmicrograph of rotavirus. Note the wheel-like appearance.

Note that gastro-oesphageal reflux, unless gross, usually produces regurgitation rather than true vomiting. This usually involves the frequent non-forceful bringing back of small volumes of milk after feeds. Small amounts of regurgitation may also occur in the absence of gastro-oesophageal reflux, especially in overfed infants. Sometimes regurgitation and vomiting may be difficult to distinguish.

Management of infant vomiting involves treating the underlying cause. Antiemetics should only be used for drug-induced vomiting (e.g. after chemotherapy) and sometimes as part of a combination of drug treatments for gastro-oesophageal reflux.

Causes of persistent vomiting in infancy are listed in Information box 3.15.

Information Box 3.14

Hypernatraemic dehydration

- Plasma sodium >150 mmol/L, often with raised urea and creatinine and raised blood glucose levels.
- Clinical signs of dehydration, such as reduced skin turgor, may be less obvious as a relatively high proportion of fluid is lost from the intracellular compartment.
- Drowsiness or coma may be present.
- Rehydration with very hypotonic solutions can lead to rapid influx of water into (brain) cells producing cerebral oedema.

Surgical causes of vomiting should not be missed. Pyloric stenosis (see Chapter 11) results in forceful vomiting (classically projectile, but not always) in a baby who often looks lean and hungry. The vomiting never contains bile. Bilious vomiting in an infant should always raise the possibility of intestinal obstruction. Malrotation is the most important diagnosis to exclude since delay may lead to massive gut necrosis. Sometimes vomit may contain blood (Practical box 3.6).

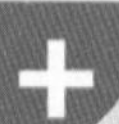

Practical Box 3.6

If an infant's vomit contains blood consider the following:

- Swallowed maternal blood from mother's cracked nipples
- Late-onset haemorrhagic disease of the newborn
- Small streaks of fresh blood may represent a minor mucosal tear from vomiting or a mild gastritis.

Information Box 3.15

Causes of persistent vomiting in infancy

Causes		Notes
Surgical	Pyloric stenosis	Projectile, never bilious
	Gastro-oesophageal reflux	Not true vomiting: regurgitation
	Obstruction, e.g. malrotation	Bilious
Infection	Gastroenteritis	
	Urinary tract infection	
	Meningitis	
	Otitis	
	Food poisoning	Not always a true infection
Metabolic	Inborn errors	
	Diabetes	Rare to have onset in infancy
Neurological	Raised intracranial pressure	
	Cerebral irritation	
Respiratory	Excessive coughing	Infection (especially pertussis) Asthma
Cardiac	Heart failure	
Hepatic	Hepatitis	
Drugs	Chemotherapy	
	Opiates	
Miscellaneous	Overfeeding	Usually not true vomiting
	Poor feeding technique	
	Lack of 'winding'	

The infant with constipation

Breastfed babies tend to have rather loose yellow stools while those on formula feeds have more formed and usually less frequent stools. However, infants bowel habits, whichever way they are fed, vary enormously and, particularly during the weaning period, they will be very much influenced by the diet. Constipation in children can be defined as a bowel habit producing stools which are infrequent and/or excessively hard, to the extent that the baby's wellbeing is affected. In milder cases the symptoms will include irritability, straining at stool and sometimes anal fissuring leading to bleeding upon passage of stool.

When blood is present in the stool as a result of constipation it is always fresh in appearance and sits on the surface of the stool. (Blood mixed into the stool is suggestive of bleeding from higher up.) Anal fissuring can also lead to pain and therefore reluctance to pass stool. In severe cases of constipation there may be gross faecal loading with abdominal distension and vomiting.

The history and examination should address the points listed in Information box 3.16. Delayed passage of meconium beyond 48 hours after birth is suggestive of Hirschsprung disease, which can be excluded or confirmed by the relatively straightforward technique of suction rectal biopsy, which is examined for the presence or absence of ganglion cells.

Potent laxatives should be avoided in very young infants. Increasing the fluid intake with extra water may help. The traditional method of adding brown sugar to feeds is to be deprecated: it can lead to obesity. Lactulose is a relatively safe 'osmotic' laxative.

The infant with skin problems: rashes

Inherited skin conditions such as naevi or epidermolysis bullosa will have been diagnosed in the neonatal period.

Acquired rashes include seborrhoeic dermatitis with cradle cap and rash over the face, neck and upper trunk. This commences early, within a few weeks of birth.

Atopic eczema usually starts later, at around 8 weeks. Although this and seborrhoeic dermatitis are separate conditions they may overlap and 'blend into' each other.

Napkin dermatitis is a common problem; it may be irritant (ammoniacal) or due to candidal infection or both. Irritant rashes tend to spare the skin folds (which are less exposed to urine) while candida concentrates in these areas (Fig. 3.27). However sometimes the two are not easily distinguishable. Persistent severe ammoniacal rash raises the possibility of poor parenting/neglect.

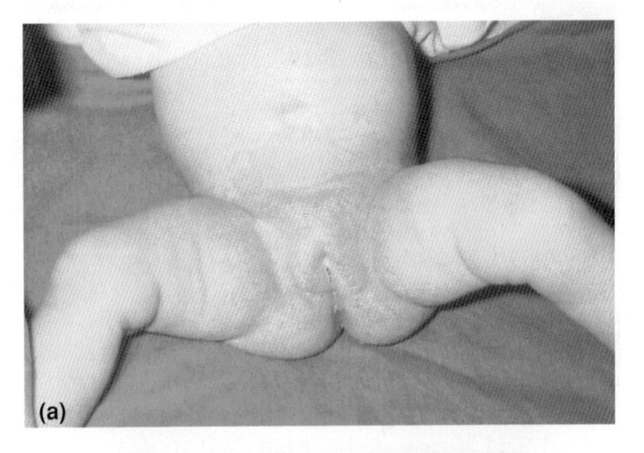

(a)

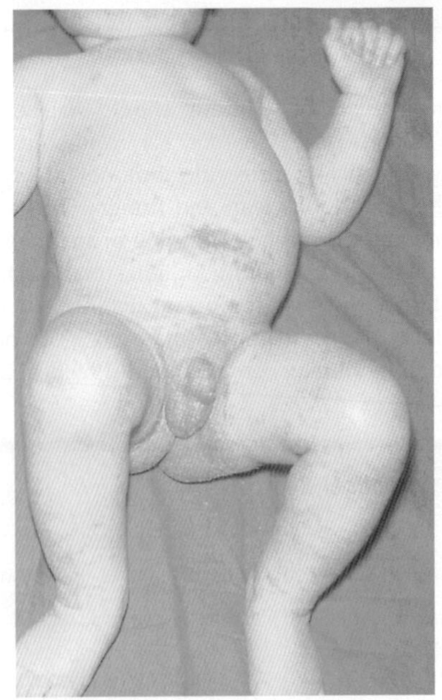

(b)

Fig 3.27
Napkin rashes: (a) ammoniacal, and (b) candidal (courtesy of Dr Richard West).

> **Information Box 3.16**
>
> **Some associations of constipation in infants**
>
> - Too low a fluid intake
> - Family history of 'lazy' or irritable bowel
> - Endocrine disorder: hypothyroidism
> - Intestinal disorder: Hirschsprung disease

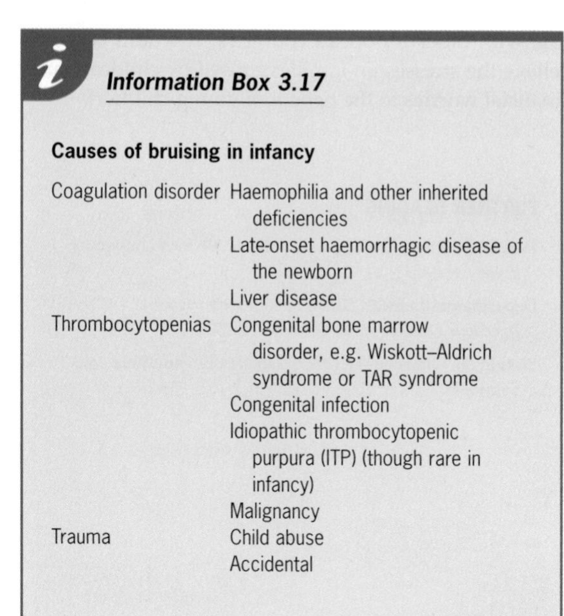

Information Box 3.17

Causes of bruising in infancy

Coagulation disorder	Haemophilia and other inherited deficiencies
	Late-onset haemorrhagic disease of the newborn
	Liver disease
Thrombocytopenias	Congenital bone marrow disorder, e.g. Wiskott–Aldrich syndrome or TAR syndrome
	Congenital infection
	Idiopathic thrombocytopenic purpura (ITP) (though rare in infancy)
	Malignancy
Trauma	Child abuse
	Accidental

The infant with bruising/bleeding

For most of infancy children are relatively immobile and therefore not prone to the normal bruises and scrapes found in toddlers and older children. Bruising should therefore be taken seriously (Information box 3.17, see also Chapter 13).

The causes of bleeding are much the same as those of bruising. Minor bleeding of the gums with teething, and from an anal fissure due to constipation, may occur without any haematological abnormality.

The pallid infant

Pallor in infants does not always signify anaemia. It may be a nonspecific indicator of an unwell child or be a feature of other problems such as hyponatraemia or hypopituitarism. When it is due to anaemia a number of causes should be considered including inherited disorders of bone marrow and red cells, which have escaped detection in the newborn period, and acquired disorders including haematinic deficiencies (from malabsorption or lack of dietary intake), and bone marrow depression secondary to malignancy or infection. It should be borne in mind that the normal haemoglobin value varies considerably during the first six months of life (Table 3.3).

Careful examination of the infant may provide clues to the diagnosis. Splenomegaly is suggestive of haemoglobinopathy. Hepatosplenomegaly, with or without lymphadenopathy, suggests malignancy or infection (or, rarely, a storage disorder). Signs of malabsorption and failure to thrive may be indicative of intestinal disease.

Table 3.3
Haemoglobin values (g/dl) in the first 6 months of life (from Behrman, R E et al (1999) *Nelson's Textbook of Paediatrics*, 16th edn. London: WB Saunders)

Age	Mean	Range
Cord blood	16.8	13.7–20.1
2 weeks	16.5	13.0–20.0
3 months	12.0	9.5–14.5
6 months	12.0	10.5–14.0

New horizons

Reducing the incidence of first-year deaths

There is still much to be done in this age group in terms of preventative child health. The initiative on sleeping position has reduced the incidence of SIDS. There are already health education initiatives to increase awareness of severe life-threatening infections such as meningococcal infection, and hopefully the result will be earlier diagnosis and treatment with a resultant fall in mortality.

New vaccines

New vaccines currently under early development offer exciting prospects for the future. As for the Hib vaccine, the process of polysaccharide–protein conjugation greatly enhances the immunogenicity of bacterial vaccines and this makes them effective in young infants (which is not the case with the current polysaccharide vaccines). A conjugated group C meningococcal vaccine was introduced to the normal schedule in 1999. In the UK group C organisms previously accounted for 30–40% of meningococcal disease and since the vaccine was introduced there has been a significant reduction in cases. A vaccine against group B disease (which accounts for 55–60% of cases) would be even more useful. However this is still a long way off because the important antigen in the polysaccharide capsule of the organism mimics a human antigen thus making it non-immunogenic for humans. Current research work is concentrating on using other protein antigens for vaccine development.

Conjugated pneumococcal vaccines against the most common disease-causing serotypes have shown great promise in clinical trials. These vaccines offer the prospect of preventing not only serious invasive disease such as meningitis caused by this organism but also less severe common infections such as otitis media. With the increasing concern over the emergence of antibiotic resistance amongst pneumococci this is a potentially

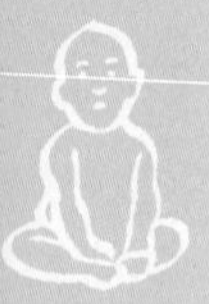

very important development. These developments offer the prospect of continuing the decrease in incidence of bacterial meningitis which commenced with the introduction of the conjugated Hib vaccine in 1992.

Looking further ahead, the successful development of a vaccine against respiratory syncytial virus would greatly reduce respiratory morbidity, and possibly mortality, in young children.

Sociological change

A much needed sociological development would be an initiative to greatly increase the provision of childcare facilities in the workplace. This would bring the UK into line with other European countries. It would serve to relieve the stresses on families caused by childcare and financial worries to the benefit of young children.

FURTHER READING

Hall DMB (1996) *Health for All Children*. Oxford University Press

Department of Health (1996) *Immunisation against Infectious Diseases 1996*. London: HMSO.

Plotkin SS, Orenstein W (1999) *Vaccines*. Philadelphia: WB Saunders.

4 The young child from 1 to 5 years

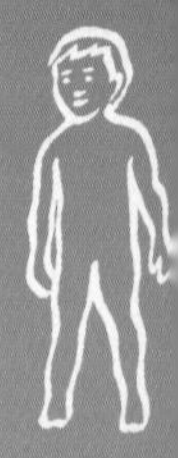

Introduction

Using this chapter

In this chapter, we review the development, main illnesses and health problems that are specific to preschool children. Emphasis is on the common; much reference is made to parenting skills and the needs of young children that have to be supplied by both the family and society at large.

The child from 1 to 5 years

By the first birthday the infant has started to develop a highly individual pattern of behaviour, parents are more experienced and the demands they make on health services start to change. Maternal immunity which protected the younger infant from infections such as measles and mumps has waned. Infections, especially those affecting the upper respiratory tract, middle ear and gastrointestinal tract are common. Doctors need to understand and manage the common and often under-researched 'minor' disorders: coughs, colds, earaches, rashes, feeding upsets and temper tantrums whilst recognizing the rarer 'major' conditions, such as meningitis and other serious infections, epilepsy and asthma. They should ensure that timely and appropriate management is undertaken. Some children will have undergone surgery for severe congenital malformations and others will have survived as a result of neonatal intensive care.

During the second year the infant should start to walk and talk. Mobility enables them to explore their environment, but they become vulnerable to household dangers. Ever-increasing independence is accompanied by rebellion against the parents and a search for boundaries of what is and is not permissible. Between 2 and 3, children discover that they can control what happens around them by their actions and by talking – especially saying 'no'. This period is often referred to as the 'terrible twos'. Parents may feel unable to cope and seek support elsewhere; the consultation rate with general practitioners for under 4 year-olds is the highest of any age group until age 75 is reached. Gradually, children begin to establish their own identity and use the pronoun 'I'. Most have worked out the functions of their surroundings and familiar adults and gained confidence to deal with new situations.

By the age of 4, children have acquired such

confidence that they become self-important. In familiar situations, children join in complex games with other children. Parents can actively encourage this growing independence in preparation for school by enrolling them in playgroups and making opportunities for play with other children. New situations are still frightening and may cause unexplained fears or changes of mood. The conventional age of compulsory school entry is 5 years but many start school or playgroup much earlier. If a child's initial experiences are happy and secure, they are better able to cope with the discipline and learning environment of school.

Our birth is but a sleep and a forgetting:
The soul that rises with us, our life's star,
Hath had elsewhere its setting,
And cometh from afar:
Not in entire forgetfulness,
And not in utter nakedness,
But trailing clouds of glory do we come
From God, who is our home:
Heaven lies about us in our infancy!
Shades of the prison-house begin to close
Upon the growing boy,
But he beholds the light, and whence it flows
He sees it in his joy;
The youth, who daily farther from the east
Must travel, still is Nature's priest,
And by the vision splendid
Is on his way attended:
At length the man perceives it die away,
And fade into the light of common day.

W. Wordsworth

Epidemiology

Over the 10 years leading up to 1999 there was a 35% decrease in the mortality rate for children aged 1–4 years (Office of National Statistics (ONS) data (Table 4.1). Children in developed countries should no longer die from vaccine-preventable infectious diseases such as pertussis, polio, *Haemophilus influenzae* type b and measles. Due to improved surgical techniques or more accurate antenatal diagnosis and selective termination, fewer children are dying of congenital abnormalities. Deaths from injuries and poisoning have also decreased. Infectious diseases (particularly meningococcal sepsis) wax and wane in incidence; 'new' infectious diseases such as HIV/AIDS have appeared. Cancer, despite massive improvements in management remains a major problem.

In 1995 the death rate for this age group was 0.3 per 1000 children. The majority of deaths (19%) are still due to accidents, mostly traffic accidents, and burns (5%).

Table 4.1
Causes of death in children aged 1–4, 1995 (Office of National Statistics data)

Cause of death	Number of children
Injury and poisoning, including accidents	172
Congenital abnormalities	117
Neurological disease	90
Infections and parasitic disease	88
Neoplasia	88
Respiratory disease	54
Cardiovascular disease	37
Endocrine, metabolic, nutritional, immunological causes	23
Gastrointestinal disease	19
Blood disorders	10
As a result of perinatal problems	7
Genitourinary disease	3
Connective tissue disease	2
Skin disease	1
Other	26
Total	737

(From: Mortality Statistics, ONS. © Crown Copyright 1995. Reproduced with permission)

(see Table 4.1). Infection remains a common cause of mortality (12%) and children still die after the first year as a result of congenital abnormalities (16%), congenital heart disease being the commonest. Other major causes of death in this age group are neoplasia (12%), particularly lymphoma and leukaemia and acquired neurological problems (12%) especially after head injury.

Social, cultural and environmental factors affecting child health

Between 1 and 5 years as the child becomes less reliant on his parents and increasingly independent, his mother may have returned to work or had a further child. Genetic factors and early experiences powerfully influence child development. Some toddlers are clearly brighter than others as shown by their play, speech and alertness. To make the most of their potential, toddlers need a good deal of one-to-one nurture and opportunity. In their early stages they need expensive playthings less than playtime with loving adults and then playmates to socialize with.

Social factors

Over one-third of children in Great Britain come from families where the breadwinner is a skilled manual worker (social class III M); a quarter where the breadwinner is a managerial 'white collar' worker (class II); 6% higher professional (class I), and 5% unskilled manual (class IV). The major factor that greatly affects the child is poverty, which is at its extremes where there is unemployment, with rates varying according to the economic circumstances of the country from 5 to 10%, and among children in single-parent families. Mortality rates are 2.6 (girls) and 3.4 (boys) times greater for children aged 1–4 years in social class V compared with those in social class I. These differences start at birth and continue throughout life. More children in industrialized societies are living in relative poverty than was the case a generation ago. In Scandinavian countries there is less difference in child health between these groups.

At all ages, boys have higher mortality and morbidity rates than girls for acquired conditions, especially accidents and infections, though for some conditions such as epilepsy, the excess is marginal. There is no clear reason for these differences. Girls may be subject to more powerful role-modelling from their mothers that protects them from accidents. Having two X chromosomes protects against otherwise lethal conditions such as haemophilia, but there are some rare conditions where only females survive fetal life, e.g. Rett syndrome (see p. 323).

Preparation for school

In the UK, children must by law start school at 5 years of age. Many children now attend some preschool group activity such as playgroup or nursery school. Early education is particularly important for children with disabilities. Their special needs make a longer period of learning essential if they are to fulfil their potential. A minority of children have either physical or learning problems which make it impossible to profit from normal schooling, unless they receive special help. National policy now expects all children to attend mainstream schools unless there is need for a type of education that could only be provided in a special school with appropriate facilities (e.g. for children with blindness or severe autism). For a child to receive special educational help a *Statement of Special Educational Need* has to be drawn up, under the 1981 and 1993 Education Acts. This is compiled by the local education authority and includes descriptions of the child's problems and needs as seen from the perspective of the parents and those professionally involved with the child's care.

Critical learning periods

Children tend to develop new skills in relatively discrete time bands, for example becoming dry by day between 18 months and 2½ years. If the child fails to gain a developmental skill at an appropriate age, it can be assumed that some process interfered with development at a critical point or learning period and that it might not be possible to catch up. Untreated bilateral congenital cataract or squint may cause blindness through such a mechanism. Does the same apply to children who have been hindered by illness from learning to walk, feed or speak at the usual time? There have been many debates around the concept of critical learning periods, but no agreement that this concept applies to all aspects of development.

Clinical approach

(The key points in the paediatric history are shown in Practical box 4.1.)

As in the first year of life there are important differences from the approach used in adult medicine. When talking to the parents, get the child's sex, age and name right. Young children assume that everyone knows their name and sex, and they and their parents will be insulted if you refer to them incorrectly. Let the child see that his parents have confidence in you; older children will then join in and may be the only ones who know the answers. For this age group, a full family and social history is very important and a past history of contact with the medical profession will yield useful information. Most preschool children in the UK have a parent-held *Child Health Record* (usually in a red cover, see p. 67); ask to see it, get as much information as you can from it and always update it (Fig. 4.1). Remember that the past medical history of a child begins with the pregnancy, and concerns that the mother may have about her child may stem from otherwise undisclosed problems, which occurred during pregnancy and birth. Finally, determine what the parents (and often grandparents) are really worrying about (Fig. 4.2) and their expectations of the outcome of the consultation.

In preschool children, understanding the presenting

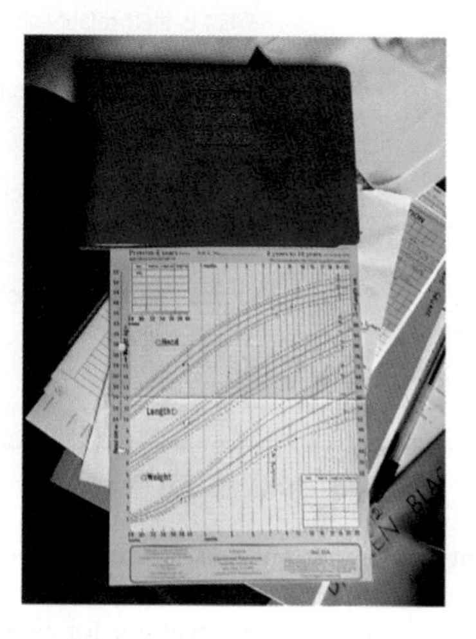

Fig 4.1
A parent-held Child Health Record.

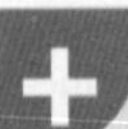

Practical Box 4.1

Key points in the paediatric history

Name:	
Age/sex:	
History from:	
Complaining of:	Symptoms and duration
History of presenting complaint:	When was the child last well? Precise order and progression of symptoms Treatment already given
Activity/apathy:	
Feeding/appetite:	Estimate of food intake
Previous medical history:	Pregnancy, including maternal illness and drug ingestion Antenatal problems Birth, place of birth, birthweight Neonatal problems including jaundice Previous illness, hospital admissions, surgery Contact with infectious illness Allergies
Immunizations:	List. If any omitted, why?
Feeding:	Duration of breastfeeding Change to artificial milk Weaning
Developmental history:	Appropriate milestones reached in gross motor, fine motor and vision, social, speech and hearing Current level of development
Family history:	Family tree with ages of parents and siblings List health problems in the family Stillbirths, miscarriages and childhood deaths
Social history:	Who does the child live with? What is their relationship? House or flat? Number of bedrooms, condition (e.g. dampness) Parental occupations Financial problems and benefits claimed School or playgroup Who else looks after the child or helps the mother? Travel abroad

complaint is all important and it may not be easy to get to the heart of the problem which may be many-layered. The fact that the parent is speaking for the child can compound difficulties. You will learn a great deal from letting the child speak to you, not necessarily through language but by play, behaviour and willingness to separate from parents (Fig. 4.3).

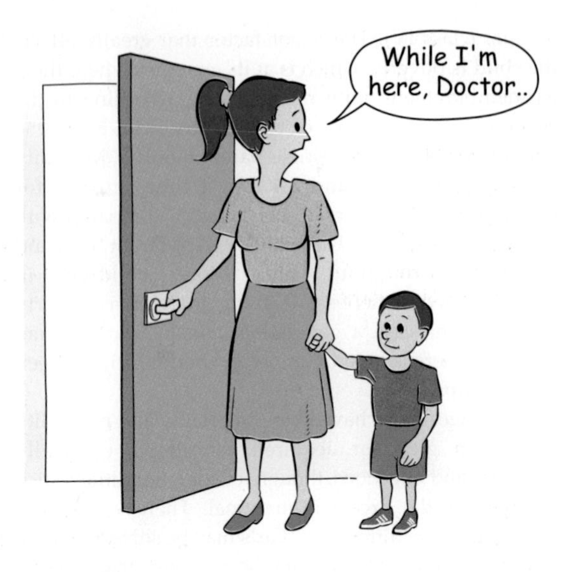

Fig 4.2
Try to determine what parents are really worried about.

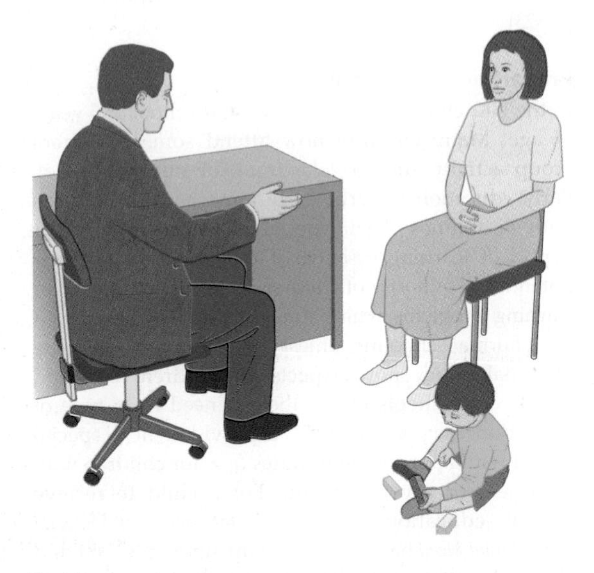

Fig 4.3
Much can be observed while the history is being taken.

Physical examination

The key points in the paediatric examination are summarized in Practical box 4.2.

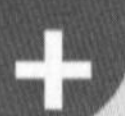

Practical Box 4.2

Key points in paediatric examination

Weight:	Centile
Height:	Centile
Head circumference:	If under 2 years
Temperature:	Where measured
General inspection:	Appearance and demeanour Dysmorphic features Nutritional status State of hydration Jaundice, pallor, cyanosis, clubbing, oedema, fetor Lymphadenopathy
Skin:	Distribution, colour and character of rash Hair
Respiratory system:	Cough, wheeze, stridor, whoop Respiratory rate Chest shape, chest expansion Signs of respiratory distress Percussion note Breath sounds, added sounds
Cardiovascular system:	Pulse: rate, rhythm, volume Blood pressure Thrill or parasternal heave Mediastinum: apex, trachea Heart sounds, added sounds, position and radiation Femoral pulses
Abdomen:	Scaphoid/distended? Masses, tenderness, guarding, rebound Size of liver, spleen, kidneys Ascites Bowel sounds Hernias, testicular size Inspection of perineum Rectal examination if indicated (rarely)
Central nervous system (CNS):	Level of consciousness Head shape Fontanelle (if under 18 months) Posture, abnormal movements Signs of meningitis Cranial nerves Motor: power, tone, coordination Reflexes: knee, ankle, plantars, persistent, primitive Gait Sensation (if possible)
Skeletal:	Deformity, tenderness, swelling of bones and joints Range of movement and pain on movement Kyphosis, scoliosis, torticollis Limb deformities Muscle wasting, hypertrophy
Ears, nose and throat (ENT):	Ears – tympanic membranes, external auditory canals Throat Tonsillar lymph nodes

General examination

Nappies will cover 20% of the body and beneath them may lurk abnormal genitalia, inguinal hernia and impalpable femoral arteries. The skill comes in making friends with children, even the most truculent – if they cry are you the cause? Sometimes it may not be possible to do the whole examination first time and it may be better to repeat later. Paediatricians have to become good at looking at eardrums and optic discs, even when it feels like doing it in a rowing boat (Fig. 4.4).

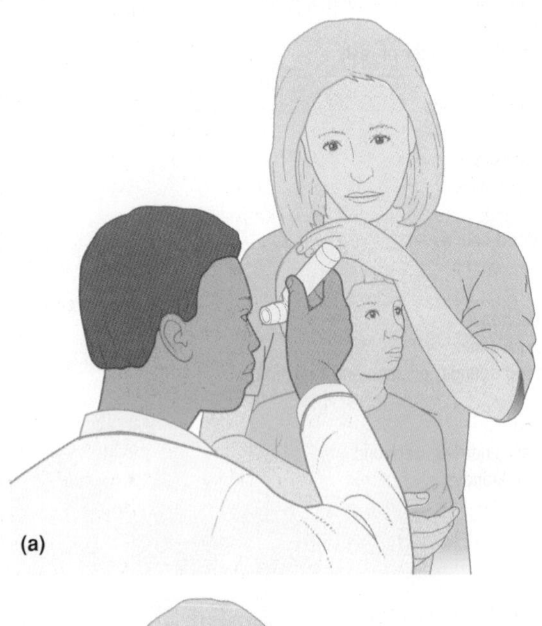

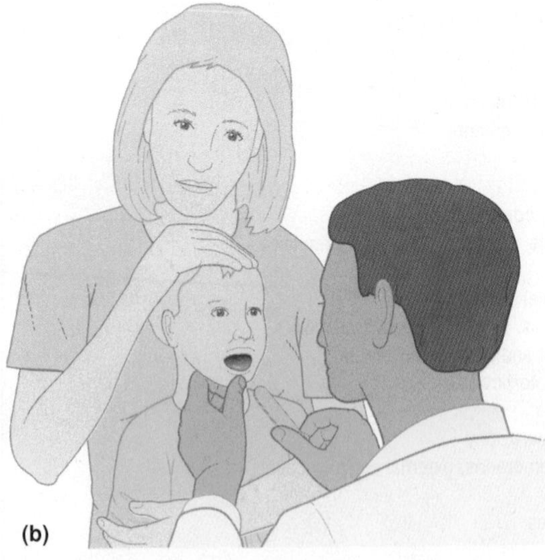

Fig 4.4
Examining a young child. (a) For examination of the ear with an auriscope, the mother has one hand on the child's head, the other holds the child's upper arm. (b) Examining the throat. The mother has one hand on the head and the other across the child's arms. The same position is used for examining eyes and chest.

The majority of diagnostic information can be obtained from the history and general inspection, so watch the child out of the corner of your eye whilst taking the history. Have plenty of age-appropriate toys around the floor or with you at the bedside. Observe how the child is dressed and interacts with his/her parents and other people and plays with toys. Form a general impression of the fully dressed child running around and at play. Eventually you will need to see the child undressed though not all clothes need to come off at once. Whilst the genitalia need to be examined, appreciate that most children, whatever their age, do not like this.

Examining a child requires empathy, patience and understanding. A friendly and gentle approach is usually the most productive. The least traumatic part of the examination should be performed first.

Height, weight and head circumference (using a nonstretch paper measure) need to be recorded accurately and entered on a *centile chart* (p. 76). Whilst it is 'best practice' to examine a child in the classic order taught in adult medicine, there are times when one has to grab signs in whatever order you can get them. Even so one has to try to be systematic; otherwise it is all too easy to forget to examine the child adequately – this is the way to making mistakes. Sometimes one has to start at the head and work downwards, getting the socks off at the last moment. Paediatrics is never dull.

Skin and systemic conditions

The skin can only be examined fully if the child is completely undressed right down to removal of socks. Skin lesions may be dramatic and affect most of the body surface or be small and localized (Fig. 4.5). (See Ch. 15 for exanthems and Ch. 9 eczema.)

Skin rashes in children are common and can usually be diagnosed from the description, distribution and associated features. Some conditions, such as warts, require only brief examination, whereas others need a more systematic approach.

Decreased turgor indicates dehydration, and a swollen pitting skin indicates oedema. Feeling the skin can be as informative as looking at it. Birthmarks and other congenital skin abnormalities can cause great concern and need accurate diagnosis – conditions such as neurofibromatosis or tuberose sclerosis (see p. 325) may be readily apparent. Acute skin lesions can lead to an instant diagnosis in meningococcal septicaemia, measles or chickenpox (see Ch. 15). Eczema may be variable in appearance and is commonly associated with asthma. Fungal conditions are difficult to diagnose and may require scrapings for confirmation by microscopic examination and culture.

Note the distribution of the rash. Does it blanch on pressure? Is it palpable? Does it exhibit the Koebner

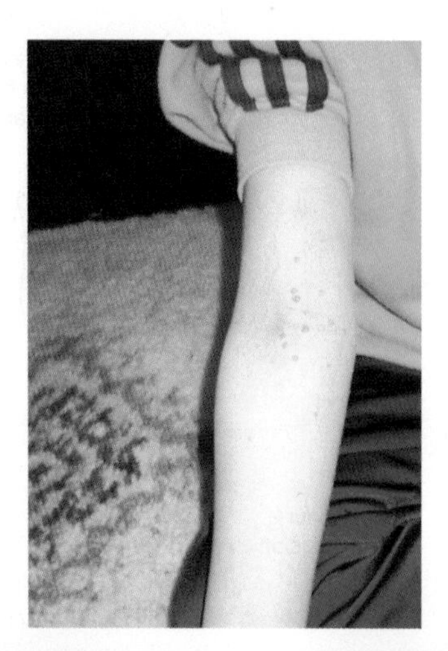

(a)

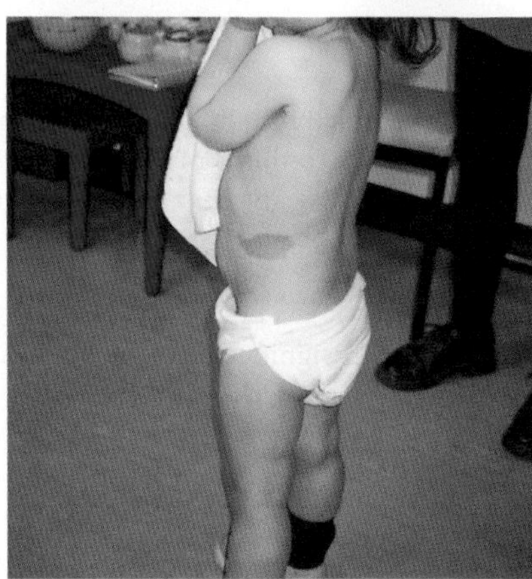

(b)

Fig 4.5
Common skin lesions. (a) Molluscum contagiosum; (b) large café-au-lait patch.

phenomenon, i.e. develops at sites of skin damaged by injury or trauma? Examine for other physical signs such as hepatosplenomegaly or lymphadenopathy.

The scalp hair should be examined for ringworm (which gleams under Wood's light), head lice and alopecia. The latter may be due to plucking out in behavioural disturbance or constant head rubbing, iron-deficiency or it may be a side-effect of cytotoxics and sodium valproate. Long lists of congenital abnormalities are associated with sparse or unusual hair. Nails should be examined for clubbing, cyanosis, white transverse lines suggesting recent illness (Fig. 4.6), or koilonychia of iron-deficiency. A low hairline is seen in some syndromes (e.g. Turner XO).

Purpuric rash. Purpuric lesions are caused by haemorrhage into the skin and do not blanch on pressure. They are either due to low platelet counts, as in idiopathic thrombocytopenic purpura (ITP) or leukaemia, or due to vasculitis as in Henoch–Schönlein syndrome (HSS) (see p. 209) and meningococcal disease (see p. 280–283). HSS is the commonest cause of purpura in childhood; the rash has an extensor distribution and may be associated with haematuria and joint pain. In contrast, the child with ITP can be expected to remain otherwise well apart from the rash. If the child is systemically unwell you need to consider meningococcal disease and leukaemia. The child with meningococcal disease will have a short history of being ill, may or may not have signs of meningitis, will be feverish, drowsy, irritable and shocked; they need immediate treatment with penicillin. The child with leukaemia may have lymphadenopathy, hepatosplenomegaly, joint pain, fever, and anaemia and has usually been unwell for several days. Diagnosis requires examination of the bone marrow and treatment with chemotherapy. Drugs such as antibiotics, antiepilepsy drugs, antihistamines and nonsteroidal anti-inflammatory agents may cause thrombocytopenic purpura; so remember to take a drug history.

Maculopapular rash. Macules are discrete, flat, erythematous lesions which blanch on pressure. Papules are palpable. Discrete tiny pink macules appear in rubella, associated with suboccipital lymphadenopathy. In roseola, the rash appears as the fever subsides. Measles is a more confluent maculopapular rash, associated with cough, nasal discharge and conjunctivitis.

Maculopapular rash occurs in viral infections including glandular fever when the patient has been given ampicillin; in other patients an ampicillin rash may occur about 10 days after starting the drug. Perhaps the commonest cause of such rashes are enteroviruses including Coxsackie and ECHO viruses.

Urticarial rash. There are many causes of urticarial rashes, including allergy, viral infections, insect bites and cold. Chronic papular urticaria is usually due to sensitivity to insect bites.

Vesicles are caused by collections of fluid within the skin. In chickenpox, vesicles occur in crops and are diagnostic. In *Herpes zoster* infection, vesicles may be preceded by itching and occur in a dermatomal distribution. *Herpes simplex* infection occurring around the mouth tends to have a honey-coloured crust.

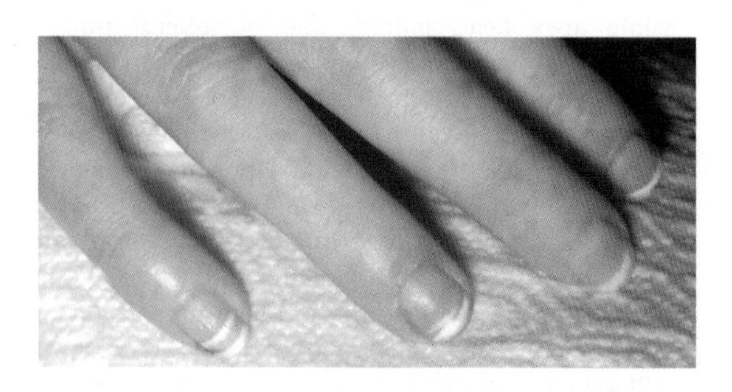

Fig 4.6
Nails showing signs of recent serious illness.

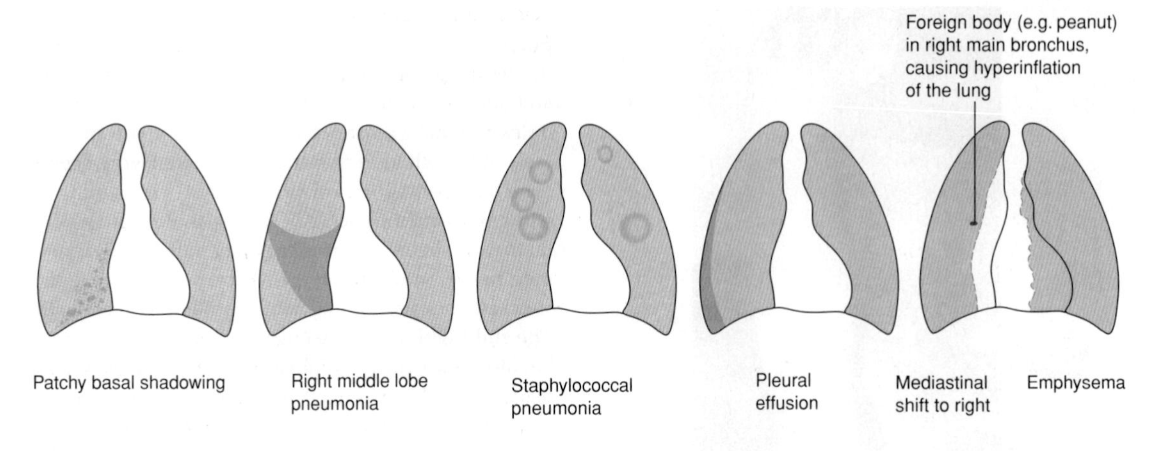

Fig 4.7
Appearance of chest X-ray with different respiratory disorders.

Respiratory system

Tachypnoea may be defined as a respiratory rate greater than 40 in children less than 2 years old and a rate greater than 30 in children over 2 years of age. Asymmetry, chest deformity and recession can be detected on observation. The anteroposterior diameter of the chest should be less than the lateral diameter and is increased in asthma and cystic fibrosis. The trachea is very mobile in young children and readily displaced by cervical masses or lung collapse. Percussion should be light and may suggest effusions or consolidation. Auscultation is easier in a quiet child but can be performed on a crying child during inspiration. Listen for breath sounds, which sound harsher than in an adult, and then for the presence of added sounds, such as inspiratory stridor or expiratory wheeze. Chest X-ray often aids diagnosis (see Fig 4.7).

Foreign body aspiration is discussed on page 168.

Cardiovascular system

Note the skin colour; does the child look pale, cyanosed or anaemic? Examine the chest for cardiac bulges or a visible apex beat; palpate the peripheral pulses, parasternal area and apex. The heart rate of a preschool child normally varies between 75 and 120 beats per minute. Finally listen for murmurs. Murmurs heard in children are usually systolic and the position of greatest intensity should be recorded. Don't forget to listen to the back where a patent ductus, coarctation and pulmonary stenosis will radiate, and to check the femoral pulses, which are reduced or absent in coarctation (Fig. 4.8).

Blood pressure measurement is time-consuming, but important (Fig. 4.9). The systolic pressure in a quiet preschool child should not be over 105 or the diastolic over 75. Use a correctly calibrated sphygmomanometer with a cuff at least two-thirds of the length of the upper arm. Undersized cuffs give a spuriously high reading (p. 181).

Innocent murmurs

Most children with significant congenital heart disease will have been diagnosed before their first birthday.

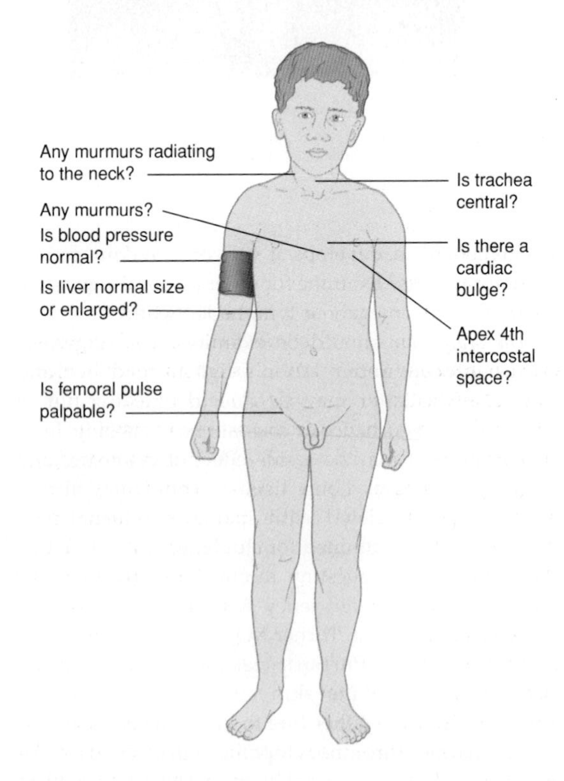

Fig 4.8
Cardiovascular examination.

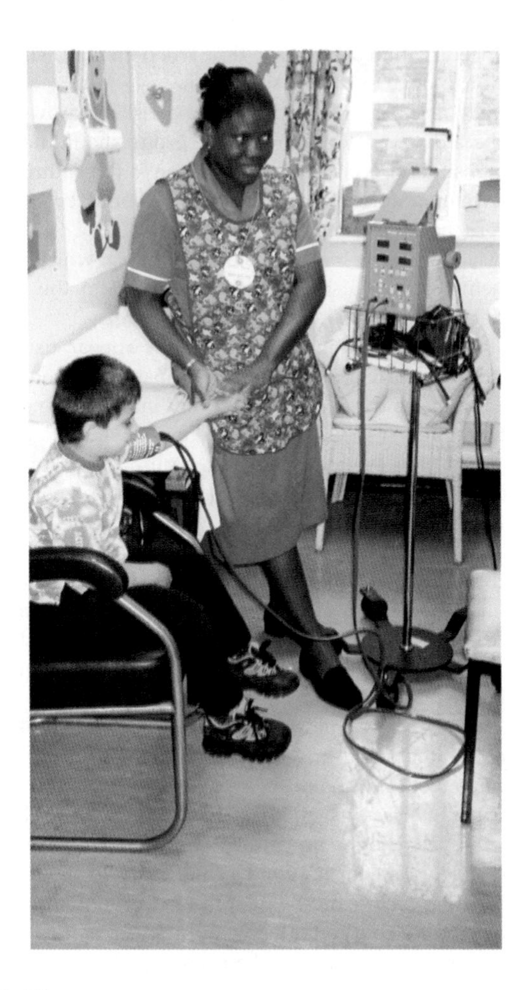

Fig 4.9
Blood pressure measurement by Doppler technique.

Functional or innocent murmurs are by far the most common type to present later. One in five preschool children has a systolic murmur and one in two may develop a transitory innocent murmur during a febrile illness. Fever, exercise, anxiety and anaemia all increase cardiac output and accentuate innocent murmurs which appear to be related to flow velocity in the great arteries. The child's past medical history will usually be uneventful, and the child is pink with normal precordial activity, pulses and second heart sound. Innocent murmurs are soft to medium in intensity, systolic, and crescendo–decrescendo in quality. The murmur is best heard along the left sternal border and does not radiate up into the neck. Manoeuvres that transiently decrease venous return such as squatting will decrease the intensity of innocent murmurs while pathologic murmurs will persist unchanged.

Management is targeted at reassuring the parents that the child's heart is normal, that the murmur will eventually disappear, and avoiding expensive investigation.

Pathological murmurs

Inflammatory conditions that involve the heart such as acute rheumatic fever, myocarditis and endocarditis are now thankfully rare in developed countries but remain a serious problem elsewhere.

A child with serious heart disease might have no murmur because the pressure in both ventricles is the same whilst the left heart fails. Where there is suspicion of structural heart disease investigation is most likely to reveal an abnormality in those with poor growth, breathlessness, central cyanosis or family history of cardiomyopathy. A small ventricular septal defect (VSD), pulmonary stenosis and aortic stenosis also produce systolic murmurs, although they tend to be louder and can be diagnosed from the position of maximum intensity (see p. 174).

A cautionary note. Despite infant sceening, heart problems may be missed, only to present late as a medical emergency with congestive cardiac failure: big liver, rapid breathing, central cyanosis. Include palpation of femoral vessels in routine examination. Be prepared to take the blood pressure in both arms.

Digestive system

Teeth and gums are the start of the digestive system

Teeth should always be inspected (Fig. 4.10) and certain diseases can be diagnosed from the mouth, e.g. aphthous ulcers of Crohn's disease (see Information box 5.24, p. 146 and p. 233–234). Gross dental decay is now rare and its occurrence suggests poor care. Yellow

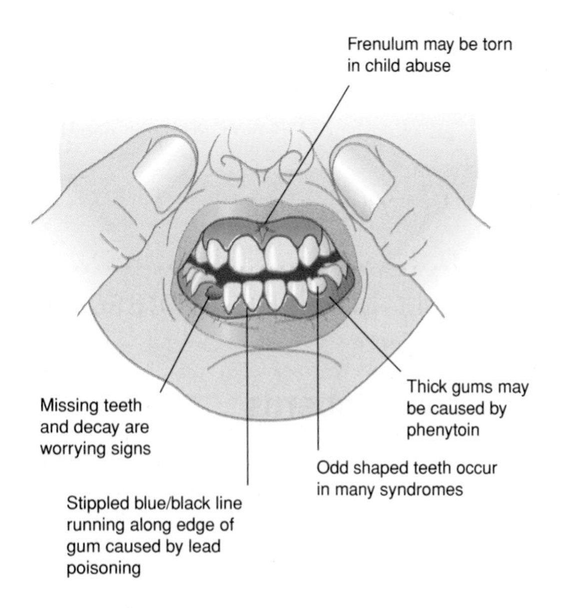
Frenulum may be torn in child abuse
Missing teeth and decay are worrying signs
Thick gums may be caused by phenytoin
Odd shaped teeth occur in many syndromes
Stippled blue/black line running along edge of gum caused by lead poisoning

Fig 4.10
Examination of the teeth and gums.

teeth suggest tetracycline administration in infancy or kernicterus, now rare in developed countries. Teeth are abnormally formed in conditions such as ectodermal dysplasia. Dental disease should be specially sought in children with congenital heart disease, who are at risk of subacute bacterial endocarditis, and in boys with haemophilia. Missing teeth prior to normal shedding of first dentition and rupture of the upper buccal frenulum is indicative of child abuse. Gross crowding of teeth and malocclusion need orthodontic advice. Examination of the gums may reveal the black lines of lead poisoning or thickening following chronic treatment with phenytoin (and other antiepilepsy medications to a lesser extent).

Note. When you examine the mouth use the opportunity to spread messages about good dental care.

Abdominal inspection

This may reveal an abdomen distended due to air swallowing, organomegaly, ascites or intestinal obstruction, or a scaphoid (sunken) abdomen in a child who has lost weight. Palpation can be performed with the child lying either on a couch or across the mother's knee. Gentle palpation of the whole abdomen for tenderness and masses should be followed by palpation of the organs. The tips of the fingers or side of the index finger, on expiration, gently advancing towards the costal margin can palpate a liver edge. The size of the liver can be estimated by percussion. Palpation of the spleen should start in the right iliac fossa and be repeated starting in the left flank. The spleen can be just felt in a small proportion of normal children; in an enlarged spleen the notch may be palpable. The kidneys are often ballottable in normal children, and faeces may be felt in the left iliac fossa. Avoid rectal examination if possible, but there are times when it becomes mandatory if surgical diagnoses are being considered, or in severe constipation. It should be done by an experienced person and not needlessly repeated.

Behaviour problems in preschool children

Common concerns

As families get smaller and more fragmented, fewer and fewer parents come to the task of child-rearing with previous day-to-day experience. Parents who once sought advice from relatives tend to seek it from doctors and health visitors who must be well versed in the arts and science of childcare. In 1- to 5-year-olds this particularly applies to concerns about feeding, cleanliness, toileting, sleeping and behaviour – particularly punishment at a time when there is a strong national move to outlaw smacking.

Bath-time. The bathroom poses a risk of drowning and scalding. Children in this age group should not be left unsupervised in the bath or alone in the bathroom. The temperature of the bath water should be tested before the child is put in.

Many children have dry skin or eczema, which may benefit from emulsifying ointment, used in the bath water, and added oils.

Teeth need cleaning as soon as they appear, using a soft toothbrush and fluoride toothpaste. Discourage poking in the ears with cotton wool buds and fingers; external debris should be washed away with a flannel. Earwax can be loosened with pure olive oil or proprietary wax softeners dropped into the ear with the child on one side.

Accident prevention in the home. Kitchen hobs, stoves and kettles pose obvious dangers as do inflammable clothes, household cleaning materials and medicines. Medical staff who see the results of injuries have a duty to advocate means of avoiding these tragedies through primary public health measures.

Bedtime. Many children are frightened of the dark or use bedtime as an opportunity for 'playing up' their parents. Bedtime should become an enjoyable routine; reading stories instead of watching TV should be encouraged. Stories need to be short, not too exciting and appropriate for the child's age. The child should be left feeling secure and be discouraged from getting up again. Young children often want to get up earlier than their parents; they need to be encouraged not to wake them up and have a supply of toys to keep them occupied in the bedroom.

Dressing. Children should be encouraged at an early stage to help with dressing and undressing even if it means the whole process takes longer. Children readily become overheated; they should not have too many bedclothes or be overdressed.

Social behaviour

Children vary enormously in their behaviour; 'crabby' infants can transform themselves to placid toddlers and vice versa. Toddlers have a short attention span and easily become bored; they need a great deal of stimulation. Until 3 years of age they will play alongside other children, sometimes grabbing and distracting them. Beyond 3, they will start to play constructively with other children. Learning to socialize is a key requirement before the child starts school; this is best learnt in an appropriate playgroup. Behavioural problems such as temper tantrums can be dealt with by the parents' setting boundaries which are to be kept to on both sides; sometimes the parents need the support of another person such as a health visitor or extended family member to enforce these boundaries. Sibling rivalry can become a problem with the arrival of a second child and the parents may need advice about spending time with both children. Think about the potential for exhaustion of parents who bring up multiple birth children.

Referral to child and family psychiatry

Professional opinions are increasingly sought about unacceptable child behaviour but it is impossible to determine whether child behavioural problems are really becoming more common than they were in the past. The patterns of psychiatric problems seen in young children are very different from those that affect adolescents and adults. It is important to distinguish:

- The psychological problems that affect children with disabling conditions, particularly learning disorders, from those that that are secondary to the environment
- Behavioural problems that are secondary to other disease states
- Idiopathic behavioural problems.

Child psychiatry is normally taught in conjunction with child health but has its own textbooks. In this section we concentrate only on the more common problems, particularly those that will be seen often in paediatric practice; many of these children will need to be seen jointly with other professionals.

Some of the commoner problems in preschool children

Sleep

Some children develop bizarre sleep patterns; they may be very reluctant to go to sleep and can greatly disturb their parents who may become dysfunctional from chronic lack of sleep. Sometimes a straightforward review of home life can lead to simple modifications that help the child and family through a very difficult stage. There are now voluntary organizations which help families with sleep-disordered children. The key is to help the child feel relaxed at bedtime. Parents may need a list of do's and don'ts to help them and their child develop a robust sleep rhythm which helps to keep the child out of the parental bed.

Enuresis and encopresis

See page 153, 155, 219.

Temper tantrums

No one knows why young children have such variable patterns of behaviour. Some have a low threshold for self-control and may, often for no apparent reason, appear to lose control of their senses and start to have rages. The best treatment is to help the child feel secure. Some develop attention-seeking behaviour that can be very unsettling such as biting or head banging to the extent of causing self-injury. These children need to be referred to a child psychiatrist.

Attention deficit/hyperactive behaviour

This serious pervasive problem is described on p. 158.

Screening and health promotion (Fig. 4.11)

In order to ensure that children are growing and developing normally, it is necessary to have a policy for regular assessment for detection of problems and to allow parents the opportunity for informed discussion and health education. Increasingly in the UK this work

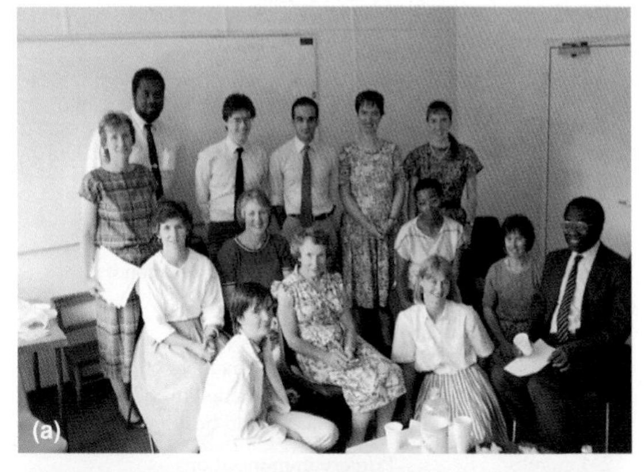

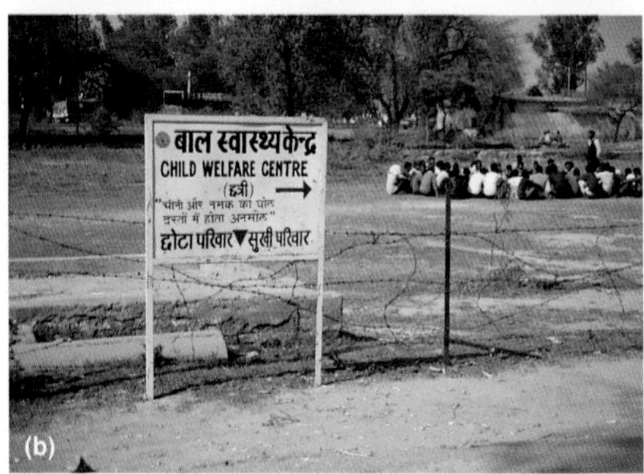

Fig 4.11
Community paediatric teams in (a) London and (b) India.

is being done by family doctors, nurses and health visitors (Fig. 4.12).

The Hall Report (*Health for All Children*, 3rd edition, 1996) outlines the rationale and basic schedule of childhood developmental testing. It recommends that child health surveillance should be a component of a Child Health Promotion Programme and suggests the routine surveillance programme shown in Table 4.2.

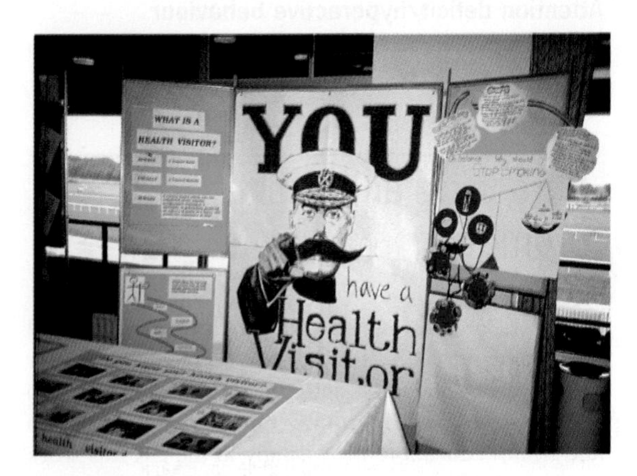

Fig 4.12
Multidisciplinary working: you have a Health Visitor!

Table 4.2
Recommended core surveillance programme (Hall Report (1996) *Health for All Children*, 3rd edn. Oxford University Press)

Neonatal examination	By GP or hospital staff
First 2 weeks	Further physical examination if appropriate. Health education
6–8 weeks	Examination by member of primary health team trained in child surveillance and health education
2–4 months	Primary immunizations
6–9 months	Examination by doctor and health visitor together, including distraction hearing test Health education
13 months	Measles, mumps, rubella (MMR) vaccine
18 months–2 years	Parental guidance and education by health visitor
$3\frac{1}{4}$–$3\frac{1}{2}$ years	Preschool assessment by doctor and health visitor Preschool booster (DT and MMR) Health education
5 years	School entry medical by school health service, usually of children selected through concerns raised by parents, teachers or the preschool medical Height, vision and hearing to be checked in all children

By the first birthday most of the important congenital disorders should have emerged either from routine screening checks or because sudden deterioration has brought them to urgent medical attention. Relatively crude testing during the first year should have determined how the child is seeing or hearing but repeated follow up is needed to establish whether the condition is permanent, transient or remediable. This involves both careful history taking and examination.

Children may develop sensory problems later in life, having had normal test findings in the first year.

Hearing, speech and vision

Ear, nose and throat examination

Examination is incomplete without a look at the eardrums and throat; they should be examined last as they can upset the child. A good auriscope and light source are essential. To examine the ears, the child must be gently held (see Fig. 4.4 in Physical examination). Observe whether wax or foreign bodies obscure the drum, if it is visible, whether you can see a light reflex, inflammation, fluid level, perforation, grommets or scarring. A drum which is dull and retracted and the light reflex reduced or absent suggests secretory otitis media or 'glue ear' (p. 119–120). Finally, look at the throat for inflammation, exudates, membranes, the size and appearance of the tonsils and palpate the tonsillar lymph nodes below the ears. The size of the tonsils does not correlate with the frequency of infection.

Hearing

About 4.5 in 1000 preschool children need extra help on account of hearing loss at some stage. About 1 in 1000 will need a hearing aid at least temporarily and about 1 in 10 000 have profound hearing loss, delayed speech and will need special education.

Although children are entitled to routine evaluation of their hearing during their first year, some instances of profound deafness get missed. Other children acquire permanent deafness later from meningitis or encephalitis, ototoxic drugs, head injury, or late presentation of congenital abnormality, and many more develop severe but usually transient deafness associated with chronic secretory otitis media.

The key to detecting deafness is intensive history taking and observation of the child. Some severely deaf children learn to lip-read at an early stage. Turning up the TV very loudly and not noticing that the telephone is ringing are important clues. Even astute observers, however, may fail to suspect that all-important high tone frequency loss has occurred, so that low tone noises are readily heard but not the full components of speech and music. Such loss may make the child appear to be unintelligent.

Examination of the eardrums before undertaking a hearing test is important as it may reveal secretory otitis media and ear wax or foreign bodies in the external auditory meatus (Fig. 4.13). Deafness is usually due to secretory otitis media, leading to a conductive pattern of hearing loss with loss of lower frequencies. If chronic secretory otitis media is excluded, other causes of congenital or acquired abnormality of the conductive mechanism must be sought. Other children may have a sensorineural problem (see Information box 4.1), which causes a predominantly high frequency hearing loss.

Any child who is not hearing adequately will speak poorly and may appear mentally slow, disobedient and start to lip-read. Such children should have their hearing checked (Information box 4.2). The techniques can only be learnt by spending time with an audiologist who modifies their technique according to the child's stage of development. Initially they may use a recognized toy test in which the child is asked to recognize standardized toys and repeat lists of specially chosen words, which incorporate the full range of speech sounds, spoken at a standardized distance from the child. Eventually both ears should be checked separately. If such tests cannot be done locally or there is any doubt about the results, the child should be referred

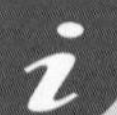

Information Box 4.1

Causes of high frequency hearing loss

- Prenatal viral infection; cytomegalovirus is now more common than rubella
- Kernicterus due to hyperbilirubinaemia (rare)
- Congenital abnormality of the inner ear
- Administration of aminoglycoside antibiotics
- Bacterial meningitis and viral encephalopathies, including measles and mumps
- Following head injury
- Genetic condition (e.g. Pendred syndrome)

Information Box 4.2

Indications for audiology assessment

- Significantly impaired language development
- History of chronic or repeated middle ear infection or upper airway obstruction
- Developmental delay or behavioural problems
- A family history of childhood deafness
- Parental concern, e.g. child not paying attention or turning the television sound up

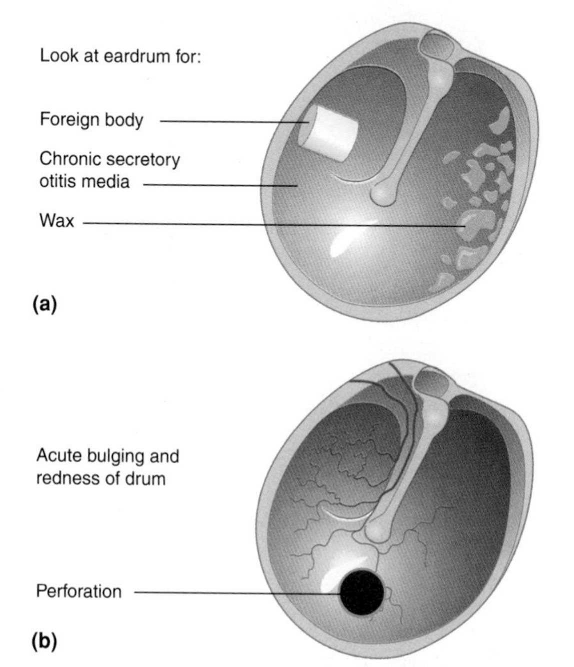

Fig 4.13
Examination of the eardrum.

for pure tone audiometry and possibly further tests including brain stem audiometry. This involves fitting earphones to the child. Sounds of varying pitch and loudness are transmitted to the child who is asked to make a very definite movement, say putting a toy in a box, each time they hear the sound. This is very skilled work and will only be carried out on selected children. The majority of children will have the chance to have their hearing re-checked on school entry in the course of a simplified audiometry 'sweep test' undertaken on the whole class at that time.

Speech and language

Normally children start to put meaningful words together at around 18 months and by 30 months they are making simple sentences. Speech delay beyond these key ages needs rapid action. Multidisciplinary review establishes that the child is seeing and hearing normally, has no global delay, and is exposed to spoken language. A speech therapist will then initiate treatment, often in a group. Speech delay is a priority for nursery admission; if there is no rapid improvement

Information Box 4.3

Causes of speech and language problems

- Deafness
- Dysarthria (defective quality of speech)
- Developmental delay
- Dysphonia (difficulty in speaking)
- Dysrhythmia (disturbed rhythm)
- Deprivation (social)
- Defective vision (the child cannot see items that are being discussed)
- Delayed or poor repair of cleft palate (or underdiagnosed submucous cleft)
- Disorders of the facial nerve (weakness)

the child may need to attend a speech and language unit. It is always best to initiate treatment rather than wait. Many children hear more than one language at home, but they should soon pick up English once they are exposed to it at school. Those with true speech delay may also have problems with understanding their parent's language. There are many causes of speech and language problems (Information box 4.3).

Examining the eyes

Many systemic and developmental disorders can be diagnosed by examining the eyes (see Fig. 4.14). The following signs are obvious:

- Purulent discharge.
- Abnormal shape of eyelids or pupils. In gross cases this is obvious, but minor squints are common (see Ch. 3). A late-onset squint suggests new origin of a cranial nerve disorder.
- Examining the optic disc in active infants whose pupils have not been artificially dilated can be very difficult, but abnormal findings are so important that this is a skill that must be learnt by constant practice. Is the disc edge sharp? If not is there evidence of raised intracranial pressure?

The harder question involves squint (Fig. 4.15). The easiest test is to determine whether distant window-panes reflect symmetrically on the cornea. If there is any doubt an ophthalmic specialist opinion is needed.

Visual handicap is common. Its prevalence is probably underestimated as it is very difficult to test vision accurately in young infants, and even more so in those with developmental delay who particularly need to have their vision assessed.

Watch the child for reaction to visual clues. Blind and partially sighted children tend to have hyperacute hearing and may react to auditory rather than visual clues. The STYCAR series of visual awareness tests are useful in skilled hands. Preliterate children from about 3 onwards can be tested by using Sheridan–Gardiner letter matching test cards, or the more recently introduced Silver–Sonksen test which uses crowded letters as in normal printed material. By 5 years of age

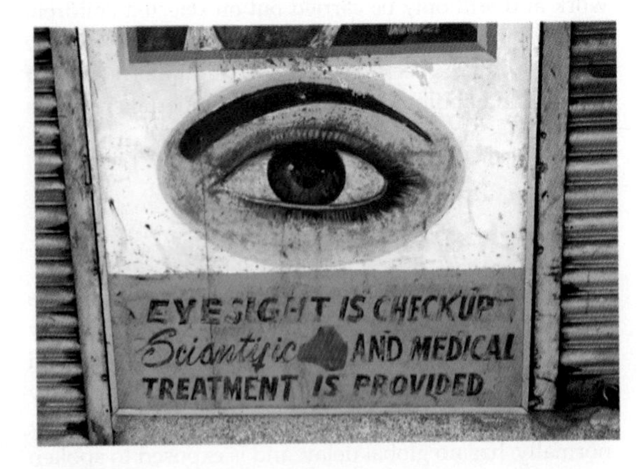

Fig 4.14
Eye examination is vital for spotting many ophthalmic and systemic disorders.

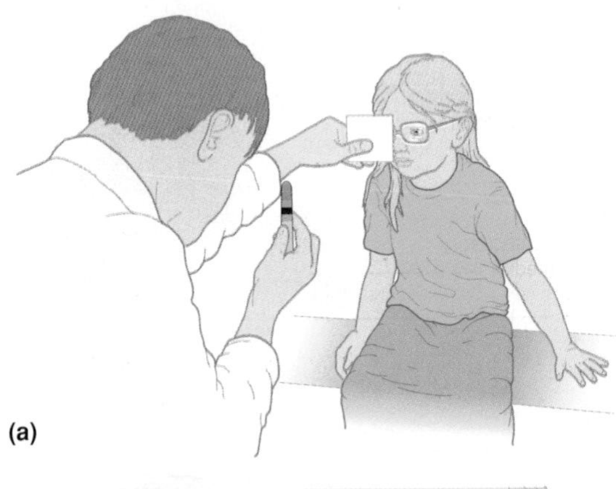

(a)

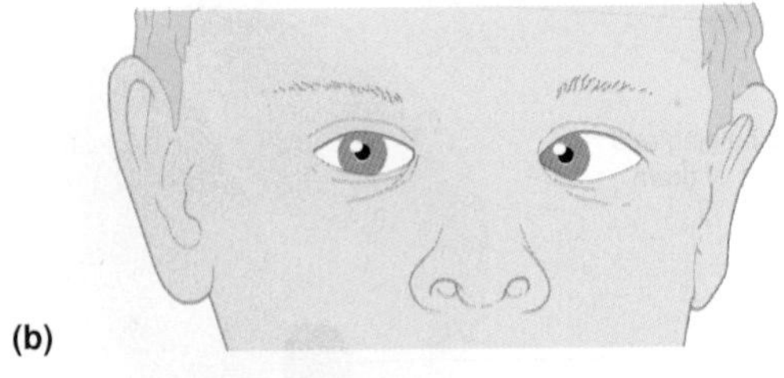

(b)

Fig 4.15
Examination for squint. (a) If the eye follows the stick as it is moved from side to side then the child is fixing on the stick. (b) The angle of the squint stays the same: if the right eye is straight then the left one will squint and vice versa.

Information Box 4.4

Causes of blindness

- Retinopathy of prematurity
- Cataract
- Retinoblastoma
- Optic atrophy
- Congenital, e.g. optic nerve hypoplasia
- Syndromic, e.g. septo-optic dysplasia
- Brain malformation or acquired brain problem, e.g. cerebral haemorrhage in neonates
- Albinism
- Retinal degeneration
- Severe myopia
- Untreated amblyopia

many children can use a simplified Snellen chart. It may be necessary to use a half-sized chart at a 3-metre distance or, preferably, a full-sized chart with reversed letters reflected in a mirror, in order to relate to the child. Both eyes are tested separately to detect unilateral problems. If there is the slightest doubt about the child's visual acuity or the presence of a squint, an ophthalmic opinion is needed.

To be registered blind, visual acuity in the better eye must be 3/60 or worse; those with visual acuity between 4/60 and 6/24 in the better eye are 'partially blind'. Visual handicap can mask the true intellectual ability of the child and appear to make developmental delay worse. Causes of blindness are presented in Information box 4.4.

Immunization

See also the Immunization section in Chapter 3 and Table 3.1 (p. 68).

Immunization schedules are liable to change and vary between countries. In the UK a government publication *Immunisation against Infectious Disease* is issued every few years and contains up-to-date information (Table 4.3). Worldwide, measles, pertussis and tuberculosis kill up to 1.5 million children a year; all these deaths are preventable through immunization. In the UK and other developed countries these infections, which are theoretically entirely preventable, still occur though thankfully in tiny numbers. Immunizations must be affordable and the reasons for administration must be understandable by and acceptable to the community. Vaccines must be of good quality, delivered in a safe and effective form and the cold chain, the means by which vaccines are always kept at the correct temperature, must be scrupulously maintained.

The British schedule in 2000 for children between 12 and 60 months comprised the following.

1. *Measles, mumps, rubella (MMR) vaccine.* This is usually given by a trivalent injection at ages 13–15 months (after passive immunity has waned). These are attenuated live virus vaccines. Although monocomponent measles vaccine had been available in the UK 20 years earlier, the national uptake rate had never been adequate to control the disease. Rubella vaccine was previously given to girls only just before puberty. MMR vaccine was introduced to UK practice in 1988. Uptake rates with the combined vaccine rose and the three diseases have largely come under control, but there are no grounds for complacency as scattered cases and small epidemics still occur. In 1994 there were signs that measles epidemics were starting to occur among older unimmunized young people. The decision was taken to advise that a second dose of MMR should be given prior to starting school, in order to boost immunity and give a second chance to immunize children who might have been missed the first time round. This policy having been established, much media attention was given to a report that inflammatory bowel disease and autism might be associated with measles vaccine. This hypothesis was

Table 4.3
Immunization uptake in the UK. Completed primary vaccinations (all antigens) by 12 months and 24 months, January to March 1996. (From Salisbury DM Begg N T (eds) (1996) *Immunization against Infectious Disease*. London: HMSO) © Crown copyright

	% coverage at 12 months	**% coverage at 24 months**	**% Health authorities reaching at least 90% coverage by 24 months**	**% Health authorities reaching at least 95% coverage by 24 months**
Diphtheria	93	96	98	75
Tetanus	93	96	98	75
Pertussis	92	94	91	43
Polio	93	96	98	73
Haemophilus influenzae b (Hib)	93	95	95	70
Measles, mumps, rubella (MMR)	N/A	91	73	9

not confirmed from other studies in Britain or abroad, but led to much parental confusion and a small drop in immunization levels.

2. *A single repeat injection of diphtheria and tetanus toxoid vaccine.* This is given before school entry, plus one dose of oral attenuated live trivalent (three types of poliovirus) *polio vaccine*. This is known as the 'pre-school booster'.

3. Those children who did not receive *Meningococcus* C vaccine in infancy are being given a single catch-up dose.

Care of the preschool child

Children with chronic illness and disability

Disabled or chronically sick children place great extra responsibilities on parents (see Information box 4.5), and every family will react differently. Some families find the emotional resources to cope with distressing problems whereas others are devastated by less severe disabilities. Some parents reject medical terms that imply disability or handicap, feeling that such terms and formal therapy may stigmatize the child. Other parents may eagerly seek a medical label, in the belief that modern medicine must have an answer to their child's problems if only the right doctor can be found. Parental suffering may be worse at times when they realize that the child is unable to walk or talk at the usual time or is unable to attend a mainstream school.

Parents may recognize the effects of disability or chronic illness at different rates. This can lead to conflict and disharmony which can be reduced if both parents are seen and counselled together. In a mutually supportive marriage, the relationship may be strengthened, but unstable relationships often collapse under the strain. Other members of the family take longer to accept the situation, particularly grand-parents, who may insist that the child is normal despite the evidence. Siblings will reflect their parents' emotions as well as having problems unique to themselves. They are likely to feel neglected and ignored and may express neurotic or antisocial symptoms. Their own social life may be disrupted or they may be embarrassed to bring friends home. Some hospitals organize 'siblings' groups' for brothers and sisters of children with chronic illnesses such as leukaemia, to make them feel important too.

The problems of the child who is disabled or has a chronic illness are complex and multiple. For the young child the judgement that he is disabled is not one that he makes himself, but is made by those around him, initially parents and professionals. Later, the child may or may not feel that he is disabled. In the early years, a programme to help the child achieve his maximum potential should be based on the normal development of daily living skills, such as feeding, dressing, mobility and language, although progress may be slower.

Parents and child may need breaks from each other. It can be very difficult for parents of a disabled child to make informal arrangements with friends and relatives for childminding. A limited amount of respite care is available in most parts of the UK usually via social services. Mostly this is for children with chronic disabilities such as severe learning difficulties. Children with life-threatening disorders tend to attract more sympathy and there are imaginative schemes supported by charities which supply home-visiting nurses and home-care workers in collaboration with major cancer-treating hospitals.

Information Box 4.5

Problems faced by children with disabilities and their families (From Dunn M, Kaufmann M, 96/97 Factfile. London: NCH Action for Children)

The Social Policy Research Unit (SPRU) undertook a national survey of over 1000 parents to explore the needs and circumstances of families caring for a severely disabled child. The researchers found that:

- Severely disabled children of all ages are highly dependent upon parents to meet their basic care needs. Older children are likely to have social, communication and behavioural problems.
- One in two children in the study were dependent upon at least one piece of medical equipment.
- On average, household incomes are lower among families with children with disabilities. Nine out of 10 lone parents in the study and over a third of two-parent families had no income other than benefits.
- Four out of 10 families live in unsuitable housing.
- Only half of those taking part described their relationship with professionals as positive and supportive.
- The most common unmet needs of parents were financial resources, help in planning for the child's future, help with care and knowledge of available services. The most common unmet needs of the children related to their physical needs, learning skills and someone with whom discuss their disability.
- Families from ethnic minorities, lone parents and those caring for the most severely impaired children had particularly high levels of unmet needs and tended to be living in the poorest circumstances.

Source: Expert opinions: a national survey of parents caring for a severely disabled child. Bryony Beresford, SPRU: 1995

Death and bereavement

It is impossible to take away the grief that comes from the loss of a child, but careful and sympathetic management of the death can help to avoid unnecessary pain for all concerned. Poor management will always be remembered and resented.

Some deaths are sudden and unexpected. Collapsed children will be brought into hospital by ambulance with 'suspended breathing' if there are no obvious signs of life. All doctors must know how to resuscitate children. Careful documentation is important. After death the child should be restored to as normal an appearance as possible by removing drips and ET tubes, before being handed to the parents with as much care as if he were alive. The parents must be given time, space and privacy to say their goodbyes. They need advice about the necessary formalities, including explanation about postmortem examinations that are legally required in sudden death. Parents need opportunities to talk over the reasons for their child's death. They may blame themselves or others including medical staff and much skilled help will be needed, sometimes repeatedly. Detailed postmortem histology, particularly of the brain, may not become available for several weeks. The retention of postmortem tissue has become a key issue and the need for parental consent has come to the fore. Genetic counselling may need to be offered particularly if the parents decide to have more children or are worried about the genetic implications for their other children.

TERMINAL CARE AND DEATH OF THE CHRONICALLY SICK CHILD

The terminal care of a chronically sick child should begin long before the child becomes moribund. Naturally parents wonder how long a child with a severe illness will survive. It can be disastrous to give specific predictions, which usually turn out to be wrong. Parents should be warned that estimates of survival are based on statistical data and may not be predictive for what will happen to a specific child. It is important to find out what the parents would wish to be done in the event of a life-threatening illness, and to negotiate a policy before the child reaches the terminal stage. Ideally, the same doctor who had previously been responsible for the child's general care should manage life-threatening medical problems in the severely disabled child. The doctor who knows the family well is more likely to be able to gauge their feelings as to appropriate management.

Ethical issues surrounding the maintenance of life in severe disability cannot be avoided; it is not desirable to have rigid rules derived from one's own personal beliefs, but to be guided by the parent's conscience. The medical responsibility is to determine what course of action is most acceptable in terms of the family's personal beliefs and then share the burden of that decision. When confronted with difficult situations, the views of colleagues may be helpful. All such consultations and the decisions reached should be carefully documented in the notes.

Sometimes it is difficult to decide when a child, who has been sick for a long time, is terminally ill. The parents may wish to care for the dying child at home, and arrangements should be made to support this wish. In hospital, the parents should be allowed access and privacy at all times and should be encouraged to touch and hold the child. Religious beliefs should be respected and appropriate arrangements made. Useful medications for terminally ill children include morphine for distress, hyoscine for excess salivation and midazolam for sedation and fit control. These can be combined and given by a continuous subcutaneous infusion through a syringe pump.

After death

After death, the death certificate needs to be completed. General practitioners and medical records departments should be informed of the death and pending outpatient appointments cancelled. Social workers, educational psychologists and teachers need to be notified promptly. Parents may appreciate practical help in managing funeral arrangements; they usually appreciate the request for donation of tissue for transplantation or research, even if only to decline it. They may need help over discussions with siblings or with how to organize a memorial for the child. Staff who know the child often wish to attend the funeral; this should be encouraged if the parents wish it.

The child's experience of death in others

A child's understanding of death develops gradually. Below 5 years, children see death as a temporary, reversible state, not unlike sleep in another place and continuous with life. They assume that life goes on, but under changed circumstances. A child can understand more than he can articulate. Toddlers and young children are exposed to death (of pets, for example) before they can talk about the experience, but can express their feelings through play. It has been estimated that the average child has seen about 10 000 killings on TV by age 10 as well as much murder and mayhem on news broadcasts.

If a sibling or parent dies, children are the least demanding members of bereaved families. They fear that other people in the family or even they themselves may disappear. They may express themselves in play or drawings or behaviour that others are unable to understand. There is a longing for the dead person, a wish to talk about them and a persisting sadness. Their grieving relatives may be unable to give them the attention they normally receive.

Protecting children from abuse

Preschool children are very vulnerable to abuse. During 1995, 8900 children between 1 and 4 years old were added to the Child Protection Register in England (Department of Health statistics); most were registered because of physical abuse, the next most common category being neglect (see Table 4.4).

Abuse may be perpetrated by either parent, acting alone or together, or by a member of the extended family without parental knowledge, or by outsiders. There has been much recent concern about instances in residential childcare 'homes', where children had been sent because of impossible parental circumstances.

Much thought has been given to the reasons why children are abused. This is not a new problem but it is getting ever more attention. Some parents lack self-esteem and expect much more of their children than they can give them. They appear to lack insight and the ability to nurture. Excessive crying may be interpreted as bad behaviour, which requires punishment. This can take a variety of forms. Any child who is disabled or has to rely excessively on caretakers becomes particularly vulnerable to abuse. Problems of mobility prevent escape and problems of communication may prevent disclosure; thus disabled children are at increased risk. Very rarely, parents have sadistic tendencies and wish to dominate or sexually assault children. The child can be abused as a result of a deliberate act or by a failure to provide adequate care. A small proportion of these children will die as a result of their injuries.

The key to protection is awareness of early clues. Dealing with the problems requires much skill gained through training and experience and constant vigilance. One of the most important skills is the ability to listen to children. For a discussion of the diagnosis and management of a child where there is suspicion of abuse, see Ch. 8 pp. 183–186.

Table 4.4
Children added to the Child Protection Register in England during the year ending 31 March 1995, aged 1–4, by category under which recorded

	Numbers/percentages of children
All	8900 children
Physical	44%
Neglect	35%
Sexual	15%
Emotional	12%

Some children were registered under more than one category

Accidents and the preschool child

Accidents are the most common cause of death in preschool children (see Table 4.1). Mobile children soon learn how to copy parents and reach household cleaning materials such as bleach or garden pest poisons and carelessly stored medicines. Drowning becomes a hazard in the bath and paddling pool; two-thirds of drowning accidents in the under-5s occur in and around the home. Falls from stairs and windows readily occur. The incidence of road accidents increases from 15 months, once children start walking independently in public. Cuts and bruises occur in imitative play, as children try to copy adult behaviour. Falls are common. Accidents also occur through breaking glass in windows, patio doors and greenhouses where safety glass is not installed. Of childhood burns and scalds, 70% occur in children under 5, although the number is decreasing thanks to less flammable clothes and better kitchen design.

The preschool child needs appropriate supervision inside and outside the home, and a safe environment with appropriate fastenings for doors and windows. Household cleaning materials and medicines should be stored securely and children should have safe areas for play, protected from traffic. (See also Section 2, p. 165.)

Growth and development

Normal growth

Growth is closely related to health and nutrition. Single measurements can mislead and are only of value if plotted on a centile chart. Serial measurements are the most important way of measuring growth. It is good practice to record the preschool child's height and weight at least annually on a growth centile chart (which is printed in the Child Health Record) and whenever the child is seen at the surgery or hospital, especially if there is concern about the child's growth or if a parent or teacher is concerned about the child's development. In the healthy child, growth and development go hand in hand and the final result is relatively predictable. In the disabled child, growth and development become dissociated from each other and the result is a mismatch between the two processes.

The maximum rates of increase in height, weight and head circumference have already occurred during the first year of life. By 1 year, most children weigh three times their birthweight and by 5 years they are usually twice their weight on their first birthday. Height measurement becomes more important once the child is

MEDICAL SCIENCES BOOKSHOP
Medical Sciences Building
University Road
LEICESTER LE1 7RD

MS01:000007-02 20th Jan 2007 11:34

RESPIRATPRY PHYSIOLOGY
1 * 9780781757485 @ 18.95 18.95
DIGESTIVE SYSTEM
1 * 9780443062452 @ 20.99 20.99
CLINICAL PAEDIATRICS AND CHILD
1 * 9780702017261 @ 31.99 31.99

Total at 0.00% VAT 71.93

Total 3 items 71.93

Visa Delta 71.93
Card 4929429608763018 Exp 04/08

Amount Tendered 71.93

Change Due 0.00

Thank you for your custom
'phone number: (0116) 252 3456
VAT number: GB 115121526

Please retain as proof of purchase

Information Box 4.6

Causes of short stature

Constitutional/familial	3% of normal children will lie below the third centile; check parental heights
Endocrine	Growth hormone deficiency Insensitivity to growth hormone (Laron syndrome) Hypopituitarism
Prematurity	Some infants who were extremely premature continue to grow poorly
Intrauterine growth retardation	The effects may continue after birth
Genetic disorders/ syndromes	Down syndrome Russell–Silver syndrome
Brain tumours	Craniopharyngioma Diencephalic syndrome
Malabsorption	Cystic fibrosis Coeliac disease
Poor feeding/gross neglect	
Emotional deprivation	
Bone growth disorders	Achondroplasia
Renal disorders	Renal tubular acidosis
Congenital heart disease	
Chronic respiratory disease	Cystic fibrosis Asthma (undertreated) Bronchiectasis
Iatrogenic	Corticosteroid treatment

able to stand. Roughly, the height at 24 months is half the final adult height.

Short stature

Causes of short stature are listed in Information box 4.6. Investigations of short stature are presented in Information box 4.7.

Nutrition

Worldwide, childhood malnutrition is still the most important cause of preventable death (Fig. 4.16) and vitamin A deficiency is the most common cause of blindness. In high income countries overnutrition has led to obesity becoming the commonest nutritional disorder. By the age of 1 year most children in high income countries have been weaned off the breast. In low income countries breastfeeding often lasts well into the second year. For children of this age breast milk

Information Box 4.7

Investigations of a child with short stature

Baseline investigations	Full blood count Erythrocyte sedimentation rate (ESR) Urea and electrolytes Creatinine Liver function tests Calcium/phosphate Urinalysis Urine culture Bone age Chromosomes in females, to exclude Turner syndrome Thyroid function Ferritin, iron, folate Coeliac antibody screen
Further investigations	Sweat test Chest radiograph Midnight and 9 a.m. cortisol Prolactin Growth hormone stimulation test Luteinizing hormone-releasing hormone (LHRH) stimulation test

contains inadequate iron and vitamins C and D and supplements are needed. Preschool children need a diet rich in calories in order to grow. The diet should also contain fruit, vegetables and fibre in moderation. Low fat versions of foods, particularly dairy products, are

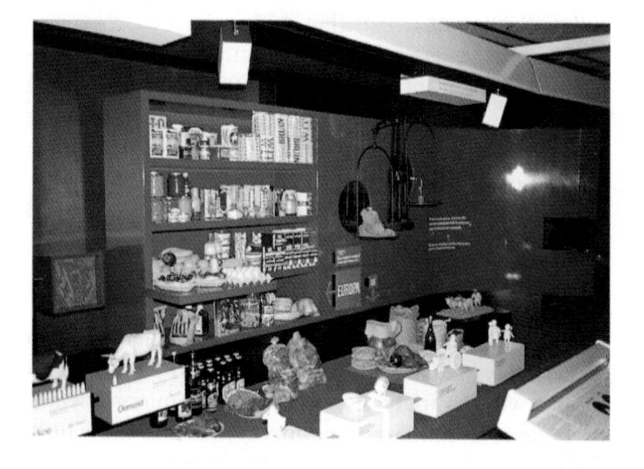

Fig 4.16
Food for a month: behind, for an adult in a high income country, and on the counter for an adult in a low income country. Note that the food from the low income country is largely dried and fibrous, with minimally expensive packaging but readily contaminated.

discouraged, as are excessive sugar and salt. Semi-skimmed milk can be introduced after 5 years of age. An increasing proportion of parents are vegetarian and expect their children to be likewise. Vegan diets are particularly low in iron, vitamin D and essential amino acids, fat-soluble vitamins and calories.

Iron-deficiency anaemia

Children fed solid diets inadequate in iron or vitamins will eventually develop severe anaemia and rickets, which can still be found in the UK.

Infection appears to deplete iron stores (see also Section 2, p. 250). Low haemoglobin is related to poverty and ethnic origin, with a prevalence of up to 30% in at-risk populations (e.g. Asian, African and Caribbean) in the second year of life. It is associated with reversible psychomotor delay and behavioural disorders in those most severely affected. High risk populations should be screened and individuals with a haemoglobin between 8 and 11 g/dl should be treated with a 6–8-week course of iron supplements and given dietary advice. Those with a haemoglobin of less than 8 g/dl or those who are resistant to treatment need further investigation for malabsorption or occult blood loss from the gut. Iron-deficiency is also found in toddlers who are excessive milk drinkers. This places responsibilities on primary and community health. Paediatric dieticians trained in multicultural dietary practices have an important role in the UK as advisor both to families and to health education programmes.

Rickets (Fig. 4.17)

Photoactivation of 7-dehydrocholesterol to pro-D_3 is the chief source of vitamin D in humans but dietary sources are also important. Poor sunlight absorption in African and Asian children in the UK can lead to inadequate vitamin D availability causing inadequate bone mineralization or rickets (Fig. 4.18).

Treatment is with oral vitamin D (1500–5000 IU/day) or intramuscularly (600 000 IU as a single injection) where compliance may be poor. Following treatment most of the bony deformities eventually heal. Not all cases of rickets are due to lack of vitamin D. Other causes include metabolic abnormality and renal disease.

Excessive cow's milk

By the end of the first year, most children will have been successfully weaned onto solid foods and have learned to cope with a variety of food textures. A minority want to continue to take large amounts of milk and show little desire for solid food. The mother, worried about the child's calorific intake may offer excessive quantities of milk. Once this is recognized as a problem, the amount of milk offered should be limited to 500 ml per day and the rest of the diet should be offered as regular meals. Although the child may initially complain, hunger usually results in eating a more balanced diet.

Transition to table foods

By the end of the first year, most children will be experimenting, with varying success, with finger foods.

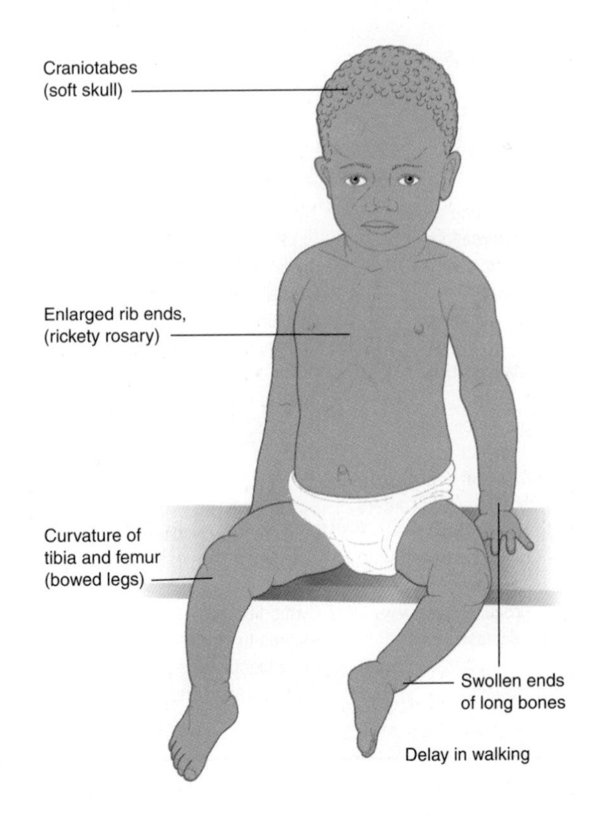

Fig 4.17
Clinical appearance and presentation in rickets.

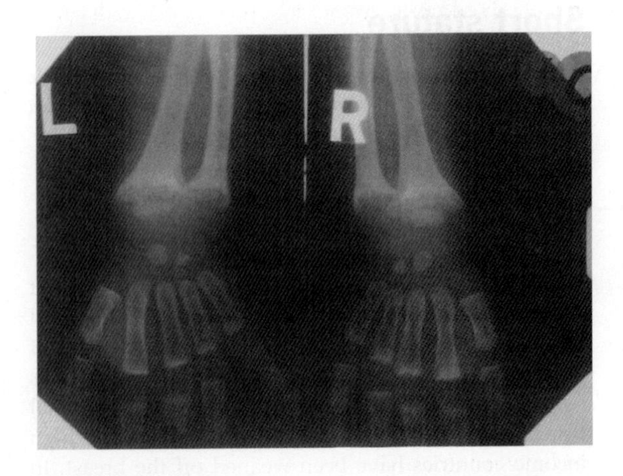

Fig 4.18
Wrist X-ray of a child with rickets showing widened irregular epiphysis.

Families should be encouraged to eat together at set times, so that the child can learn that mealtimes can be enjoyable social occasions free from television or toys. The child may be slow to eat and it is important that the meal should not drag on for longer than about half an hour. The child should be encouraged to feed himself, be offered foods which let him do this, and be allowed to make a reasonable mess.

Picky habits

Many children go through phases of refusing to eat certain foods or at times even refusing to eat anything at all as a way of showing independence – a normal part of growing up. The parents need to offer regular meals rather than letting the child pick through the day. A child should never be forced to eat and parents should try to appear indifferent rather than annoyed. Make sure that he isn't being filled up with fizzy drinks, squash, crisps and biscuits between meals. Small portions of food should be offered at mealtimes, and more offered if these are eaten up. Alternative foods should not be offered if the child refuses what is offered initially.

Food intolerance

Food intolerance is a reproducible adverse reaction to a specific food. The term food allergy should only be used when there is evidence that the reaction is due to an immunological response and not for more trivial indications.

Children who are allergic to cow's milk, eggs, nuts and fruit develop a variety of reactions from urticaria, through swelling of the mouth and lips, to full blown anaphylaxis. Children who are intolerant of cow's milk may also develop vomiting and diarrhoea; some will also be intolerant of soya milk. A high proportion of children who are intolerant of cow's milk or egg will become tolerant with time, usually by the third birthday. Their reactions tend to be less severe and parents should be given advice about total exclusion of the offending foodstuff.

Nut or fish intolerance is more likely to persist. Peanut intolerance maybe lifelong and potentially fatal in older children. Peanuts are not true nuts; they are widely used in manufactured foods. They may be used to bulk out other nut products and machinery may become contaminated. Patients who are intolerant of peanuts should thus be advised to avoid true nuts as well. It may be necessary for parents of children who have had severe peanut reactions to carry an injectable form of adrenaline in case of an emergency. It will be necessary to instruct everyone looking after the child, including teachers and playgroup leaders, about what a reaction looks like and how to give the injections (see Anaphylaxis, p. 353).

The growth of children on exclusion diets must be carefully monitored to ensure that they are getting enough calories and a correct balance of nutrients. Such patients need to be referred to a state-registered dietician. There is an increasing tendency for parents to follow bizarre diets which they may impose on their children; these can lead to severe deficiency states.

Obesity

Childhood obesity is becoming increasingly frequent in western countries. The ponderal index that applies to adults does not allow for age, making formal calculation and definition of childhood obesity difficult. Around 20% of preschool children can be regarded as overweight, and when followed up it is found that they tend to remain fat. Onset of obesity before the age of 2 years has a better prognosis than obesity of later onset.

Obesity is an easier problem to prevent than solve. It is essential when treating the obese child that the whole family's way of eating is changed. Parents need to understand that whatever they think caused the obesity, weight can only be lost by the child eating less than is actually needed. Parents must take full responsibility for their child's weight, as it is they who have bought and served up the food which has made the child fat. Cans of 'regular' fizzy drinks may contain the equivalent of ten lumps of sugar. Rather than losing weight, the child is encouraged to 'grow into' their current weight. Adequate nutrients must be ensured for longitudinal growth. Hunger is avoided by regular meals; even low calorie snacks between meals should be avoided. All the family are encouraged to increase their exercise.

Food fads and pica

Some children develop bizarre eating habits; sometimes they are conscious attempts to exert authority or to copy behaviour seen elsewhere. Other children can be very choosy from an early age and reject food that parents know to be nutritious. Most of these fads are harmless and most disappear if the family can bring themselves to ignore them.

Pica, the eating of non-food substances is another matter. Children may pick at old flaky paint or plaster containing lead or other noxious substances and poison themselves. These children may be iron-deficient and subconsciously seeking iron. Such children need investigation and steps should be taken to remove the harmful substances.

Neurodevelopmental evaluation

Developmental paediatrics is a specialty in its own right. Knowledge of the major developmental milestones from informed study of the wide range of normality equips one to recognize the child with developmental delay.

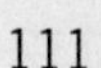

At 1 year of age, most children are near to walking, or at least standing upright holding on to furniture, can self-feed and can pick up small objects with a pincer grip movement. They speak in single words, have a brief attention span, self-centred lifestyle and are still incontinent of urine and faeces. By 5 years of age the normal child can run, climb, hop, dance and walk up and down stairs in an adult manner. They should be able to speak in complex sentences, sometimes in more than one language, be continent of urine and faeces (although some still wet at night), use a spoon, feed, dress and have a concept of right, wrong and argument. Some can read and understand numbers; all love drawing and being read to.

Developmental milestones (or stepping stones)

Aspects of development can be separated into sequences which are achieved at similar ages, known as 'developmental milestones' (Table 4.5). There is a wide natural variation in rates of normal child development, but in health the outcome should conform to a predictable pattern. Delayed development should not be missed. Even though this may be obvious to an outsider, parents or grandparents may at least temporarily deny its presence. Health professionals must know enough about normal development to

Table 4.5
Developmental milestones between 1 and 5 years of age*

15 months	
Motor	Walks alone: crawls up stairs
Adaptive	Makes tower of 3 cubes; makes a line with crayon; inserts pellet in bottle
Language	Jargon; follows simple commands; may name a familiar object (ball)
Social	Indicates some desires or needs by pointing; hugs parents
18 months	
Motor	Runs stiffly; sits on small chair; walks up stairs with one hand held; explores drawers and waste baskets
Adaptive	Makes a tower of 4 cubes; imitates scribbling; imitates vertical stroke; dumps pellet from bottle
Language	10 words (average); names pictures; identifies one or more parts of body
Social	Feeds self; seeks help when in trouble; may complain when wet or soiled; kisses parent
24 months	
Motor	Runs well; walks up and down stairs, one step at a time; opens doors; climbs on furniture; jumps
Adaptive	Tower of 7 cubes (6 at 21 months); circular scribbling; imitates horizontal stroke; folds paper once imitatively
Language	Puts 3 words together (subject, verb, object)
Social	Handles spoon well; often tells immediate experiences; helps to undress; listens to stories with pictures
30 months	
Motor	Goes up stairs alternating feet
Adaptive	Tower of 9 cubes; makes vertical and horizontal strokes, but generally will not join them to make a cross; imitates circular stroke, forming closed figure
Language	Refers to self by pronoun 'I'; knows full name
Social	Helps put things away; pretends in play
36 months	
Motor	Rides tricycle; stands momentarily on one foot
Adaptive	Tower of 10 cubes; imitates construction of 'bridge' of 3 cubes; copies a circle; imitates a cross
Language	Knows age and sex; counts 3 objects correctly; repeats 3 numbers or a sentence of 6 syllables
Social	Plays simple games (in 'parallel' with other children); helps in dressing (unbuttons clothing and puts on shoes): washes hands
48 months	
Motor	Hops on one foot; throws ball overhand; uses scissors to cut out pictures; climbs well
Adaptive	Copies bridge from model; imitates construction of 'gate' of 5 cubes; copies cross and square; draws a man with 2 to 4 parts besides head; names longer of 2 lines
Language	Counts 4 pennies accurately; tells a story
Social	Plays with several children with beginning of social interaction and role-playing; goes to toilet alone
60 months	
Motor	Skips
Adaptive	Draws triangle from copy; names heavier of 2 weights
Language	Names 4 colours; repeats sentence of 10 syllables; counts 10 pennies correctly
Social	Dresses and undresses; asks questions about meaning of words; domestic role-playing

* Data are derived from those of Gesell (as revised by Knobloch, Shirley, Provence, Wolf, Bailey, and others). After 5 years the Stanford–Binet, Wechsler–Bellevue, and other scales offer the most precise estimates of developmental level. In order to have their greatest value, they should be administered only by an experienced and qualified person.

detect abnormalities and act on suspicions when unsure. Constant vigilance is needed in order to detect newly presenting physical and psychological signs. Every time you examine a child remember to ask whether this child can hear, see, think, behave and perform at an age-appropriate level. Always take seriously any comment from the parent that the child is not hearing or behaving normally; great harm can be done by inappropriate reassurance.

A child may be behind in one modality of development but not in others, so detailed assessment of all modalities is needed. Schedules of developmental observation and testing have been drawn up in the UK by Griffith, Sheridan and Bellman, and in the US as the Denver and Bayley developmental scales. These are systems whereby the developmental achievements of children can be charted chronologically. These are time-consuming and special training is needed to use them to the full. Useful clinical information can be collected by simpler means such as jigsaw puzzles.

The average girl takes two consecutive steps at 13 months and the average boy at 14.5 months. The normal range is from 10 to 18 months, with racial differences: many children of African and Caribbean origin walk with one hand held at 7 months. Hence a black child of 16 months who does not walk may present more cause for concern than a white one. Late walking occurs for many reasons; it depends on the maturity of the central and peripheral nervous systems and the strength of the muscles and bones. Whilst the majority of 'late walkers' give no cause for concern, the question of muscular dystophy will need to be considered in boys who do not walk during the latter part of the second year. Typically they have difficulty in rising from the floor and 'climb up their legs' (Fig. 4.19). A greatly raised creatine phosphokinase is the key biochemical test, prior to referral to a muscle clinic for fuller investigation.

Developmental testing requires a thorough knowledge of paediatrics and developmental psychology, tempered with experience in working with children. Often it is not possible to make one's mind up on a single occasion, especially if the child is tired or unwell, so be prepared to repeat the examination later. Developmental assessment gives contemporary information, which can lead to a diagnosis, but unless a clear-cut syndrome is found, it cannot predict the future. It aims to detect problems at a stage when remedial action can be taken or, if this is not possible, early, accurate advice and realistic planning for therapy, education and genetic counselling. The results allow sensible advice to be given to the parents and a suitable treatment programme drawn up. Assessment which does not lead to practical help is of little value.

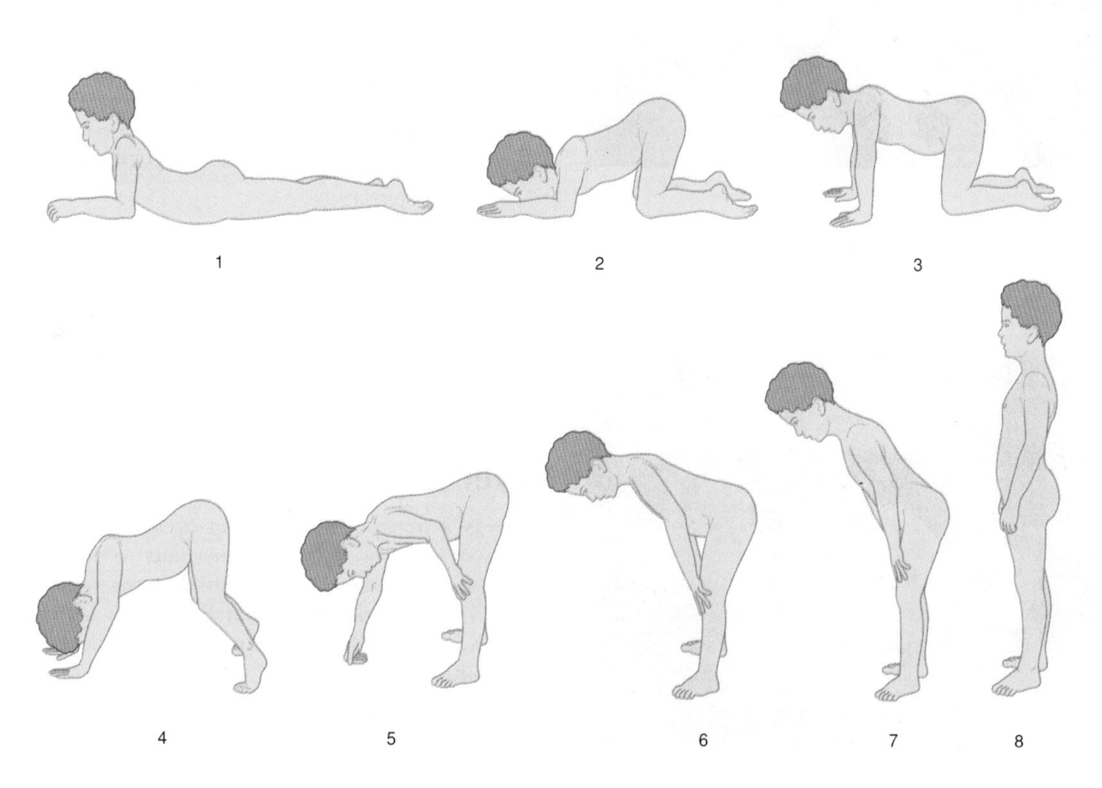

Fig 4.19
A child with muscular dystrophy 'climbing up his legs' to raise himself to a standing position.

Assessment must be multidisciplinary and may involve children's nurses, therapists (physiotherapy, speech, occupational and psychological), geneticists and surgeons, as well as paediatricians with special skills in neurodevelopment and psychiatry. Nearly all children with disabilities need careful audiometry and visual assessment. Professionals and voluntary organizations work together with parents as a Child Development Team, based in a Child Development Centre (Fig. 4.20) where diagnostic assessments and treatments can be carried out. These centres may also form a powerful focus for teaching and research.

Voluntary organizations may be involved at a local or national level. The latter tend to concentrate on single disabilities (Fig. 4.21). They usually organize local meetings and produce newsletters as well as stimulating interest and research into 'their' condition.

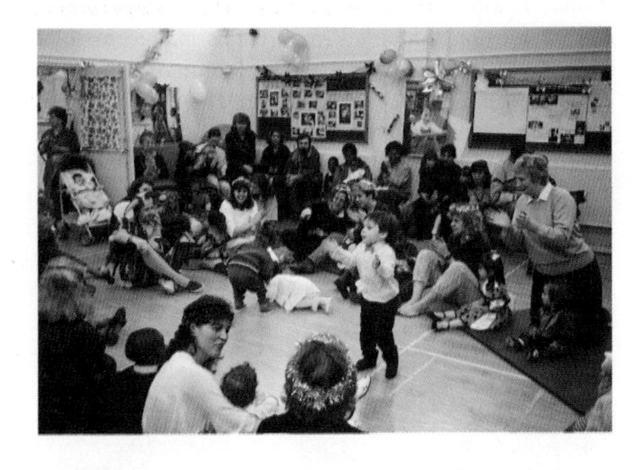

Fig 4.20
Party time at the Child Development Centre.

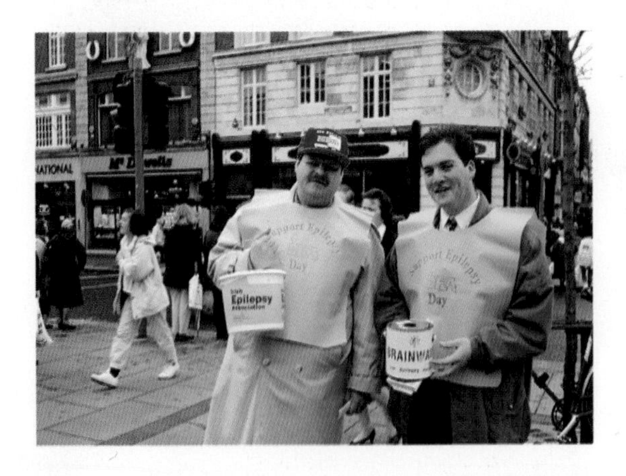

Fig 4.21
Collecting money for epilepsy research, Dublin.

Problems in children with syndromes and other globally disabling disorders

Children with genetic disorders have a greatly increased prevalence of behavioural problems. Sometimes the behavioural problem is recognized first and then a search is made for a syndrome. In some instances, e.g. fragile X syndrome the main problem is short attention coupled with decreased intelligence. There are many other instances where behavioural characteristics plus low intelligence run together; Prader–Willi syndrome is another example.

The majority of children with psychological problems are of normal intelligence. They may present with a somatic symptom such as enuresis or encopresis (see p. 155, 219); physical examination and routine blood studies usually reveal nothing but the history may well reveal complex social problems. The difficulty is knowing whether the latter are causal, and how commonly similar social problems occur among the nonaffected.

Whilst history taking is particularly important in child psychiatry, it is important to remain strictly nonjudgmental and not to seek simplistic causes for problems which can lead to victim blaming. Social deprivation and poverty underlie a great many behavioural problems. Sometimes the poverty is not financial but associated with deep-seated family problems.

Symptoms of acute illness in young children

Recognizing whether a child is seriously ill or has a minor illness can be very difficult, especially in the early stages. Much experience is needed, yet the most experienced paediatrician can readily be humbled.

Fever

Fever is a nonspecific sign that occurs in a huge variety of illnesses. A thermometer must be used for temperature assessment. Circadian rhythms, exercise, stress, disease, and individual thermostat settings in the hypothalamus influence normal body temperature.

Axillary temperatures are often the method of choice for parents and medical staff. The normal axillary temperature range for young children is between 35.2°C and 37°C. Fever is an axillary temperature above 37°C or a rectal temperature above 38°C.

Axillary temperatures are roughly 1 °C lower and oral temperatures 0.5 °C lower than rectal temperature measurements.

Physiological effects of fever include increased metabolic rate, tachypnoea, tachycardia, malaise, irritability, and vasodilatation leading to flushed, moist and warm skin. Differentiating serious bacterial illness from viral illness, especially in children less than 2 years of age, is a major challenge. A fever greater than 38 °C, leukocytosis (WBC count >15 000), absence of focal findings on examination and a relatively 'well' appearance are typical of occult bacteraemia. It is important not to miss these signs as they may progress to more serious problems such as meningitis. Sepsis or septicaemia, by contrast, implies a severe illness with signs of widespread infection and a 'toxic' appearing child. High fever, agitation or profound lethargy, unresponsiveness or inconsolability are ominous features.

The history taken on a febrile child should focus on changes in behaviour, activity level, eating, drinking and eliminating patterns. Are there any CNS, urinary, ENT, respiratory, gastrointestinal, musculoskeletal or dermatological symptoms? Has the child been exposed to anyone at home, school or playgroup with similar symptoms? A thorough physical examination looking for a focus of infection is mandatory, but observation of a toddler's behaviour frequently provides the best clues regarding severity of illness. Reassuring signs include spontaneous eye contact, interest in the environment, playing, vocalizing or talking, smiling, interacting with parents or the examiner and being easily comforted. Adequate doses of antipyretics should be given early in the illness, since children who initially appear quite ill may dramatically improve permitting a more accurate assessment of their condition.

Investigations of fever in toddlers without a focus of infection include blood culture, full blood count (FBC) with differential and film, urinalysis and urine culture on a clean catch specimen. A chest X-ray especially in children under 2 may be needed since chest physical signs can be unreliable. Lumbar puncture (LP) is performed when the possibility of meningitis cannot be excluded, bearing in mind that the classical sign, neck stiffness, may not be present in toddlers (see p. 280).

The following febrile conditions in preschool children are highly likely to be due to bacterial infection and will warrant antibiotic treatment:

- Otitis media (OM)
- Pneumonia
- Urinary tract infection (UTI)
- Follicular tonsillitis.

In about 40% of incidents of febrile illness a virus can be demonstrated if thorough investigation is instigated; with improving techniques this proportion is likely to rise, though in everyday clinical practice virological studies are reserved for cases where making a diagnosis is considered essential. In every recent decade more and more pathogenic viruses have been recognized. Fevers above 42 °C are rare and usually result from CNS trauma or heat stroke rather than infection. Other noninfectious causes of fever include collagen vascular disorders, e.g. systemic onset juvenile idiopathic arthritis, and neoplasia, e.g. leukaemia and Wilms' tumour, and drug reactions.

Note. Always ask about recent foreign travel and never forget malaria.

FEVER MANAGEMENT

Not all fevers require treatment. It is important to treat the patient rather than the temperature. If the temperature is below 38.5 °C, the child is comfortable, drinking well and not irritable and there is no sign of neck stiffness or a nonblanching rash it is appropriate to watch and wait. Fever is a normal physiological response to infection. If the child is uncomfortable, or known to be at risk of febrile seizures or has a condition such as congenital heart disease where the increased metabolic demand associated with even mild fever may aggravate the situation, symptomatic fever reduction is indicated (See Practical box 4.3)

Educating and reassuring parents is important. They need to know how to treat fever, what to expect from treatment and when to seek medical attention. Since parents worry about 'brain damage' from high fevers,

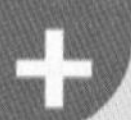

Practical Box 4.3

Symptomatic fever reduction includes:

1. Adequate oral hydration with clear cool liquids, ice-lollies, etc.
2. Sponging with tepid water to enhance evaporation from skin surfaces. NB. If the child begins to shiver, sponging should cease since shivering is a physiologic response to cold and results in increased body temperature.
3. Removing clothing or blankets to minimize heat retention.
4. Medications such as paracetamol 10–15 mg/kg 4-hourly or ibuprofen 5–10 mg/kg 6-hourly. Aspirin should not be given to children because its administration, especially to those with chickenpox and influenza, has been associated with the development of Reye syndrome (see p. 260).

A one- to two-degree centigrade drop in fever within 1 hour of treatment with either paracetamol or ibuprofen should occur, but the child's temperature may not return completely to normal. Antipyretics need to be given at appropriate intervals to be effective.

advice that neurologic damage does not occur from fever below 41 °C should be reassuring. Parents should be instructed to seek medical attention: if the fever does not respond to symptomatic treatment; if it persists beyond 48 to 72 hours; if the child has a nonblanching rash; if the child is refusing fluids, becomes less responsive or more irritable, or has a chronic health problem associated with immune deficiency where even minor fever could signal life-threatening infection.

Abdominal pain

'Tummy ache' is a common problem in preschool children. A detailed history is essential to diagnosis; you will need to know how long the child has had abdominal pain and about its nature. If the pain is intermittent, ask about the frequency and duration and how the child reacts when the pain occurs. Enquire about the site; it is said that the further the pain is localized away from the umbilicus, the more likely the pain is to be organic in nature. Similarly, if the site of the pain varies, it is less likely to be due to organic disease (but beware appendicitis, which begins in the umbilical region then localizes to the right iliac fossa). A pain associated with pallor or vomiting and followed by sleep may be abdominal migraine, especially if other members of the family have migraine too. Always ask about precipitating and relieving factors. A stabbing pain may be pleural or peritoneal in origin and the child may be holding his abdomen stiff like a board to protect it; the commonest cause of peritonitis is a perforated appendix. Abdominal pain associated with diarrhoea suggests a gastrointestinal cause, although urinary tract infection may present in this way. Any child presenting with abdominal pain should have urine examined for infection. Examine for masses, site of maximum tenderness, rebound tenderness or guarding, and never forget to check the hernial orifices and the scrotum.

Some of the commonest causes of abdominal pain are listed in Information box 4.8; the acute abdomen (p. 207), acute appendicitis (p. 208), and intussusception (p. 209) are discussed in Ch. 11. Chronic recurrent abdominal pain is defined as more than three attacks of pain occurring over 3 months and is also discussed in Ch. 11.

Cautionary note. Acute diabetic ketosis can present with acute abdominal pain. Check urine for glucose and ketones before operating.

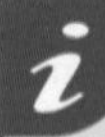

Information Box 4.8

Causes of abdominal pain in childhood

Intussusception
Volvulus
Strangulated hernia
Appendicitis
Meckel's diverticulum
Referred pain from pneumonia
Renal tract disease, especially urinary tract infection (UTI)
Diabetes mellitus
Gastroenteritis
Migraine
Recurrent abdominal pain

Vomiting (see also p. 234)

Young children vomit much more readily than adults do. The vomiting is more likely to have an organic cause if it is sudden in onset or if there is weight loss. The commonest organic cause of vomiting is infection, particularly urinary tract infections (p. 297) and meningitis (see p. 280, and Information box 4.9). Recurrent vomiting may be due to the periodic syndrome, recurrent volvulus or herniation, recurrent urinary tract infection or migraine. Bile-stained vomiting usually indicates intestinal obstruction and warrants a surgical opinion, but may also occur after prolonged vomiting. Unexplained vomiting may be due to drugs or poisons. Vomiting because of psychological factors, such as excitement, fear or attention seeking, is common; the child will be well between attacks.

Cautionary note. Be aware of brain tumour being the cause of daily effortless morning vomiting.

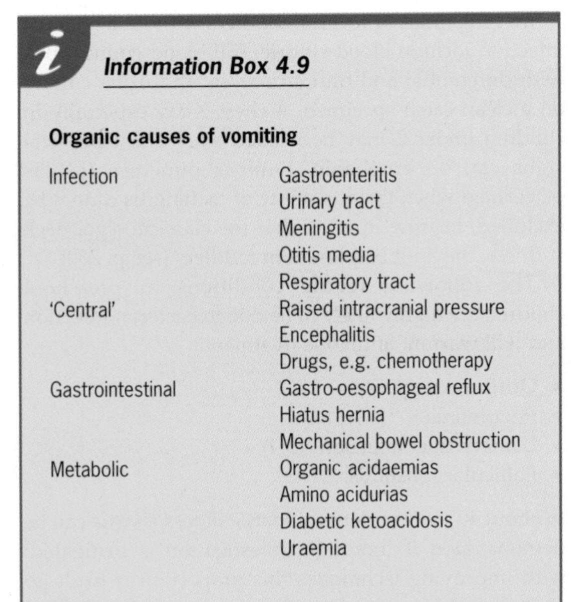

Information Box 4.9

Organic causes of vomiting

Infection	Gastroenteritis
	Urinary tract
	Meningitis
	Otitis media
	Respiratory tract
'Central'	Raised intracranial pressure
	Encephalitis
	Drugs, e.g. chemotherapy
Gastrointestinal	Gastro-oesophageal reflux
	Hiatus hernia
	Mechanical bowel obstruction
Metabolic	Organic acidaemias
	Amino acidurias
	Diabetic ketoacidosis
	Uraemia

Diarrhoea

Diarrhoea can be regarded as more than three loose stools per day and continues to be a problem in this age group, although less so than in the first year.

The commonest cause of acute diarrhoea is infection, usually due to food contamination or viral gastroenteritis. The degree of hydration needs to be assessed and fluids replaced either by an electrolyte solution given orally or by intravenous fluids. Acute diarrhoea needs no further treatment and should resolve on its own (see p. 221).

Diarrhoea is regarded as chronic if it lasts longer than 2 weeks. Chronic diarrhoea in developing countries usually follows acute diarrhoea and can result in malnutrition due to persisting damage to the gut lining. Specialized diets based on locally available foods are being devised to manage chronic diarrhoea. In developed countries the commonest cause of chronic diarrhoea in children up to 3 is 'toddler diarrhoea' (see p. 230), which contains altered food particles, such as peas and carrots, and is due to rapid gut transit. The child will have normal weight gain. Exclude carbohydrate intolerance (sucrose and lactose) and giardiasis (see p. 228–230).

The next task is to convince the parents that their child is healthy, albeit with loose stools. Loperamide (a drug which must be used with caution due to the danger of overdose and retention of toxic bowel products in enteric disease) can be helpful when stools are very loose. Diets high in fats can decrease intestinal transit time and reduce stool frequency. Toddler diarrhoea usually improves with age.

Constipation (see p. 219)

Regularity of bowel movement is a cultural fixation and children cannot escape parental anxiety about their bowel habits, which in perfectly normal health may vary from motions several times a day to two to three times a week. Parents need to know that children differ in the frequency with which they naturally have their bowels open. Food containing fibre is important and the trick is to encourage children in appropriate eating habits from an early age.

For more severe cases of constipation treatment with large doses of laxatives is required (see below). A decision may have to be made concerning whether a child has a behavioural disorder combined with inappropriate defecation. Input from child psychiatry may be needed. There are also rare, but very important, organic causes of constipation which include Hirschsprung disease (ask about delay in meconium passage after birth), mechanical abdominal obstruction, hypercalcaemia and hypothyroidism.

In the absence of one of these serious causes, management depends on the degree of constipation. In mild cases, encourage a high fluid and fibre diet with regular lactulose and senna. In more severe cases where there is obvious faecal overload and a palpable descending colon, the bowel needs to be evacuated with suppositions; the help of sodium docusate or sodium picosulphate; enemas may also be needed, but should only be administered to children under sedation. This should be followed by a programme of regular laxatives and careful follow up. In most cases the constipation will resolve within months. The laxatives must be gradually reduced, to prevent relapse, sometimes over a period of a couple of years. Relapse is common and may be due to either inadequate evacuation or too rapid reduction in therapy.

Failure to thrive

Failure to thrive (FTT) is a key concept in paediatrics. It can be defined as a decline in weight gain crossing two centiles on the child's growth chart. Height and head circumference may also be involved. FTT is common and accounts for about 1–5% of referrals to paediatric outpatient clinics. More than 80% of cases reflect normal variants or environmental problems and are the focus of this section. In general poor weight gain reflects inadequate calorie intake, poor absorption or increased losses of nutrients. A reduction in height velocity with minimal change in weight or head circumference is frequently of endocrine origin and a primary decline in OFC reflects a CNS problem. These children are usually under 3 years of age at presentation and there is an equal sex incidence.

Environmental failure to thrive

The differential diagnosis of FTT includes early onset growth deceleration. A child may be born with height, weight and occipitofrontal circumference (OFC) on the 75th centile and slowly adjust to ultimately grow along the 50th or 25th. This is usually achieved by 13 months of age and reflects genetic potential. In approximately 20% of cases FTT results from organic disease. These are discussed in greater detail on pages 77, 227. Social factors contributing to FTT are summarized in Information box 4.10.

The history and findings on examination will influence the choice of laboratory investigations. Simple screening tests include full blood count, urea and electrolytes (U&Es), urinalysis and culture, and thyroid function. Children who continue losing weight as outpatients, those who are at risk of abuse or who are severely malnourished should be admitted to hospital. The outcome for children with environmental FTT is generally good if therapy is directed at optimizing nutrition and assisting the family to ameliorate social, emotional and financial stresses.

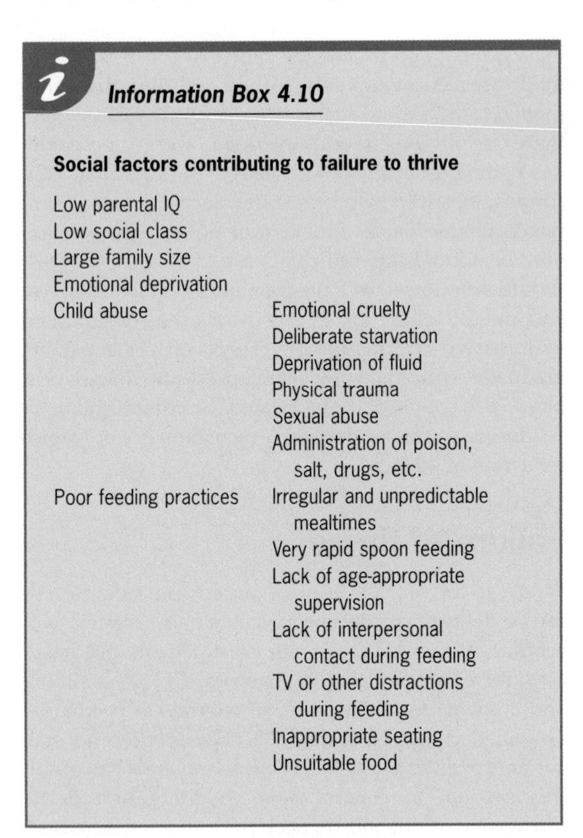

Information Box 4.10

Social factors contributing to failure to thrive

Low parental IQ	
Low social class	
Large family size	
Emotional deprivation	
Child abuse	Emotional cruelty
	Deliberate starvation
	Deprivation of fluid
	Physical trauma
	Sexual abuse
	Administration of poison, salt, drugs, etc.
Poor feeding practices	Irregular and unpredictable mealtimes
	Very rapid spoon feeding
	Lack of age-appropriate supervision
	Lack of interpersonal contact during feeding
	TV or other distractions during feeding
	Inappropriate seating
	Unsuitable food

Unfortunately, up to one-third may have permanent deficits in growth, intellectual achievement and social functioning.

Fatigue

Fatigue in toddlers is often fleeting. Fatigue prompting a paediatric visit is infrequent and deserves careful consideration. It may present as irritability, excessive sleepiness and tiredness despite adequate rest, inability to keep up with playmates or lack of interest in playing. Questions regarding onset and duration of fatigue, associated symptoms, timing of symptoms and medications may assist in determining the cause. There may be few physical signs other than poor growth, but pale conjunctivae or skin tone, petechiae or excessive bruising, lymphadenopathy, wheezing, crackles or a new murmur may be clues.

Infectious causes include bacteraemia, hepatitis, TB and intestinal parasites. Poorly managed asthma, presenting as fatigue with chronic nocturnal cough is not unusual. Endocrine disorders such as hypothyroidism and adrenal insufficiency will usually have been diagnosed in infancy but Cushing syndrome may present with fatigue, obesity and short stature. Previously undiagnosed congenital heart disease, congestive heart failure, renal failure, renal tubular acidosis and juvenile rheumatoid arthritis may all present with fatigue as the major symptom. Malignancies such as acute lymphocytic leukaemia, lymphomas or solid tumours may present with fatigue as an early symptom. Chronic intermittent upper airway obstruction manifesting as snoring, fatigue and lethargy may be due to anatomic abnormalities or adenotonsillar hypertrophy. Finally, side-effects from medications such as anti-epilepsy drugs and antihistamines are always a possibility.

Simple investigations may include FBC, erythrocyte sedimentation rate (ESR) or C reactive protein (CRP), U&Es, urinalysis, and Mantoux test with more extensive testing directed by the clinical condition.

Note. Bottles of tonic or their latter day replacements are not the answer.

Headache

Headache is an uncommon complaint in young children since their ability to express it verbally before 3–4 years is limited. It may manifest as irritability, lethargy, nausea and vomiting, and the child may point to or hold his head. History is directed at frequency, timing and associated symptoms. Most often headaches in childhood are benign and may accompany minor infectious illnesses. Rarely they signal a more ominous process. There may be a history of head trauma with concussion. A pattern of headaches on waking or early morning vomiting must be taken seriously, as they could be associated with raised intracranial pressure due to brain tumours or other causes of raised intracranial pressure which should be considered.

Physical examination includes measuring blood pressure to rule out hypertension, and careful neurologic and ocular examinations (Fig. 4.22). Hydrocephalus and brain tumours may result in raised intracranial pressure with blurred optic discs, changes in visual fields or ataxic gait. Meningitis and encephalitis may present with photophobia and general irritability as a sign of meningeal irritation. Neck stiffness and Kernig's sign may be absent in children under 2. Rarely, lead intoxication may present with headache, muscle weakness and ataxia in toddlers. Refractive errors are often cited as causes of headache but rarely prove to be the whole answer. Occasionally referred pain from ear or throat infections may present as headache and become evident upon ear, nose and throat (ENT) examination.

If the child's neurologic, ocular and ENT examinations are normal, investigations are generally not required and paracetamol should provide adequate pain relief. If the neurologic examination is abnormal or the history is suggestive of intracranial haemorrhage or raised intracranial pressure, a CT or MRI scan is appropriate. A lumbar puncture is indicated on

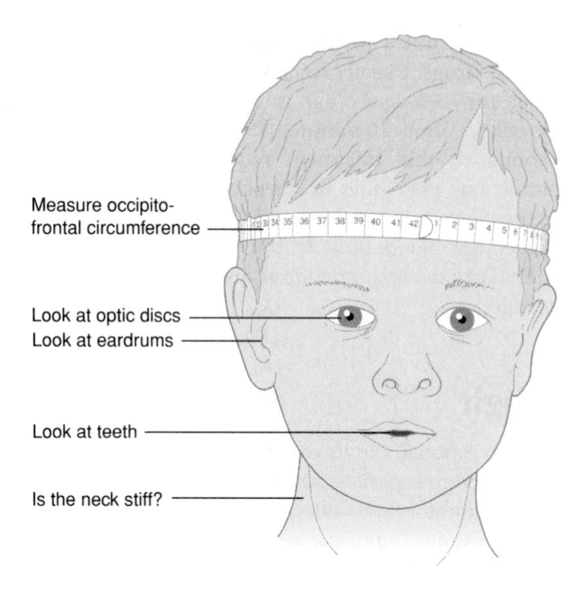
Measure occipito-frontal circumference
Look at optic discs
Look at eardrums
Look at teeth
Is the neck stiff?
• Check blood pressure
• Check growth
• Does child mind light?
• Vomiting?
• Time of day of headaches
BEWARE
Headache every morning = raised intracranial pressure

Fig 4.22
Examination of a child with headache.

suspicion of CNS infection, provided there is nothing to suggest raised intracranial pressures, and skull radiographs if head trauma is suspected. Sinus X-rays are rarely helpful in preschool age children since only the ethmoid and sphenoid sinuses are aerated.

Ear pain

Ear pain, most often due to otitis media (OM), accounts for up to 20–40% of young child consultations with general practitioners. The peak prevalence occurs in the 6- to 36-month age group with two-thirds of all episodes occurring before the third birthday. A third of children will experience three or more episodes of OM and overall, 15–20% of children will develop OM with effusion, increasing their risk of recurrent middle ear disease. The incidence is higher in boys than in girls, higher in children with craniofacial defects including cleft palate and Down syndrome, and higher in children who use dummies beyond their first birthday. Inflammation causing abnormal eustachian tube function and transient obstruction frequently precedes the onset of OM.

Classic symptoms of acute OM include fever, otalgia and diminished hearing during a cold. Crying, irritability, anorexia, loose bowels and pulling on the ear are additional nonspecific symptoms. Diagnosis depends on direct examination of the tympanic membranes, which are red and dull, with distorted landmarks and a diminished light reflex. Colour alone is insufficient to diagnose OM, as children who are upset, crying or febrile may have red, infected tympanic membranes. The eardrums may bulge or there may be otorrhoea if the eardrum ruptures, discharging fluid into the external canal. Tympanograms demonstrate reduced movement of the tympanic membrane in the presence of middle ear effusion.

The clinical diagnosis of OM is usually straightforward. The differential diagnosis of ear pain includes otitis externa or swimmer's ear, mastoiditis, impacted wax or foreign body, barotrauma or direct penetrating trauma. Referred pain from pharyngitis, peritonsillar abscess, sinusitis, parotitis or teeth may also cause otalgia.

The most common organisms causing OM are viruses but bacterial causes such as *Streptococcus pneumoniae* and *Haemophilus influenzae* are clinically indistinguishable. Management of acute OM includes analgesia with paracetamol and a broad-spectrum antibiotic such as amoxycillin or a macrolide (e.g. azithromycin). Many children still have middle ear effusions after antibiotic treatment. In the majority the fluid will spontaneously clear, but up to 10% may still have effusions 3 months later. Management with prophylactic antibiotics shows mixed success. Tympanostomy tubes or 'grommets' (Fig. 4.23) are usually reserved for children with chronic OM with effusion or 'glue ear' who demonstrate conductive hearing loss, have delayed language development or have specific conditions such as Down syndrome or cleft palate which predisposes them to recurrent OM. The indications and thus readiness to insert grommets varies; their insertion usually improves hearing rapidly but there is uncertainty about whether they lead to longer-term benefit.

Seizures

At least 7% of children have at least one episode of altered consciousness. Many parents on seeing their child fitting for the first time think that the attack may be fatal. Correct management depends on diagnosis, which in turn relies on a good eyewitness account.

- Many young children have episodes of breath-holding and temper tantrums which to the uninitiated can be confused with fits; these are benign. Reassurance via explanation is the treatment.
- About 3% of children have febrile convulsions with

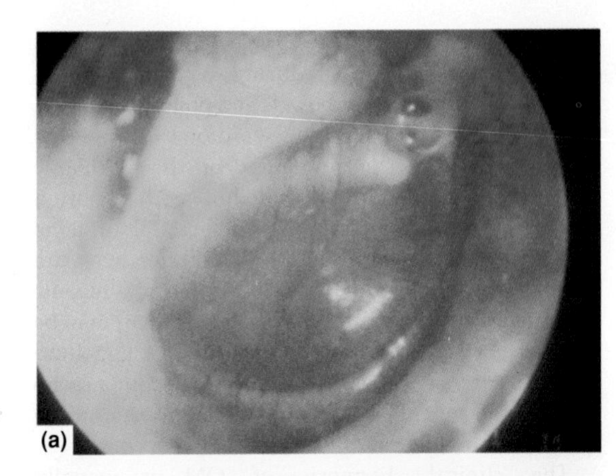

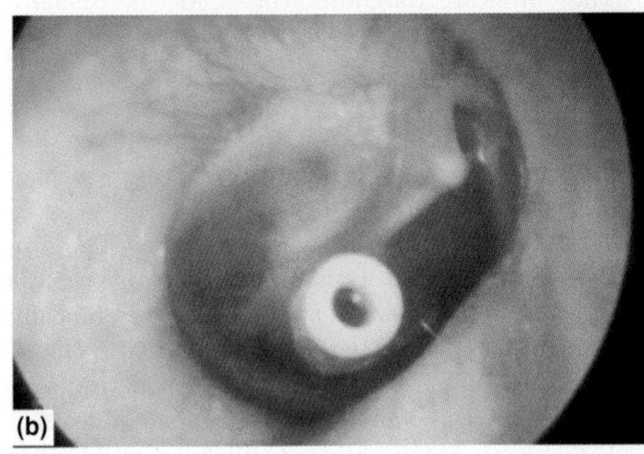

Fig 4.23
(a) Acute otitis media. (b) Appearance of grommet in situ to treat chronic secretory otitis media.

a peak between 1–2 years. Two-thirds have them only once; one in five has them repeatedly.
- These should be distinguished from true epilepsy that affects about 4 per 1000 children. About 80% of children with epilepsy have grand mal (tonic–clonic) seizures.

Other forms of epilepsy seen in this age group include the following:

- Absences lasting around 10 seconds, associated with a 3-Hz spike and wave pattern on the EEG.
- Myoclonic epilepsy, usually associated with developmental delay and an underlying brain abnormality.
- Complex partial seizures, where an aura is followed by a bizarre, disjointed complex action. See page 317–319 for further discussion about these and other types of epilepsy, and investigations that may be needed.
- Breath-holding attacks or syncope can produce nonepileptic convulsions (see p. 316–317).

Most fits have ceased by the time the child has reached medical attention. A seizure that is continuing and has lasted 10 minutes justifies the prompt use of anti-epilepsy drugs. Usually rectal or intravenous diazepam (5 mg for 1–5-year-olds) is given and repeated if necessary after 10 minutes. Seizures that do not respond to this treatment require treatment with intravenous phenytoin or phenobarbitone. In extreme circumstances, thiopentone and ventilation are used to protect the blood flow to the brain. Certain areas, particularly the temporal lobes, are at risk of ischaemic damage.

Cough

Asthma, especially in its early stages may present with chronic cough especially at night. Other causes include upper respiratory tract infection (URTI), foreign bodies, chronic rhinitis, sinusitis, croup and irritation of the airway by environmental pollutants such as cigarette smoke. Pertussis is now rare, thanks to immunization, but one must be able to recognize its characteristic whoop.

The type, pattern and timing of the cough usually provide important diagnostic clues. A dry, hacking cough occurring at night may be due to asthma. Physical examination may be normal except for the cough, and a trial of bronchodilators before bedtime is often therapeutic. A dry cough also occurs secondary to irritation from passive smoking and from the postnasal drip associated with seasonal allergies or URTIs. A history of parental smoking, the appearance of itchy watery eyes and a family history of atopy or symptoms of fever, sore throat and rhinorrhoea are evident.

A loose or productive cough is associated with lower respiratory conditions, usually asthma, but bacterial pneumonia needs to be considered. Fever, shortness of breath, malaise and respiratory distress are additional presenting features. Vomiting may occur following a prolonged coughing episode since most young children are unable to expectorate and may gag on the mucus. Examination reveals tachypnoea, recession, and localized crackles or diminished breath sounds. If the chest X-ray demonstrates an area of pneumonia and the child is not in marked respiratory distress, outpatient management with oral antibiotics is usually sufficient.

A chronic cough associated with recurrent pneumonia after antibiotics are discontinued suggests the presence of a foreign body. In up to 50% of children who inhale foreign bodies, the initial choking episode is unwitnessed. The usual age at presentation is 6 months to 3 years and the most common inhaled object is a peanut. The child presents with a history of persistent cough, and with asymmetric wheezing and diminished breath sounds on examination. The chest X-ray may be clear in up to one-third of cases. In the remainder an area of atelectasis, pneumonia or air trapping may be apparent. In only 15% of cases is a radioopaque object seen. If the history and examination suggest a foreign body, rigid bronchoscopy is required for both diagnosis and treatment. Chest physiotherapy should be avoided in suspected foreign body aspiration since it may dislodge the object and result in increased respiratory distress.

A harsh barking cough, worse at night and associated with low grade fever, hoarse voice and respiratory distress suggests laryngotracheobronchitis or croup (see Stridor). A chronic barking cough (like a seal) may have a psychogenic cause. Rarely conditions such as prolonged gastro-oesophageal reflux, cystic fibrosis, undetected vascular rings or other structural airway anomalies may exist and result in chronic or recurrent cough.

Note. Pulmonary tuberculosis is still around and should be sought in unexplained cough.

Wheezing

Wheezing results from airway narrowing of the lower respiratory tract. Common causes in children under 5 include asthma, pneumonia, foreign body aspiration, vascular rings, congestive heart failure and cystic fibrosis.

The most common cause of wheezing in children is asthma. Between 5 and 10% of children are estimated to suffer from asthma and the incidence is rising. About half will be diagnosed before age 5. Asthma is characterized by reversible airway obstruction, inflammation and increased airway reactivity to a variety of stimuli. A child with asthma may have had recurrent wheezy episodes as an infant following respiratory syncytial virus (RSV) bronchiolitis or viral URTIs, intermittent eczema or a strong family history of atopy. Triggers for asthmatic exacerbations include URTIs, changes in the weather, vigorous exercise, or exposure to environmental allergens, such as house dust mite, mould and animal dander or irritants, such as passive tobacco smoking. Many children present only with a chronic nocturnal cough as noted above.

Examination focuses on the child's colour, respiratory rate, work of breathing, alertness and breath sounds. Most will be tachypnoeic, using accessory muscles and will have a bilateral expiratory wheeze. An alert playful toddler with audible wheeze is less worrying than the anxious or listless child too breathless to speak. A chest X-ray may show evidence of hyperexpansion. There are no specific diagnostic tests for asthma and diagnosis depends on the presence of chronic and recurrent symptoms, identifiable triggers, family or personal history of atopy and response to bronchodilators. It is difficult to ensure that inhalers are correctly used by young children, and much thought has been given to their design. Incorrect use means that the child will not be appropriately treated and may explain circumstances where they seem to be ineffective.

Management is targeted at minimizing exposure to triggers (hard floors, and mattress covers, keeping away from longhaired animals, irritant dusts and moulds). Prophylaxis is with inhaled steroids, and acute treatment with inhaled bronchodilators and short courses of oral steroids. Maintenance therapy with inhaled sodium cromoglycate is an alternative. Measuring peak flow becomes possible by the age of 4 or 5 and is a useful way of regulating therapy. Parents should be educated about the signs and symptoms of a worsening attack and instructed to seek immediate medical attention if the child is unable to feed or speak due to dyspnoea, or develops respiratory distress, cyanosis, restlessness or excessive sleepiness. Further details are found on page 354.

Stridor

Stridor (described on p. 85, 358) is still seen in this age group. It is an inspiratory noise created by air passing through a narrow larynx or trachea. (Remember Poiseuille's law – on the flow through tubes being proportional to the radius to the power of four.) Viral croup, acute epiglottitis, bacterial tracheitis and foreign body aspiration are the major causes of stridor in young children.

Viral croup is the most common cause of upper airway obstruction in children under 3 years. It is usually caused by the parainfluenza virus although influenza and RSV are also common. There is a seasonal incidence with the peak period between October and April, and boys are affected twice as often as girls. The symptoms are worse at night, may be transiently relieved by exposure to cool moist air and normally resolve in 5–7 days. The child usually presents after several days of mild coryzal symptoms and low grade fever, with a classic barking cough, stridor and some respiratory distress. The child may be anxious and tachypnoeic with variable intercostal and suprasternal recession. Examination of the mouth and throat is not advised since it may precipitate complete airway obstruction. Management in mild cases includes keeping the child calm; using humidified cool air, and encouraging cool oral fluids and antipyretics. Educating the parents about the time course of the illness and signs of worsening respiratory distress, so that they know when to seek additional medical attention is vital. In more severe cases the child may be treated with nebulized budesonide or adrenaline in hospital.

Acute epiglottitis has significantly decreased in incidence since the widespread use of the Hib vaccine. The history and severity of symptoms distinguish acute epiglottitis from viral croup. The onset of illness is hours rather than days; the child usually has a high fever, looks very ill, has marked stridor, may be drooling excessively and appears frightened. He may be leaning forward in an attempt to keep his airway open. If confronted with such a child the most appropriate thing to do is keep the child calm by *not examining* him. The anaesthetist and ENT surgeon should be called and the child kept with his parent on the way to theatre for intubation and examination of his airway under anaesthesia. *H. influenzae* type b is treated with a third-generation cephalosporin and the child usually improves dramatically after treatment and may be extubated and running around the ward within a day or two.

Bacterial tracheitis also presents with stridor and may start with mild URTI symptoms like croup. Instead of getting better over several days however, the croup progresses and the child develops a high fever, thick purulent secretions and increasing respiratory distress which may rapidly progress to complete airway obstruction from accumulated secretions. Management includes antibiotics that cover *Staphylococcus aureus*, the most frequently isolated organism, and intubation with frequent suctioning to maintain the airway if necessary.

Cautionary note. It has been known for a child to suck the spout of a hot teapot and scald the larynx, leading to respiratory obstruction.

Dysuria

This is pain on passing urine, especially in association with urinary tract infection. After the first birthday, urinary infection is three to four times more common in girls. Young children cannot localize their urinary symptoms; for example, a very young child may cry or draw the legs up when passing urine. When presented with this problem, ask about associated symptoms including fever or vomiting and check the perineum for ulceration or napkin rash. Examine the abdomen for loin tenderness and always take a urine sample for microscopy and culture.

See page 299, for management.

Leg pain and limp

Pain in the leg may arise from the joints, bone or muscle or be referred from the spine or abdomen. It may be complained of directly by an older child or present with limp or failure to weight-bear in a younger child. It may be due to a minor injury that will recover spontaneously in a few hours or be a presentation of a more serious condition. The accurate diagnosis of the cause of a limp may be very difficult and sometimes impossible. If no diagnosis can be made, the child should be observed until fully recovered. A full history and examination is essential. Enquire about a history of minor trauma or upper respiratory tract infection that may indicate a reactive arthritis. Vigorous playing in the back garden may have caused a sprain. Some children have unexplained pains in the calf and thigh muscles, which occur at night; the causes of these are unknown. The examination should start with the shoe for a protruding nail or tightness and the foot for verrucas and foreign bodies. Then examine the limb for warmth and tenderness and the joints for restriction of movement and swelling. Examine the inguinal region for lymphadenitis.

Pain in the leg may be referred from the hip or spine and these joints should also be thoroughly examined and X-rays performed if necessary. Ultrasonography is the best method of detecting a joint effusion. Nonaccidental injury may cause a limp or leg pain. A low threshold for performing an X-ray of an unexplained sore leg is wise. Any patient with recurrent pain or pain which doesn't settle within a few days deserves further investigation. Transient synovitis of the hip (irritable hip) is common, occurring after a viral infection, usually in boys. There may be a raised ESR. Bed rest and traction relieve the symptoms; some go on to develop Perthes' disease (see p. 348). Juvenile chronic arthritis is a seronegative arthropathy which may present in this age group with joint pain and fever; one or more joints (particularly the ankle joint) may be affected and it may be associated with a salmon pink rash. Acute rheumatic fever (see p. 180) is now rare but should not be forgotten and is much more likely to be seen in developing countries.

Causes of limps are presented in Information box 4.11.

Information Box 4.11

Causes of limp

'Irritable hip'	A transient synovitis of unexplained origin of the hip joint
Osteochondritis	Such as Perthes' disease (see p. 348)
Osteomyelitis	May take 2 weeks to show up radiographically and bone scanning is needed for earlier diagnosis
Bone tumour	e.g. osteogenic sarcoma
Missed fracture	Consider abuse
Juvenile idiopathic arthritis	
Soft tissue injuries	e.g. sprains or sores on feet
Haemoglobinopathy	Sickling crisis in an at-risk patient
Scurvy, rickets	
Neuromuscular dysfunction	
Leg inequality	
Leukaemia	
Psychological disturbance	

Cautionary note. Osteomyelitis may have a negative X-ray appearance in the first 2 weeks. Be very chary about ascribing joint pains to 'growing'.

New horizons

The length of hospital stay is shortening due to new advances in diagnostic techniques. Length of admission is now more often dictated by circumstances at home rather than medical needs. Many complex treatments such as respirators and parenteral feeding can be provided through hospital outreach schemes and community paediatric services, for use at home or school.

The introduction of conjugated meningococcus B vaccines is eagerly awaited.

In the UK accidents are still the largest cause of death in this age group; most are avoidable, and more work needs to be done on accident prevention and improving safety on the roads. The incidence of cancer is increasing and the improvement in survival for childhood cancers needs to be continued. Equal challenges lie in developmental paediatrics, the care of disabled children and in paediatric psychiatry, where the causes, and thus rational treatment, of problems such as autism remain obscure.

Global concerns

Despite recent advances in the care of infants, on a global scale the greatest needs are so simple in theory – clean water, good food, immunization. Preventing war, and simple health education would vastly improve health and save millions of children's lives each year.

Transplantation

Complex and expensive transplant operations involving the bone marrow, kidneys, heart, lung and liver have become available in national centres in developed countries. Such transplants are often performed in very young children. Indications for bone marrow transplantation have expanded in recent years (see Information box 4.12). New techniques, better immunosuppression, improvement in anaesthesia, and comprehensive monitoring of patients during the operation, and on intensive care units postoperatively, have helped advance this rapidly growing field. Careful early selection of patients and their families is essential. Education and support must be provided for the whole family who undergo enormous stresses during the peri- and postoperative stages. Careful follow up in hospital and subsequently at home is important to ensure that any problems are detected and managed early. The goal is to improve the child's quality of life.

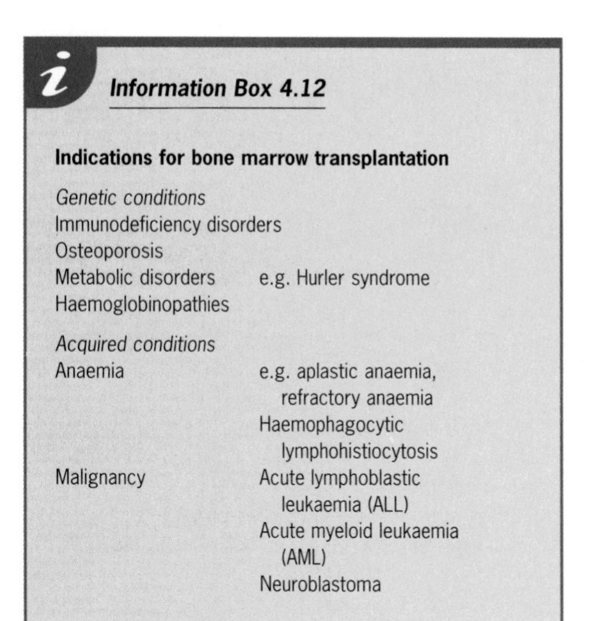

Information Box 4.12

Indications for bone marrow transplantation

Genetic conditions	
Immunodeficiency disorders	
Osteoporosis	
Metabolic disorders	e.g. Hurler syndrome
Haemoglobinopathies	
Acquired conditions	
Anaemia	e.g. aplastic anaemia, refractory anaemia Haemophagocytic lymphohistiocytosis
Malignancy	Acute lymphoblastic leukaemia (ALL) Acute myeloid leukaemia (AML) Neuroblastoma

FURTHER READING

Meadow R (1997) *ABC of Child Abuse*, 3rd edn. London: BMJ Publications.

5 The older child from 5 to 16 years

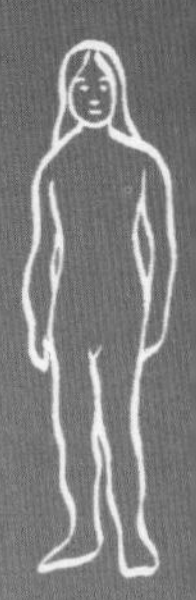

Introduction

In this chapter we discuss the health and development of children through their school years till their care is handed over to services for adults. We have concentrated on the main acute and chronic health problems, both physical and psychological, and ways of promoting healthy lifestyles. We have tried not to describe again conditions also encountered in younger children or already studied in adult medicine. Detailed descriptions of diseases are in Section 2 of this book.

Episodes of severe illness become less frequent as the child gets older. Most of the congenital problems have declared themselves by now. Accidents are the major cause of death. Behaviour-related and social problems tend to crowd out purely physical disease. Having said this, physical disease can greatly blight a time that should be the healthiest of one's whole lifespan and doctors who care for school children need very special skills. Few secondary school children will be found on hospital wards.

There is no hard and fast age at which children should leave paediatrics for adult specialist care; increasingly we talk about transition from child- to adult-based health services and appreciate that it is not always done well. Most of the services for adults are designed to meet the needs of the elderly, and the young disabled child may easily lose out once they are too old for child-centred services.

In the UK children must by law start school once they reach 5 years. Although they can leave at 16, economic prospects are poor without further secondary and increasingly tertiary education. Disabled children are entitled to educational provision from 2 to 19 years of age.

For most children their school years are the healthiest in their lives and the time in which permanent attitudes to health, eating habits, sex and behaviour are formed. It is also the time when some adult disorders and diseases may originate from the acquisition of undesirable social habits and lifestyles (see Information box 5.1). Accidents and self-harm rather than acute illness are the major problems that present to accident and emergency departments. These problems are much influenced by lifestyles.

Information Box 5.1

Undesirable social habits and lifestyles in adolescence

- Drug abuse
- Alcohol
- Smoking
- Lack of sporting activity or exercise
- Engaging in early and unprotected sex
- Poor dietary habits, junk food
- Dangerous activities especially by males
- Violence

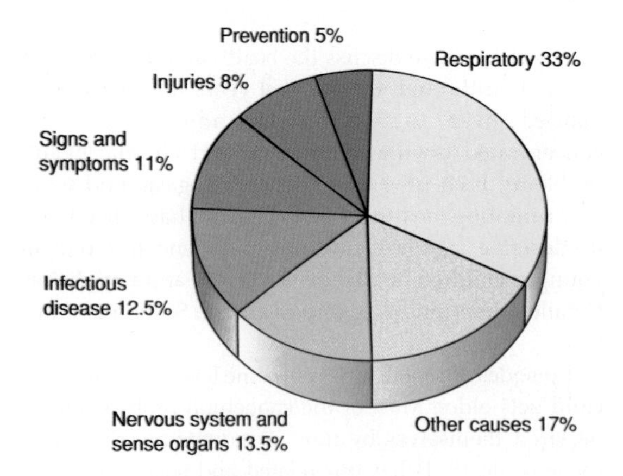

Fig 5.1
Reasons for general practitioner consultations, children aged 4–14 years. (Source: Office of Population, Censuses and Surveys (OPCS) MB5/1, London: HMSO). © Crown copyright

Reasons for consulting the doctor

Data from the *Fourth National Survey of Morbidity in General Practice 1991–1992* show that, on average, children aged 5–15 years are seen by their general practitioners about twice a year. Infections are still a frequent reason for visiting doctors (Fig. 5.1). Other common reasons include abdominal pains, headaches, 'growing pains', behaviour problems and enuresis.

Increasingly, adolescents visit their doctors for advice on contraception. New law enshrined in the Children Act 1989 made it permissible to prescribe the contraceptive pill to teenage girls, provided that their doctor is satisfied that their young patient is mature and understands the issues involved. Though it is preferable to involve the parents in such issues, this is not a prerequisite (Gillick v. West Norfolk and Wisbech Health Authority 1986, Appeal Cases 112–207, p. 34). It is required that the patient's confidentiality is respected. At the end of the day it is up to the doctor and patient to work out a mutually acceptable solution. This may not be easy.

Key issues in school-age children

Important issues in this age group include the following:

- The use of the school educational system and curriculum to teach children about health matters, including nutrition, sports, bullying and accident prevention, sex education and living a healthy lifestyle.
- The use of the computer-based school health recording system:
  1. to ensure full coverage of immunization and other screening programmes, e.g. vision screening
  2. to ensure that children about whom teachers are concerned are seen by the school doctor, with the permission of the parents.
- Child abuse – though physical abuse and neglect becomes less common as children get older, it does not disappear. In adolescence, child sexual abuse continues to be a problem. It is also important to be

aware of the needs of siblings in such families and engage in multidisciplinary teamwork. Follow up is essential as recurrence of previously reported abuse does occur. (For further details on child abuse see p. 183, and for Munchausen by proxy syndrome see p. 185.)

Origins of adult disorders and diseases

Most medical conditions of adults have their roots in childhood; we think especially of hypertension, furred arteries and the environmental causes of many cancers. These hazards keep changing.

Keeping school children healthy

This section starts with drug abuse because it is so clearly a major own goal against health.

Drug abuse

Really accurate data are not available but it is believed that the average age at which adolescents start drug taking is now around 13–15 years (Information box 5.2). Earlier illicit drug abuse is often associated with heavier subsequent drug abuse, more persistent abuse, and the abuse of 'harder' drugs. These children are particularly likely to get involved in later delinquency and develop severe psychiatric disorders and antisocial problems. Drug abuse is notoriously influenced by social and cultural fashion, availability and legislation. Abuse of volatile substances (lighter fuel and petrol) accounts for about 100 deaths each year in the UK.

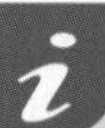

Information Box 5.2

Facts on drug abuse (in the UK)

- 5–20% of school-age children have 'never tried' an illegal drug/substance
- 2–5% of school-age children use drugs at least weekly
- Peak prevalence of drug abuse in school-age children is at 14–16 years
- Boys are more likely to abuse drugs and start earlier than girls, but girls' drug abuse is more committed
- Newly introduced illegal drugs keep appearing; strengths, purity and means of administration keep changing

Use of cannabis, amphetamines, hallucinogenic substances, and 'pills', such as tranquillizers and hypnotics is commonly associated with higher rates of alcohol use and cigarette smoking.

Whilst most adult 'addicts' begin taking drugs in their teens, only a small proportion of teenage drug abusers progress to addiction. The extent of future abuse is influenced by prior abuse and peer pressure.

If drug abuse remains untreated there is a risk of continued (and possibly dangerous) use together with high rates of psychiatric and social problems, where aggression, antisocial behaviour, occupational and marital problems are most common. There is also an increased risk of HIV infection associated with contaminated needles. Adolescent drug abusers are also more likely to have unprotected sexual intercourse after drug use. Adverse effects of the commoner drugs of abuse are shown in Information box 5.3.

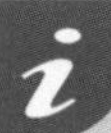

Information Box 5.3

Adverse effects of the more common drugs of abuse

Causes of deaths in volatile substance abuse
- Anorexia
- Cardiac arrhythmias
- Respiratory depression
- Trauma

Consequences of chronic volatile substance abuse
- Central nervous system (CNS) depression
- Upper respiratory tract infection
- Persistent cough
- Laryngitis
- Liver damage
- Cardiomyopathy
- Renal damage

Adverse effects of amphetamine and other stimulants
- Increased arousal
- Sleep disturbances
- Weight loss
- In toxic doses: confusional state and psychosis

Adverse effects of cannabis
- Sweating
- Tachycardia
- Peripheral vasodilatation
- Psychosis

Adverse effects of opiates
- Clouding of consciousness
- Nausea and vomiting
- Respiratory depression
- Bradycardia
- Constipation

With drug abuse increasing to pandemic proportions, attempts at prevention should be aimed primarily at discouraging individuals from adopting the habit at all and secondarily to advise abusers against using increasingly more hazardous substances or from continuing the habit into adult life. This is much easier said than done. Children's doctors need to be informed about these matters and involved in this vital form of health protection.

Alcohol (Fig. 5.2)

Alcohol is another contributor to unnecessary mortality and morbidity in children and adolescents (Information box 5.4). Its sensible use is greatly influenced by example from family life. Adolescent drunkenness appears to be a marker of social unrest.

There are pronounced differences in drinking patterns between young men and women, and differences according to social grouping. Higher socioeconomic groups tend to experiment and drink regularly but lower socioeconomic groups have higher consumption levels. The consumption of alcohol is influenced by availability, price, and, in part by advertising. Moreover, a significant correlation between unemployment (especially for longer than 6 months) and an increased risk of heavier drinking has been shown among men in the 1958 Birth Cohort study.

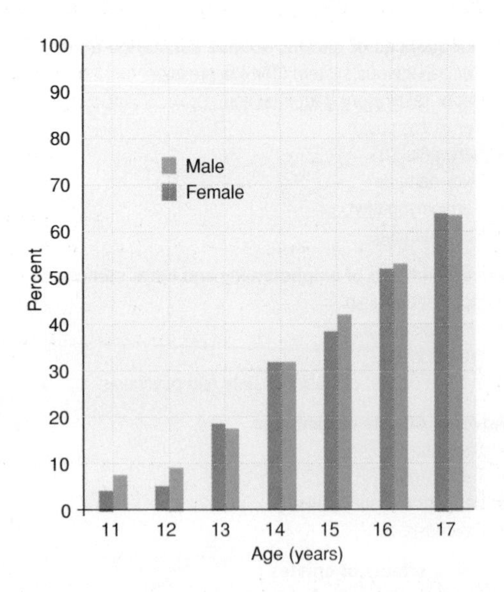

Fig 5.2
Percentage of children, aged 11–16 years, who had an alcoholic drink in the week before interview; England 1990. (Source: Lader & Matheson (1991). Smoking among secondary school children in 1990. London: OPCS; Goddard, E (1991) Drinking in England and Wales in the late 1980s. London, HMSO. Derived from an original graph in: Woodroffe et al. © Crown copyright (1993) Children, Teenagers and Health; The key data. Buckingham: Open University Press.)

Information Box 5.4

The health consequences of alcohol consumption

1. Accidents, including road traffic accidents, at lower alcohol blood levels compared with adults
2. Poisoning
3. Violence
4. Crime
5. Dependence and psychiatric illness
6. Gastritis
7. Association with some cancers, fatty liver and cirrhosis, pancreatitis, hypoglycaemia (especially in young children)
8. CNS depressant effect; convulsions (especially in those with a low convulsive threshold); peripheral neuropathy

There is also an association between adolescent drinking and smoking.

Smoking

Smoking is a key health risk. The resultant adverse effects, such as respiratory disorders, are not confined to older individuals but are also a concern for young people. The earlier in life that individuals start smoking, the less likely they are to give it up. This means that the duration of exposure to the harmful effects of tobacco will increase. Young people soon become parents themselves and damage their own offspring in utero; thus the problem cycles through the generations. Since the risk of lung cancer is related to the length of time of smoking, and not only the total exposure, this can have serious consequences: consumption of 20 cigarettes per day for 30 years produces a greater risk than 40 cigarettes per day for 15 years.

The more immediate health effects of smoking during childhood include increases in respiratory symptoms and reduced physical fitness. Passive smoking can also have adverse effects on health.

In 1990 16% of children aged 11–15 were regular or occasional smokers in England; comparable figures for Scotland and Wales were 20% and 15% respectively. By age 16–19 years, 30% of Britain's young people smoke. This has not changed since 1982. Moreover the percentage of children who had tried smoking before the age of 11 decreased from 23% of pupils in England in 1982 to 13% in 1990. Whilst recent surveys are showing a higher prevalence of smoking in young women (the reverse of the pattern observed 20 years ago), male smokers appear to have heavier consumption levels.

The possible influences on starting to smoke seem to

be numerous, and range from individual characteristics, family, school and peer groups, through socioeconomic environment and availability, to the price and promotion of tobacco.

One of the stated aims of the Government White Paper of 1992, *The Health of the Nation*, was the reduction of the prevalence of smoking in children at least up to the age of 14 or 15. The need is for soundly reasoned concerted action to influence tobacco promotion, price and fashionable nature, and the availability of cigarettes to children.

Back pain

Back pain is an uncommon problem in childhood and deserves investigation when it is persistent. In childhood, musculoskeletal injury to the back is usually caused by trauma secondary to sports injuries, fights, road traffic accidents or abnormal strain caused by inappropriate carrying and lifting, awkward seats and desks at school or home. For other causes of back trouble see Information box 5.5.

While many causes of back pain in childhood can be treated, chronic degenerative changes caused in childhood may surface later in adult life. Such problems have no specific cure except for analgesia and surgery. Hence prevention is an important issue, for instance by means of good design of chairs and desks at home and school, and policies to ensure safe sports facilities, measures to reduce school fights and avoid road traffic accidents. Children need to be taught the best ways of lifting and carrying in order to reduce the burden of later back trouble.

Information Box 5.5

Some causes of childhood back trouble

1. Congenital and developmental spinal deformity (p. 344)
2. Inflammatory diseases, e.g. discitis, vertebral osteomyelitis, spinal epidural abscess (p. 346)
3. Rheumatic diseases, e.g. juvenile idiopathic arthritis (p. 361)
4. Developmental disorders, e.g. scoliosis, Scheuermann syndrome, spondylolisthesis (p. 348)
5. Mechanical
   - hip/pelvic anomalies
   - overuse syndromes, e.g. in athletes
   - vertebral stress fractures
6. Neoplastic diseases: tumours (primary and metastatic) (p. 333)
7. Systemic conditions, e.g. renal abscess, pancreatitis, sickle cell disease (p. 252)

Physical fitness

Physical activity and fitness are recognized as having powerful benefits on physical and mental health. During childhood, exercise has positive effects on growth and development, while at older ages protective effects have been documented, particularly in preventing cardiovascular disease, but also in the treatment of diabetes, protection against osteoporosis and in the reduction of hypertension. Habits and skills acquired in childhood influence habits later in life.

While levels of physical activities can be high in childhood and adolescence, many become much less active after the age of 15 years, especially in girls. By the age of 16 to 24 years it is estimated that over one-third of men and over a half of women do not take regular exercise. Reasons given include work commitments and lack of relevant interesting activities, dislike of team games, inadequate and expensive community facilities, money and personal transport. (Question: where do all the many bicycles bought every year go?)

Sexually transmitted diseases (STDs)

The pattern of STD in adolescence has greatly changed during this century. Syphilis has become rare and gonorrhoea much less common than it was, thanks to antibiotics, but viral diseases have become rampant, especially human papilloma virus which causes cervical cancer, chlamydia which blocks fallopian tubes, and genital herpes.

These conditions are likely to remain prevalent unless a sea-change in attitudes to promiscuous intercourse occurs. Infected individuals act as reservoirs from which these infections spread. HIV and AIDS-related diseases are likely to remain a major source of problems. Much effort is going into initiatives aimed at limiting these problems, especially sex education in school and advocacy of barrier contraception.

School and health issues

The school health service: aims and objectives

The aim of the school health service is to promote health.

The school health team of nurse, doctor and therapists is drawn from the local NHS community child health service. It is closely involved in health education both as part of the school's policy and as adviser to the individual parent and child. School health teams should also have a role in educating teachers about health matters; in general teachers receive little education on health matters during their training and may have incorrect information about conditions such as AIDS/HIV or epilepsy.

Some problems, such as enuresis, are so frequent that it may be worth running special clinics. As children grow up they should be expected to take an interest and be 'in charge' of their own health. Health professionals can assist here by explaining the nature of illnesses and resulting anxieties to children and indicate how they or their parents can be helped. Psychosocial problems are now more common than the previously undetected heart or lung disorders that were commonly found in the past. The school health service is thus becoming more involved in counselling and health promotion.

Screening: school medicals

Children starting school should have already had an examination at around 4 years and their immunizations brought up to date at that time. Only where this has not been done, or the results suggested a continuing problem, is repeat examination on school entry justified. Parents, children and teachers should be encouraged to seek advice about health-related matters from the service.

Universal screening

The school health service has a duty to promote health in school children. Its original purpose was to detect and correct health problems in school children through repeated school medical examinations. Gradually the incidence of detectable disorders has fallen, making regular full examinations less necessary.

Selective screening

Selective screening may be prompted by teachers, parents or school health service personnel. As teachers get to know children, they may request selective medical examinations so that appropriate advice can be given. Where parents are worried and feel that they would like their child examined, they can request a medical. The school nurse and doctor scrutinize the parent-held record and other information about children before they start school. When the school doctor and nurse feel either that the existing information is inadequate or that there is cause for concern, they will ask the parent to bring the child, for discussion and examination, if necessary. The aim of this selective medical examination is not so much to detect problems as to interpret them for the benefit of the child, parents and educational staff at school, so that an appropriate policy can be made. Epilepsy and attention deficits are examples. It is vital that the local hospital-based paediatricians and child psychiatrists keep in close touch with the school health service over mutual patients.

Special screening and special education needs

The school health service has a responsibility, shared with teachers, parents and social workers, to identify those children with problems which are likely to interfere with their capacity to learn, e.g. deafness, partial sightedness. When problems are suspected and extra educational help or resources are needed, the provisions laid down by the Educational Act 1991 (applicable to England and Wales, other legislation applies elsewhere) have to be followed. Parents and all those professionally involved are asked to write a description of the child's needs as seen from their perspective. It is essential that these be clearly written without medical jargon. These are assembled and a *Statement of educational need* is derived from them. This entitles the child to extra help, either from within his or her own school, or by transfer to a special school. There is a statutory duty to revise this statement on a yearly basis. About 3% of children receive a statement though there is all too often a long wait for the process to be completed.

Policy is now aimed at educating these children as far as possible within 'mainstream' schools with appropriate extra provision. 'Extremists' tend to advocate that all disabled children should be educated in mainstream schools, but it is obvious that there are some children who need specialized education because of severe hearing or visual impairment, severe emotional problems or severe learning disability.

In general, these children need small, dedicated schools which can concentrate on their particular needs. An alternative is to run a special unit within a larger school. Schools for these very disabled children need extra medical facilities; the school should be able to cope with a wide range of problems, including seizures and severe behaviour difficulties. It may be more appropriate to hold consultant clinics in the school rather than to take the children to hospital outpatient clinics. The schools need a great deal of input from specialist speech therapists, psychologists, occupational therapists and physiotherapists.

Disabled children, especially those in mainstream schools, need encouragement and inspiration in order to take part in everyday activities. For example, a boy severely affected by a progressive neurodegenerative condition (Friedreich's ataxia, see p. 319) may be able to bat at cricket from a wheelchair, and play snooker. Advice on sports for disabled children can be obtained from the Sports Council.

Bullying

Bullying is unprovoked, repetitive activity, carried out by a stronger child with the intent of hurting the recipient, who is usually weaker. It can take many forms including stealing, blackmailing, threatening, physical aggression, name-calling, victimizing, and so on. Its prevalence ranges from 10 to 30% of children and probably half the cases are not reported.

All the warning signs (Information box 5.6) are nonspecific but, in the absence of medical causes, the clinician should enquire about change of school, teacher, or unhappiness at home.

Bullies get gratification from using power, verbal and/or physical. They choose their victims carefully. Victims tend to be weak, loners and unassertive. Children with disabilities or ethnic minorities are at increased risk, as are short children and new immigrants.

Management of bullying includes behaviour modification and changes in school policies, such as encouragement to report such incidents. Both schoolteachers and parents play an important role in primary prevention and management of bullying and have a key role in working with both the bullies and their victims, with the aim of preventing long-term adverse psychological sequelae.

Information Box 5.6

Warning signs of bullying include:

- School refusal
- Bruising
- Behaviour change (anxiety)
- 'Losing' money and possessions repeatedly
- Nightmares
- Abdominal pain
- Enuresis

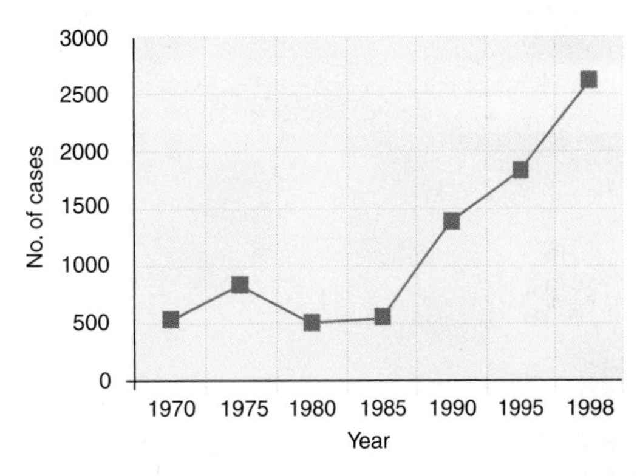

Fig 5.3

Notifications of meningococcal infections in England and Wales, 1970–1998. (*Note*: Figures are for meningococcal meningitis from 1970–1998. From 1989, figures also include meningococcal septicaemia with or without meningitis). (Source: Public Health Laboratory Service. More detailed information is available from: http://www.phls.co.uk/. Similar information for Scotland is available from the Scottish Centre for Infection and Environmental Health. web site: http://www.show.scot.nhs.uk/scieh/.)

Infections in school

By the time a child reaches school age, the immune system has developed enough to enable them to handle most infectious agents. Schools are ideal breeding grounds for epidemics; immunization has prevented the old ones but diarrhoeal and respiratory illnesses are common. Many schools have poor toilets and handwashing facilities; it is up to the teachers and health professions to get action to remedy this. Formal quarantine for postinfectious children has been abandoned, but sense dictates that children who are overtly infectious should not be at school. In particular, children with active chickenpox should be kept away from those who are on immunosuppressive treatment. In a large school there may be several such children.

Meningitis causes much anxiety among health professionals, teachers and parents, and has public health implications as some forms of it can result in death in susceptible individuals. It is a statutory requirement to notify meningococcal infections at diagnosis (Fig. 5.3). For further details see page 280.

Tuberculosis is becoming more prevalent in some regions of the UK after a long period of decline (Fig. 5.4). Resistance to treatment is becoming a problem. Because of the earlier decline, today's doctors have little experience in diagnosing and managing the condition (Fig. 5.5), which has a reputation for virulence in

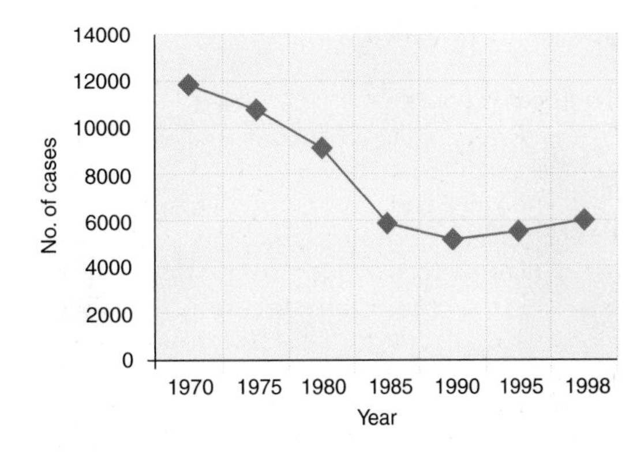

Fig 5.4
Notifications of tuberculosis (respiratory and non-respiratory) in England and Wales, 1970–1998 (Source: Public Health Laboratory Service. See relevant web sites mentioned in Fig. 5.3 for more detailed information.)

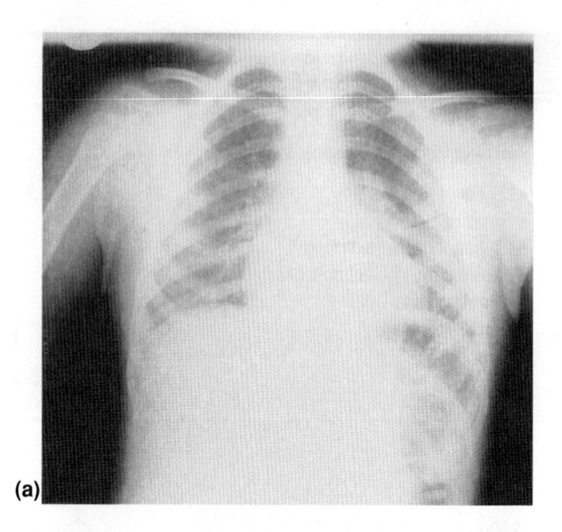

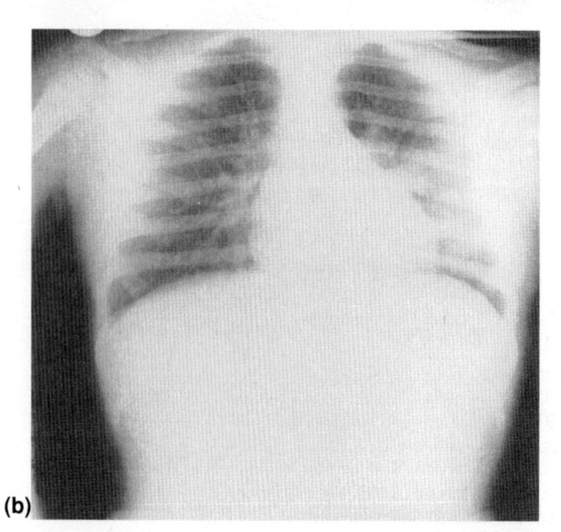

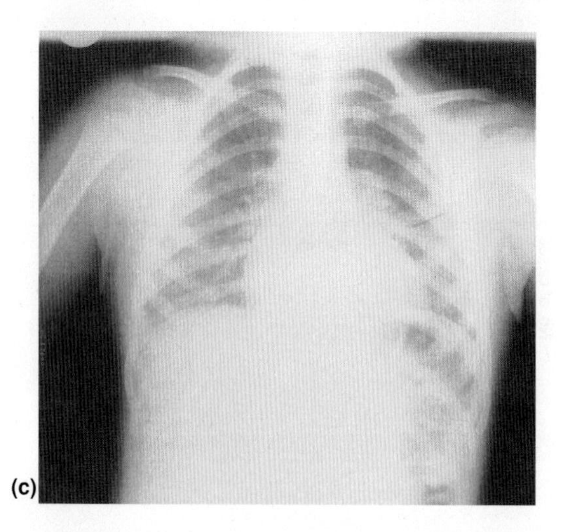

Fig 5.5
Chronic cough due to tuberculosis. (a) The X-ray shows left perihilar consolidation. (b) 5 months later there is increased consolidation on the left. (c) Another 6 weeks later, there is lingular volume loss with consolidation of the left upper lobe.

teenagers. TB is a notifiable disease and contact tracing is essential to treat the asymptomatic cases. Bacillus Calmette-Guérin (BCG) vaccination should be offered to contacts with no evidence of disease after testing. It is normally offered to all skin test-negative secondary school children via the school health service.

Epidemiology

Accidents

Accidents, i.e. unintentional injuries, are the commonest cause of death and hospital admission in children aged 5–16 years in the United Kingdom. Accidents cause nearly one-half of all deaths between the ages of 1 and 19 years, and hospital admission rates for child accidents continue to rise.

In the United Kingdom mortality rates for pedestrian road traffic accidents among children are the second highest in Europe. Fires are the major cause of accidental deaths at home. Other potentially preventable causes of accidental deaths in the 5–14-year-old age group include drowning and suffocation (Information box 5.7). In the USA a significant number of deaths occur in teenagers due to fights involving firearms and knives.

The direct costs to the NHS of accidental injury in childhood are estimated at over £200 million per annum. Injuries result in many other costs beyond those to the NHS.

There have been reductions in the child accident mortality rates in England and Wales over the last 20 years. There are major international differences in accident mortality rates, with the USA, Canada and Australia having higher rates and Sweden and the Netherlands having relatively lower rates. Mortality rates are higher amongst children from disadvantaged socioeconomic groups. There is a striking variation within regions in England and Wales, child accident death rates being highest in the north.

Information Box 5.7

Common causes of fatal accidents in childhood

- Road traffic accidents
- Fire and burns
- Drowning and suffocation

Sports injuries

Sports injuries account for 3% of the workload of a paediatric accident and emergency department, with a slight male predominance, but these injuries tend not to be severe. Many sports injuries are seen in hospital departments and data are not recorded. Seasonal variation exists in relation to both the sports involved and the nature of the injuries. Upper limb soft tissue injuries and fractures are particularly common types of injury, followed by lower limb soft tissue injury.

The sports implicated include football, gymnastics, basketball, netball, and rugby. Good refereeing and proper training are important. (For more details about accidents and injury, see p. 165. Details about poisoning can be found on p. 170)

Disability

In 1985/1986 the Office for Population, Censuses and Surveys carried out a major survey of disability, particularly looking at prevalence and diagnoses. It was found that 3% of children had a high level severe disability, with a higher prevalence amongst boys. The prevalence was higher in the 5–9 and 10–15 age groups than in younger children and infants, probably reflecting increasing survival of disabled children due to better health provision.

Behaviour disability was most common (2% of children surveyed); 1% of children had a locomotor disability; 1% were incontinent of urine or faeces; 1% had problems of intellectual function; 0.6% had hearing difficulties; and 0.2% had a visual disability (see Fig. 5.7). Disability seldom occurred in isolation. (For further details of cerebral palsy and learning disorders, see p. 313 and p. 322 respectively.)

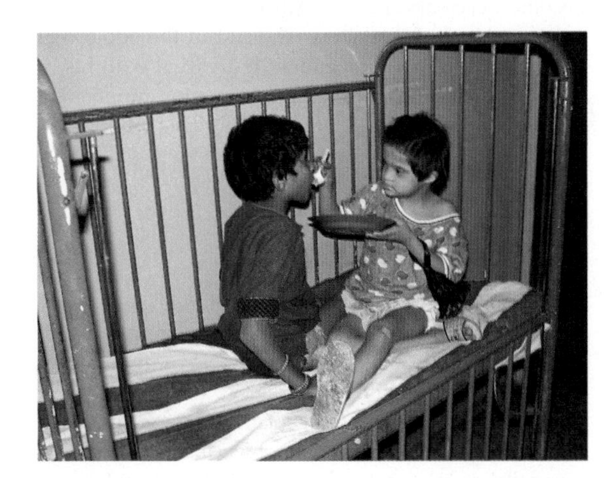

Fig 5.6
Disabled children in Pakistan.

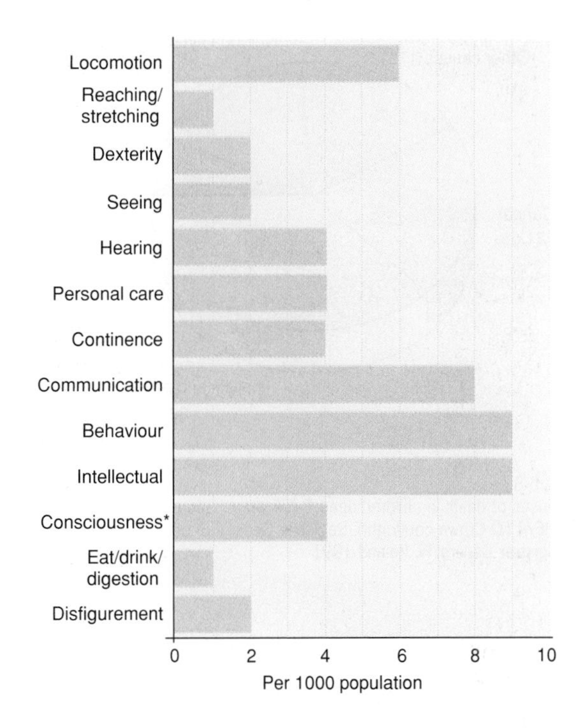

Fig 5.7
Disabilities by functional category in young people aged 16–19 years in Great Britain; *includes fits and convulsions.
Source: Bone M and Meltzer H (1989). The prevalence of disability among children: OPCS Surveys of disability in Great Britain, report 3, London, HMSO. © Crown copyright

Pregnancy

The teenage pregnancy (see Information box 5.8) and abortion rates in Britain are among the highest in Europe and more than five times higher than those in the Netherlands, despite the similarity in the level of teenage sexual activity.

Overall there has been a decline in teenage conception rates between 1969 and 1991. This has not been a steady decrease; fluctuations have occurred, especially among 16–19-year-olds. In 1991 the

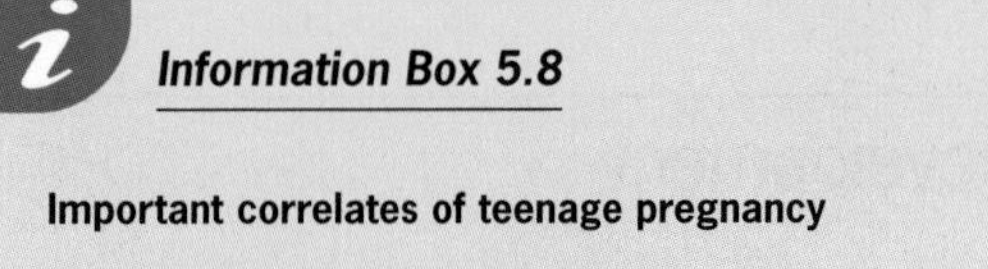

Information Box 5.8

Important correlates of teenage pregnancy

- Poor attendance for antenatal care
- Poor socioeconomic circumstances
- Single marital status
- Increased risk of abortion
- Increased risk of low birthweight
- Behaviour and educational problems in the offspring

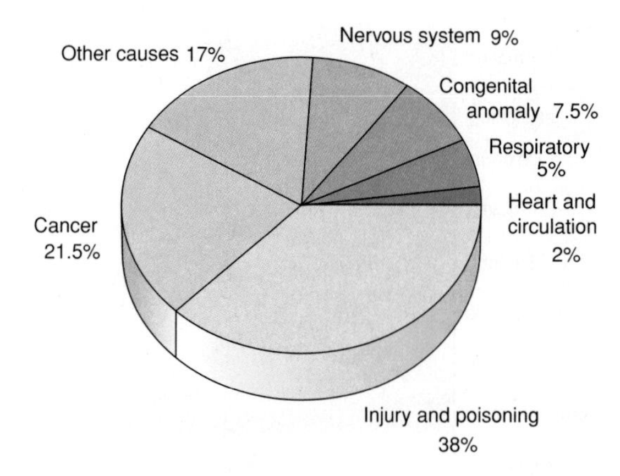

Fig 5.8
Causes of death in children aged 5–14 years. Source: OPCS DH2/17; DH6/4 (© Crown copyright), Registrar General Scotland 1990; Registrar General N. Ireland 1991

conception rate in England and Wales was 9.3 per 1000 women aged 14 and 15 years, and 51% of these ended in abortion.

Adolescence is a stage when sexual behaviour can be influenced. A reduction in unwanted pregnancies and sexually transmitted infection requires radical social action based on sound research.

Mortality (Fig. 5.8)

Death rates for school children are at historically low levels. At all ages in childhood there is an increased risk of mortality, especially in children in lower socioeconomic groups; boys are consistently at a higher risk than girls. During the teenage years, the risk of dying for boys and girls increases rapidly with age, the increase for boys beginning at the age of 12, which is a year earlier than for girls. In 1991, the childhood mortality rate per 100 000 population for children aged 5–14 years was 44 for boys and 31 for girls.

The role of the doctor in the event of the death of a child is discussed in detail in Chapter 4 (p. 107); similar principles apply for this age group.

Development

Developmental milestones

Although the concept of 'developmental milestones' is generally applied in relation to preschool children, development naturally continues throughout the school years, for example, of hand–eye coordination or the ability to master complex ideas of right and wrong. Speed of reaction and muscular strength continue to develop. Some skills, such as speed swimming, reach their peak by the later school years.

Psychological and emotional development

As the school years start, the child looks outside the home for models of development and behaviour. During the early school years children learn to be more responsible and independent and have an increasing sense of personal identity. Children develop hypotheses about life and death, religion, past, present and future, good and bad. Peer group activities also begin, widening the child's experience and developing the mind.

During early adolescence the child learns to be more independent from the family, and wants greater privacy. Peer group activity is common, with members of the same sex. The cognitive gap between boys and girls widens: girls appear to be more mature and their school performance tends to be better than that of boys in the same age group.

By mid-adolescence, boys are striving for more independence and achievement, while girls tend to aim at improving personal skills. Loyalty and intimacy are valued, but at home communication with parents may be poor and relationships are sometimes fraught.

Complex abstract thought and reasoning develops. Self-image is strongly influenced by the physical changes of puberty. Fatness becomes an important issue for girls, causing poor and negative self-image. Peer group activities expand, and social groups now include members of the opposite sex. Dating and relationships with the opposite sex begin. Unintended pregnancy and sexually transmitted diseases become important health issues in this age group.

In late adolescence career and employment decisions become necessary. Loyalty, trust and support become valued traits in friendships. The end of the adolescent years produces an independent individual with his or her own ideas and personality. Decreasing numbers of individuals go directly into employment, while more continue in higher education.

Psychological testing

Whilst many scales and tests of aptitude and ability have been marketed, there is a natural reluctance to make known the results of these tests to individuals for fear of the 'self-fulfilling prophecy'. Such tests cover motor coordination, intelligence, language, memory, and writing. The use of school performance tests is normally restricted to child psychologists who will carry them out when there is concern about whether a child is achieving his or her potential.

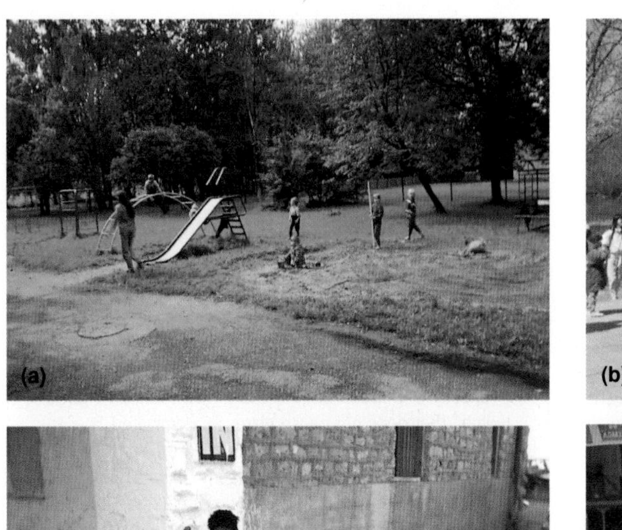

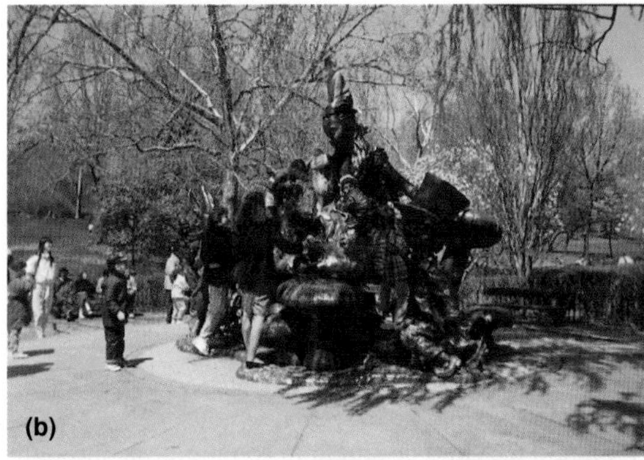

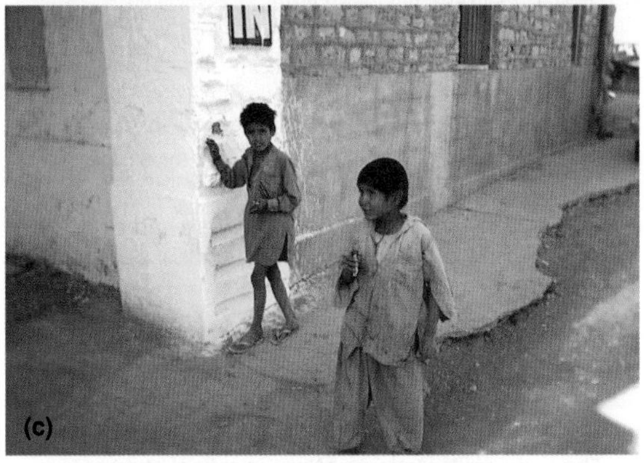

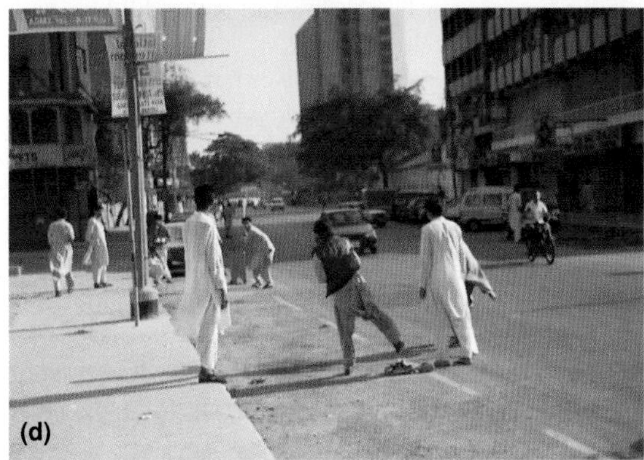

Fig 5.9
Playtime in (a) Estonia, (b) New York, (c) & (d) Pakistan.

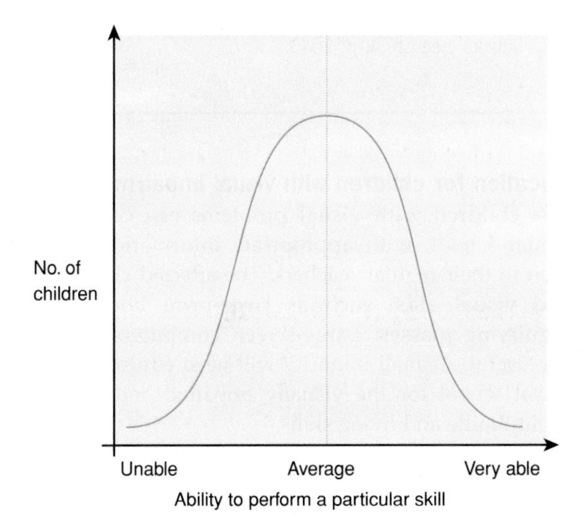

Fig 5.10
The bell-shaped range in ability, for any given skill, in a population of children.

Normal and abnormal development

As in younger children, there is a wide range of ability: a bell-shaped or Gaussian curve will describe the distribution of most abilities (Fig. 5.10). There will be two populations at the left of the scale: those who have naturally poor ability, plus those who are disabled.

Disabilities

There are many types of disabilities (see Fig. 5.7).

As disabilities are usually multiple and complex, it is essential that a full examination is carried out when a child is assessed for disability. Multidisciplinary assessment is usually necessary so that all potential problems are sought and if present, fully documented. This will enable effective planning in the light of the individual child's specific needs.

Special senses: hearing

Although for most children hearing loss will have been detected prior to school entry, in some it will have been missed, and a few children will lose their hearing during their school years, following accidents (usually with unilateral loss), meningitis or progressive ear pathology, including congenital otosclerosis, that may present in the late teens. Immigrant or travellers' children may arrive at school without prior screening.

One per 1000 school children can be expected to have a hearing problem severe enough to warrant special educational provision, and 1 in 10 000 will be profoundly deaf. Important decisions for these children must be made as early as possible:

- Should the child go to special school?
- Should the child be taught to communicate through sign language or lip reading and is the child expected to develop speech?
- Is the hearing problem stable or liable to deteriorate?

In most schools regular 'sweep' hearing tests are carried out on all children by a visiting audiometrician. Those who are repeatedly absent from school may be overlooked, as may those with fluctuating partial hearing loss caused by 'glue ear'. The education of many children is greatly hampered by intermittent deafness. Where there is doubt about a child's hearing, urgent referral for specialist assessment is imperative.

Note. Deaf child + hearing aid does not = normally hearing child. Hearing aids often get lost, or are not used, and the batteries often fail.

Special senses: vision

For most children with a visual problem this will have been recognized before they enter school; however in a few, problems will not have been detected. If there is any doubt, the child's sight should be tested (Practical box 5.1).

Note. A newly appearing squint is an important neurological sign that must be investigated straightaway by an ophthalmologist or paediatric neurologist.

Routine school eye tests are usually done by orthoptists when children are aged 5, 9 and 13 years, so that changes in visual acuity can be identified. Information box 5.9 shows the main ophthalmic problems found in school children.

Glasses tend to be overprescribed for minor visual defects. Slight defects do not need treatment, and wearing glasses does not cure optical defects. If a child is prescribed glasses, yet will not wear them, professional advice is needed. The lenses may have been incorrectly ground. In older children who are self-conscious contact lenses may be the answer, but these and their cleaning fluids are expensive. Contact lenses must be cared for properly in order to avoid eye infection.

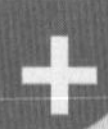

Practical Box 5.1

Testing eyes in school children

1. Ask the child about his/her eyesight. Have the child or parents noticed any problem?
2. Examine for a squint, as in the preschool child (Ch. 4, p. 104).
3. Examine for distant vision. A standard Snellen letter chart, without serifs (plain unembellished letters) is needed; picture cards should not be used. The floor must be accurately measured so that the child is exactly 6 metres from the chart. There must be 'good light' that does not cause glare. An illuminated Snellen screen is best. Do not let bright children learn the screen letters before the test (some cheat!). Test each eye separately. As long as the child manages a visual acuity of 6/6 by both eyes, sight should be regarded as satisfactory. Many children can read the smallest (6/4) letters and most can manage 6/5.

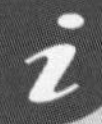

Information Box 5.9

The main ophthalmic problems in school children

1. Myopia (short sight) often develops around the time of puberty.
2. Astigmatism. The eyeball is an irregular (imperfect) sphere, thus shapes and edges are distorted.
3. Hypermetropia. Long sight impairs near vision.
4. Eye infections are mainly bacterial (usually staphylococcal) or viral.
5. Allergic conjunctivitis is usually associated with hay fever.
6. Eye injury readily occurs; eyes must be protected by goggles in laboratories and in workshops.
7. Squints (see Ch. 4, p. 104.)

Education for children with visual impairment

Most children with visual problems can cope in a normal school, with appropriate information being given to their regular teachers. The affected child may need visual aids, such as large-print books and magnifying glasses. Large-screen computers can be very useful. A small minority will need education in a special school for the visually impaired and will be taught Braille and living skills.

Communication disorders

One percent of children come to school with marked language disability and a further 4–5% may also show

Information Box 5.10

Classification of language disorders

- Impaired language input
  - (a) Hearing loss
  - (b) Environmental influences:
    - Stressful family life
    - Large family
    - Multiple births
    - Bilingualism
    - Parental mental health disorder
- Language processing
  - (a) Hearing problems
  - (b) Specific social and affective problems with cognitive impairment (autism)
  - (c) Functional brain abnormalities, e.g epilepsy following head injury
  - (d) Specific language or speech problem
- Language output
  - (a) Structural abnormalities of the palate
  - (b) Disorders of oromotor control, e.g. dysarthria

Information Box 5.11

Outcomes of language disorders

- Most children with mild language delay improve.
- Children with severe delay in expressive speech are likely to have continuing problems of word finding and language formulation in school.
- Children with problems in understanding language are particularly likely to have continuing problems.
- Those with other learning and social problems are at high risk of persisting language problems which result in lasting difficulty.

the sequelae of earlier language difficulties (mainly in speech and expressive language).

Language delay implies the acquisition of language along normal lines but more slowly than expected.

Language disorder implies a pattern of development not seen in normal language acquisition. For a classification of language disorders see Information box 5.10.

There is a strong male predominance for language problems; the male : female ratio is 4 : 1. There is often a positive family history of language impairment, reading or spelling difficulty. There is an increased incidence of language problems in children with sex chromosome disorders; the fragile X syndrome should be excluded.

Causes of language delay

- Brain injury causing cerebral palsy can cause impaired language output, or problems with processing of information.
- Families with several children, multiple births, parental depression, or low intelligence. Social problems leading to neglect can cause delayed language acquisition.
- Deafness. Sensorineural deafness is a very important cause of language delay and must always be looked for in children with language disorders, as well as otitis media with effusion – though the latter is not usually the sole cause. Sometimes poor vision denies the child the visual cues which they need in the initial stages of speaking.

Many children with language impairment have subtle difficulties in high level problem solving and thinking; sometimes there is impaired control of mouth movements, chewing and swallowing and an increase in dribbling; they may show slowness on other movement tasks and mild generalized clumsiness. Frustration and distractibility are also associated with language difficulties.

The assessment of a child with speech and language impairment is often multidisciplinary. If the problem is confined to speech and language the child is usually managed by the speech therapist. Outcomes in language disorders are shown in Information box 5.11.

Reading problems – ‘Might it be dyslexia?’

‘Dyslexia’ is a term applied to children who read significantly below the expected level for their age yet appear to be making adequate developmental progress in other areas. It is a lifelong difficulty and its nature changes with maturation and development, e.g. reading can improve but spelling may worsen. A diagnosis of dyslexia should not be made lightly, nor used as a ‘kindly’ explanation for low intelligence. In dyslexia there is usually a speech-processing deficit, especially phonological processing.

There may be a family history of dyslexia, especially in either parent. No cause for dyslexia is known but functional imaging techniques which relate structure to function, such as PET scanning, are likely to be of diagnostic value in the near future.

A child’s reading difficulties should be discovered by teachers, though these are sometimes detected in the course of neurological examination. An assessment by a specialist teacher or psychologist should be arranged to confirm the extent and the severity of the child’s difficulties, and to initiate an intervention programme.

It is good practice to ask a child of school age to read in the course of physical examination; this tests visual function, mental state and ability.

Severe learning difficulties

The prevalence of severe learning difficulty (IQ <50) in the general population is 3–4 per 1000. Identification of the aetiology (see Information box 5.12) is usually a great help to all concerned because a rational plan for the future can be developed. It is very difficult to discuss the prognosis meaningfully when one does not have a diagnosis. The latter is also helpful in determining recurrence risks. It is also important to look for associated disorders (Information box 5.13).

In a significant proportion of children no cause can be found. It is important that the child remains under specialist supervision because frequently advances are made and new techniques are developed, and opportunities for making a diagnosis may become available later. It is vital that the family is informed about possible special educational measures for the affected child.

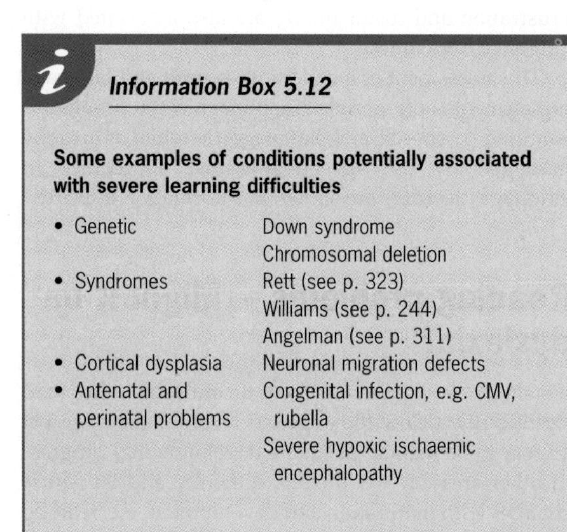

Information Box 5.12

Some examples of conditions potentially associated with severe learning difficulties

• Genetic	Down syndrome Chromosomal deletion
• Syndromes	Rett (see p. 323) Williams (see p. 244) Angelman (see p. 311)
• Cortical dysplasia	Neuronal migration defects
• Antenatal and perinatal problems	Congenital infection, e.g. CMV, rubella Severe hypoxic ischaemic encephalopathy

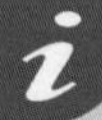

Information Box 5.13

Associated disorders in children with severe learning difficulties

- Cerebral palsy
- Epilepsy
- Severe hearing or visual impairment
- Autism
- Severe psychiatric problems

Rehabilitation (Fig. 5.11)

The aim of rehabilitation is to help an individual achieve their maximum potential following a severe injury or chronic illness. This particularly applies to head injury, where children may experience a great deal of overprotection and hence lose confidence. It can be very difficult to sort out psychological from organic factors.

An assessment of the situation before the trauma is needed, so that the present condition can be understood in the light of previous development. Depending on the severity of the brain damage, children may be left with convulsions and various degrees of memory and learning deficits. This can become a litiginous area and very careful record keeping is needed. Some children develop a temporary post-traumatic state with headaches, personality change and memory loss. This should settle and normal function usually returns with the passage of time and the post-traumatic state should not be allowed to develop into a psychological overlay and a focus for unconstructive grievance. If the child had seizures after the accident, there is an increased risk of development of a continuing tendency to epilepsy.

Children who cannot walk require a wheelchair. These may be pushchairs, self-propelled or electric. Selection of the chair and fitting it is a skilled process, which will need to be repeated frequently as the child grows. The chair must be safe, robust, comfortable, and adaptable to allow growth. It should be sufficiently manoeuvrable to get through doors and traverse various surfaces, transportable and foldable to get into cars, and affordable. Electric battery-operated chairs are heavy and expensive, but give great freedom to those with the ability to use them. Self-propelled chairs have to be relatively light, and give exercise as well as

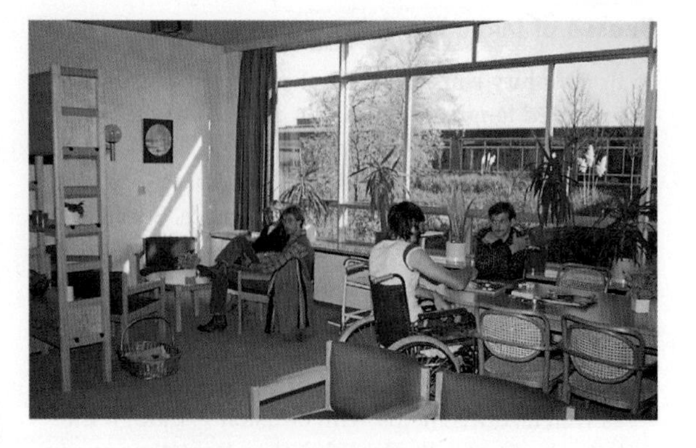

Fig 5.11
A rehabilitation centre in Holland for adolescents in wheelchairs.

mobility. Several types may be needed for different purposes at home and at school.

A multidisciplinary team, involving a paediatrician, physiotherapist, appliance fitter, occupational therapist, speech therapist, specialist nurse and health visitor, must work together with the family doctor, parents and social worker to make the rehabilitation programme succeed.

Growth

Growth and the mechanism of puberty are key paediatric subjects. James Tanner undertook much of the pioneering work that led to present day knowledge. His book *Growth at Adolescence* is the classic text. Other useful texts include Wales JK et al (1995) *Color Atlas of Pediatric Endocrinology and Growth* (see Further reading).

Growth is determined by a complex interplay of genetic, health and environmental factors (see Information box 5.14). Growth starts at conception, being greatest in the second trimester. In the first 2 years of life it is dependent on nutrition; thereafter hormonal influences become important, especially growth hormone in early childhood.

The endocrine factors that underlie the onset of puberty and its physical changes are gradually becoming clearer. During the 1–3 years before the first pubertal changes are seen, gradually increasing levels of luteinizing hormone are released during sleep. This appears to be a marker that gonadotrophin-releasing hormone (GnRH) is being produced by the hypothalamus. Once a critical level is produced, the physical changes of puberty begin to appear. By mid-puberty GnRH is also being produced by day, in pulses every 90–120 minutes. This is necessary for full pubertal development, menarche and ovulation. Growth hormone in conjunction with the sex steroids leads to acceleration of body growth and skeletal maturation. Pulsatile GnRH secretion starts later in boys, by an average of 2 years; their peak growth rate is greater but the period of fast growth is shorter. The net result is that boys eventually become, on average, taller than girls by 12.5 cm. Growth, influenced by sex steroids, stops when the epiphyses fuse. Fusion of the epiphyses occurs from the feet upwards and is only complete when the clavicles stop growing at about 25 years.

Information Box 5.14

Factors affecting measured growth/height

- Parents' current height and the age of onset of their puberty
- Birthweight
- Social factors (e.g. deprivation)
- Bone age
- Exercise
- Time of day when measurements are done (morning height is greater than the afternoon height as the vertebral discs become flatter in the upright posture)
- The equipment used
- The operator's experience

Growth assessment

A stadiometer (an accurate measuring device) is used to measure sitting and standing heights. The head is held in a standard position with the external auditory meatus and the outer eye canthus being on the same horizontal plane. Other important measurements include weight and head circumference; in males testicular volume is evaluated using an orchidometer (see p. 142).

An assessment of the pubertal stage is important. This is done by comparing the development of pubic hair, female breasts and penile growth with standard photographs originally published by Tanner.

All growth measurements must be plotted on a growth chart. Revised charts that reflect increasing child rates of growth were produced in the early 1990s. Male and female charts are available. The charts are reproduced in Appendix 3, pages 373–381. The parents' heights should also be plotted, subtracting 12.5 cm from the father's height when plotting it on his daughter's chart, while adding 12.5 cm to the mother's height when plotting it on her son's chart. This is done to allow for the difference in height between the sexes.

Abnormal growth

Where there is concern about a child's growth pattern, further measurement and reassessment in 3 or 6 months' time is vital. It is usually the rate of growth that is important, and this can be plotted on special growth velocity charts, available for males and females; these are reproduced in Appendix 3, pages 375–376. Disparity between height and weight measurements, abnormal growth velocities and measurements crossing height centiles need to be investigated (Fig. 5.12). A single height measurement below the 3rd centile is unlikely to be abnormal on its own but must be followed up in order to establish a growth trend and interpretation in the light of the parental growth pattern.

Some causes of short and tall stature are shown in Information boxes 5.15 and 5.16, respectively.

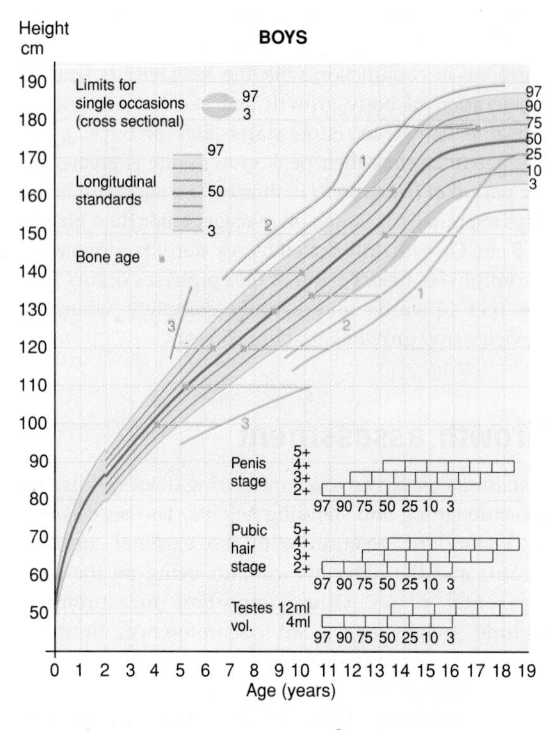

Causes:
Constitutional tall stature
Advanced growth
Endocrine disease (usually)
growth hormone excess
hyperthyroidism
sex steroid excess
hypocortisolism

Causes:
Constitutional short stature
Delay in growth
Endocrine disease
hypopituitarism
hypothyroidism
cortisol excess

Fig 5.12
Various patterns of abnormal growth and their causes.

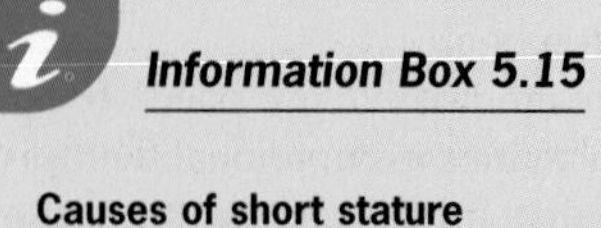

Information Box 5.15

Causes of short stature

Proportionate short stature
Growth delay, i.e. delayed puberty
Genetic/constitutional
Endocrine
- Growth hormone deficiency (see p. 203)
- Hypothyroidism (Fig. 5.13) (see p. 202)
- Hypogonadism (see p. 205)
- Hypopituitarism (see p. 204)
- Long-term consequences of Cushing syndrome

Chronic systemic disease
- Cystic fibrosis (see p. 352)
- Inflammatory bowel disease (Crohn and ulcerative colitis and short-bowel conditions)
- Cardiac: pulmonary hypertension, chronic cardiac failure
- Respiratory: severe asthma
- Renal failure (see p. 304)
- Chronic infection, e.g. AIDS, TB, tropical parasites and worms, giardiasis
- Emotional deprivation
- Starvation
- Syndromic, e.g. Down syndrome (see p. 241) but there are many other syndromes

Disproportionate short stature

Short limbs, short stature	Turner syndrome (see p. 240) Achondroplasia (see p. 244)
Short trunk, short stature	Mucopolysaccharidoses (see p. 289, 291) Metaphyseal dysplasia (see p. 345) Extreme pubertal delay Spinal irradiation

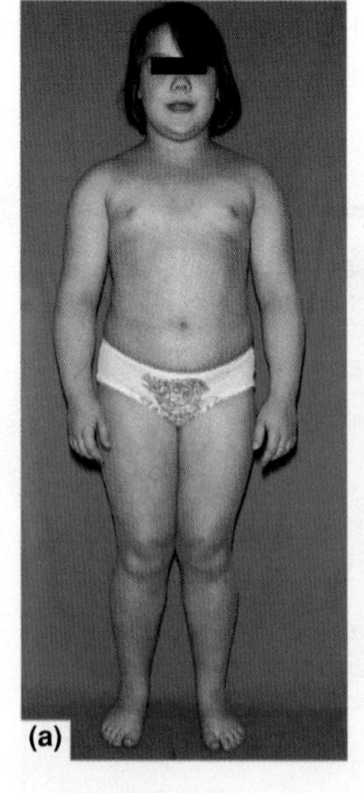
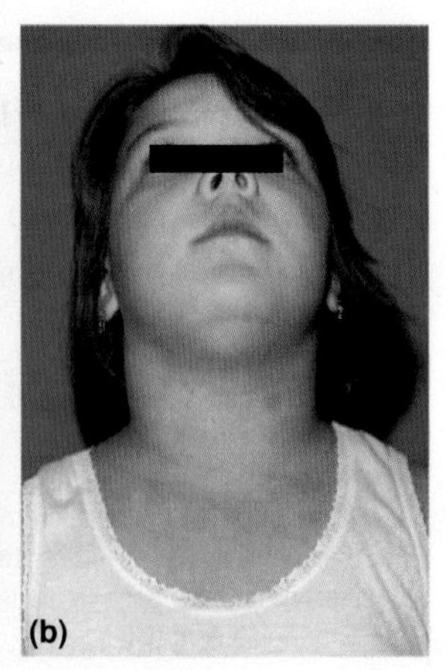
(a) (b)

Fig 5.13
Hypothyroidism in a young girl.

Information Box 5.16

Causes of tall stature

Proportionate tall stature	Familial tall stature Advanced growth, e.g. early puberty, precocious puberty Endocrine: hyperthyroidism, growth hormone excess, sex steroids excess, short-term consequence of Cushing syndrome Syndromic: Sotos (see p. 205)
Long-limb tall stature conditions	Marfan syndrome (see p. 245) Homocystinuria (see p. 288) Klinefelter syndrome (see p. 241)

Special growth charts have been produced for children with Down syndrome and girls with Turner syndrome (who tend to be short).

Puberty and its assessment

Female puberty

Tanner divided breast development into five stages (Fig. 5.14): B1 (prepubertal) to B5 (adult). Puberty starts with breast development (B2) at an average age of 10.5 years (range 8–13 years). Breast buds develop first followed by the development of smooth breast contour. Pubic hair follows 6 months later (Fig. 5.14). By stage B3 the uterus has doubled in size. Menarche (B4) occurs relatively late, at an average age of 12.8 years (range 11–15 years). Menstruation is often irregular for 1–2 years and early cycles are usually anovulatory. At stage B5 the uterus has enlarged fivefold.

> ***Information Box 5.17***
>
> **The normal sequence of puberty in females**
>
> - Breast bud (B2) followed by onset of pubic hair development
> - Growth spurt
> - Breast contour development (B3)
> - Menarche (B4)
> - Adult pattern breast (B5), and complete pubic hair

The average time from B2 to B5 is 4 years (range 1.5–5 years). For a summary of the normal sequence of female puberty see Information box 5.17.

Breast and pubic hair development

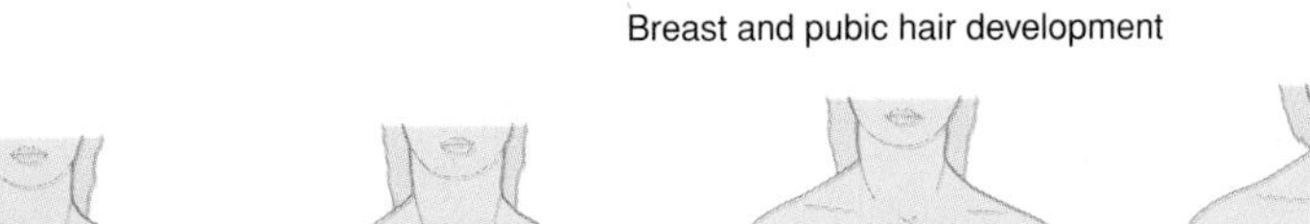

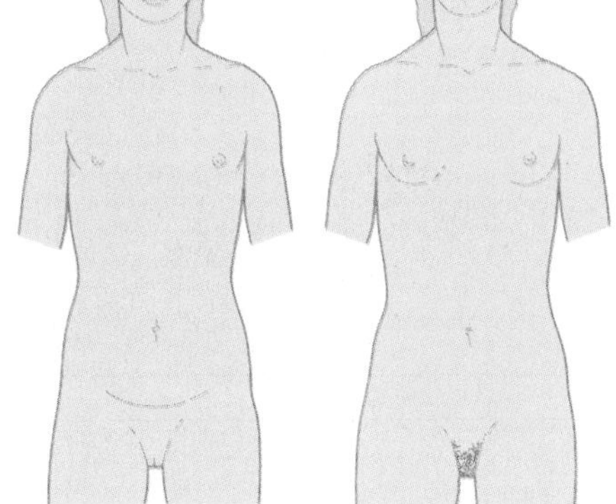

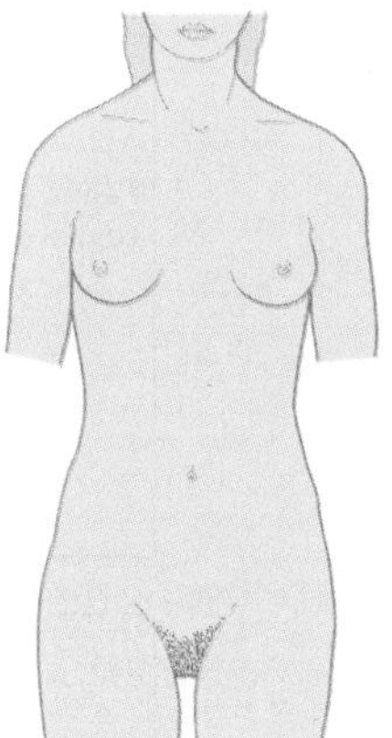

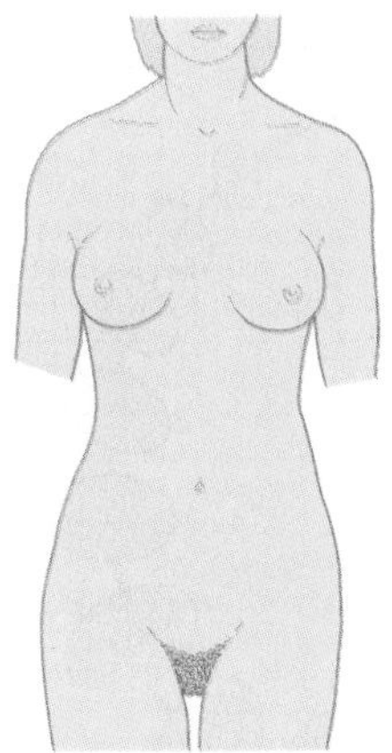

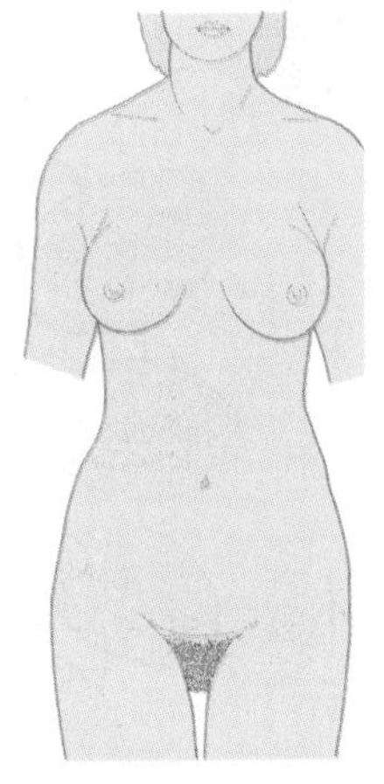

Breast development

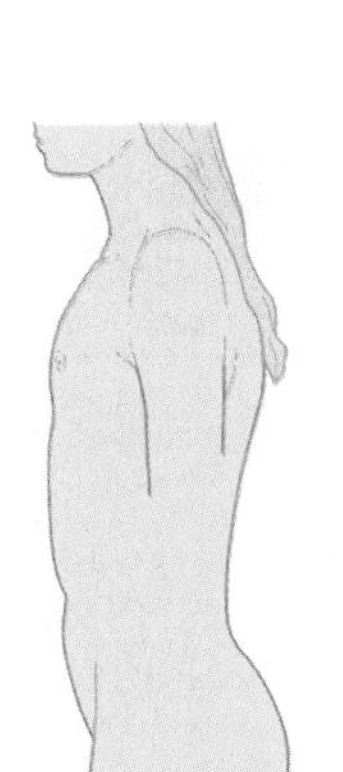

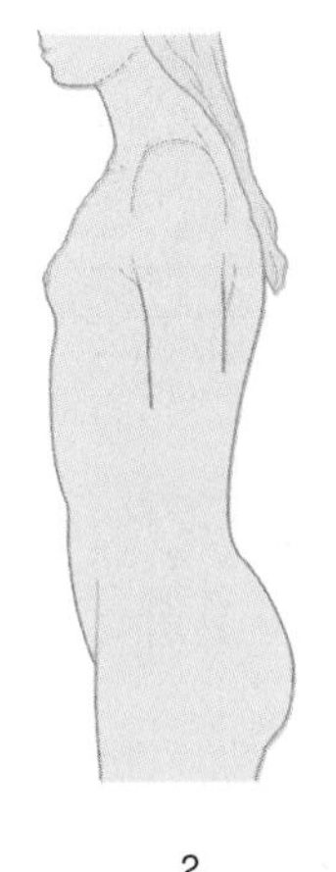

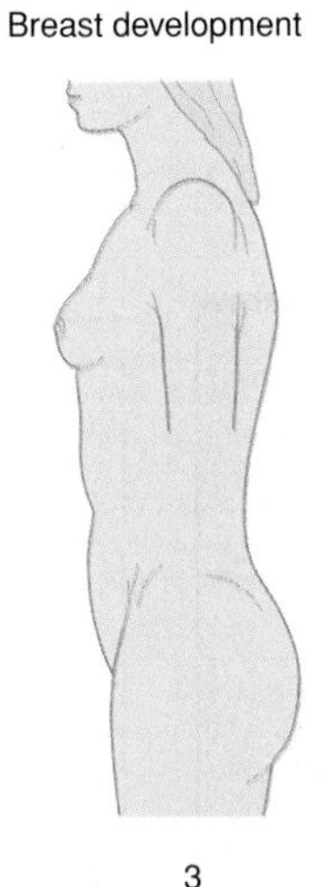

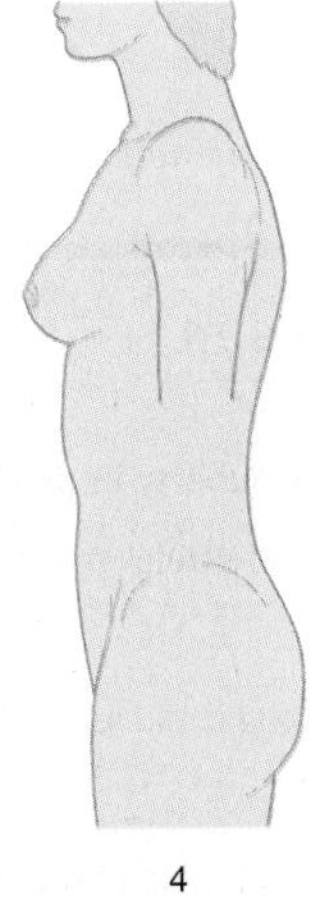

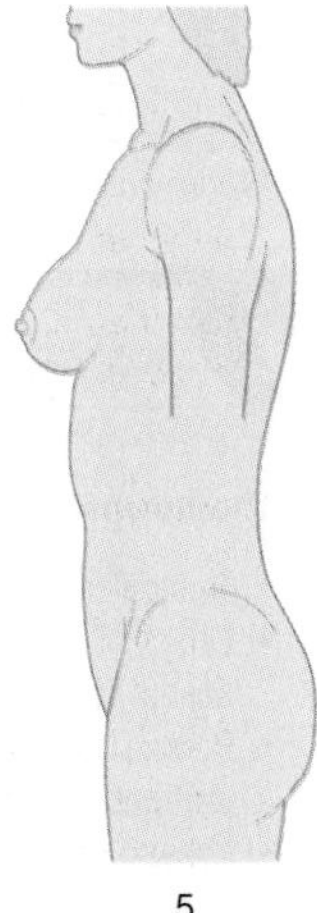

Fig 5.14
Female pubertal changes.

Male puberty

Boys start puberty later than girls. The first sign is testicular enlargement. A volume greater than or equal to 4 ml indicates the beginning of puberty. The testicular volume can be measured using an orchidometer; this uses beads of increasing sizes (Fig. 5.15).

Penile enlargement starts at mean age 11.5 years with a range 9.5–13.5 years (Fig. 5.16) and the male growth spurts occur 2–3 years later, with peak velocity occurring when testicular volume is about 12–15 ml. Axillary and facial hair develops late, as does the breaking of the voice.

Usually pubertal changes occur over 3 years. For a summary of the normal sequence of male puberty see Information box 5.18.

There is no fixed age at which the onset of puberty is abnormal, and the onset of puberty at a time within the normal range does not exclude pathology. In the UK, 3% of boys and girls will have started puberty by 9 and 8 years respectively, and only 3% will have no signs of puberty by 13.8 and 13.4 years respectively.

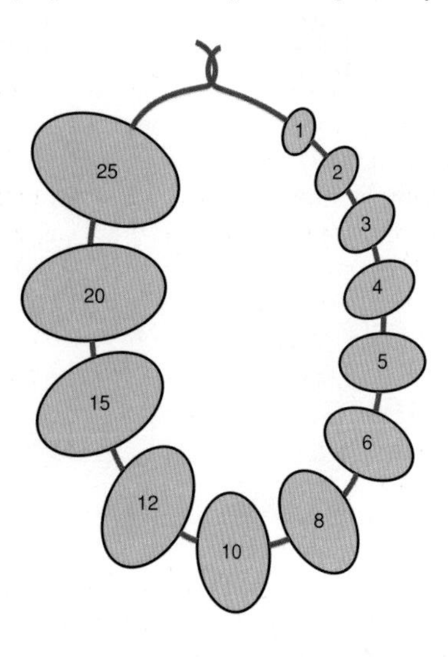

Fig 5.15
The Prader orchidometer (numbers are volumes in millilitres).

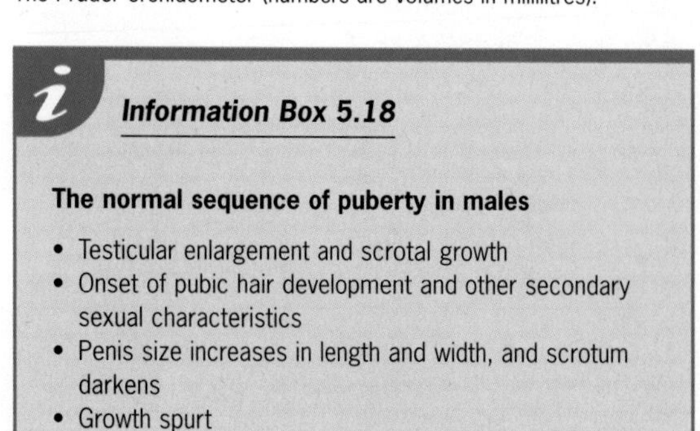

Information Box 5.18

The normal sequence of puberty in males

- Testicular enlargement and scrotal growth
- Onset of pubic hair development and other secondary sexual characteristics
- Penis size increases in length and width, and scrotum darkens
- Growth spurt
- Established adult pattern of pubic hair and axillary and facial hair

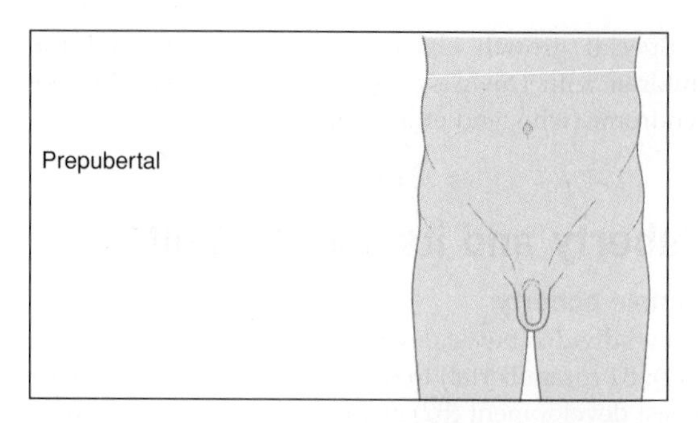

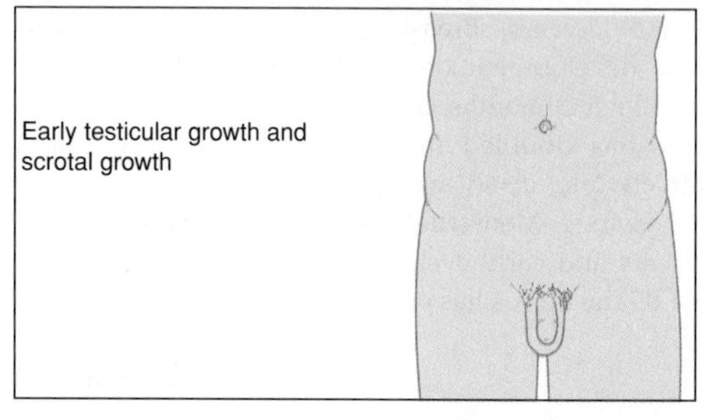

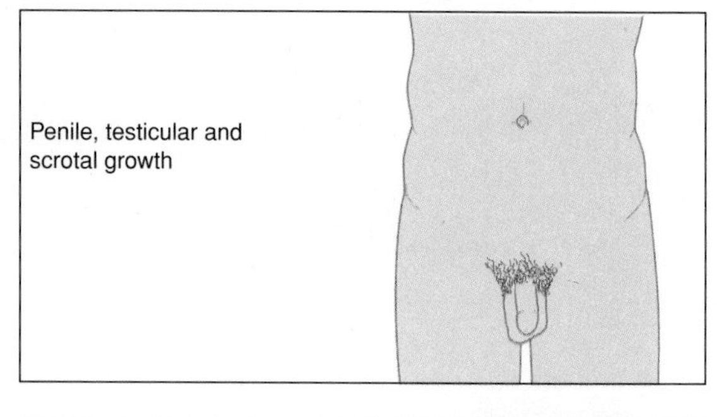

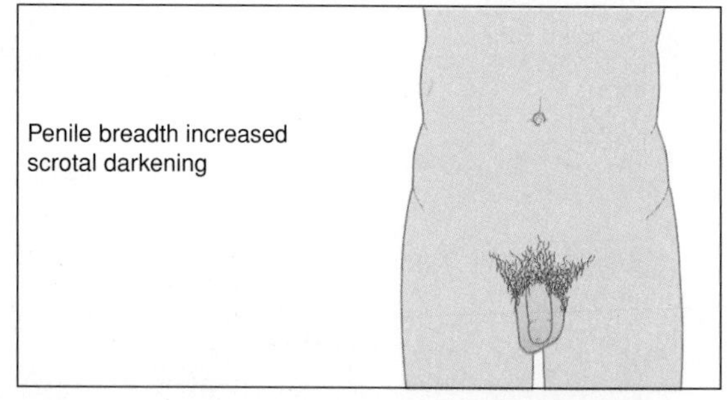

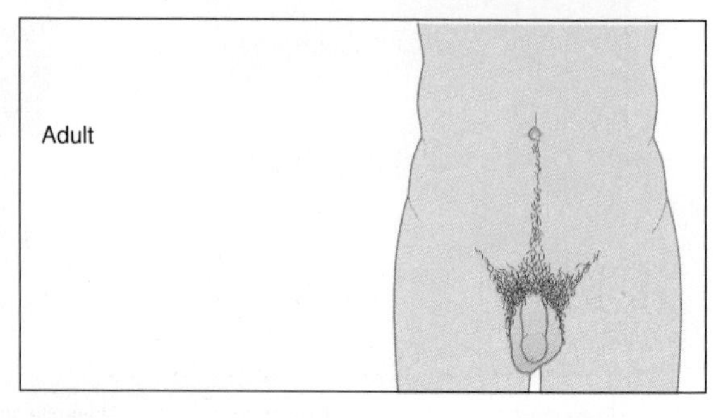

Fig 5.16
Male pubertal changes.

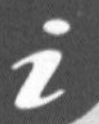

Information Box 5.19

Causes of precocious puberty

Early with normal pubertal sequence	Central precocious puberty: early activation of the hypothalamic–pituitary–gonadal axis, either idiopathically (especially in girls) or secondarily to intracranial pathology (especially in boys) Excess gonadotrophins, e.g. testotoxicosis
Early with abnormal pubertal sequence	Isolated premature thelarche: occurs in the first 2 years of life where the only abnormality is mild breast development; it is usually self-limiting Adrenal pathology, e.g.: – Adrenal hyperplasia (see p. 197) – Tumours – Cushing syndrome Gonadal causes, e.g. tumours Sex steroids ingestion Primary hypothyroidism McCune–Albright syndrome (see p. 204)

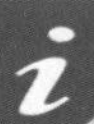

Information Box 5.20

Causes of delayed puberty

Late, with normal pubertal sequence	Constitutional, common especially in boys Chronic systemic disease Hypogonadotrophic hypogonadism, e.g.: – Kallman syndrome (see p. 204) – Cranial irradiation – Panhypopituitarism – Primary hypothyroidism
Late, with abnormal pubertal sequence	Turner syndrome Ovarian agenesis Polycystic ovaries Anorchia, i.e. absent testes (see hypogonadism, p. 205)

Abnormal puberty

A child should be investigated if there is an abnormal sequence of pubertal changes or if signs of puberty are outside the age limits mentioned above. For causes of precocious and delayed puberty see Information boxes 5.19 and 5.20 respectively.

Nutrition (Fig. 5.17)

Surveys of British children and adolescents suggest that the majority are well nourished, although average intake of fruit and vegetables is lower and fat intake higher than is currently recommended. Obesity is the most common nutritional problem.

There are wide variations in the diets of British children and a concern remains that some children have deficient diets. Dietary surveys have consistently shown that children from lower socioeconomic backgrounds have poorer diets, reporting more consumption of fats, sweets and sweet drinks, and less high fibre and first class protein foods. Some groups of children, especially in some Asian communities, receive too little dietary iron and vitamin D. The great majority of children do not need iron and vitamin supplements but there is real difficulty in detecting the few who do. Thus taking dietary histories is important; there are great differences in the vitamin and iron content of vegetarian diets. Those who eat a great deal of unrefined grain in chapatis are at risk of malabsorbing vitamin D due to the effect of phytates in the flour. 'Stop rickets' campaigns are run in areas where there are known to be children at dietary risk. Rickets is commonly found in Pakistan where there is abundant sunshine but children wear clothes that shield them from the sun.

Note. Do not think of children from Asian backgrounds as a homogeneous group; they come from a huge geographical territory with great differences in customs, religion, diet and degrees of assimilation of European cultural patterns.

There is a key place for health education, which must underpin the achievement of good nutrition: this should be aimed at both the parents and the children at school.

Junk food

Food availability, influence of the peer group, boredom, and pressure from advertising are major influences on quality and quantity of food intake.

The concept that mealtimes should be a family event is tending to fade. More foods are bought either 'oven-ready' or 'take-away'. In order to make these foods tasty and relatively economic to produce they are usually

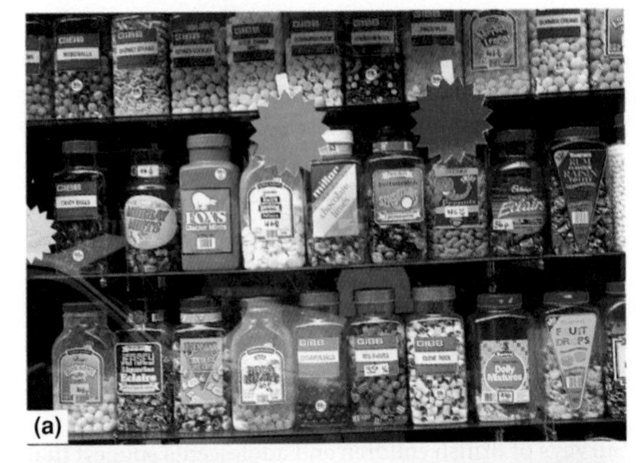

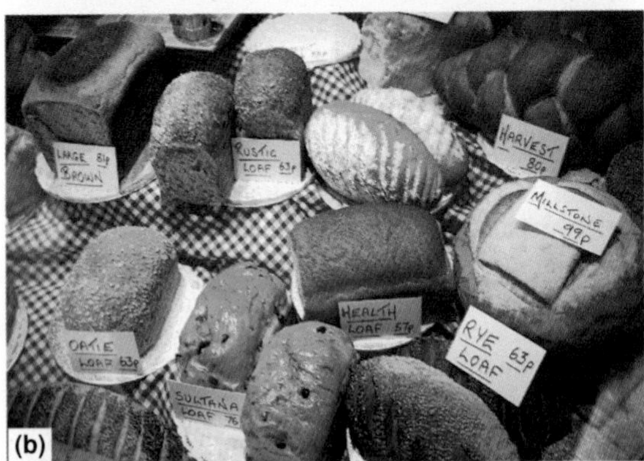

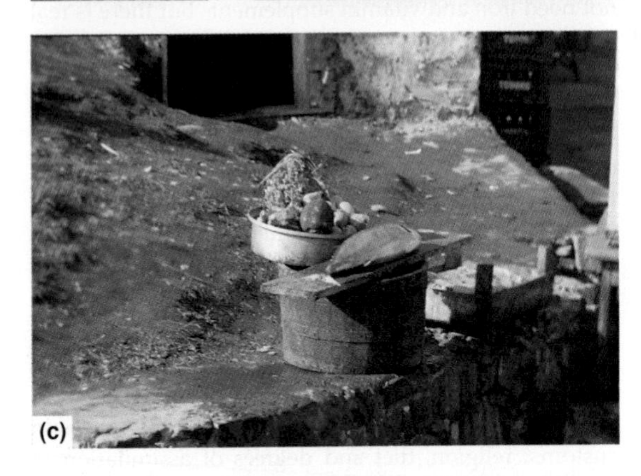

Fig 5.17
Food from different countries, (a) Bad for teeth in Scotland. (b) Good Scottish bread. (c) Healthy food in Turkey.

high in fat, starch and total energy, with little nonstarch polysaccharide. When meals are not eaten as a family there is little need for children to eat the same as the rest of the family.

Faddiness (selective eating) can originate even at weaning. 'Fussy' children may have been determined toddlers whose food refusal was greeted by carers as an indication that the children did not like these foods, while it is usually an expression of independence in response to new tastes and new textures. These feeding habits can lead to either underfeeding or obesity, depending on the quantity of food ultimately consumed by the fussy child.

Management revolves around educating parents on better weaning practices and discouraging high fluid intake after the first year of life. Children should be encouraged to eat with the family. The family meals must be of good quality, containing protein, fruit and vegetables, and must be low in saturated fats. On a wider scale, public health education and socioeconomic changes are needed to influence the bad eating habits of children.

Obesity

The proportion of children who are regarded as overweight is continuing to rise in the UK and other industrialized countries. Obesity is a public health problem, although it is in later life that the most adverse effects on morbidity and mortality become apparent (Information box 5.21). Nevertheless, fatness in childhood is a predictor of adulthood obesity in populations and individuals, and affected children can be badly teased (see Fig. 5.18).

Factors influencing weight are both genetic and environmental (Information box 5.22). In general, fat children come from fat families, and changing long established feeding patterns is very difficult because one has to encourage the whole family to change their lifestyle. Management starts with education: explaining where calories lurk in sweets, fizzy drinks, etc; the importance of eating only at mealtimes and not between; and the importance of exercise (Practical box

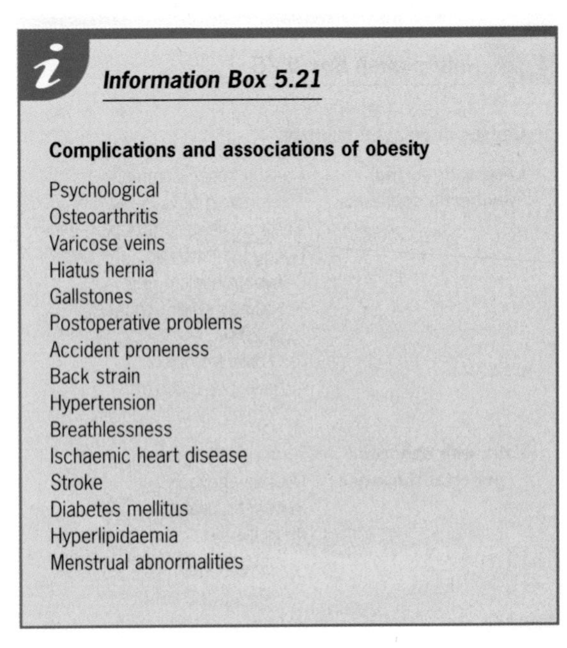

Information Box 5.21

Complications and associations of obesity

Psychological
Osteoarthritis
Varicose veins
Hiatus hernia
Gallstones
Postoperative problems
Accident proneness
Back strain
Hypertension
Breathlessness
Ischaemic heart disease
Stroke
Diabetes mellitus
Hyperlipidaemia
Menstrual abnormalities

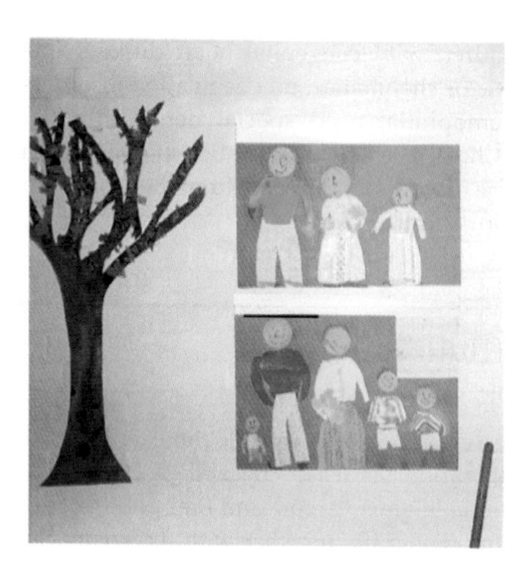

Fig 5.18
Self-portraits by an obese child, showing a perception of themselves as thin.

5.2). Strict diets usually fail; the child should be encouraged to keep their weight stationary whilst they grow in height and get more active. Notice how slowly and how little some children walk.

The rare physical causes of obesity should be excluded (Information box 5.23).

Prevention

This should be aimed at the population as a whole, with education concerning sensible eating and to encourage the choice of low fat foods and unrefined carbohydrates. Prevention requires socioeconomic changes in policy, aimed, for example, at better play and sports facilities, greater opportunities for walking within cities and discouragement of sloth and excess time spent with computers or watching TV.

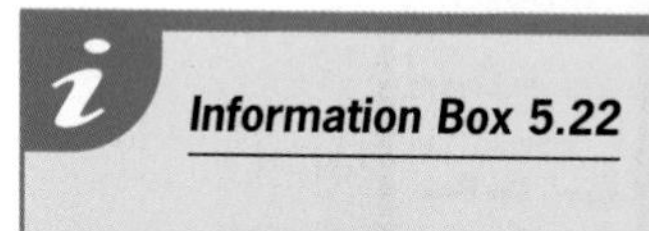

Information Box 5.22

Factors influencing weight

- Sex
- Ethnicity
- General health/illness/treatment
- Behaviour: diet, exercise
- Cultural 'norms'
- Self-concept: perceptions
- Psychosocial stress
- Parental height and weight
- Parental behaviour, e.g. diet, exercise

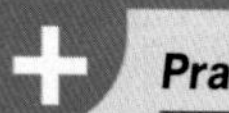

Practical Box 5.2

Principles of the management of childhood obesity

- Motivation
- Diet modification
- Encourage physical activity

Information Box 5.23

Medical causes of obesity

Endocrine:	Cushing syndrome, growth hormone deficiency, hypothyroidism
Syndromic:	Prader–Willi syndrome, Laurence–Moon–Biedl syndrome
Drugs:	Steroids, sodium valproate (which can increase appetite)
Apparent:	Oedema (any cause)
Neurological:	Hypothalamic disorders, e.g. due to trauma, tumour
	Hydrocephalus with spina bifida

Eating disorders

Anorexia nervosa and bulimia declare themselves during adolescence and, whilst not unknown, are rare before then. The incidence of anorexia nervosa peaks in the late teens with girls up to ten times more likely to be affected than boys. Whether the problem is really becoming more prevalent is unclear, Victorian girls certainly starved themselves, yet amongst some sixth-form girls in Eastern Europe recently, none had heard of the problem and did not recall any anorexic classmates. Children with eating problems which meet the full diagnostic criteria of anorexia in the UK are rare. Most studies suggest a prevalence of around 2 per 1000 in women and girls, with rates being highest (at about 10 per 1000) in middle-class schoolgirls; the problem is much less common but not unknown in boys.

There is a tremendous variation in the presentation of anorexia nervosa in children. The danger of overlooking the diagnosis is that the eating disorder becomes more entrenched; it may become more difficult to engage the patient and the family in appropriate treatment, and the longer term risks, for emotional and physical health, of a period of prolonged starvation become more substantial. Clear communication within the team responsible for the child's management, and with the family, is essential, as is a consistent approach to treatment.

Teeth

Toothache is largely a preventable problem. The principal factor in keeping children's teeth healthy is health education. Children need to understand the basis of plaque and how it causes tooth decay. Understanding that sugar coating on teeth leads to their decay empowers them to prevent it. Whilst tooth brushing morning and night with fluoride toothpaste is to be recommended, they need to appreciate that 'acid attack' on the tooth enamel between brushing times is the main problem. Eating sweet food and fizzy drinks between meals is particularly damaging. They need to eat vegetable fibre foods which naturally clean the teeth and to know that 'cheese is good and sweets are bad'.

The number of fillings carried out in children is now decreasing rapidly. At last it is being realized that much mild decay is self-healing. Payment for children's dentistry has been reorganized, so that in the UK it is now based on dental health maintenance.

Overcrowded irregular teeth cause great distress. Children need to know that orthodontic procedures at the right time, usually around the age of 15, can correct this.

Information Box 5.24

Certain diseases diagnosable from the mouth

- Yellow-stained teeth suggest tetracycline administration in infancy, or kernicterus (now rare in developed countries).
- Teeth are soft and decay readily in disorders such as osteogenesis imperfecta. Teeth also decay readily in cyanotic heart disease; all children with heart disease need expert dental care because they are at risk of subacute bacterial endocarditis.
- Missing teeth prior to normal shedding of first dentition and rupture of the buccal frenulum of the upper lip is indicative of child abuse.
- Black lines in the gums above the teeth suggest lead poisoning.
- Teeth may be damaged by intrauterine infection, e.g. syphilis.
- Thick gums occur following chronic treatment with phenytoin, and to a lesser extent with other antiepilepsy drugs.
- Recurrent oral ulceration may be a feature of Crohn's disease.

Children with congenital heart disease, especially cyanotic or rheumatic, and coagulation disorders, such as haemophilia, need special dental attention (see p. 99, Ch. 4). The key is prevention of dental decay.

Some diseases diagnosable from the mouth are given in Information box 5.24.

Immunization

Before or immediately after school entry children's immunization status is checked. A booster dose of diphtheria-tetanus vaccine and oral polio is advised at this time (Fig. 5.19), together with the second measles, mumps and rubella (MMR) vaccine.

Rubella vaccination

This vaccine is no longer offered to teenage girls as the MMR vaccines given at 1 and 3.5 years have replaced it. It is vital that young people understand about these diseases, why they were immunized and know which immunizations they have had. As these illnesses become rarer, people tend to fail to understand why protection is needed.

Polio, tetanus and diphtheria vaccination

School leavers require a repeat dose of oral polio vaccine, plus a booster injection of tetanus and adult strength diphtheria vaccine which has a lower dose of diphtheria toxoid and is advised for those over 10 years.

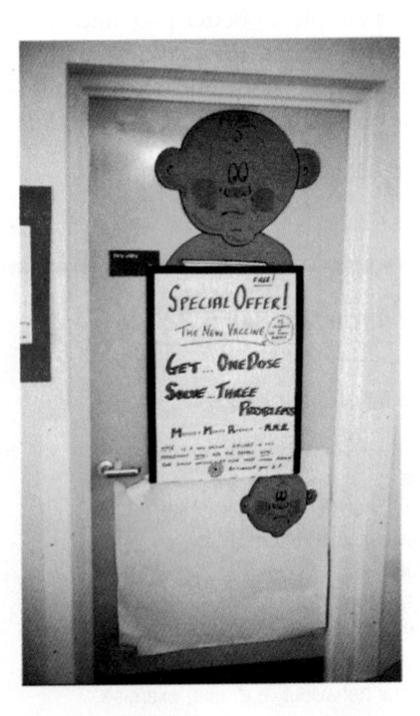

Fig 5.19
Poster advertising the MMR vaccine.

Bacterial meningitis vaccines

School children should have been vaccinated against *Haemophilus influenzae* b in infancy. In Autumn 1999 conjugated meningococcus C vaccine was introduced. Initially it was offered to school children until a new generation entered school who had the immunization in infancy with their other primary immunizations. There are hopes that meningococcus B and a pneumococcal vaccine for all will also soon become available.

Tuberculosis – BCG vaccine

TB is on the increase; sporadic cases occur, particularly in poor inner city populations. In populations where the disease is uncontrolled there is a peak in presentation in late adolescence. The key to diagnosis is chronic cough, unexplained loss of weight and night sweats, but TB can present with meningitis, ascites and arthritis.

The UK policy is to undertake detection of previous infection, usually around the ages of 13–14 years. This is done by means of skin testing, with a low dose of tuberculin given as either a Mantoux test (the more reliable test) (Fig. 5.20) or a modified Heaf test gun using a disposable magnetic needle plate. The dose is intradermally injected into the palmar aspect of the forearm and inspected 3 days later. It is explained that BCG vaccine will not be offered if the skin test is positive (grade 3 or 4).

Those with a negative response are offered BCG vaccine. This should be injected intradermally at the level of the insertion of the deltoid into the outer aspect of the upper arm. Explain that it will leave a small scar; there are no good alternative sites. Scars tend to be larger in those with a tendency to keloid formation, and this should be pointed out.

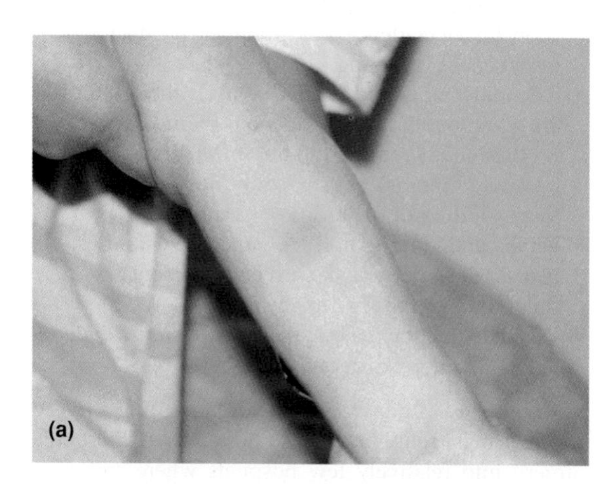

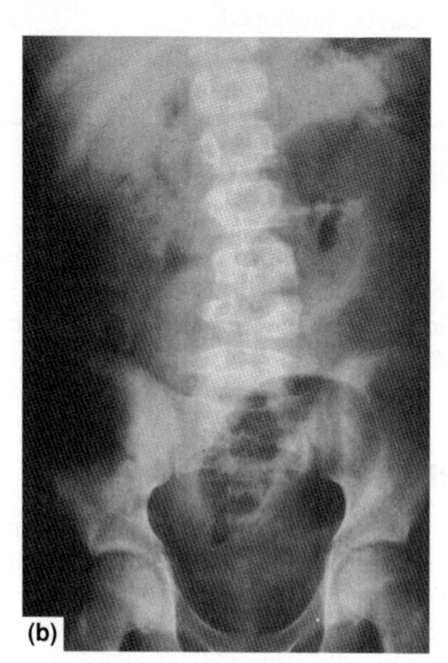

Fig 5.20
(a) Positive Mantoux test. (b) Tuberculosis of the spine in a child.

Clinical approach

History taking

Progressive involvement of the child

Young children need to be seen with their parents. The older school child will want to take a major role in giving their history. They are often inhibited in the presence of a parent and it may be necessary to ask parent(s) and staff to leave the room so that the child can talk freely.

The Children Act gives the right to confidentiality to children. It is left to health professionals to decide when children are mature enough to take responsibility for decisions regarding themselves, rather than sticking to precise ages. The emphasis now is on informed consent. (See page 126 in this chapter, concerning 'Gillick competence'.)

The parents may also feel the need to talk to the doctor without the child present. Either way, it is important that the absent party is told the substance of the discussion, and that there is no feeling that the doctor and parents are conspiring together.

Other aspects of history taking

When taking the history, pay particular attention to the health of parents and siblings: is there a subtext of illness and unhappiness at home? Whether working in hospital or GP surgery, it is important to ask about the child's school and its location. Try to gauge how the child is progressing and his/her best and worst subjects in schoolwork and out of school hobbies and sports. These points should be considered:

- Is the child aware of the outside world? Does the

child live a life that is confined and repressed or do they radiate confidence and optimism?
- Do they have real friends? Popularity is a good sign of psychological integration.
- What about school performance and relations with teachers and fellow students?
- Are they getting reasonable educational opportunities; social factors such as poor housing can play a crucial role. Are the parents together or not? Are the grandparents involved?
- Home amenities, location, crowding: is the child getting any pleasure out of life?

It can be difficult to ascertain whether one is dealing with a psychological or physical disorder, and details about the family background will help.

Physical examination

There is no substitute for a full physical examination, and shortcuts can lead to disasters. The examination must be conducted with respect for the dignity of the child, and he or she should understand the objective of the examination. The school-age child will be even more shy than the preschool child about being physically examined yet, competently done, it may give great assurance. Remember the often-heard complaint against doctors – 'I was never examined!' When examining the genitalia, explain what one is doing to the child and parents. It is wise to have a chaperone.

Children should not be asked to take all their clothes off at once for examination. Keep underclothes on for removal later if needed. If you explain why you need to examine children, they will be much more likely to be cooperative. A full central nervous system examination including fundoscopy and inspection of eardrums can usually be done without difficulty in most children in this age group. Some physical problems can only be discovered on inspection, especially birthmarks. Most of these should have been picked up by school entry, but there can be surprises.

Cardiac murmurs may be picked up for the first time; many, but not all, are innocent. Heart sounds must be carefully listened to. The murmur site, loudness, radiation, how it changes with respiration and positioning of the child, its timing within the cardiac cycle, are all important.

Remember to examine the rest of the cardiovascular system. This must include pulse, BP measurements and palpating for femoral radial delay: an important sign in coarctation (narrowing) of the aorta. As hypertension is usually asymptomatic it is important to measure blood pressure routinely whenever seeing a new patient. Unlike adults, hypertension in children commonly occurs secondarily to disorders affecting the renal tract (see p. 304) or the endocrine system (see p. 180, 198). For details on congenital heart disease, see page 174.

Preparing a child for surgery

In the event of surgery becoming necessary, school children need to be properly informed. They are entitled to an explanation of what is to happen, and unless surgery is an absolute emergency they should not suddenly be confronted, unprepared, with hospital admission. They need to be welcomed by staff trained in the needs of school children and accompanied by their parents to admission and recovery rooms.

The commonest indication for acute surgery is trauma. Elective surgery may be needed for:

- Squint correction.
- Orthopaedic disorder, including scoliosis.
- Grommets to treat chronic secretory otitis media. (Conclusive evidence that grommets have a long-term benefit is lacking.)
- Adenoidectomy and tonsillectomy. Although these are going out of fashion, adenoidectomy on its own is occasionally required to treat sleep apnoea, because of the risk of pulmonary hypertension in long-standing upper airway obstruction.
- Undescended testes and hernia. These would usually have been dealt with before school age, though they may arise at any age.
- Dental extractions, particularly for overcrowded teeth and for gross decay.

Since the overall numbers of children needing surgery are few, it is good practice to concentrate children's surgery into relatively few hospitals where sufficient expertise can be developed.

The symptomatic child

In this section the main presenting symptoms in school children are listed. In order to save repetition, discussions of the more common problems are given in Ch. 6–12.

Fever

This is usually defined as a peripheral temperature greater than 37.5°C or a central temperature greater than 38°C. The reading should be taken after at least 2 minutes.

Fever is usually caused by infections including otitis media, pneumonia, tonsillitis, urinary tract infections and meningitis. Less common causes include:

- TB, brucellosis, endocarditis, osteomyelitis, Lyme disease, leptospirosis
- Malaria and typhoid fever (always ask about foreign travel)
- Unusual cases of fever include autoimmune disorders (e.g. juvenile rheumatoid arthritis, systemic lupus erythematosus)
- Malignancy (e.g. leukaemia, lymphoma)
- Kawasaki disease.

Fever should be investigated by careful history, examination and investigation especially if it is persistent.

Fever should be treated with paracetamol or ibruprofen and plenty of fluid. The cause must be treated.

Fits and faints

Faints are many times more common in adolescents than epilepsy and are usually easily explained by transitory hypotension when standing in the sun, nausea or overexcitement. If they keep happening, consider cardiac arrhythmia. 'True' epilepsy affects about 4 per 1000 school children. Of these about half have had no fits in the previous 2 years. The other half have 'active epilepsy': at least one fit in the past 2 years. About 1 in 2000 have severe and largely drug-resistant epilepsy. There are many different types of epilepsy. In school children, two-thirds of epilepsy sufferers are in mainstream education, and one-third have epilepsy as part of a complex neurological disorder, often including learning difficulties. Epilepsies and their management are described in more detail elsewhere (p. 317). Three types that are almost exclusive to school children are described here:

1. *Absence seizures*. This is an uncommon form of epilepsy. Affected children have momentary episodes of altered consciousness lasting only a few seconds, often with eye staring and blinking; it is more common in girls. Rapid deep breathing may precipitate attacks. EEG shows a classic 3-Hz spike and wave pattern (Fig. 5.21). This condition tends to have abated by puberty.

The differential diagnosis includes daydreaming, poor night sleep and temporal lobe epilepsy. Drug treatment is based on regular daily antiepilepsy drugs, e.g. sodium valproate, ethosuximide or lamotrigine.

2. *Benign focal nocturnal seizures (Rolandic seizures)*. These are simple partial seizures affecting facial or oropharyngeal muscles. They tend to occur during sleep; some progress to brief generalized tonic–clonic seizure. The EEG shows abnormality in the centrotemporal regions of the brain.

Usually the condition is benign. Antiepilepsy drugs may not be needed. The condition should clear up spontaneously. If medication is needed, then carbamazepine is the drug of choice.

3. *Juvenile myoclonic epilepsy (JME)*. This usually starts around puberty. Seizures tend to occur in the early morning and include jerks of the head and upper limbs. Things held in the hands may be dropped; hence the description 'flying cornflakes' syndrome. Photosensitivity is common and will be demonstrated by the EEG. This is an example of an epilepsy which can be readily misclassified unless an expert in paediatric epilepsy sees the child. There is a known gene locus on chromosome 6 of great interest to geneticists. Antiepilepsy medication is needed to control the condition and may need to be continued in the long term.

Nonepileptic seizures

Some children can act out seizures very convincingly, yet if an EEG is recorded at the same time a normal wave pattern is seen. Some children who have nonepileptic seizures have had epilepsy in the past or have witnessed other children having fits and realize how much they worry onlookers. Non-epileptic seizures are very dramatic; the affected child is unlikely to sustain personal injury, and the type of seizure is not characteristic of genuine attacks. Accurate diagnosis is essential.

Headache

Headache is a common symptom from age 5 or 6 onwards. Very careful history taking (see Practical box 5.3) and examination is needed in order to detect the very occasional child with a severe pathology out of the many with so-called tension headaches and the few due to migraine (which is usually associated with a positive family history).

Rarely, the headache is due to raised intracranial pressure due to blockage of cerebrospinal flow, e.g. by brain tumour. Similar symptoms can be due to idiopathic 'benign' intracranial hypertension in which the headache is due to the raised intracranial pressure which wakens the patient in the morning. Continuously raised intracranial pressure can lead to optic atrophy and blindness in this condition.

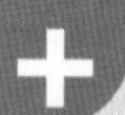

Practical Box 5.3

Questions to ask a child with headaches

- Where is the ache? Where does it start? Is it always the same?
- What times of the day and night does it occur?
- Does anything make it better or worse?
- Are there any aches elsewhere in your body?
- Are you ever sick with them?
- Is your sight affected?

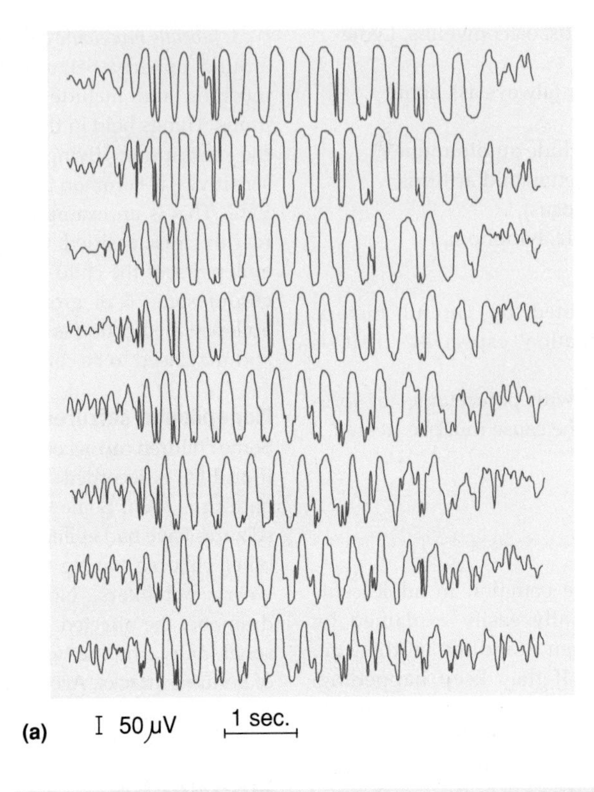

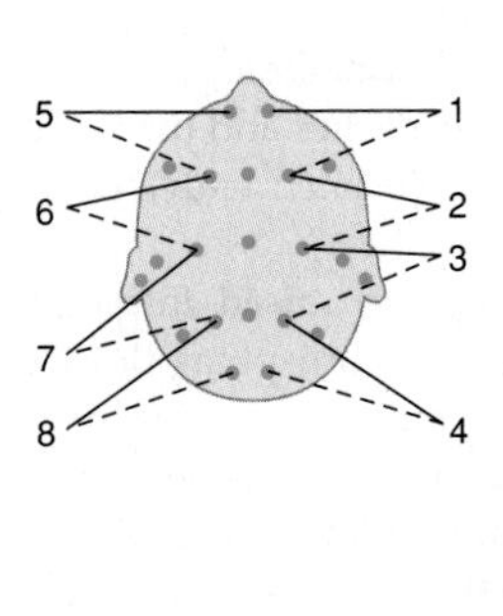

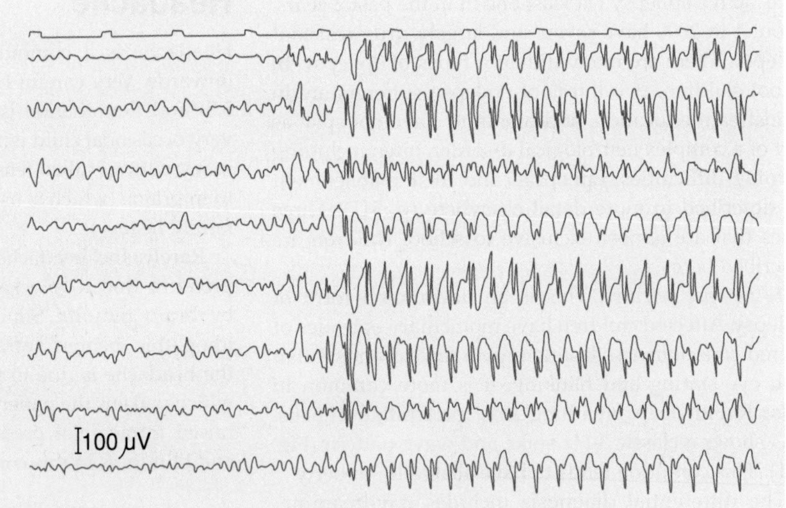

Fig 5.21
(a) EEG showing 3-Hz spike and wave discharges, typically seen in petit mal epilepsy. (b) EEG of boy aged 11 years and awake with eyes open showing generalized bilaterally synchronous spike–wave complexes at 3 Hz occurring during hyperventilation.

Be sure to examine the gait and the fundi during your examination.

DIFFERENTIAL DIAGNOSIS

This should include:

1. Febrile illnesses causing headaches, e.g. meningitis, encephalitis, otitis media and tonsillitis
2. Ophthalmological disorders (not mild visual defect)
3. Sinusitis
4. Dental diseases
5. Jaw joint dysfunction (e.g. dislocation or arthritis)
6. Hypertension, both systemic and intracranial
7. Trauma.

MANAGEMENT

Symptomatic treatment with analgesia is given, while appreciating that 'drug rebound headache' frequently occurs and excess analgesic consumption may make headache worse. Treat the underlying cause (if any); many worry that the child might have a brain tumour or other serious cause. Give a clear explanation to parent and child. This can break a vicious cycle.

Earache and sore throat

The child can usually localize pain to the ear, which is usually due to infection and consequent blocking of the eustachian tube. Diagnosis is by inspection of the eardrum, using an auriscope, and the pharynx for inflammation. Most cases soon clear up. Otitis media (see p. 119) may be due to a recognizable bacterial or viral infection. Severe long-lasting sore throat may be due to glandular fever.

Cough and wheeze

For the more common causes of cough and wheeze see Information box 5.25.

Asthma is a major health problem of school children. It poses severe management problems in relatively few children, but troubles parents and teachers who can easily find it difficult to strike a balance between understanding the affected child, and not allowing the condition to become a reason for underachievement. There is hardly a school class without a child who does not use some type of inhaler. For details on asthma and its management see page 354–356. Details about cystic fibrosis can be found on page 352.

Information Box 5.25

Causes of cough and wheeze in childhood

- Respiratory infections: bacterial, viral, mycoplasma, etc. (including pertussis)
- Asthma
- TB
- Cystic fibrosis
- Inhaled foreign body (see p. 168)
- Psychological

Bruising

Bruising (Information box 5.26) indicates subcutaneous bleeding. All cases should be fully investigated. A detailed history, including family history, social history and associated symptoms is needed.

Information Box 5.26

Causes of bruising

- Trauma: accidental (Fig. 5.22(a)) and nonaccidental
- Bleeding diathesis, e.g. idiopathic thrombocytopenia purpura, haemophilia (Fig. 5.22(b)), von Willebrand disease, liver disease
- Bone marrow failure or infiltration, e.g. aplastic anaemia, leukaemia
- Infection: disseminated intravascular coagulation, seen particularly in meningococcal sepsis
- Haemolytic uraemic syndrome
- Vasculitis, e.g. systemic lupus erythematosus (SLE), Henoch–Schönlein purpura

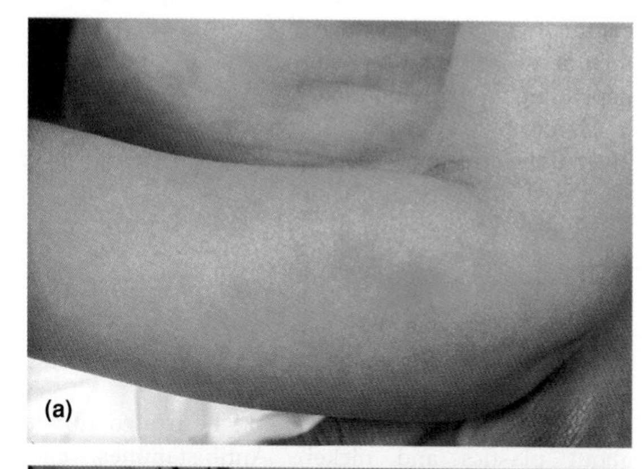

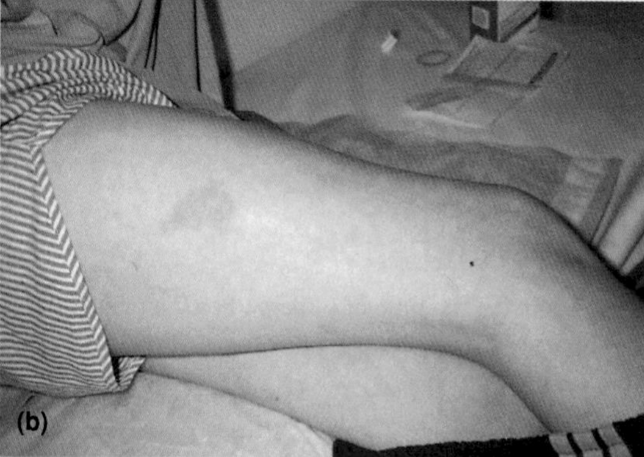

Fig 5.22
(a) Petechial rash on the left arm due to trauma. (b) Bruise on the lateral surface of the right thigh due to haemophilia.

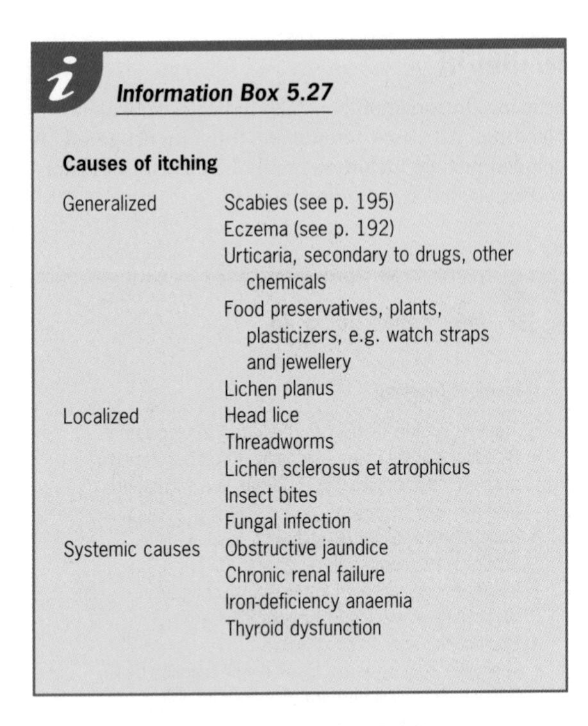

Information Box 5.27

Causes of itching

Generalized	Scabies (see p. 195) Eczema (see p. 192) Urticaria, secondary to drugs, other chemicals Food preservatives, plants, plasticizers, e.g. watch straps and jewellery Lichen planus
Localized	Head lice Threadworms Lichen sclerosus et atrophicus Insect bites Fungal infection
Systemic causes	Obstructive jaundice Chronic renal failure Iron-deficiency anaemia Thyroid dysfunction

On examination bruises do not blanch with pressure. The distribution of bruises and their shape, size and colour must be documented. Investigations must include FBC, clotting studies, and other tests, depending on the symptoms.

Management depends on the cause. Analgesia is given if the bruising is severe and painful.

Itchiness

This is a cutaneous sensation provoking a desire to scratch or rub. For causes of itching see Information box 5.27.

The cause of the itching should be treated (think about plastics and nickel). Antihistamines, e.g. chlorpheniramine, may be given, but these drugs can act as sensitizers. Nails can be clipped short and gloves may be needed.

For further details on eczema see page 192–193.

Rashes and spots

Acne begins at the time of puberty. For the majority it is a temporary phase, but for a few it is the beginning of a lifelong problem (see p. 187).

Causes of rashes include:

- Eczema (see p. 192–193)
- Psoriasis
- Contact dermatitis; plastics and nickel ornaments
- Artefactual dermatitis

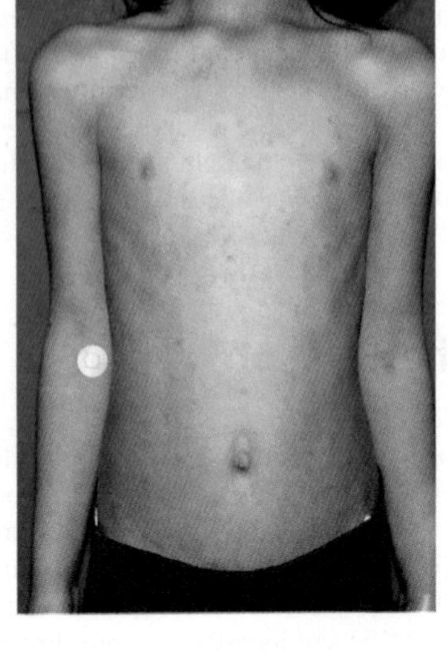

Fig 5.23
Nonspecific enteroviral rash.

- Warts on hands, feet and genitalia (warts on genitalia may be due to sexual abuse)
- Allergies to drugs, plants, food, soap, shampoo, domestic bleach and washing powders (? urticaria)
- Infection:
  - Viral, e.g. enteroviruses (Fig. 5.23), measles, chicken-pox, 5th disease (slapped cheek syndrome)
  - Parasites, e.g. scabies.

For further details on exanthema see page 271.

Vomiting

This is a nonspecific symptom and a full history and examination is important.

Possible causes include gastroenteritis, excessive coughing, reflux oesophagitis, bowel obstruction, drugs, increased intracranial pressure and migraine.

The cause should be treated. Antiemetics may be given in certain instances, e.g. after chemotherapy, but note that oculogyric crises can occur in children given antiemetics, such as metoclopramide.

Diarrhoea

See page 221–230 for full details.

This is a common reason for consulting the doctor in this age group. Causes include gastroenteritis and food poisoning. Diarrhoea lasting more than 2 weeks needs further evaluation for chronic inflammatory bowel disease, e.g. Crohn disease and ulcerative colitis. Other causes include infectious agents, e.g. Giardia, and coeliac disease. Allergic causes are less common as a new presentation in this age group.

Look for evidence of dehydration, muscle wasting, pallor, evidence of perianal fissures, fistula, aphthous mouth ulcers associated with Crohn's disease, which also has extraintestinal manifestations including erythema nodosum, arthritis and iritis.

In most cases, the diarrhoea is self-limiting. Encourage fluid intake. If the child is 10% dehydrated give intravenous fluids until oral fluids can be tolerated and the dehydration corrected. Investigate chronic (i.e. >2 weeks) diarrhoea and treat accordingly.

Coeliac disease is discussed in more detail later (p. 224).

Constipation

Constipation is usually due to a faulty bowel opening habit associated with some upset in the child's care or routine at critical phases. (p. 219 for full details.) Organic causes include:

- Hypothyroidism
- Hirschsprung disease which has usually been recognised by the time the child reaches school age (see p. 220–221)
- Hypercalcaemia
- Anal stenosis.

Most other cases involve psychosocial factors.

A distended abdomen with palpable colon in the left iliac fossa is found. Management involves correction of the upsetting home factors, if possible. The child is encouraged to eat a diet high in fibre, and oral laxatives may be given. Occasionally suppositories and, as a last resort, enema may be needed. This should be as part of a planned regime.

Encopresis

See pages 219–220 for full details.

This refers to the deposition of stools in inappropriate places and signals deep-seated emotional/ psychiatric problems. It becomes less prevalent as the child grows and enters the teenage years.

Organic causes for faecal incontinence must be excluded, e.g. constipation with overflow incontinence, lax anal sphincter, child sexual abuse, or neurological disorders affecting bowel control and anal sphincter tone, e.g. spina bifida or lower spinal cord anomalies.

Management is usually aimed at behaviour modification and family therapy, depending on the underlying psychological cause. Constipation, if present, must be treated sympathetically. Family support is important. See page 219 for further details.

Information Box 5.28

Causes of abdominal pain in childhood

- Gastroenteritis (see p. 221)
- Mesenteric adenitis (see p. 208)
- Constipation (see p. 219)
- Urinary tract infection (see p. 297–300)
- Strangulated hernia (see inguinal hernia, p. 215)
- Appendicitis (see p. 208)
- Peptic ulceration (see p. 212)
- Pancreatitis (see p. 237)
- Hydronephrosis and other urological problems
- Gynaecological problems include mid-cycle pain, menstruation, pelvic inflammatory disease, pregnancy, and torsion of an ovarian cyst
- Other causes: diabetic ketoacidosis (see p. 198), sickle cell disease (p. 252)
- Rarer causes: porphyria, volvulus, intussusception (see p. 209), lead poisoning, inflamed Meckel diverticulum

Abdominal pain

This is a common symptom especially in this age group. For causes of abdominal pain see Information box 5.28.

Abdominal pain can be caused by repeated violent vomiting, pneumonia and abdominal distension (see below).

Management includes analgesia and treatment of the cause.

See pages 207 and 210 for full details about abdominal pain.

Abdominal distension

This may have benign causes e.g. flatus, constipation, pregnancy, 'obesity'. More serious causes include ascites, bowel obstruction (e.g. strangulated hernia), visceromegaly and tumours.

Ask about the period of onset and associated symptoms, e.g. vomiting, pain or constipation. Examination must be complete: look for ascites and visceromegaly; feel for fluid thrill, and listen to bowel sounds; check the hernial orifices.

The management depends on the cause.

Jaundice

Jaundice refers to the yellow discoloration of the body, particularly well seen in the conjunctival mucous membranes. Important questions are listed in Practical box 5.4.

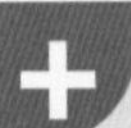

Practical Box 5.4

Important questions concerning jaundice

- Ask about the colour of urine/stools
- History of foreign travel
- History of blood transfusion, sexual contacts and drug abuse (in teenagers)
- Previous medical history and family history of jaundice
- Other symptoms: appetite, weight loss, itching, abdominal pain and distension

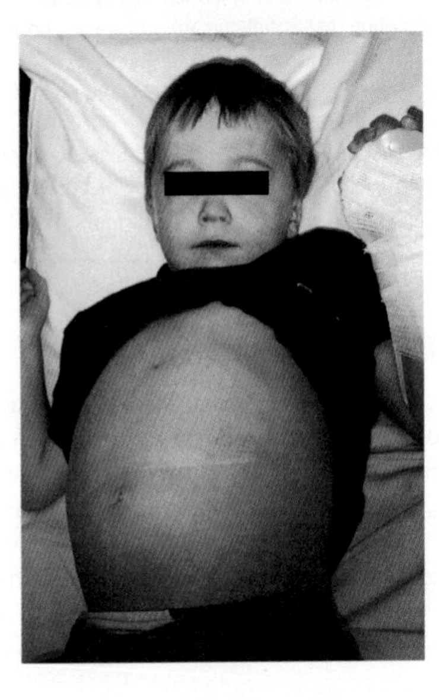

Fig 5.24
The abdomen of a 12-year-old boy with chronic liver disease, showing abdominal distension, jaundice, a surgical scar and distended abdominal veins.

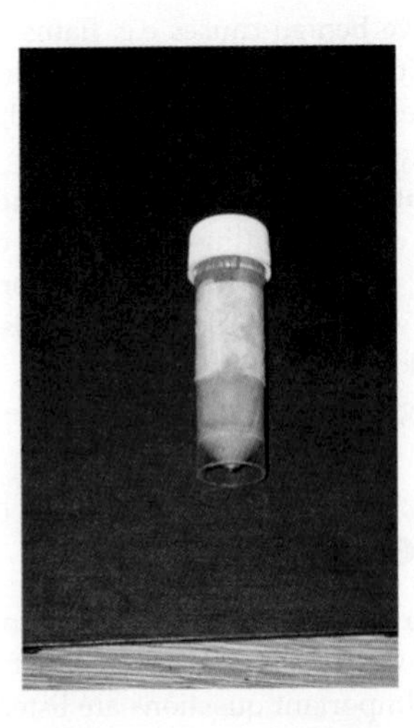

Fig 5.25
Abnormal stools – pale colour caused by high fat content.

On examination, look for pallor, stigmata of chronic liver disease (Fig. 5.24) and hepato-splenomegaly. Test the urine for bilirubin; inspect the stools (Fig. 5.25).

Management depends on the cause (see p. 257).

Dysuria

This is painful micturition and is often associated with vulval irritation in girls and balanitis in boys. Urinary tract infection can be the cause (p. 297). Other uncommon causes include traumatized urethra, either secondary to injury or due to passing a stone. Ask about other associated urinary symptoms including frequency, haematuria, and nocturia.

The diagnosis can be established from the history and examination and by urine microscopy, culture and sensitivity.

Dysuria secondary to urinary tract infection usually resolves with antibiotic treatment, but long-term follow up is needed to ensure that the condition does not become chronic and cause hypertension.

Haematuria

This is blood (haem) in the urine. It can be microscopic or macroscopic (Fig. 5.26(a)). For causes of haematuria, see Information box 5.29.

Differential diagnosis of haematuria

Haematuria must be distinguished from:

1. Haemoglobinuria, usually caused by intravascular haemolysis
2. Myoglobinuria caused by crush injury
3. Beetrooturia (Fig. 5.26(b)) and dyes from cheap sweets
4. Rifampicin therapy.

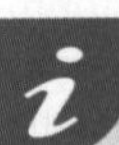

Information Box 5.29

Causes of haematuria

- High fever
- Urinary tract infection (see p. 297–300)
- Bleeding diathesis
- Renal stones
- Renal disease, e.g. Berger disease (IgA nephropathy)
- Nephritis
- Tumours of the renal and urinary tract
- Trauma to the renal tract

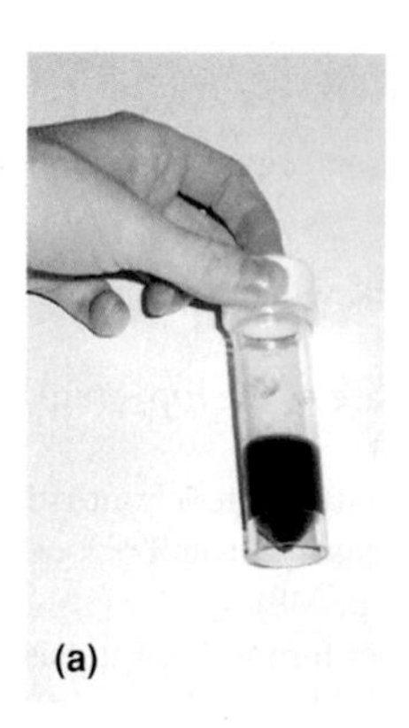

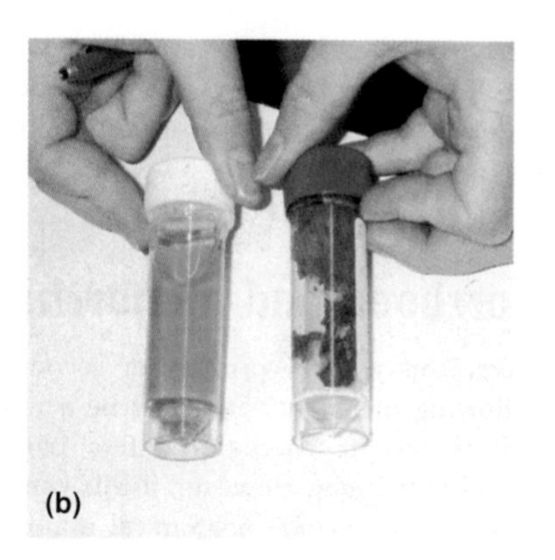

Fig 5.26
(a) Haematuria. (b) Beetrooturia (left-hand sample) with beetroot in the stools (right-hand sample).

Management depends on the cause. Persistent haematuria must be fully investigated.

Enuresis

Daytime lack of bladder control may be associated with chronic renal tract infection, diabetes, malformation and neurological disorders; specialist advice is usually needed. Nocturnal (only) bedwetting affects about 7% of 7-year-old boys and 2% of girls, and is defined as at least three wetting accidents per month.

If the symptom persists much after 5 years of age, consider investigations to exclude urinary tract infections, diabetes and spina bifida especially if the child was dry before or if they are enuretic during daytime as well. Some children become dry once some fuss is made, such as starting a 'star chart' (Fig. 5.27), or giving an enuresis alarm (a buzzing device which wakes the child as soon as wetting starts). We have little enthusiasm for drugs, e.g. imipramine, or hormone treatment such as desmopressin nasal spray, for enuresis; relapses after stopping desmopressin occur commonly. It is a popular method for short-term control of enuresis, for example, during school camp.

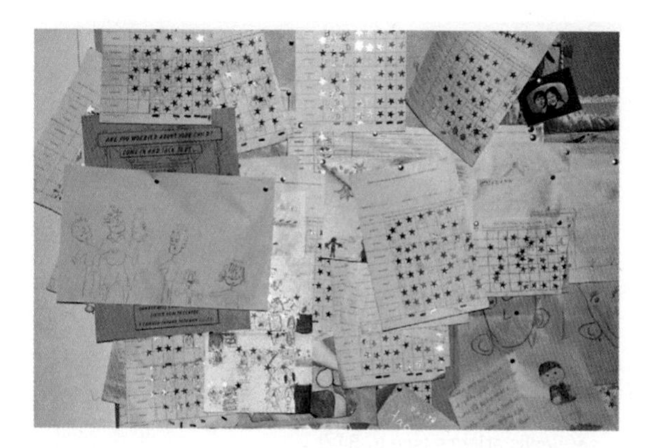

Fig 5.27
Enuresis 'star charts'.

Lethargy

This is a nonspecific symptom. If it is severe and persistent or associated with other clinical problems, then it warrants investigation. It can be the first symptom of many chronic diseases especially those with an infective or inflammatory aetiology (see Information box 5.30). A full history and examination is important including urinalysis, weight and height measurements. Investigations should be guided by the clinical findings.

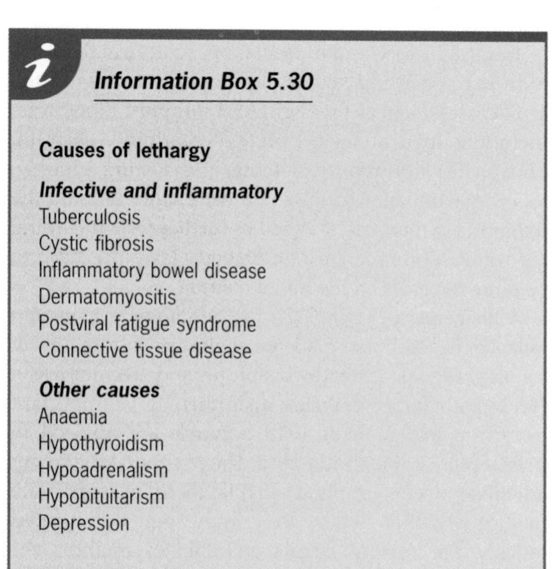

Information Box 5.30

Causes of lethargy

Infective and inflammatory
Tuberculosis
Cystic fibrosis
Inflammatory bowel disease
Dermatomyositis
Postviral fatigue syndrome
Connective tissue disease

Other causes
Anaemia
Hypothyroidism
Hypoadrenalism
Hypopituitarism
Depression

Management depends on the cause. It may be worth exploring other factors including family life, schooling, etc, as external factors and stresses commonly cause lethargy.

Amenorrhoea and menorrhagia

Amenorrhoea. This may be primary or secondary (i.e. occurs following menarche) and may be a temporary physiological variant, as the first few periods are irregular and infrequent. However, if this continues to be a problem then exclude anatomical abnormalities, such as imperforate hymen or endocrine disorders, such as polycystic ovarian disease or chromosomal conditions (Turner syndrome) or testicular feminization syndrome. Pregnancy needs to be excluded.

Management should include full history and examination, focusing on growth and puberty stages. Height should be plotted. Referral to a gynaecologist is appropriate if no obvious reason is found.

Menorrhagia is usually not common in pubertal girls. It may be due to hormonal imbalance. It is important to check for anaemia which occurs if the periods are heavy and frequent. If menorrhagia persists, referral to a gynaecologist is made for further evaluation, for example to look for polyps, etc.

Polydipsia and polyuria

This is a common manifestation of diabetes mellitus. Other rarer causes include chronic renal failure, hypercalcaemia and diabetes insipidus (nephrogenic and hypothalamic, see p. 198, 303). Excessive habitual drinking, also called psychogenic polydipsia, can cause polyuria.

Careful history and examination, with urinalysis for reducing sugar and ketone, are important steps in the initial assessment of this symptom complex. Blood tests including urea and electrolytes, creatinine, calcium, phosphate, albumin, osmolality and fasting glucose, together with urine sodium and osmolality will aid the diagnosis in most cases. Whether further tests including the water deprivation test for diabetes insipidus need to be done depends on the initial results.

Management depends on the aetiology, e.g. insulin will be needed for diabetes mellitus, indomethacin for nephrogenic diabetes insipidus and desmopressin for hypothalamic diabetes insipidus. It is important to ensure that patients with polyuria are advised to drink plenty of fluids and they should have an adequate water supply available to them, especially in hot weather when they may get dehydrated quickly. For further details on diabetes mellitus see page 198.

Limping

Acute limp requires urgent assessment. It may be due to:

- Osteochondritis, which presents in three main forms:
  - Perthes disease of the hip – rare before the age of 5 (see p. 348)
  - Osgood–Schlatter osteochondritis of the upper tibial epiphysis and Kienböck osteochondritis in the foot (see p. 348)
  - Slipped upper femoral epiphysis is a cause of acutely painful hip and limp in older children, particularly in obese 10–15-year-old boys
- Sprain: ligamentous injury secondary to trauma
- Osteomyelitis (see p. 346)
- Arthritis of the lower limbs from any cause
- Bone disease, e.g. rickets (see p. 110, 329)
- Lesions on the feet (tinea, tight shoes, bunion, etc)
- Central nervous system disorders
- Primary tumours of the bone or bone metastasis, e.g. from neuroblastoma
- Previously undetected fractures, e.g. marching fracture of foot bones.

Joint pains

These are often transitory; some are fleeting hypersensitivity to common bacterial and viral illnesses including infectious mononucleosis. Often nothing is cultured and the condition is never adequately explained. SARA – sexually acquired reactive arthritis – is creeping in to the news as an explanation why so many expensive young footballers go off sick with joint pains. Avoid the lay term 'growing pains'. See Information box 5.31 for other causes of joint pains.

Information Box 5.31

Causes of joint pain in childhood

See causes of acute limp above, particularly osteomyelitis and osteochondritis.

Also consider:

- Henoch–Schönlein Syndrome (Fig. 5.28; p. 157, 209)
- Juvenile idiopathic arthritis (see p. 361)
- Haemoglobinopathy: sickle cell disease and thalassaemia (see pp 252 and 251)
- Rheumatic fever
- Septic arthritis (see p. 347).

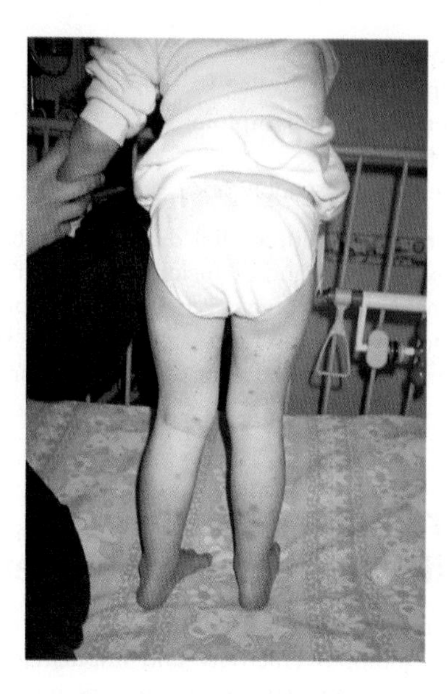

Fig 5.28
Henoch–Schönlein Syndrome associated with mild arthritis.

Management is with analgesia, e.g. ibuprofen, and the cause is treated.

Poisoning

This is common in childhood (see also p. 170). In the later school years it can be deliberate as part of an attention-seeking cry for help or in the course of intended suicide. Drugs include iron, paracetamol, co-proxamol, benzodiazepines, antidepressants, antihistamines, opiates, and illegal drugs. Clinically the symptoms and signs depend on the drug taken.

MANAGEMENT

If vital functions are supported and if complications, particularly aspiration pneumonitis, are avoided, then most seriously poisoned patients can recover, unless serious irreversible damage has been sustained.

Psychological and psychiatric problems

Mental health problems in childhood range from relatively transitory emotional and behavioural difficulties to severe pervasive developmental disorders, such as autism. Epidemiological studies suggest that between 14 and 20% of children will be affected by some level of psychiatric disturbance, with conduct and emotional disorders making up the great majority of those figures.

It is vital to determine whether a child's symptoms are organic or not; often children with physical problems develop psychological problems as well. Children and their parents must not be dismissed out of hand as being 'neurotic'. They must be handled sympathetically and their histories, however bizarre, must be heard in detail.

It is often difficult to be sure whether a child has psychological problems, which can be regarded as 'medical', or a social disorder. Social disorders can range from truancy from school, to delinquency of many forms through to serious crime. School-age children undertake most of the burglaries in Britain and much of the car crime. It is at this age that addiction to drugs, including alcohol and tobacco, usually starts. Some children are bullies; two-thirds of children are bullied at some stage. Sometimes the behaviour of carers is deviant and health professionals may be the first to appreciate this. The pattern of psychological illness in children changes with the advent of puberty. The prepubertal child is most likely to present to the child psychiatrist with enuresis, encopresis, school refusal, 'bad behaviour', sleeplessness and hyperactivity. In the older schoolchild, suicide begins to take an appreciable toll. With puberty come excessive shyness and more serious conditions including anorexia and bulimia. Some will show depression and early signs of schizophrenia. A few pose such great problems to society that they need to be segregated into special treatment units or young offenders' institutions.

Bad behaviour

British studies have found that behavioural difficulties were the most common disabling problems of childhood, affecting 2% of under-16-year-olds. They occur more commonly in children with learning disabilities.

Conduct disorders manifest as aggression, destructiveness, and cruelty or antisocial behaviour, lying, stealing, truancy and, at the extremes, criminal and delinquent behaviour. They are commoner in boys. Often the parents, school or police bring such children to medical attention, in the search for an explanation or treatment of the child's problem.

It is important to look for associated organic diseases including neurodegenerative disorders and subtle seizure disorders (Information box 5.32), though in most instances no organic cause is found. Usually a history of dysfunctional family life is obtained. A thorough history of development and intellectual performance (school reports) is essential, as is a detailed psychosocial history. Other associated behaviours

Information Box 5.32

Differential diagnosis of psychological and psychiatric problems

- Organic
  - Subacute sclerosing panencephalitis
- Hypoglycaemia
- Epilepsy
- Drug and alcohol abuse
- Neurodegenerative disorders (Batten disease), or sex chromosome disorder, such as fragile X or Klinefelter syndrome
- Brain tumours

Information Box 5.33

Important underlying risk factors for depression

- Chronic organic disorders
- Eating disorders
- Drug abuse including alcohol
- Dysfunctional family
- Problems at school

worth enquiring about include alcohol, drug abuse and smoking.

Management includes counselling, referral to a child psychiatrist and a multidisciplinary team approach to the presenting problems.

Depression

Overt depressive disorders are rare in childhood, but by adolescence they become more common and show a female preponderance. Childhood depression is associated with a significantly increased risk of affective disorders in adulthood. For risk factors for depression see Information box 5.33. Clinical manifestations include the following:

- Physical: sleep and appetite disturbance
- Psychological
  - Sadness
  - Worthlessness
  - Hopelessness
  - Helplessness
  - Overt psychotic symptoms
- Others
  - Deteriorating schoolwork.

The diagnosis and differential diagnosis are based on history, examination and exclusion of organic disorders. Management may involve psychological therapies, such as psychotherapy, antidepressants, such as tricyclic antidepressants and treatment of the underlying cause (if any).

Hyperactivity (attention deficit–hyperactivity disorder)

This disorder is characterized by poor ability to attend to a task, motor overactivity and impulsivity. These children are fidgety, have a difficult time remaining in their seats in school, are easily distracted, have difficulty following instructions and sustaining attention, shift rapidly from one uncompleted task to another, and often seem not to listen to what is being said.

The diagnosis is mainly based on the history. The differential diagnosis may involve neurological diseases, learning disabilities, conduct disorders, or side effects of drugs, e.g. anti-epilepsy drugs.

MANAGEMENT

Psychological management involves a programme that gives structure to the child's environment, decreases the effects of the handicap, and helps in academic and social learning.

The prescription of drugs such as methyl phenidate is a controversial matter. Although this has been licensed, it is essential that treatment is closely supervised by a paediatrician and child psychiatrist working together. This drug may have adverse effects on growth and appetite and cause insomnia if given in the evening.

Truancy and school refusal

These disorders are important causes of absence from school. The two disorders are compared and contrasted in Information box 5.34.

Suicide and parasuicide

In children under the age of 12 years suicide and parasuicide are rare. From the age of 14 years onwards

Information Box 5.34

Features and risk factors in truancy and school refusal

Truancy	**School refusal**
Conduct disorder	Emotional disorder
(Poor prognosis)	(Better prognosis)
Risk factors	
Disorganization at home	Separation anxiety
Personality disorder	Depression
Parental rejection	Parents keeping their children at home (e.g. parental overprotection)
	Fear of peers or teachers
Large family	Small family
Social class IV, V	Social class I–III
Boys > girls	Boys = girls

during the teenage era, the rate of recorded suicide rises each year. Whilst the incidence of suicide among teenagers is lower than in any adult age group, it is one of the most important causes of death in 15–24-year-old males. Conversely parasuicide is mostly an adolescent and early adult phenomenon; 70% or more of teenage hospital admissions for self-poisoning are by females who tend to take tablets, e.g. paracetamol, antidepressants, antibiotics and oral contraceptives.

Between the late 1970s and the 1980s rates of suicide amongst males aged 15–19 increased by almost 45%. Over the same period comparable rates for teenage girls fell by 23%. The suicides rate in 1992 per 100 000 population for males aged 15–19 years was about 6. The figure for females in the same age group was about 2. There was an increase among males of hanging, strangulation and suffocation, use of firearms, explosives and poisoning by exhaust fumes, between the early 1970s and 1980s. Affective disorders, substance misuse and personality disorders were important diagnoses in such individuals.

New horizons

Development of services for adolescents

In most developed countries the technical aspects of children's health services are now relatively satisfactory. By contrast, adolescent or teenage medicine is not well served in the UK.

Teenagers are the only age group in the UK whose health is known to have deteriorated in the past decade. This is due to accidents, suicides, violence, drugs and HIV. Unfortunately, when children get to the end of the 'paediatric' age range at around 16 years, the intensive services provided by children's specialists tend to disappear. In developed countries the amount of illness in young adults is decreasing and specialists in 'adult' conditions tend to focus on the elderly where the vast majority of their work lies. Such specialists, therefore, may have little knowledge of the health needs of young people, though there are pioneering adolescent clinics, particularly in psychiatry. There is a tendency for young people with conditions such as diabetes, milder forms of cerebral palsy, cystic fibrosis, chronic inflammatory bowel disease, epilepsy, muscular dystrophy, psychiatric disorder and mental subnormality to receive less than appropriate care when they reach adult life because services are not geared to their particular needs.

This problem has come to the fore because survival rates through childhood have greatly increased and service provision has not kept up with this. Too often, teenagers when admitted to hospital are either put in adult wards where most of the fellow patients are much older than they are, or confined to children's wards where most of the patients are infants and babies. There is a need for much more special provision for this group. Family doctors looking after adolescents thus need to carefully select specialists to whom they can hand on the young person after they become too old for services for young people.

Most physicians for adults are not specifically trained to deal with young people. More recently, however, some have begun to run joint clinics with paediatricians to give much-needed specialist services for adolescents and young adults. Such moves also promote the sharing of information and the development of new areas of experience and research interests between paediatricians and physicians.

Improved outcome in cystic fibrosis

Survival from cystic fibrosis has increased substantially over the past three decades with the result that most patients alive today will live into adult life, and those born today may live well into middle age. Many factors are likely to have contributed to this improvement, especially broad-spectrum and antipseudomonal antibiotics and pancreatic enzyme supplements. Other reasons include better health care, specialist clinics and early diagnosis.

Cystic fibrosis, therefore, accounts for a diminishing proportion of childhood deaths, with the majority of severe morbidity and mortality now occurring in early adult life. Social class and region of residence influence survival.

Recent advances in cystic fibrosis treatment include the use of:

- Inhaled human recombinant DNAse
- Gene therapy
- Heart/lung transplantation.

Antenatal testing for cystic fibrosis is available, but is not used for population screening. It is currently being evaluated as a screening tool. Whether screening will be offered to everyone or to high-risk groups only remains to be seen.

Improved outcome in cancer

In Britain about one child in 600 develops cancer during the first 15 years of life. About one-third of cases are leukaemias, mostly acute lymphoblastic leukaemia (ALL), and more than one-fifth involve various types of brain tumours (see p. 333).

There have been remarkable improvements in survival and consequent reduction in population mortality rates for childhood cancers during the past 25 years. The current 5-year survival rate for all forms of childhood cancer combined is about 70%. These improvements have been achieved using a combination of modern surgery, radiotherapy and chemotherapy. The advent of better cytotoxic drugs, developed following collaborative trials, have had a great impact on childhood cancer, together with the policy of centralization of treatment. Radiotherapy fractionation techniques and the more precise localization of tumour area have also helped.

Too little is known about the aetiology of childhood cancer; this is an area of active research.

Prospects with regard to muscular dystrophy (Duchenne and Becker)

These allelic X-linked recessive disorders result from an abnormality of the dystrophin gene on the short arm of the X chromosome. In 66% of boys with the condition a deletion or duplication may be identified in a peripheral blood sample and the diagnosis confirmed without the need for a muscle biopsy. Point mutations in the gene are likely to account for the remainder.

When a muscle biopsy is necessary, immunostaining techniques demonstrate the abundance and distribution of dystrophin. These advances have enabled much more accurate detection of female carriers and prenatal diagnosis.

Unfortunately, no effective treatment is yet available but research is proceeding, particularly in the field of gene therapy with the use of viral vectors to transfer the dystrophin gene into muscle cells, or direct injection of dystrophin DNA into muscle. Other novel methods include myoblast implantation.

Advances in epilepsy treatment

Genetics. Out of all epilepsies, 20% have a genetic basis. Recent advances in molecular genetics and linkage studies in families with certain types of epilepsies have enabled us to identify chromosomes, and even gene loci, which are thought to be associated with some types of epilepsies, for example, tuberose sclerosis and chromosomes 9, 16, and familial juvenile myoclonic epilepsy and chromosome 6.

New drugs. Over the past 20 years a growing understanding of the pathophysiology underlying epilepsy has prompted novel approaches to drug therapy. It has been recognized that that neuronal hyperexcitability is pivotal for the genesis and maintenance of epileptic seizure. Gamma-aminobutyric acid (GABA) has been shown to play a major inhibitory role in many brain regions. Glutamate is an excitatory amino acid in the brain, especially found in the temporal lobe, and inhibitory drugs (e.g. lamotrigine) have been licensed for use in children over 2 years as an add-on therapy in complex partial seizures and myoclonic absence epilepsy.

Surgical treatment for epilepsy. Of the 100 000 children in the UK with active epilepsy, 25% will remain intractable to medical therapy. In about 10–20% of the latter, surgical treatment offers the potential to stop, or at least alleviate the seizure disorder.

With the recent technological advances, and using multiple methods, such as EEG, video telemetry, MRI, SPECT scanning and neuropsychological testing, in addition to the clinical history and examination, it has been possible in a selected group of patients to identify a well localized epileptogenic abnormality, which is responsible for the patient's seizures, in an area of the brain which can be removed without resulting in significant neurological deficits.

The technique is particularly useful in partial

seizures, e.g. in temporal lobe epilepsy caused by mesial temporal sclerosis, where local resection can be done, or in unilateral hemisphere damage where hemispherectomy can be done. More than 10 major paediatric epilepsy surgery series have been published, showing good outcomes. The results are dependent upon selection criteria and careful evaluation of children before surgery.

There is increasing interest in the use of vagus nerve stimulation for the control of certain forms of epilepsy. Stimulators, akin to cardiac pacemakers, inserted into the ascending vagus nerve in the neck have been shown to improve seizure control and experience in their use in children is accumulating.

FURTHER READING

Behrman RE, Kliegman RM, Jenson HB (1999) *Nelson's Textbook of Pediatrics*, 16th edn. London: WB Saunders.

Botting B (ed.) (1995) *Health of Our Children*. Decennial Supplement No. 11. London: HMSO.

Department of Health (1992) *The Health of the Nation*. London: HMSO.

Swadi H (1992) Drug abuse in children and adolescents: an update. *Archives of Disease in Childhood* 67(10): 1245–1246.

Wales JK et al (1995) *Color Atlas of Pediatric Endocrinology and Growth*. London: Mosby.

FURTHER READING

2

Paediatric conditions
a systems approach

6 Accident and emergency paediatrics

Accidents

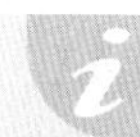

Definition

An unintentional event in which there is an abnormal exchange of energy (mechanical, thermal, chemical, etc.) which may result in injury through damage to the tissue.

Epidemiology

A global child health problem which, in the UK, is the commonest cause of death in the second year of life.

Lifestyle

Accidents are preventable and their incidence is increased by social deprivation.

As many as one-quarter of all children attend accident and emergency departments each year, one-quarter of all people attending A&E in total. While some of these attendances will be for emergency conditions, the majority, especially in inner cities, are for minor illnesses best dealt with in the primary healthcare service.

AETIOLOGY AND INCIDENCE

The definition of accidents is broad; they can have many different causes. As with infectious diseases, the host, vector and environment model is helpful in understanding the pathogenesis of injuries. Taking road traffic accidents as an example, we can apply the model as follows.

Environment

Children live in an environment that may or may not protect them from injury. Failure to separate residential areas from road areas leads to an increased risk of pedestrian road traffic accidents. The environment may be the car in which a child rides. If there are no child seat restraints, even a small collision or rapid deceleration can lead to significant head injury secondary to contracoup forces as the child's head hits the car. Socially deprived environments present greater risks to children because of poor housing.

Vector

The motor vehicle itself is the vector in the case of pedestrian accidents. Vehicle design may determine the likelihood of an accident or the nature of the injury which results. The addition of external 'extras' such as 'bull bars' may increase the force on impact at any speed. Likewise the visibility provided by mirrors of the area behind a car or lorry is a major determining factor in the likelihood of a child being crushed when a vehicle reverses. The speed at which a vehicle is driven determines the force on impact and the likelihood of death or permanent disability.

Host

A child must be considered within the context of his or her family and therefore family characteristics are also important in determining risk. The most important individual characteristics of a child or adolescent in determining the risk and the nature of injury are age and sex. The likelihood of an accident is highest in the early years, primarily because of accidents in the home. The risk drops to the lowest level in the junior school years, though the location of the accident shifts out of the home. The risk rises again in adolescence as children achieve increasing degrees of independence. Males are at much greater risk of injury throughout life.

Other important host characteristics include alcohol and smoking (Information box 6.1). Inappropriate use of alcohol is also a risk factor for child abuse, suicide and homicide.

Accidents are the major cause of mortality to children over the age of 1 year in developed countries. In developing countries, they may have a higher incidence, but infectious diseases outnumber accidents as the primary cause of death. In the United Kingdom the mortality rate from accidents to children under 15 years was 6.6/100 000 in 1990. Accidental injuries represent a significant cause of hospitalization and of long-term disability, largely due to head trauma. Apart from congenital problems, accidents and meningitis are the main causes of acquired learning disability and acquired cerebral palsy. Accidents vary by age and by development, as described above. Over time, the mortality due to accidents to children has been falling.

The leading national causes of mortality in the United Kingdom include road traffic accidents (particularly involving pedestrians), house fires, suffocation and drowning. There may be local variation in the causal patterns. Principal causes of morbidity leading to hospitalization include falls, road traffic accidents and poisonings.

CLINICAL PRESENTATION

The clinical presentation may vary from a minor contusion or a laceration to a moribund child arriving by ambulance at the Accident and Emergency Department. A small proportion of children are brought directly to a hospital, bypassing their general practitioner.

PREVENTION

Since the consequences of accidents to children may be so devastating, including death and long-term disability, the clinical emphasis should be on prevention. Prevention of injury operates on three levels, primary, secondary and tertiary, and can be characterized as 'active' or 'passive' (see Information box 6.2).

Information Box 6.1

Alcohol and smoking as key behavioural risks for injury to children (behaviour of child, adolescent and parent)

- Smoking
  - House fires
- Alcohol
  - Road traffic accidents, occupant and pedestrian
  - House fires
  - Drowning
  - Boating accidents

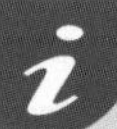

Information Box 6.2

Types of accident prevention

- *Primary prevention:* preventing an injury from occurring
- *Secondary prevention:* decreasing the severity of an injury which has occurred
- *Tertiary prevention:* decreasing the long-term consequences of the injury
- *Active prevention:* this requires repeated actions by the individual to be effective, i.e. it requires behaviour change. Examples include:
  - Seat belts
  - Bicycle helmets
  - Designated driver schemes
- *Passive prevention:* this also requires change, but once made, there is no longer the need for repetitive actions by the individual. Examples include:
  - Oven guards to reduce the possibility of scalding
  - Air bags
  - Changes to car bodies which increase protection to the occupants, and decrease damage to anyone hit by the car (pedestrian-friendly cars)
- Fences around swimming pools

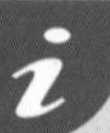

Information Box 6.3

Successful interventions

- Road traffic injury
  - Seat belts
  - Bicycle helmets
  - Traffic-calming schemes
  - Speed cameras
  - Drink-driving interventions
  - Regular car maintenance checks
- Fires
  - Smoke alarms
  - Fire-retardant night clothes and furnishings
- Poisoning
  - Medicine bottles with child-resistant caps
  - Reducing the amount of medication in any one prescription to below the lethal dose

Examples of successful interventions which lower children's risk of accident are shown in Information box 6.3.

MANAGEMENT

The management of major accidents to children is divided into three phases: pre-hospital, hospital and post-hospital. An example of such a scheme in action is the management of near drowning. The key is to maintain the airway, reducing the chance of brain damage through brain dehydration and timely surgery when indicated. Training is crucial especially in paediatric advanced life support and in paediatric trauma life support. Trauma protocols are needed to designate the equipment required and precise duties of staff. These should include liaison with the family as well as support to the child.

The pre-hospital phase involves the ambulance system. Staff must be well trained in paediatric resuscitation and the use of the appropriate equipment available, to maintain an airway and adequate respiration and to treat shock.

Cardiopulmonary resuscitation should be commenced immediately after rescue and continued during transport, as after immersion in cold water, hypothermia can protect from irreversible damage. The outlook is poor in those who are comatose and unresponsive after resuscitation, particularly if they have been submerged for more than 5 minutes in warm fresh water.

After arrival in hospital, if $P\text{CO}_2$ is normal, continuous positive airway pressure (CPAP) is given by mask to prevent alveolar collapse. If there is respiratory failure, or the patient is in coma, ventilation is required; maintaining a low $P\text{CO}_2$ helps prevent cerebral oedema. Large volumes of fluid may be swallowed, and removing these by nasogastric tube may prevent further aspiration of stomach contents. Fluid balance changes may be dramatic because of absorption of fresh water through the lungs, or, in the case of sea water, because of drawing of water and protein into the alveoli.

The post-hospital phase of injury management includes rehabilitation, which begins in the hospital phase. This should include both specific therapies, where appropriate, and re-entry into normal family and school life. This needs to be monitored by the general practitioner and often the community paediatrician or a psychiatrist, particularly after head injury.

Inhaled and swallowed foreign bodies

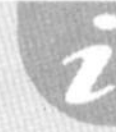

Prognosis

Inhalation of large foreign bodies is an immediate threat to life.

Button batteries must be removed to avoid tissue necrosis.

INTRODUCTION

Large inhaled foreign bodies are an immediate threat to life. Laryngeal and tracheal foreign bodies are included in the differential diagnosis of croup. The possibility of a foreign body in the respiratory tract should always be considered in a young child with persistent respiratory symptoms. By contrast most swallowed foreign bodies pass through the gastrointestinal tract.

AETIOLOGY AND PATHOGENESIS

Bronchial foreign bodies may allow air past in inspiration but not in expiration, resulting in obstructive overinflation. An obstructive foreign body causes absorption of air beyond the obstruction (atelectasis). Disc batteries can cause local tissue necrosis which may result in an acquired tracheo-oesophageal fistula.

In the normal oesophagus, ingested foreign bodies impact at regions of physiological narrowing as shown in Figure 6.1. If they stick elsewhere, this suggests coexistent oesophageal disease. Once a foreign body reaches the stomach it should usually pass through the intestinal tract. If impaction occurs there is a danger of perforation. For example small safety pins will usually negotiate the gut, whether they are open or closed but large safety pins will not.

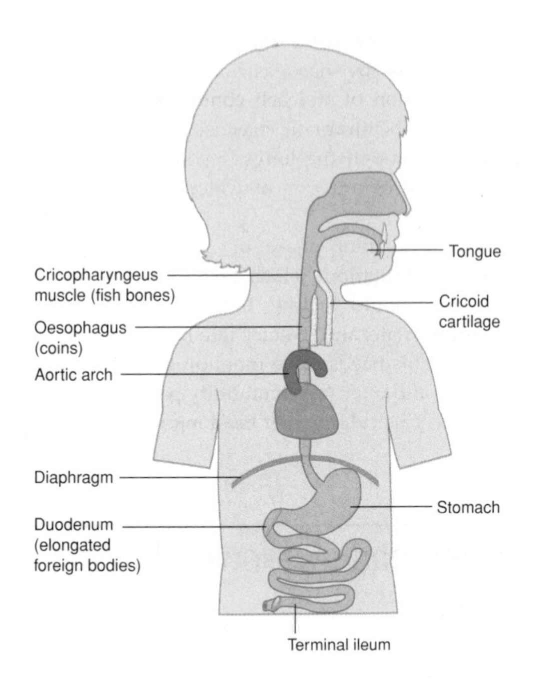

Fig 6.1
Impaction of swallowed foreign bodies.

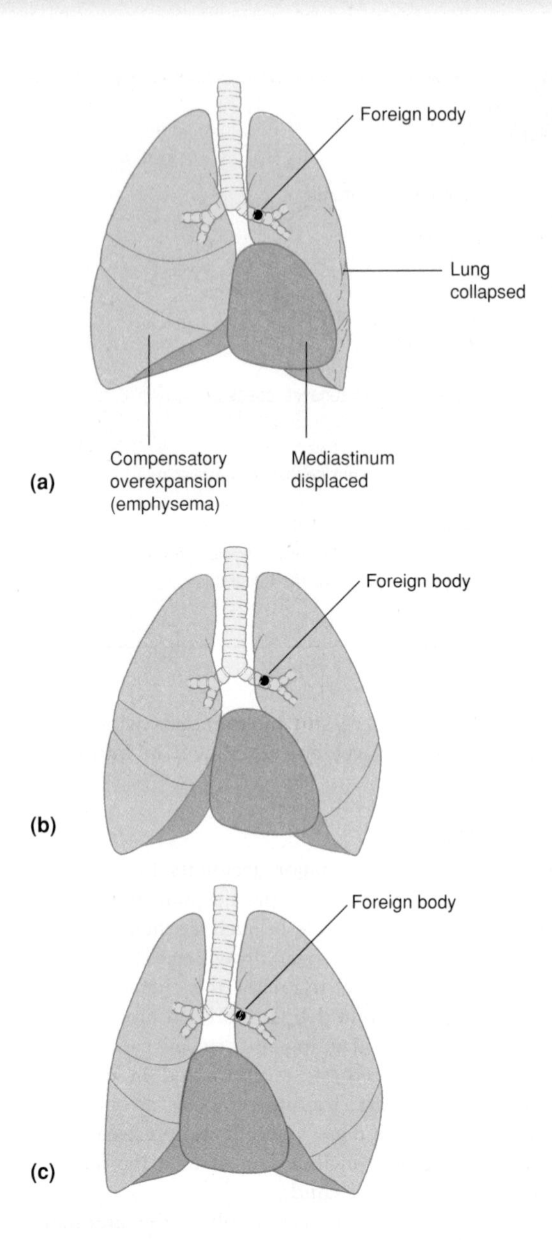

Fig 6.2
Radiological changes produced by foreign bodies in bronchi: (a) atelectasis; (b) obstructive emphysema during inspiration – relatively normal except for some mediastinal shift; (c) obstructive emphysema during expiration – foreign body acts as a flap valve, left lung overexpanded and mediastinum displaced.

CLINICAL PRESENTATION

Respiratory tract foreign bodies

A laryngeal foreign body causes hoarseness and a croupy cough. The child may be cyanosed and dyspnoeic. The symptoms of a tracheal foreign body are similar to those of a laryngeal foreign body except that wheeze is more often heard rather than croup and the foreign body may be heard moving up and down the trachea with respiration. Bronchial foreign bodies are usually aspirated into the right main bronchus, which is more vertical in relation to the trachea. Small, non-irritating bronchial foreign bodies can be tolerated for weeks before symptoms occur. A partially obstructed foreign body produces a wheeze and therefore must be differentiated from asthma. The initial paroxysmal choking episode is followed by a latent period before chronic suppuration with haemoptysis occurs. Foreign bodies that partially obstruct the bronchus produce wheezing. The obstructed foreign body may cause rapid onset of lung collapse (atelectasis) or, more commonly, overexpansion (emphysema) if there is a partial obstruction with a ball-valve effect (Figs 6.2 and 6.3). Inhaled peanuts cause a remarkably severe reaction in the surrounding lung, and there is cough, dyspnoea and fever.

Gastrointestinal foreign bodies

The swallowing of a foreign body causes choking, drooling and coughing. If the foreign body lodges in the oesophagus it produces pain and dysphagia.

DIAGNOSIS

The diagnosis of laryngeal foreign body is suggested by lateral X-ray of the neck if the foreign body is radioopaque. If the foreign body is posterior to the

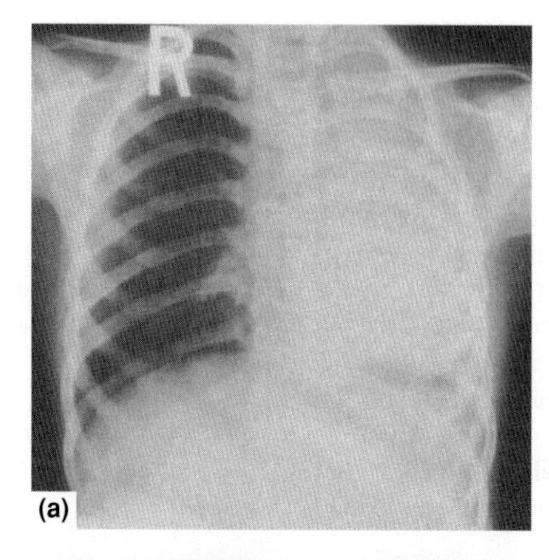

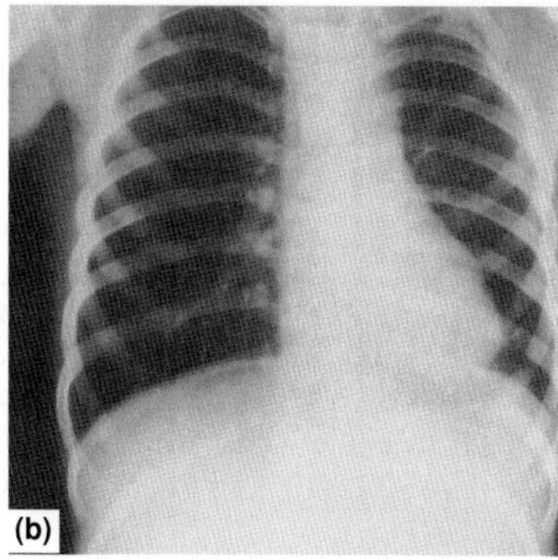

Fig 6.3
Chest X-ray **(a)** before, and **(b)** after removal of respiratory tract foreign body.

larynx it is in the hypopharynx or oesophagus. The diagnosis is confirmed by direct laryngoscopy. Tracheal foreign bodies may be seen on chest X-ray and confirmed on bronchoscopy or inspiratory and expiratory chest X-ray, and confirmed and removed at direct bronchoscopy. Partially obstructed bronchial foreign bodies may be diagnosed by the development of overaeration of the affected lung on expiration. Occasionally a bronchial foreign body is found when a lobe of the lung is removed for bronchiectasis.

A barium meal is required to detect radiolucent foreign bodies in the gastrointestinal tract.

PREVENTION

Prevention involves commonsense measures, such as keeping small objects away from toddlers, especially nuts.

MANAGEMENT

See Emergency box 6.1

Foreign bodies which have passed through the vocal cords should be removed as soon as possible.

Emergency Box 6.1

Treatment of a laryngeal foreign body

- Emergency treatment may be required for children who are unable to speak, cough or breathe.
- Blows between the shoulder blades are combined with chest compression (abdominal compression is used after infancy) (see Fig. 6.4) to try to dislodge the foreign body.
- Inspection of the pharynx to extract the dislodged foreign body.

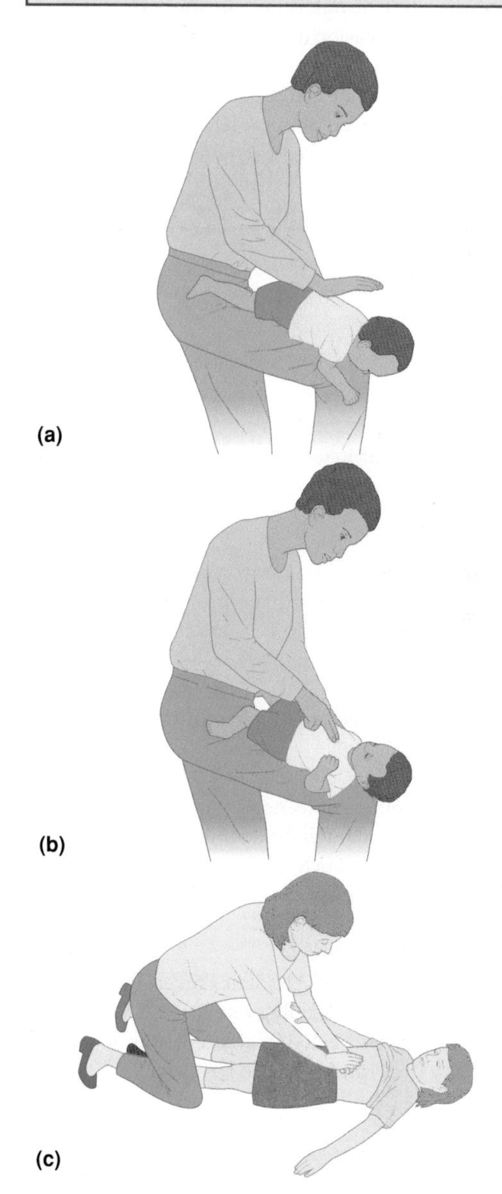

Fig 6.4
(a) Back blows in an infant. (b) Chest thrusts in an infant. (c) Abdominal thrusts in a child.

Long-standing bronchial foreign bodies, especially peanuts, may require lobectomy.

Children with oesophageal foreign bodies should be X-rayed again immediately before endoscopy to ensure that the foreign body has not advanced. When the oesophageal foreign body is a coin, attempted removal can be postponed for 24 hours if the child is asymptomatic, as many coins will pass spontaneously. By contrast, corrosive button batteries should be removed promptly, before corrosion of the oesophagus and stomach occurs.

Long foreign bodies should be removed from the stomach by gastroscope. If the foreign body negotiates the pylorus and duodenum, further progress is monitored with occasional X-rays. Perforation is unlikely if the foreign body progresses down the gastro-intestinal tract. If the object impacts for several weeks, or is long or sharp or abdominal pain develops, it should be removed endoscopically or surgically.

Poisoning

Epidemiology
Many thousands of toddlers are admitted to hospital each year following ingestion of drugs or chemicals.

Prognosis
Most are unharmed. The drugs which are particularly dangerous in overdose are tricyclics, paracetamol and iron.

Treatment
Supportive; antidotes are rarely required.

Lifestyle
Increasing numbers of teenagers are being admitted to hospital following ingestion of 'recreational' drugs such as alcohol, 'ecstasy' and LSD in combination.

Incidence
Figures from the Child Accident Prevention Trust indicate that poisoning represents 2% of accidental injuries treated in accident and emergency departments in the UK.

INTRODUCTION

Children are at the mercy of a vast array of household and industrial chemicals as well as drugs and alcoholic drinks that can be very toxic as well as causing profound hypoglycaemia. Occasionally they are administered to children as a form of child abuse – Munchausen by proxy (Meadow) syndrome. The older toddler is very prone to accidental ingestion; older children take a wide variety of substances including drugs and volatile substances both for 'kicks' and in order to cause attention-seeking self-injury.

CLINICAL PRESENTATION

See Information box 6.4.

DIAGNOSIS

Toxicology laboratories will screen blood, urine and vomitus samples for the presence of drugs.

MANAGEMENT

The management depends on the nature of the substance ingested. If this is known, but you do not know what to do there are poisons centres in the UK which are continuously staffed; they should be consulted forthwith. 'Toxbase' is a poisons database available on the internet at www.spib.axl.co.uk. Emergency box 6.2 outlines the main principles of management.

Paediatricians must support and initiate campaigns to increase awareness about existing and new drugs and chemicals, to insist that childproof containers are used, to encourage health workers to positively teach drug safety to parents and childminders, and to press for an end to industrial chemicals being in reach of children.

Information Box 6.4

Indications that a child has been poisoned

- Missing drugs or open bottles
- Being caught in the act
- Sudden onset of unexplained illness. This includes:
  - Restlessness
  - Altered consciousness
  - Fixed dilated or restricted pupils
  - Blood around the mouth
  - Diarrhoea
  - Shock
  - Hallucinations
- Confession after attempted self-harm
- Skin changes on exposure to corrosive agents

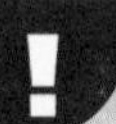

Emergency Box 6.2

Principles of management of poisoning

1. *Support vital functions* with intubation and ventilation, fluids, resuscitation, etc. Maintenance of airway and blood volume through general resuscitative and supportive measures
2. *Confirm the diagnosis* by taking a history, examination and laboratory investigation. Keep samples of any suspect substance or food.
3. *Obtain urgent advice* from the National Poisons Information Service website.
4. *Remove the poison.* This will depend on the type of poison (e.g. gas, tablets), the quantity consumed, the interval since exposure, and its effects and the part of body affected, e.g. skin, conjunctiva, stomach, etc. If the child is comatose, an endotracheal tube is passed prior to lavage, with activated charcoal to decrease absorption
   Removal of the poison can be by:
   - Dilution of corrosive skin contamination
   - Induced emesis
   - Activated charcoal
   - Gastric lavage (being aware of the danger of inhalation)
   - Induction of vomiting with ipecacuanha; this is contraindicated after corrosive ingestion
   - Whole bowel irrigation
   - Circulatory decontamination, e.g. haemodialysis, haemofiltration, plasmapheresis.
5. *Administer an antidote* (if available).
6. Adequate length of observation to allow for late effects of slow-acting drugs

Attempted self-destruction requires the involvement of child psychiatrists and social services.

Drowning and near drowning

Drowning is the third most common cause of accidental death in children in Britain (see also p. 166). The death rate is about 0.7 per 100 000 children. Older children drown in open water, and municipal and private swimming pools. In 86% of drowning accidents there is no supervision; a lack of swimming ability is another factor. An unconscious near-drowned child with fixed dilated pupils can survive, especially if hypothermia is present, as it can protect the brain. See Emergency box 6.3.

These accidents can be prevented to some extent by public education, use of safety grids in garden ponds and surveillance in public and private pools.

Emergency Box 6.3

Management of near drowning

- Waterside cardiopulmonary resuscitation should be started as soon as possible after the child has been taken from the water. Water should be cleared from the airways first. Heat loss should be prevented.
- On arrival at hospital, aspiration of water from the stomach using a nasogastric tube is important to prevent aspiration pneumonitis. In the unconscious child intubation, ventilation and slow re-warming should be commenced. Prophylactic antibiotics should be started. Resuscitation should not be abandoned until the child is re-warmed.
- Fits beyond the first 24 hours carry a bad prognosis, as does the presence of fixed dilated pupils 6 hours after hospital admission.

Water safety should be included in the National Curriculum.

Burns

Epidemiology

Fifty thousand burned or scalded children attend emergency departments each year in the UK. Ten percent are admitted and about 100 die (usually from smoke inhalation). The death rate is decreasing with improved prevention such as fireguards, flame-proof clothes and child-proof tops on bottles of flammable liquid.

Scalds are commonest in 4-year-olds. Boys are more likely to be burned and have serious scalds. There is an association with lower socioeconomic conditions.

When faced with a severely burned child it is important to adopt the protocol outlined in Emergency box 6.4.

The severity of the burn is assessed on surface area and depth of the burn (see Information box 6.5). Paediatric charts of surface area are required, because the head contributes a greater surface area in children. The palmar surface of the child's own hand is about 7% of the body surface.

Apart from facial burns, in which the airway may be compromised and the cosmetic effect of deep burns is more devastating, other important burns are to the hands and perineum. Burned hands will be functionally impaired by scarring. Perineal burns often become infected, and are difficult to manage.

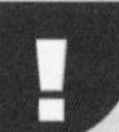

Emergency Box 6.4

Emergency treatment of the seriously burned child

- Assess for smoke inhalation
  - Exposure
  - 'Soot' around the mouth and nose
  - Darkened secretions
- Assess oedema of airway
  - Facial burns
  - Consider endotracheal intubation (easier the sooner attempted)
- Check for other injuries (e.g. cervical spine)
- Assess breathing
  - Rate
  - Apnoea
  - Colour (cyanosis is a late sign)
  - Thoracic burns may restrict breathing
  - Start high-flow oxygen
- Assess circulation
  - Shock from severe burns occurs after several hours
  - Insert two cannulae
  - Remember intraosseous (tibial) route
- Assess consciousness
  - Reduced in hypoxia (inhalational injury), shock and head injury
- Prevent heat loss
  - Warm environment
  - Sterile towels then 'bubble-wrap' or 'space blanket'

Management of burns is summarised in Practical box 6.1. Furher details of paediatric resuscitation are found in Advanced Paediatric Life Support, BMJ Publishing Group, London, 1997.

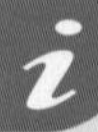

Information Box 6.5

Assessment of depth of a burn

- Superficial
  - Injury to epidermis
  - Reddened skin
  - No blisters
  - Peels and heals without scars
- Partial thickness
  - Damage to dermis
  - Blistering
  - Skin is pink or mottled
  - Scarring may not occur if deeper layers of dermis intact
- Full thickness
  - Damage to epidermis, dermis and deeper structures
  - Skin is white or charred and feels like leather
  - Painless
  - Heals by migration of skin from margins of burn or grafting – scarring results

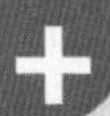

Practical Box 6.1

Emergency management of burns

- Analgesia
  - Inhalational anaesthesia (older child)
  - Intravenous morphine 0.1 mg/kg (not intramuscular, absorption unreliable in shock)
- Fluids (if >10% body surface burned)
  - 20 ml/kg fluid (plasma expander) if shocked
  - Administer basic fluid and electrolyte requirements (p. 368 and (percentage burn × weight (kg) × 4) ml/24 hours of plasma expander
  - First half of fluid to be given in the first 8 hours from time of burn
  - Subsequent therapy based on serial weighing and fluid output (hence will usually need urethral catheterization)
- Wound care
  - Leave blisters intact
  - Irrigation with cold water reduces pain but use for less than 10 minutes to avoid heat loss

Further care should be at a specialist paediatric burns centre, for >10% burns and burns to face, hands or perineum. Definitive care is best discussed with the centre.

7

Cardiology

The spectrum of heart disease in childhood is dominated by congenital heart disease. Acquired heart disease has become rare since the virtual disappearance of rheumatic fever in developed countries. However, much morbidity and mortality arises from rheumatic carditis and endocarditis in developing countries.

Functional ('innocent') murmurs

These are noises produced by a structurally normal heart, and are important in the differential diagnosis of congenital heart disease. They are very common (heard in at least 5% of the under-5 population). They are commonly found in high output states, i.e. anaemia or fever in older children, particularly those with a long slim chest shape. Details are shown in Information box 7.1.

An experienced paediatric cardiologist will make the diagnosis of functional murmur correctly on clinical grounds alone, but in practice most children if referred are investigated by Doppler or chest X-ray and ECG.

Information Box 7.1

Characteristics of an 'innocent' murmur

- Asymptomatic
- Systolic (short, soft)
- No thrill
- Mid-left sternal edge (LSE) – little radiation
- Varies with posture
- Cardiovascular system examination otherwise normal

Congenital heart disease

Epidemiology
Congenital heart disease is the commonest serious congenital malformation, affecting 1% of newborns.

Classification
Acyanotic (commoner) or cyanotic.

INTRODUCTION
By virtue of their frequency and potential to cause illness, congenital heart diseases are an important child health problem.

AETIOLOGY AND PATHOGENESIS
In most children the cause is unknown. There is an increased incidence associated with certain chromosomal abnormalities, e.g. Down syndrome or XO (Turner) syndrome, and with other familial or sporadic conditions, such as Marfan syndrome. Teratogenicity of drugs may result in congenital heart disease, such as ventricular septal defect, sometimes associated with other midline defects in the palate or lips, caused by phenytoin during pregnancy. The heart is at its most vulnerable in the 5th and 6th weeks of pregnancy when the atrioventricular septum is developing (septation). Damage can occur as a result of congenital infection, especially rubella occurring between the 4th and 8th weeks of pregnancy. As a rule, in any child with severe congenital abnormalities the possibility of associated congenital heart disease should be investigated.

Types of abnormalities

Congenital heart disease is caused by failure of septation (e.g. atrial septal defect), rotation (transposition of the great arteries) or the persistence of the fetal circulation (patent ductus arteriosus). Defects are classically referred to as either cyanotic or acyanotic. Central cyanosis is caused by deoxygenated blood gaining abnormal access to the left side of the heart or the aorta. Some lesions, e.g. the tetralogy of Fallot, may not cause cyanosis at rest. If the child exercises or cries, which increases resistance to blood flow through the lungs (pulmonary vascular resistance), the shunt across the ventricular septal defect that is normally left-to-right will be reversed and blood will shunt from right to left. This will result in clinical cyanosis. Likewise, a child with a simple ventricular septal defect is acyanotic, but a very large left-to-right shunt may eventually cause pulmonary arteriolar thickening, with increase in pulmonary vascular resistance and severe pulmonary hypertension. When the pressure in the pulmonary artery approaches that of systemic circulation the shunt reverses and the child becomes cyanosed (Eisenmenger syndrome). This syndrome is rarely seen nowadays other than in children with Down syndrome and atrioventricular canal defects (see below).

INCIDENCE
Cardiac malformations occur in 7–9 per 1000 live births. Although the incidence may be modified by termination of pregnancy in countries where high quality ultrasonography is freely available, the accurate detection of heart lesions is often difficult and these are frequently missed except in very highly specialized centres.

DIAGNOSIS
Echocardiography imaging has transformed paediatric cardiology over the last 15 years, but there is still a place for skilled clinical examination. The cardinal questions to be answered by a combination of examination, imaging, ECG and cardiac catheterization studies are:

- Is there evidence of central cyanosis?
- What is the pulmonary artery pressure?
- Is pulmonary vascular resistance raised, and if so is it irreversible?
- Is the child in heart failure? (see below).

Acyanotic lesions

Ventricular septal defect (VSD)

This is one of the commonest defects (about 2/1000 live births) and may occur in isolation or as part of a more complex malformation. In isolation it results in a left-to-right shunt during systole, and is characterized by a loud pansystolic murmur heard maximally at the lower left sternum. The murmur may radiate to the back, and may be associated with a palpable systolic thrill. A large VSD may be associated with pulmonary hypertension (see below) and heart failure. The heart failure typically develops at 6–8 weeks of age, as, prior to this time, the relatively high pulmonary vascular resistance prevents a large left-to-right shunt. The small, sometimes multiple defects (*maladie de Roger*) (Fig. 7.1) often close spontaneously during early childhood, but in any case do not warrant surgical closure. Lifelong antibiotic prophylaxis for invasive dental and other operative procedures is mandatory as long as a deficit persists.

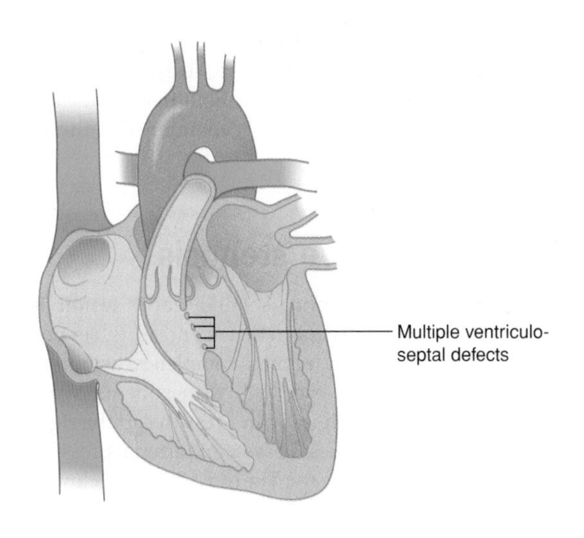

Fig 7.1
Maladie de Roger.

Atrial septal defect (ASD)

Secundum atrial septal defect is a defect in the septum secundum, which comprises 70% of congenital heart defects (Fig. 7.2). It is usually an isolated lesion, is asymptomatic, and is discovered during routine developmental surveillance in the preschool years. It is more common in girls. The classical findings are a soft systolic flow murmur over the pulmonary artery, and 'fixed' splitting of the second heart sound. When the shunt is large the hypertrophied right ventricle can be felt as a left parasternal heave and there is a prominent 'A' wave in the jugular venous pulse. The classical ECG finding is of a right bundle branch block. The chest X-ray may show an enlarged right atrium, a prominent pulmonary artery shadow, and evidence of increased blood flow through the lungs. Because this lesion does not result in a significant pressure gradient, the child is not at risk of subacute bacterial endocarditis and does not require antibiotic prophylaxis. (See below for indications for surgery.)

Primum atrial septal defect (defect of the septum primum) is a more serious defect because it affects the endocardial cushion tissue which gives rise to the mitral and tricuspid (atrioventricular) valves. It is also in close proximity to the conducting tissue around the bundle of His. The anatomical siting means that the defect produces a communication between the high pressure left ventricle and the low pressure right atrium, resulting in a very large left-to-right shunt with a high likelihood of pulmonary hypertension and raised pulmonary vascular resistance. In addition, there may be mitral and tricuspid valve incompetence, and classically the ECG shows evidence of conduction disturbances in both bundles, as evidenced by extreme left axis deviation and right bundle branch block. The clinical signs are similar to those of a large VSD (see above). This is one of the more common cardiac lesions seen in Down syndrome (see below). Early closure is advisable. The operative mortality used to be 30–50% but has decreased to below 10%. There is a small risk of inducing complete heart block.

Patent ductus arteriosus

This is the second most frequent cardiovascular defect, and accounts for 10–15% of all congenital heart disease. The ductus is an essential part of the fetal circulation. During fetal life it diverts blood from the pulmonary artery into the descending aorta to supply the lower half of the body (Fig. 7.3). It should close soon after birth in the term baby. In the preterm infant, failure of the duct

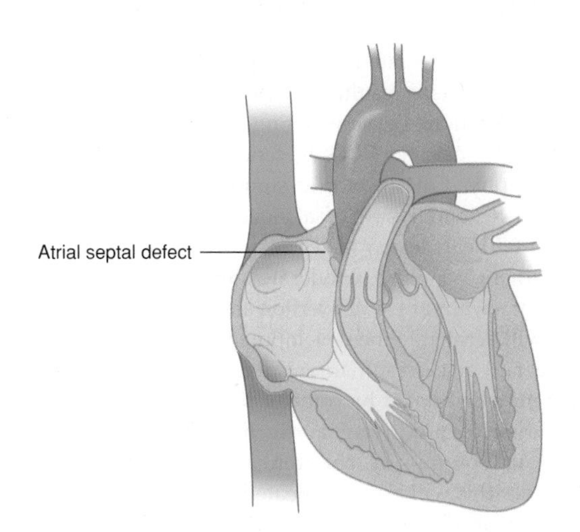

Fig 7.2
Ostium secundum atrial septal defect.

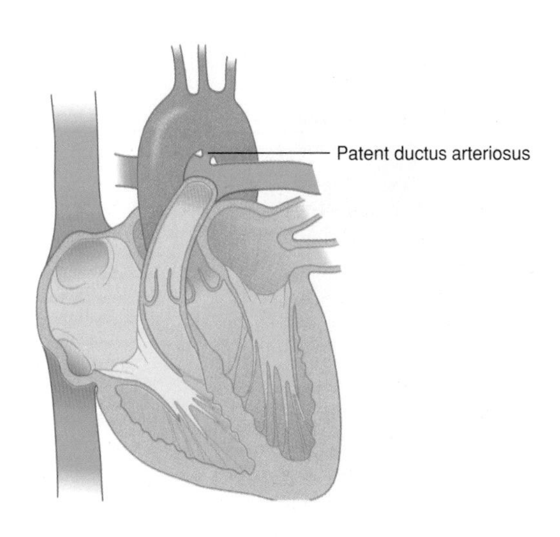

Fig 7.3
Patent ductus arteriosus.

to close is secondary to immaturity of the ductus. The relative hypoxia and acidosis associated with the respiratory distress syndrome of prematurity, tend to maintain patency of the ductus. In the term baby a patent ductus is caused by a structural abnormality of the smooth muscle and endothelium of the duct. After birth the flow through it is predominantly reversed to a left-to-right shunt from the aorta to the pulmonary artery as the ductus is not controlled by valves. Provided that the pulmonary pressure is always lower than the aortic pressure the flow will continue along the duct in both systole and diastole, leading to the characteristic ('continuous machinery') murmur. This can usually be heard over the whole of the left chest, but may be confined to the area immediately under the left clavicle.

In the preterm neonate, the ductus may be closed by the use of indomethacin; this does not succeed in the term baby because of the structural abnormality referred to above. In the older child thoracotomy and ligation has virtually been abandoned, and ducts are closed by the use of coils and umbrella devices inserted transarterially. Because of the risk of bacterial endocarditis a patent ductus arteriosus is always closed.

Coarctation of the aorta

This narrowing of the descending aorta in the region of the origin of the left subclavian artery may be associated with a previous or still patent ductus arteriosus. The arch may be interrupted (Fig. 7.4). This is the most frequent cardiac malformation to present with heart failure in the newborn period, usually around 10 days of age. Classically there is raised blood pressure in the right arm, and absent femoral pulses. The baby has not yet developed a collateral circulation to restore an absent or delayed femoral pulse. Treatment is by surgical resection and grafting. Without treatment early mortality is high. The condition is commoner in Turner syndrome.

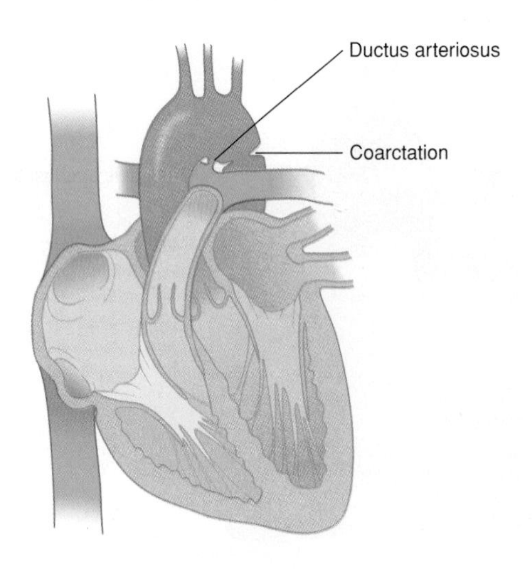

Fig 7.4
Coarctation of the aorta.

Pulmonary valve stenosis

This relatively uncommon isolated valve lesion is important because, except when stenosis is severe, affected children usually remain completely asymptomatic. The prognosis is excellent, with patients living normal lives, although those with pressures in the right ventricle which are in excess of systemic arterial pressure are at risk of premature death. The most common clinical sign is an ejection systolic murmur heard maximally at the left sternal edge in the second intercostal space. In severe stenosis, signs of right ventricular hypertrophy will also be present, i.e. a parasternal heave and a prominent 'A' wave in the jugular venous pulse. The high pressure jet coming through the stenosed, domed pulmonary valve may produce a characteristic ejection click from the wall of the pulmonary artery, similar to that heard in aortic valve stenosis, although this is often absent if the stenosis is severe. The lesion commonly occurs in Noonan syndrome, associated with atrial septal defect. Treatment is by balloon valvotomy using a transvenous approach.

Aortic stenosis

This is the commonest cause of left ventricular outflow obstruction. When present as an isolated lesion it is always congenital. Aortic stenosis can present as critical aortic stenosis in infancy or may remain asymptomatic throughout childhood, presenting on routine examination as a systolic ejection murmur radiating into the neck, associated with an ejection click. If there is fusion of the cusps resulting in aortic stenosis the pulse will be noted to be slow rising, and the child will develop clinical and ECG evidence of left ventricular hypertrophy. Calcific aortic stenosis in later life is usually the end result of a bicuspid aortic valve, a congenital heart lesion which may present in later life. When there is mild to moderate stenosis, competitive sports or severe physical exertion should be avoided as these will accelerate the development of left ventricular failure and may result in sudden death. A stenosed valve may be dilated by catheter techniques; there is a small risk of producing aortic incompetence. Open aortic valvotomy in children is best avoided as inevitably this will lead to repeated surgery as the child grows or as the prosthesis wears out. Prevention of bacterial endocarditis (see below) is of the utmost importance.

Hypoplastic left heart syndrome

This is a group of disorders in which there is underdevelopment of the left side of the heart. The right ventricle has to take over the function of the underdeveloped left ventricle. The systemic circulation is supplied by an atrial septal defect or patent foramen ovale or by retrograde flow through a patent ductus arteriosus. The condition presents with early onset heart failure and death. Cardiac transplantation may be required.

Dextrocardia

Abnormal positions of the heart are classified according to the position of the left atrium, main bronchi and abdominal organs. If the viscera are inverted (abdominal situs inversus) so are the atria. The 'left' atrium is on the right and vice versa. The ventricles are localized by determining by angiography which arteries are attached. When the heart is right-sided (dextrocardia) and the viscera normal or when the heart has normal situs (laevocardia) and the abdominal organs are inverted the heart has major malformations (Information box 7.2).

When the heart and viscera are both rotated (mirror-image dextrocardia) the heart is almost always normal. Displacement of the heart to the right (e.g. by collapse of the right lung) is called dextroposition.

Hypertrophic obstructive cardiomyopathy (HOCM)

This is hypertrophy of the left ventricle without dilatation. It does not usually present before adolescence but can occur in infancy or childhood. The right ventricle may or may not be affected, but is more frequently involved. Dominant inheritance has been described in patients who present in childhood when right ventricular outflow tract obstruction is common. Patients are usually asymptomatic and diagnosed by detection of a murmur (usually ejection systolic) or arrhythmia on routine examination. Sudden unexpected death may occur. ECG shows left ventricular hypertrophy with or without right ventricular hypertrophy. Treatment is symptomatic.

The heart muscle may also be involved in systemic illnesses such as storage disorders, muscular dystrophy, infections and collagenoses. Dilated cardiomyopathy causes congestive cardiac failure with mitral and tricuspid incompetence. Cardiac transplantation is required when the heart failure can no longer be controlled. Restrictive cardiomyopathy mimics constrictive pericarditis; cardiac transplantation is again the final outcome. Fatal arrhythmias can complicate the illness.

Information Box 7.2

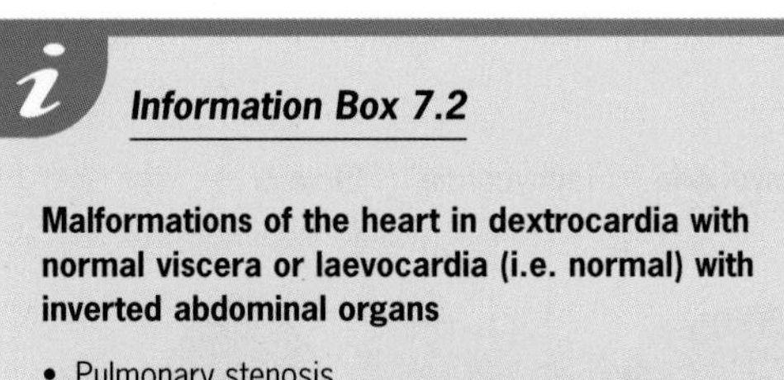

Malformations of the heart in dextrocardia with normal viscera or laevocardia (i.e. normal) with inverted abdominal organs

- Pulmonary stenosis
- Tricuspid atresia
- Transposition of the great arteries
- Anomalous pulmonary venous drainage
- Ventriculo- and atrioseptal defects
- Atrioventricular canal
- Single ventricle

Cyanotic lesions

Transposition of great arteries

This is the commonest congenital heart disease to present with cyanosis. An anteriorly placed aorta arises from the right ventricle and the left ventricle gives off the main pulmonary artery, i.e. normal figure-of-eight circulation is replaced by two separate circuits (Fig. 7.5). This arrangement is incompatible with life unless there is an adequate mixing site via an ASD, VSD or patent ductus arteriosus. The infant is severely cyanosed. Creation of an artificial hole between the atria, immediately after birth, by the procedure known as balloon septostomy, is a life-saving procedure. Early surgery consisted of complex

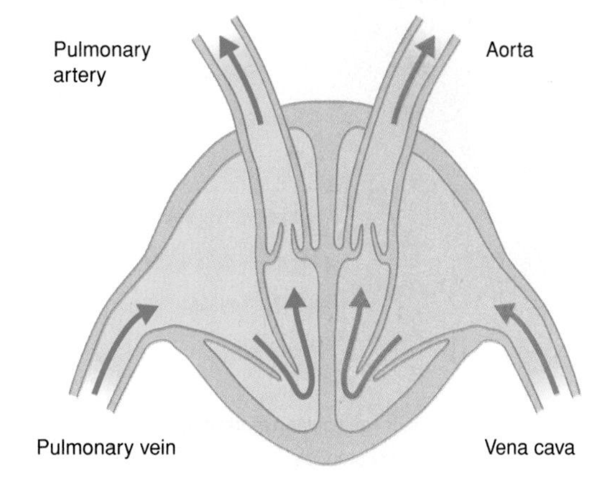

Fig 7.5
Anatomy of transposition of the great arteries.

baffle systems to redirect blood flow within the heart, but improved surgical techniques have made the obvious direct 'switch' of the great arteries the operation of choice in infancy. Long-term evaluation of this operation is awaited.

There are many more complicated versions of transposition, e.g. so called corrective transposition where the atria are also transposed, and there may be other associated cardiac anomalies. As with a number of severe cardiac malformations, there may be associated transposition of the abdominal organs (situs inversus).

Tetralogy of Fallot

This consists of:

- Pulmonary infundibular stenosis
- Ventricular septal defect
- Overriding aorta
- Right ventricular hypertrophy (Fig. 7.6).

It may be associated with moderate to severe cyanosis, but cyanosis does not usually present in the neonatal period and the child may remain completely acyanotic for several months. It is surgically correctable in infancy, with good results. In severely affected children, a palliative operation to create a shunt between the subclavian and pulmonary arteries (Blalock shunt) allows an increase in pulmonary blood flow. This should help the child to thrive prior to definitive surgical repair at a later date.

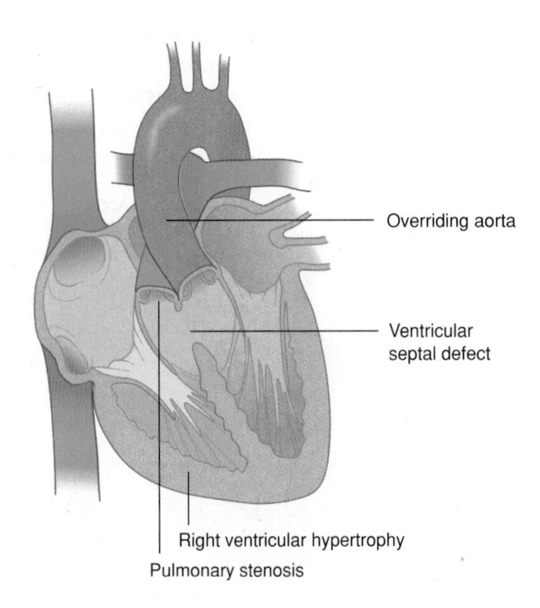

Fig 7.6
Fallot tetralogy.

Total anomalous pulmonary venous drainage

The pulmonary veins drain into the right atrium superior or inferior venae cavae, portal vein or via a persistent left superior vena cava into the coronary sinus. A patent foramen ovale is required to support life. Infants may present with cyanosis or heart failure. Surgery is required to anastomose the anomalous pulmonary arteries to the left atrium.

Tricuspid atresia

As there is no connection between the right atrium and right ventricle, venous blood is diverted via the foramen ovale into the left heart. The pulmonary circulation is perfused via a ventricular septal defect or patent ductus. Cyanosis may be present at birth. The Fontan operation is performed in which the pulmonary artery is anastomosed to the right atrium and the atrial septal defect or patent foramen ovale is closed. If the right ventricle is large enough, a conduit containing a valve is placed between the right atrium and right ventricle.

Heart failure

Some congenital heart lesions (e.g. coarctation, VSD or hypoplastic left heart) may present with heart failure. Although heart failure in the older child presents similarly to that in adults, symptoms are conspicuously absent in babies and young children so that the diagnosis is very much based on clinical history and examination. Features of heart failure are shown in Figure 7.7. Failure to thrive may be an important feature of the history, and congenital heart disease causing cardiac failure should be considered in the differential diagnosis of any child who is failing to gain weight normally. Feeding difficulties, sweating and breathlessness during feeds are other common features. On examination, dependent oedema is usually absent, and

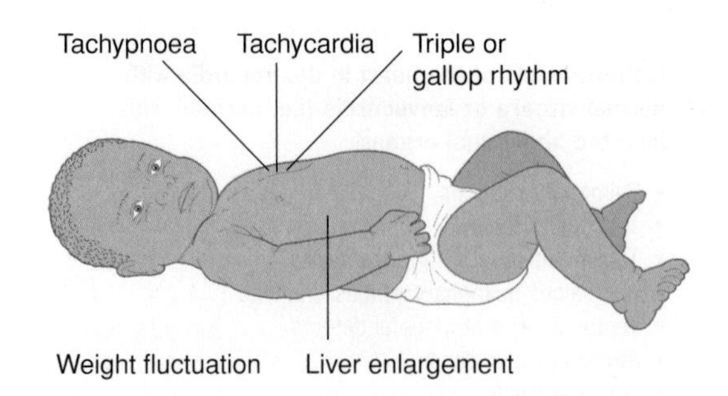

Fig 7.7
Heart failure in children.

examination of the neck veins is technically difficult. However, the soft liver of childhood reacts rapidly to changes in venous pressure, and therefore hepatomegaly is a common finding in heart failure. Changes in the size of the liver also provide a sensitive method for measuring the response to treatment.

TREATMENT OF HEART FAILURE

This follows the same principles as in adults, i.e. fluid elimination with diuretics, and fluid restriction. Digoxin has largely been replaced with drugs such as angiotensin II-converting enzyme inhibitors that are used to produce vasodilatation and thus reduce 'afterload'. Unlike adults, children cannot be made to bed rest, but will elect to do so voluntarily if significantly ill.

OPERATIVE MANAGEMENT OF CONGENITAL HEART DISEASE

The decision to operate depends on the size of the child, general medical condition, including the presence or absence of heart failure, and the operability of the lesion in terms of pulmonary vascular resistance and anatomy.

In the past even trivial ventricular septal defects were closed surgically, but this has been shown to be unnecessary. Atrial septal defects do not produce symptoms until the 5th or 6th decade, if at all. If diagnosed they are still conventionally closed before the age of 5 years because of the very small risk of paradoxical embolus. These are emboli arising from the venous circulation that gain access to the arterial circulation via the atrial septal defect.

Arrhythmias (see Information box 7.3)

Information Box 7.3

Key points regarding arrhythmias

- Relatively rare in children
- Congenital heart block
- Wolfe–Parkinson–White syndrome
- Other abnormalities of conducting tissue (e.g. prolonged QT syndrome which may be familial)
- Supraventricular tachycardias and ectopic beats
- Underlying congenital heart defect should be excluded by echocardiography

Acquired heart disease

Bacterial endocarditis

Bacterial endocarditis may be acute or subacute. Bacteria responsible for acute endocarditis (most commonly *Staphylococcus aureus*) are capable of colonizing normal valves, whereas those causing subacute endocarditis (most commonly *Streptococcus viridans*) affect only hearts with abnormal patterns of turbulence.

The most turbulent lesion of all, i.e. the patent ductus arteriosus, carries the highest risk of subacute endocarditis. Hence, patent ductus arteriosus is always closed even when the shunt through it is trivial.

Good dental care, antibiotic prophylaxis and education regarding antibiotic prophylaxis should be central to the management of a child with congenital heart disease at risk for bacterial endocarditis.

Infective endocarditis

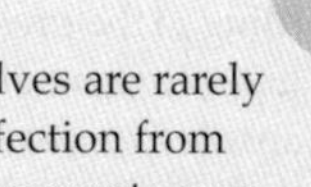

Incidence

Less common now that heart valves are rarely damaged by rheumatic fever. Infection from central lines is probably the commonest cause.

Prevention

Antibiotic prophylaxis before surgery if a high pressure cardiac shunt is present (e.g. VSD).

Streptococcus viridans and staphylococci are the commonest infecting organisms. Congenital heart lesions associated with high velocity flow, which damages the endocardium, are risk factors (e.g. VSD, patent ductus arteriosus, left-sided valvular lesions). Previous rheumatic fever is now a rare predisposing cause and it can occur in a normal heart. Dental surgery can produce the necessary bacteraemia as can an infected central venous line. Symptoms include fever, myalgia, and headache. Haematuria and splenomegaly may occur. Murmurs may change as valves are destroyed. Repeated blood cultures and echocardiographic examination of the heart for 'vegetations' at sites of endocarditis are required.

The infection is difficult to treat because bacteria at the centre of a vegetation are protected from the effects of antibiotics. Amoxycillin 50 mg/kg 1 hour before dental treatment helps prevent bacterial endocarditis in children with congenital heart lesions at risk from endocarditis. Therapy for established disease should continue for 4–6 weeks with monitoring of serum antibiotic concentrations. The choice of antibiotic is dictated by the organism isolated from blood culture (e.g. penicillin for *S. viridans*, vancomycin for *S. epidermidis*). If blood cultures are negative (which is more likely if prior antibiotic therapy has been given), then vancomycin and gentamicin are given empirically. Emergency cardiac surgery may be required, if medical treatment fails, to replace damaged valves and remove vegetations.

Rheumatic fever

Aetiology
Complication of infection with group A beta haemolytic streptococci.

Diagnosis
An elevated antistreptolysin-O titre is helpful, but the diagnosis is clinical.

This condition has become rare in developed countries over the last four decades but continues to be a serious problem in developing countries. The diagnosis is made according to the presence of two major or one major and two minor Jones criteria (see Information box 7.4).

Carditis is a pancarditis (pericardium, myocardium and endocardium) which results in permanent damage to the aortic and mitral valves. The joints are warm, red, tender and swollen in a migratory fashion. Erythema marginatum consists of pink macules that fuse. A late manifestation is Sydenham chorea: abnormal, jerky (choreoathetoid) movements, associated with emotional lability. Subcutaneous nodules 1 cm in diameter are found on the extensor surface of joints. Few cases have all these features. Evidence for preceding group A streptococcal infection would include culture or antibodies against streptococcal antigens such as antistreptolysin-O.

The streptococci are treated with penicillin. The arthritis and carditis are treated with high dose salicylates; steroids and diuretics are given for heart failure and diazepam for chorea. Penicillin prophylaxis is continued indefinitely, to avoid recurrences triggered by group A streptococci.

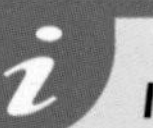

Information Box 7.4

The criteria for diagnosing rheumatic fever

Major criteria	**Minor criteria**
Carditis	Fever
Migratory polyarthritis	Arthralgia
Erythema marginatum	Previous rheumatic fever
Chorea	Elevated acute phase reactants (erythrocyte sedimentation rate (ESR), C-reactive protein (CRP))
Subcutaneous nodules	Prolonged P–R interval on ECG
	Evidence of a preceding group A streptococcal infection

Hypertension

Incidence
The genesis of essential hypertension in adult life begins in childhood.

Pathophysiology
Increased cardiac output in childhood, rather than the increased peripheral resistance of adult life.

Lifestyle
High salt intake, smoking, alcohol, lack of exercise and stress are implicated.

Diagnosis
Sphygmomanometer cuff must be tailored to the child's arm.

Techniques of measuring blood pressure (BP) in children are given in Practical box 7.1. About half of children with BP >90th percentile are likely to become hypertensive adults. Essential hypertension is, by definition, of unknown cause, but obesity, stress, sedentary lifestyle, smoking, alcohol and salt intake, are known to contribute, which are amenable to prevention. Renal disease is the commonest cause of secondary hypertension. The renal lesion may be parenchymal scarring as occurs in chronic pyelonephritis, congenital abnormalities of the kidney or vascular (e.g. renal artery stenosis). Hypertensive adolescents have a high cardiac output whereas adults have a high peripheral resistance. In common with adults, essential hypertension does not produce symptoms. The latter (see hypertensive encephalopathy below) are more likely to be associated with secondary hypertension which tends to produce more elevated pressures. Reduction of elevated blood pressure in adults reduces the risks of renal damage, stroke and congestive cardiac failure but not myocardial infarction. If preventative measures fail to decrease BP to <95th percentile, then a diuretic or beta-blocking agent should be used. If there is no response, an angiotensin-converting enzyme blocker should be added and a calcium channel blocker substituted for the beta-blocker.

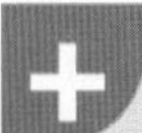

Practical Box 7.1

Methods of measuring blood pressure in children

1. Standard method. The cuff size should be **at least** two-thirds of the upper arm (too small a cuff gives a falsely elevated reading). Korotkoff phase 4 (muffling) should be used for the diastolic reading.
2. Standard cuff, using palpation of pulse and to give systolic blood pressure.
3. Flush method. Cuff is inflated to a high pressure causing blanching of the limb and then slowly deflated. Flushing of the limb indicates that the systolic blood pressure has been passed.
4. Doppler-enhanced sound measurement to give systolic blood pressure.
5. Oscillometric, using a dynamap machine.
6. Pressure transducer connected directly to an arterial line (in intensive care).

All equipment should be periodically calibrated.

Severe hypertension presents with hypertensive encephalopathy manifesting with headache, drowsiness, vomiting, visual disturbances, convulsions or hemipareses due to cerebral vasoconstriction. The underlying cause of severe hypertension in children is usually renal disease. Antihypertensive drugs that may be used for hypertensive encephalopathy include diazoxide, sodium nitroprusside, labetaol and nifedipine. They must be used judiciously since over-enthusiastic rapid lowering of blood pressure can result in infarction of retina and strokes.

Moyamoya disease

This disorder causes strokes due to narrowing of the arteries that supply the brain, especially the internal carotids. The blockage is demonstrated by angiography. Small alternative vessels, known as collaterals develop, which resemble *moyamoya*, the Japanese word for a puff of smoke. The disease was described in Japan, where other vaso-occlusive diseases appear to be much more common than in the west.

Other causes of stroke include sickle cell disease, neurofibromatosis, MELAS syndrome (see p. 324) and any disorder that causes occlusion of arteries.

8

Child abuse and child protection

Sociology
Readers of Charles Kingsley and Charles Dickens will appreciate that this is not a new problem.

Incidence
Around 25 000 children are added to the at-risk register each year. All aspects of paediatric practice are touched by child abuse in all its forms.

INTRODUCTION

The past 20 years have seen an explosion of interest in the maltreatment of children. There is nothing new about the problem and no firm evidence that it is any more common now than in the past. Public attitudes however have demanded that professional workers take responsibility for its detection, management and prevention.

In the UK the question of child death at the hands of so-called carers came to prominence following the death of Maria Colwell in the late 1960s. Following a public enquiry, new methods of coordinating the input of social work, police, paediatric and nursing services were instituted. They were instructed to abandon their professional mistrust towards each other and work in the common interests of the child. Coordination was thenceforth placed firmly in the hands of social workers.

PREVALENCE AND INCIDENCE

UK Department of Health figures show that approximately 25 000 children are added to at-risk registers (all categories) each year.

CLINICAL PRESENTATION

There are five main areas, as follows, which often overlap.

Neglect

This is usually due to a mixture of incompetence, depressive illness in the parents and gross lack of awareness of children's needs rather than being primarily due to extreme poverty. Child abuse occurs within all sections of the community and can be particularly difficult to spot in the children of the articulate middle classes. Abused children may be malnourished, dirty and withdrawn but this is not always the case. A growth chart can be most revealing when an underweight child suddenly puts on weight when looked after by a foster parent or admitted to hospital.

Emotional abuse

This includes all forms of verbal torture from mild through to systematic gross abuse. Such cruelty does not leave physical marks on the child though it may lead the child to self-injury. Mental cruelty is difficult to prove. Children may be forced to witness obscene acts or videos. They develop protective mechanisms, becoming 'mentally frozen', showing signs of terror in the company of strangers, or alternatively, aimless affection to any newcomer who shows a remote interest in the child. Another form is lack of stimulation that retards development.

Physical injury

Almost any physical injury may come to medical attention. Classic signs to look for (Fig. 8.1) are:

- Late attendance for medical care – 'it happened yesterday'.
- Incompatibility of the story with reality, e.g.
  - 4-week-old baby who 'fell off a sofa'
  - Injuries which are most unlikely to happen spontaneously, e.g. rupture of the upper lip frenulum
  - Unexpectedly missing teeth
  - Conjunctival haemorrhage which is otherwise unexplained, and retinal haemorrhage
  - Rupture of eardrums and bruising of pinnae
  - Skin signs, including human teeth marks (quite different from dog bites)
  - Bruises from whips and hitting
- Burns and scalds in unusual places, e.g. caused by:
  - being doused in hot water
  - being sat on gas hobs
  - having a cigarette stubbed out on the skin.

The clue is the unusual nature of the injury (Fig. 8.2).

It is easy to be misled and vital that false accusations are not made. Even experienced paediatricians can make mistakes; beware the pitfalls.

Sexual abuse

Early in the 1980s sexual abuse became a cause célèbre. This form of abuse is readily concealed. The perpetrator can go to extreme lengths to prevent the child from disclosing it. Retrospective surveys have shown wide variation in prevalence, with between 6 to 62% in females and 3 to 31% in males reporting being abused. Under-reporting is widespread with only 2 to 6% disclosing. Most victims (77%) are girls. Sexual abuse

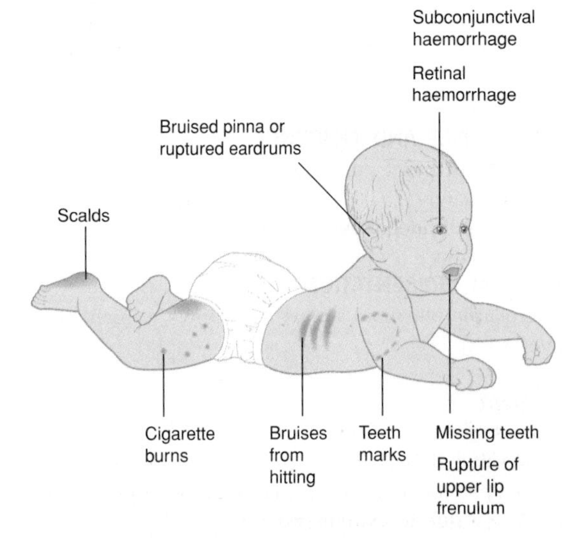

Fig 8.1
Injuries likely to be nonaccidental.

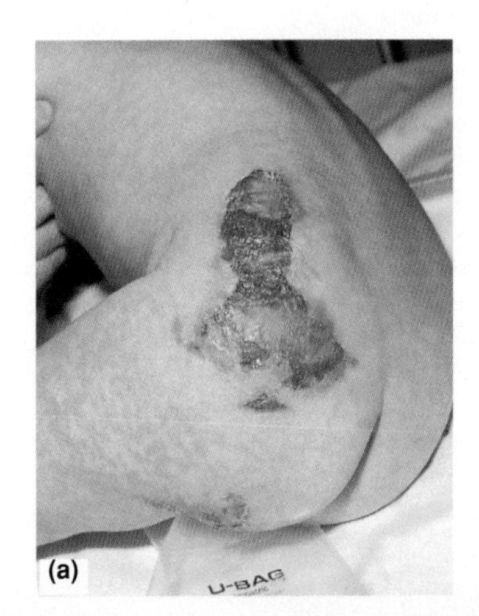

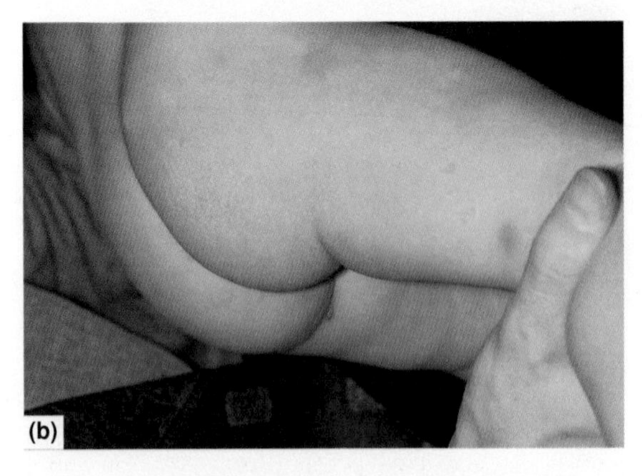

Fig 8.2
(a) Scald likely to have been caused nonaccidentally. (b) Cigarette burn.

ranges from verbal mistreatment through a wide range of acts including buggery and genital penetration. Abused children can bear lifelong mental scars affecting their whole future attitudes to sex; they are at risk of AIDS and other genital infection. Forensic detection and confirmation can be very difficult.

Munchausen syndrome by proxy

Parents and carers can do the most extraordinary things to children. Occasionally parents inflict the signs of an illness on their child; commoner examples include reports of seizures seen only by parents, or injection of insulin to cause profound and often repeated hypoglycaemia. These have to be interpreted as extreme cries for help by the parent (usually mother).

MANAGEMENT

Whenever one sees an injured child, one has to ask 'was this a true accident or am I being given a false story?' Delay in presentation is a warning sign. Children who suffer genuine accidents are usually taken to the doctor immediately. The parents are worried and sometimes feel guilty that they have allowed an accident to happen and are highly cooperative over treatment. Accurate history taking is vital; as far as possible this should be done once, by fully trained personnel coupled with an appropriate full medical examination. This starts with a conventional medical examination in which all systems are checked so that the full health profile can be drawn up before the genitalia are inspected; here there are many pitfalls. This evidence is of vital forensic importance and increasingly video recording of the disclosure interview is being required for court purposes, to spare the child from attending. Many doctors do not appreciate the normal variations of child genitalia in the penile, hymeneal, vulval and anal anatomy. Enormous problems have occurred in the recent past, including the 'Cleveland affair' in which too much reliance was placed on the appearance of the anus.

Full examination may reveal scars of earlier injuries. Sometimes a skeletal survey will show multiple old healed fractures and subperiosteal new bone formation. Small round lesions may be due to cigarette burns, rather than varicella or impetigo.

A senior professional must be consulted. They will have access to local child protection procedures and these must be followed to the letter. Although there are local variations, the following apply. Having reasonable grounds to suspect that a child is being abused, it is axiomatic that one informs social services, immediately. A 'hotline' is maintained by the local authority, day and night. On notification, the social worker is obliged to gather information. They may need a planning conference as soon as is practicable, bringing together those professionally and closely concerned with the child. In the light of the planning conference, they may need a full case conference that brings together all professionals, i.e. doctors, nurses, therapists, health visitors, teachers, and so on, who have been involved with the child. It is now becoming the practice to invite parents to these meetings. Such a meeting is fraught with potential problems and health professionals need training in their roles at such a conference.

There are many steps which can be taken to protect the child. In the UK, this is enshrined legislatively in the Children Act (1989), which clarified and reorganized the law, and came into operation in late 1991. The principles of the Children Act are as follows:

- The Act is comprehensive and consolidates earlier law dealing with children.
- It was implemented in October 1991.
- It seeks to be 'user-friendly', i.e. comprehensible.
- The upbringing of children is primarily the responsibility of parents.
- A balance between child protection and undue interference in family life is sought.
- Child protection is improved by the introduction of Child assessment orders and lower thresholds for emergency protection orders.
- Emergency protection orders may be challenged in court, after 72 hours, by parents.

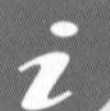

Information Box 8.1

Orders arising from the Children Act

Court orders*
- Emergency protection order
  - Lasts 8 days
  - Extended for 7 days
  - Can be challenged within 72 hours by parents
- Child assessment order
  - Lasts up to 7 days where there is a need to decide whether significant harm is likely in the absence of an emergency protection order and parental consent is withheld
- Supervision order, interim care order, full care order
  - Grounds of 'significant harm' constitutes the threshold before these orders are issued

Section 8 orders
- Residence order: where children will live
- Contact order: who will have access
- Specific steps order: determining parental responsibility
- Prohibited steps order: steps not to be taken without leave of court

*Orders by which children can be compulsorily removed from their parents or carers

- In courts, the 'child's welfare is paramount'.
- A court order should not be made unless it is better for the child than not making the order.
- A timetable will be set by the court to avoid undue delay.

The orders proposed by the Children Act are summarized in Information box 8.1.

You cannot learn from this book how to protect children and you must attend teaching sessions where this is discussed in detail. Be aware of instances when well meaning attempts to deal with child abuse have gone wildly wrong. You need to be aware of the problems in Cleveland, Orkney and Rochdale where excessive action on suspicion of child abuse has undermined confidence in the caring professions. It is extremely difficult to get the right balance. It is becoming apparent that sometimes taking children away from home in itself creates problems, and it may be better to keep the child at home and devise an effective system of supervision for the parents.

Healthcare professionals are not lawyers, and must work in harmony with their colleagues. For this reason, senior healthcare professionals, social workers and police meet on a regular basis through the Local Area Child Protection Committee. This Committee monitors the local situation, writes local guidelines and takes a role in ensuring that the various groups work collaboratively together.

Every children's doctor needs to know the local child abuse procedures, follow them explicitly and know their own duties, be aware of their limitations and whom to turn to for help.

9 Dermatology

Hormonal disorders

Acne vulgaris

Incidence
Virtually universal in adolescence, which for some individuals may be blighted by severe disease.

Lifestyle
Seems to worsen with stress but, contrary to popular wisdom, not with greater intake of fatty foods.

This is a disease of sebaceous glands which usually begins in adolescence, when sebaceous glands enlarge, and increasingly persists into adult life. The cause is not known but hormonal factors must play a part. The openings of the sebaceous glands become blocked with keratin, forming open comedones (blackheads) or closed comedones (whiteheads) in which the obstructed gland fills with keratin, lipid and bacteria. The bacterium *Propionobacterium acnes*, which colonizes sebaceous glands, releases free fatty acids from sebum, which may play a part in the inflammatory reaction. If the contents extrude into the dermis (which may occur if the lesions are squeezed) a cystic lesion develops. There is great variation in severity, and it is commoner in males. The lesions may be confined to the face or involve the shoulders and trunk.

Early treatment does not prevent the emergence of acne. It is important to meet with the parents as well as the child so that any misinformation can be corrected. Cleansing agents are ineffective because they remove lipid from the surface of the skin. The most effective topical preparations contain benzoyl peroxide, an oxidizing agent which peels the skin and suppresses *P. acnes*. If unsuccessful, topical retinoic acid should be tried, which affects the turnover of epidermal cells and softens the keratinous plug. This photosensitizes. The next step is to add long-term oral antibiotics, especially tetracycline (if older than 12 years) or erythromycin. Antibiotics are less effective when given topically than orally. Oral oestrogen may be given for young women whose acne flares premenstrually. In the most severe cystic acne (acne conglobata) oral isoretinoin is used. Because of the number of side-effects, especially teratogenicity, in the UK it is only available from dermatology clinics.

Bullous eruptions

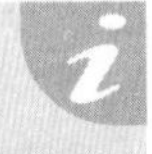

Definition

A bulla is a blister.

Aetiology

Although blisters are most commonly caused by insect bites or allergy, chronic unexplained blistering requires dermatological investigation.

Some of the commoner causes include:

- Viruses, e.g. *Herpes simplex*, *Herpes zoster* (see p. 273). Varicella are described in Exanthema (p. 271).
- Bacteria, e.g. staphylococcal scalded skin syndrome (Fig. 9.1).
- Drug reactions, e.g. erythema multiforme, Stevens–Johnson syndrome (Fig. 9.2), toxic epidermal necrolysis.

Other heterogeneous congenital blistering diseases are referred to as epidermolysis bullosa (Fig. 9.3). Epidermolysis bullosa simplex is an autosomal dominant condition in which bullae are present from birth and improve with age. Healing occurs without scarring. Junctional epidermolysis bullosa lethalis is more severe in that mucous membranes are involved. Inheritance is autosomal recessive. Dominant dystrophic epidermolysis bullosa is also mild, although scarring and nail loss occur. Recessive dystrophic epidermolysis bullosa causes oesophageal erosions and

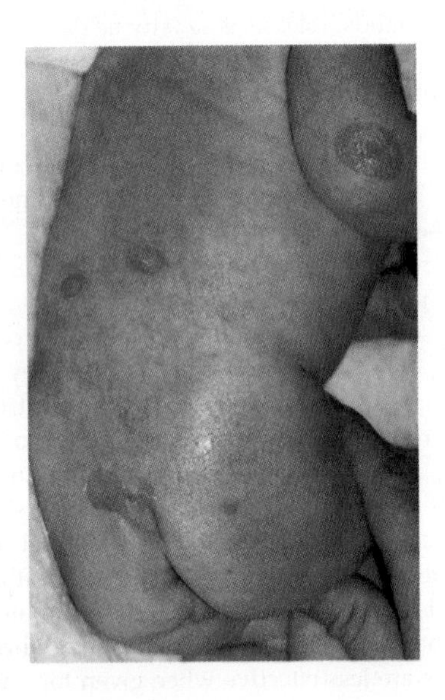

Fig 9.1
Staphylococcal 'scalded skin' syndrome.

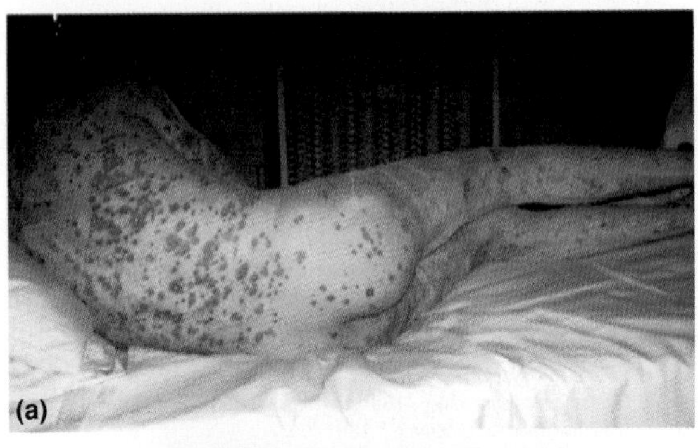

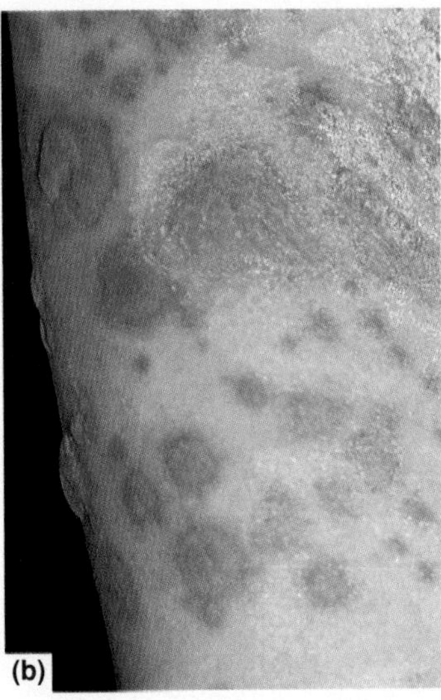

Fig 9.2
(a) and (b) Stevens–Johnson syndrome.

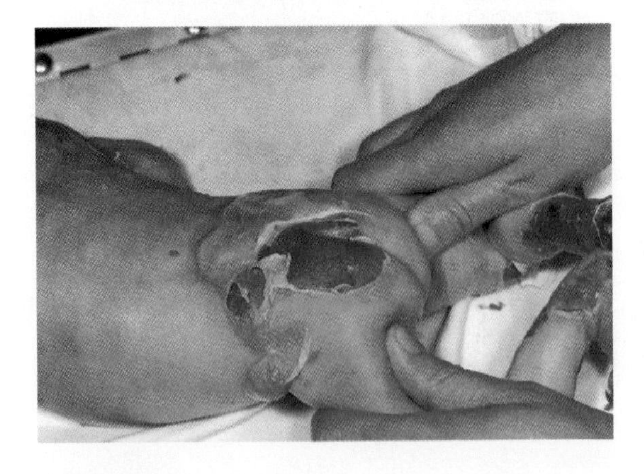

Fig 9.3
Epidermolysis bullosa.

stricture. Scarring is so severe that the digits become fused. Chronic bullous dermatosis of childhood (linear IgA dermatosis), pemphigus and bullous pemphigoid also produce blisters on the skin and mucous membranes which improve with systemic steroids. These diseases can be differentiated by light and electron microscopy examination of skin biopsies.

Congenital disorders

CHILD syndrome (congenital hemidysplasia with ichthyosiform erythroderma and limb defects)

The striking feature of this condition, which affects only girls, is a large patch of very dark thickened skin present at birth on one half of the body, with a sharp dividing line; the skin on the other side is normal. Deformity of the skeleton of affected areas may develop.

The prognosis is very variable: sometimes the skin abnormality disappears or decreases in severity.

Cystic hygroma

Cystic hygroma is a congenital disorder of the lymphatic system (Fig. 9.4). Thin-walled cysts in the head and neck region contain yellow fluid, and may extend down into the thorax and up into the tongue. Surgical removal can be a formidable challenge.

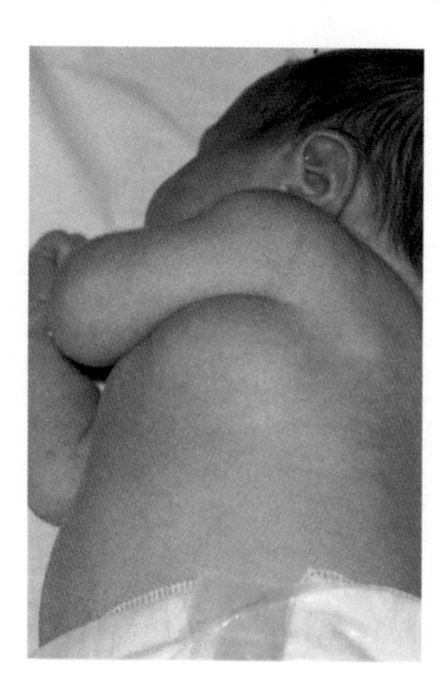

Fig 9.4
Cystic hygroma.

Dermoid (epidermal inclusion) cysts

These are nodules in the skin consisting of a cyst, lined with stratified squamous epithelium and filled with keratin. They should be treated by complete excision. Dermoid cysts containing hair follicles and hair shafts can occur on the globe of the eye and on the nose. They may have intracranial extensions and predispose to infection of the central nervous system.

Ectodermal dysplasias

These syndromes are characterized by defects in structures of epidermal origin.

Anhidrotic (hypohidrotic) ectodermal dysplasia is inherited as an X-linked recessive disorder. It presents with:

- Absent sweat and tear glands
- Wrinkled, hyperpigmented periorbital skin
- Sparse hair, eyebrows and eyelashes
- Widely spaced, peg-like or absent teeth (hypodontia or adontia)
- Hypoplastic nails.
- Recurrent infections

Affected children become pyrexial in warm environments.

If sweat glands are present the syndrome is called hidrotic ectodermal dysplasia.

Ehlers–Danlos syndrome

This is hyperelasticity and fragility of the skin. There are several clinical types depending on the features shown in Information box 9.1.

The gut, lung or major vessels may rupture.

The first sign of the condition may be premature delivery, with weakness or premature rupture of the fetal membranes.

Healing is poor, with 'cigarette paper' scars and dehiscence of surgical scars.

By contrast, in the condition known as *cutis laxa*, the skin hangs in folds, like a bloodhound's, and the joints are not hypermobile.

Giant hairy naevus syndrome

Children with large, pigmented hairy skin lesions are predisposed to the development of malignant melanoma. Widespread excision is required, with skin grafting.

Information Box 9.1

The clinical categorization of Ehlers–Danlos syndrome depends on the following features:

- Severity
- Mode of inheritance
  - Autosomal dominant
  - Sex-linked recessive
- Severity of bruising
- Presence of other manifestations
  - Softening of the cornea and sclera
  - Short stature
  - Periodontitis
  - Soft bones.

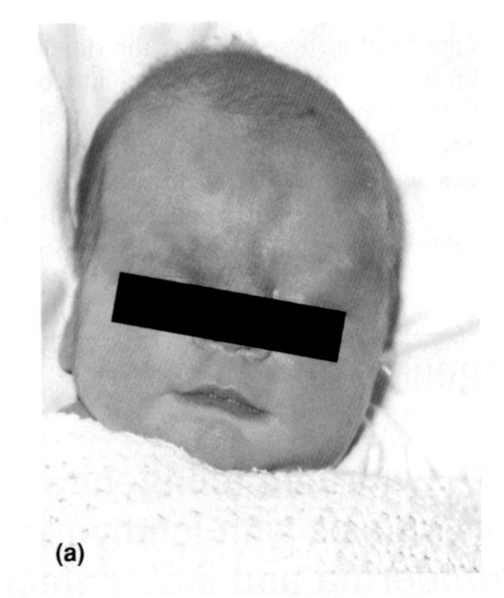

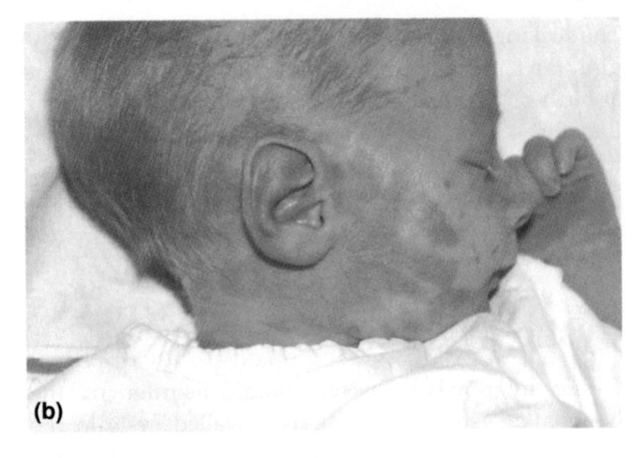

Fig 9.5
(a) Superficial capillary naevi on eyelids and forehead. (b) Naevus flammeus.

Haemangiomas

Definition
Benign tumours of blood vessels.

Prognosis
Many fade spontaneously.

They are most obvious in the skin or mucous membranes but can occur in deeper tissues. There are two main types, capillary and cavernous. Superficial capillary naevi are very common on the upper eyelids and occiput at birth; they fade with time (Fig. 9.5(a)). Naevus flammeus (port wine stain, Fig. 9.5(b)) is a vivid, permanent capillary naevus which may involve half the face especially in the area supplied by the ophthalmic branch of the trigeminal nerve, in association with glaucoma, cerebral haemangiomata, intracranial calcification, epilepsy and hemiplegia (Sturge–Weber syndrome).

Strawberry naevi are another form of capillary haemangioma. At birth they are invisible but in the early weeks they appear as red, raised unsightly marks (Fig. 9.6), reaching a maximum when the child is about 1 year old; they then tend to fade and most have gone by the time the child is 5, leaving faint speckled marks. They look alarming and parents may demand treatment, but for the great majority they should be left strictly alone as natural cure gives a much better result than treatment. Occasionally they occlude tissues such as the airway and urgent decompression or bypass by tracheotomy is needed. Steroid drugs can be useful in decreasing the size but long-term treatment carries severe side-effects so these drugs tend to be kept for emergency use.

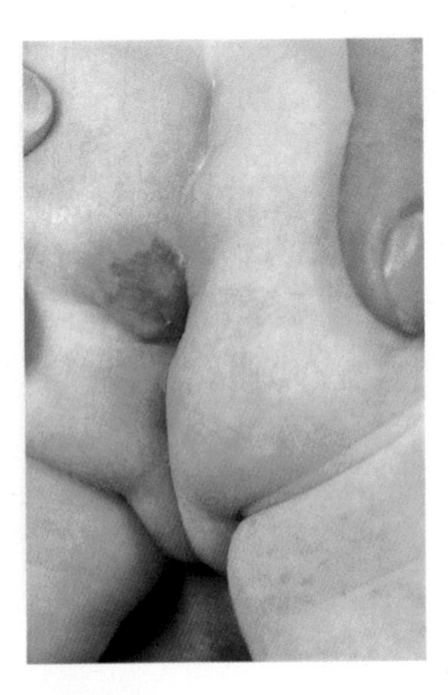

Fig 9.6
Strawberry haemangioma.

Cavernous haemangioma involves larger blood vessels. The overlying skin can be normal or discoloured bluish. If the haemangioma is situated in deeper tissues the only external sign may be a rubbery swelling or enlargement of internal organs such as the liver. Although cavernous haemangiomata also tend to subside spontaneously, this may not be as complete as in capillary haemangioma. They pose a problem if they entrap platelets (Kasabach–Merritt syndrome) and destroy erythrocytes. Steroids and embolization are used to hasten resolution. Laser therapy is also employed; the blood vessels of the haemangioma are thrombosed when the red cells passing through them absorb the laser energy.

Ichthyosis (see also Eczema)

Ichthyosis represents a group of inherited defects of keratin. The name, from ichthys, meaning 'fish' in Greek, attests to the scaly appearance of affected skin.

The most severe type is called 'collodion baby'. In this autosomal recessive disorder the skin of affected infants is covered with a membrane of keratin which eventually sheds. An X-linked variety due to steroid sulphatose deficiency is associated with corneal opacities.

The commonest type is ichthyosis vulgaris, an autosomal dominant condition in which the skin of the extensor surfaces becomes dry and scaly. Moisturizing creams are applied to affected areas.

Hypomelanosis of Ito (incontinentia pigmenti achromia)

This condition is characterized by bizarre patches, whorls, and streaks of hypopigmented skin. As with many other skin conditions, there are associated CNS defects.

The appearance of the skin improves with time.

Incontinentia pigmenti (Bloch–Sulzberger syndrome)

This X-linked syndrome is very rare but serious. Affected males usually undergo spontaneous abortion so the condition is mainly seen in females.

It usually presents in early infancy, with red streaky marks especially on the limbs (Fig. 9.7). Later, chronic blistering occurs followed by a wide variety of skin eruptions. In some lesions black pigment is deposited, giving the condition its name.

Although the skin problems often improve with age, many children with this disorder have other handicapping disorders, particularly in the nervous system, causing severe motor disorder and epilepsy.

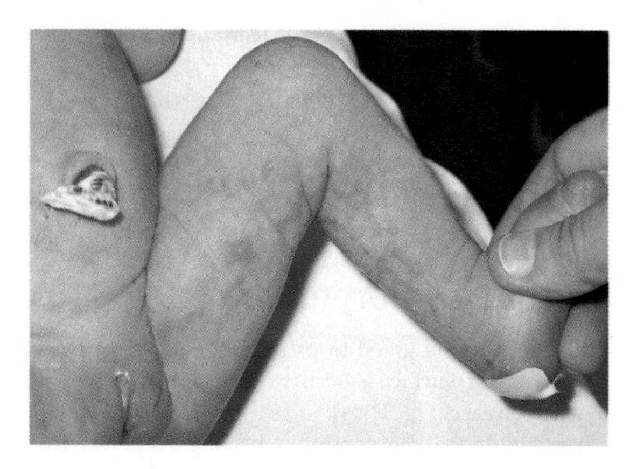

Fig 9.7
Incontinentia pigmenti. Note whorls of pigmentation.

Milroy disease (congenital lymphoedema)

This was first described by the American surgeon, William Milroy, in 1892. The unsightly condition, of unknown cause, is present from birth. Parts of the body, particularly limbs, are swollen due to a congenital failure of development of lymphatic channels, which in normal health collect the lymphatic fluid exuded from tissues and return it to the circulation. The affected skin is prone to cellulitis.

There is no specific treatment for Milroy disorder, although support hose will help.

Another congenital cause of swollen hands and feet is associated with Turner syndrome, though other tissues are not affected and with time the swelling decreases.

Acquired lymphangiopathies occur in some tropical disorders such as elephantiasis where lymphoid vessels are choked with parasites or in tumours where malignant tissue blocks the nodes.

Immunological disorders

Contact dermatitis

Saliva, transferred to the skin by dribbling or licking, is a common cause of contact dermatitis in children, and citrus fruit and detergents may also irritate the skin.

Nappy rash is a specific form of irritant contact dermatitis. Another specific form is juvenile plantar dermatosis, which occurs in children whose feet sweat excessively (hyperhidrosis) and who wear shoes made from synthetic materials.

Contact dermatitis can also be caused by an allergic reaction to, for example, jewellery, shoes, clothing, ointments and cosmetics. The distribution may give a clue to the cause.

The rash resembles eczema (see below).

The key to treatment is identification and removal of the irritant or allergen. If necessary, 1% hydrocortisone may be administered.

Dermatitis herpetiformis

This is the name given to pruritic bullae occurring on the extensor surfaces, occurring in association with coeliac disease (Fig. 11.14).

In childhood the condition usually responds to a gluten-free diet. In adult life dapsone may be required.

Eczema

> Incidence
> A very common skin disorder.
>
> Aetiology
> A cutaneous manifestation of the atopic state.

The cause of eczema is ill understood. It can be regarded as an intrinsic type of hypersensitivity reaction in the skin, probably involving at least type I and type IV hypersensitivity reactions. In some eczematous children type I hypersensitivity reactions can be demonstrated to food antigens, particularly milk and eggs. Indeed withdrawal of these substances from the child's diet often results in improvement in the eczema. However in many cases food allergy cannot be demonstrated. The majority of affected children are sensitive to the house dust mite, and in children over 2 years of age this is probably the most relevant allergen.

INCIDENCE AND CLINICAL PRESENTATION

Atopic eczema is most common in infancy and early childhood. It is more common in British children of Caribbean extraction, but the incidence is increasing in all racial groups. It has been estimated that 3–5% of children develop this before the age of 5 years and most of them have a first-degree relative family history of atopic disease, though not necessarily of eczema. Between one-third and one-half of children with eczema will at some stage develop other atopic disease such as rhinitis or asthma.

The rash of eczema is protean in its manifestations. The skin eruption may be simple erythematous, vesicular, scaling, crusting, or weeping in appearance. In acute eczema the skin is red, with papules and vesicles, which may weep. In more chronic disease, the skin becomes thickened, dry and scaly. Almost always the skin is dry (xerosis) and intensely itchy, and rubbing and scratching serve to exacerbate the findings and create a 'vicious cycle' effect. In infants the rash usually first appears at around 2 months of age and may be very extensive, but it particularly involves the face and extensor surfaces. In older children the pattern tends to change, with less widespread rash particularly localizing to flexural areas such as the antecubital and popliteal fossae. The child may appear miserable and irritable from the itching and may exhibit disturbed sleep patterns for the same reason. Extensive areas of erythema and weeping are suggestive of secondary bacterial infection usually due to staphylococci, which is very common (Fig. 9.8(a)). More serious secondary infection may occur with herpes simplex virus, leading to eczema herpeticum (Fig. 9.8(b)) which may be life-threatening, resulting in a profound illness with fever and widespread vesicular eruption.

DIAGNOSIS

The main differential diagnosis is from seborrhoeic dermatitis, or cradle cap, in early infancy but the distribution of this condition is usually helpful in

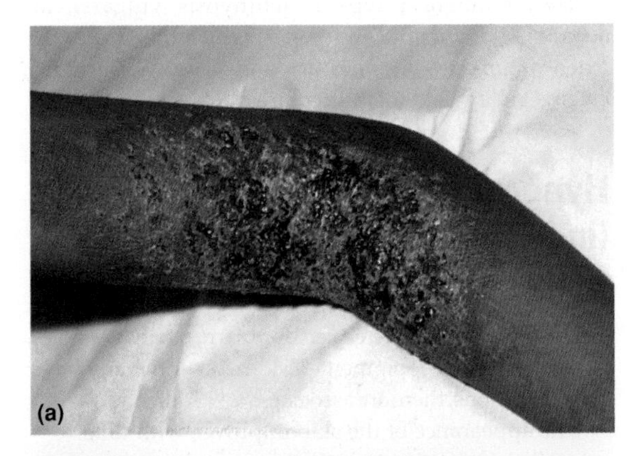

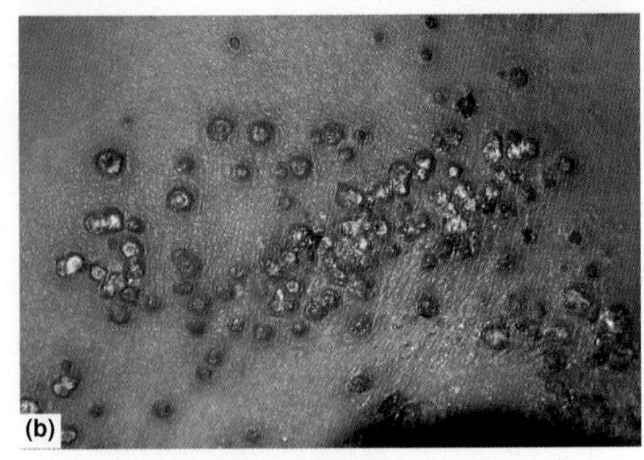

Fig 9.8
(a) Infected eczema. (b) Eczema herpeticum. Note vesicular lesions.

differentiation from eczema. It is predominantly concentrated on the cranium with the rash 'spilling' down over the face and upper trunk and back. It is also much more scaly in appearance and the child is well and happy, not irritable and itchy. In older children with localized skin disease the possibility of a contact dermatitis should be considered. Scabies infestation with eczematoid response should also be considered.

MANAGEMENT

Although eczema is not a life-threatening condition it is chronic, disfiguring and distressing for the child and the family who will need a sympathetic and supportive approach. In most cases infantile eczema improves or disappears with age and this may be reassuring for the family. The mainstays of treatment are the topical use of agents designed to lessen dryness and pruritus, and thus prevent further skin damage from scratching and spontaneous fissuring. This is called emollient treatment. Secondly, the inflammation is lessened, usually with topical corticosteroid treatment.

The first of these approaches is perhaps the most important. A variety of emollients are available and include creams and ointments designed to hydrate and maintain hydration of the skin as well as oils and soap substitutes to be used when bathing. The use of an emollient in itself seems to reduce the pruritus. Additional measures may include avoidance of itchy clothing such as woollens in direct contact with the skin. Systemic antihistamines need to be used in high dosage, particularly at night when they will not only act locally on the skin but also act as a sedative for the child. In severe eczema affecting the limbs, occlusive dressings that involve liberal emollients sealed in with bandaging of the limbs are very effective at providing intensive emollient treatment and protection from possible scratching.

Topical corticosteroids are another mainstay of therapy. They come at three levels of potency: low potency, e.g. hydrocortisone; medium potency, e.g. clobetasone; and high potency, e.g. beclomethasone. As a rule one should use the lowest potency preparation that will control the symptoms. The high potency fluorinated steroids should not be used on the face.

Other therapies will include the use of systemic antibiotic treatment when secondary bacterial infection occurs. In severe cases which are unresponsive to standard therapy it is worth exploring dietary control measures. Skin prick testing or serum radio allergosorbent testing (RAST) may reveal specific food allergies but are unreliable in small children. An alternative approach is to put the child on an oligoantigenic diet before reintroducing foods one by one over a period of time. This is quite a difficult undertaking and will involve close input from a paediatric dietician. In a very small percentage of atopic eczema sufferers, systemic corticosteroid therapy on a long-term basis is the only way to control the disease. An alternative form of therapy which is popular at the moment is the use of Chinese herbal remedies, and dramatic successes have been reported. However, great care needs to be taken as some of these therapies are toxic, and in particular hepatotoxicity has been described.

Erythema nodosum

The lesions of erythema nodosum resemble bruises on the shins. The condition is associated with chronic inflammatory bowel disease, reactions to sulphonamide drugs, collagenoses, sarcoidosis, TB and other infections. Improvement follows treatment of the underlying disorder.

Seborrhoeic dermatitis (cradle cap)

This crusting of the scalp (cradle cap) occurs during the first year of life. It often also involves retroauricular, nasolabial, axillary and perineal skin.

Erythematous, scaly dermatitis may persist into adolescence, with severe dandruff and skin changes (marginal blepharitis) on the medial aspect of the eyelids and the external auditory canals.

Scalp changes require a shampoo containing selenium. Topical corticosteroids may be applied to the skin lesions.

Stevens–Johnson syndrome

(see also Bullous eruptions, p. 188)

This is a hypersensitivity reaction to infection by *Herpes simplex*, *Mycoplasma pneumoniae* or group A streptococcus, for example. It may also be caused by drugs, such as antibiotics (sulphonamides) or anticonvulsants. The blistering rash involves the skin, mouth and conjunctiva, and new crops of blisters form for several weeks.

There is no specific treatment.

Urticaria

This presents as raised circumscribed skin lesions (hives) which may be itchy. When oedema of the skin occurs, the condition is referred to as angioedema. The upper respiratory tract may be involved.

It is caused by release of histamine when an antigen interacts with IgE molecules bound to mast cells or when complement is activated. The reaction can be triggered by a wide variety of inhaled, ingested or contact allergens and by unexplained physical causes as with cold urticaria.

Treatment is with antihistamines.

Infective disorders

Erysipelas

This infection of the skin with group A beta-haemolytic streptococci and staphylococci produces red, indurated skin with a sharply demarcated border. The lesion may progress rapidly in spite of therapy.

Herpetic whitlow

This painful infection of the fingers with ulceration of the skin is due to *Herpes simplex*, and may occur in association with herpetic gingivostomatitis.

Impetigo (Fig. 9.9)

Impetigo is caused by group A beta-haemolytic streptococci and *Staphylococcus aureus*. Flaccid blisters form on infected skin, then rupture and form crusts. Impetigo is highly infectious. It resolves spontaneously, but topical mupirocin and antibiotics such as flucloxacillin hasten resolution.

Severe impetigo occurring in infants is known as staphylococcal scalded skin syndrome (see Fig. 9.1, p. 188).

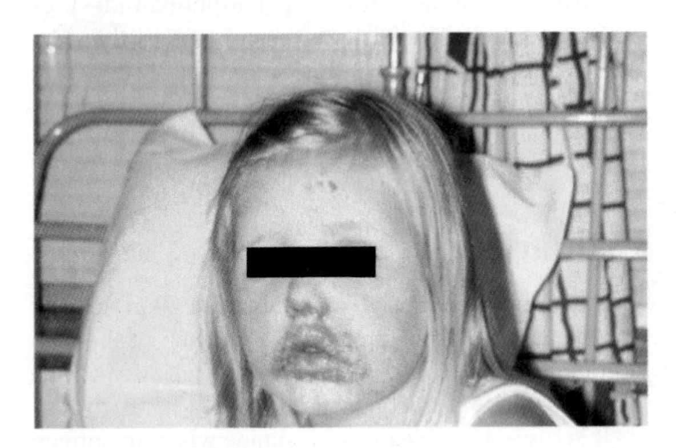

Fig 9.9
Impetigo. Note 'golden' yellow crusts.

Fig 9.10
Molluscum contagiosum. Note umbilication.

Molluscum contagiosum (Fig. 9.10)

This virus infection of the skin is acquired by direct contact. The 1–5-mm papules have a central dimple (umbilication). A core composed of virus-infected skin cells can be expressed. The infection may persist for years, and immunodeficient children and those with atopic eczema may develop a severe infection.

Lesions can be treated by brief application with liquid nitrogen.

Papillomatosis

This occurs most commonly in childhood and adolescence. Lesions are found on the hands, feet and face, and spread by direct contact then autoinoculation. The papules have a roughened, keratotic surface. Plantar warts are flush with the skin because of pressure from walking.

The lesions may be extremely painful, and may be treated by the application of liquid nitrogen.

Genital warts (condyloma acuminata)

This is a sexually transmitted disease caused by human papilloma virus. Young children may have acquired them at birth from an infected mother, but child sexual abuse should be considered.

Laryngeal papillomatosis

The wart-like tumours are caused by the same papillomavirus that causes genital warts. They can be acquired at birth, and may grow so profusely in the lumen of the larynx that they cause airway obstruction. Recurrence is common until puberty, and malignant change is a rare complication.

Various treatments have been advocated, including surgery, bleomycin or interferon.

Pediculosis

Epidemiology
Head lice are common in the majority of infant schools.

This is skin infestation by three species of insects called lice, namely, crab or pubic lice (*Phthirus pubis*), body lice (*Pediculus humanus corporis*) and head lice (*Pediculus humanus capitis*).

Phthiris pubis may be acquired by adolescents, in whom they produce intense pruritus in the inguinal area as a result of taking a blood meal. Insect eggs called nits, or occasionally 1–2-mm insects resembling crabs may be seen clinging to pubic hair and other hirsute areas of the body such as eyelashes. Topical pyrethrin or lindane are effective, the nits being removed with a fine tooth comb. Towels, bed linen and clothes require frequent laundering.

Body lice live and deposit their nits in the seams of unhygienic clothing. They cause itching when feeding. Laundering of clothes is the mainstay of treatment, and applying gamma benzene hydrochloride or permethrin to scalp hair.

Head lice deposit nits on scalp hair and cause intense pruritus. The treatment is permethrin, pyrethrin or gamma benzene hydrochloride, repeated after 2 weeks. The nits are removed with a fine tooth comb. Laundering of clothes and bed linen is required, and brushes and combs must be disinfected.

Scabies

This infection with the mite *Sarcoptes scabei* var. *hominis* produces burrows, and itchy eczematous skin lesions, especially in the interdigital spaces, extremities and perineal region.

Mites can be detected by applying a drop of mineral oil to the skin lesion, scraping with a blunt instrument and examining the scrapings suspended in oil under the microscope for the presence of the mite.

Treatment is by general application of 1% gamma benzene hexachloride, 5% permethrin (less toxic) or 10% crotamiton cream (for infants). Carers are also treated.

Tinea

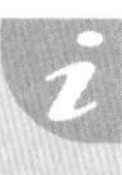

Aetiology
Fungal infection of the skin.

Tinea versicolor is caused by the yeast *Pityrosporon orbiculare* (*Malassezia furfur*). It produces reddish brown macules in white skin and hypo- or hyperpigmented lesions in black skin, on the thorax and upper arms. Skin scrapings and examination under ultraviolet light (producing a gold fluorescence) are diagnostic. Topical selenium sulphide or oral ketoconazole are effective, but the illness is likely to recur.

Tinea capitis is a fungal infection of the scalp due to *Microsporum canis* or *audouini* (blue green fluorescent) or *Trychophyton tonsurans* (nonfluorescent). *M. canis* can be acquired from cats and dogs, the other species from humans. Multiple patches of alopecia develop as the hair becomes brittle and broken. Large inflammatory masses called kerions may develop. Treatment is with oral griseofulvin or ketoconazole for up to 12 weeks.

Tinea corporis is a fungal infection of the body due to *M. canis*, *T. rubrum* and *T. mentagrophytes*. The skin lesion is a circular ring; hence the name 'ringworm'. Skin scrapings are required to differentiate from other skin lesions such as granuloma annulare or discoid eczema. Most clear spontaneously or with topical miconazole; griseofulvin is reserved for lesions that fail to improve.

Vulvovaginitis

The commonest cause is poor perineal hygiene. The vagina becomes colonized by coliform organisms of faecal origin or by upper respiratory tract-type flora such as beta-haemolytic streptococcus or *Staphylococcus aureus*. Bubble baths and tight fitting clothes have also been implicated. There is a brown or green offensive discharge. Foreign bodies in the vagina produce bleeding as well as discharge.

Hygienic advice is given, and a broad spectrum antibiotic such as amoxycillin may be used. Topical oestrogen cream may help.

Disorders of unknown cause

Lichen sclerosus et atrophicus

This is an uncommon skin disease. The vulva is commonly involved, raising questions of sexual abuse. The papules coalesce into atrophic plaques. Topical steroids, oestrogen and laser therapy have been used. The condition commonly improves at puberty.

Lipodystrophy

This is the disappearance of adipose tissue. Partial lipodystrophy is of unknown cause. It usually begins in the first decade with loss of subcutaneous fat from the upper half of the body. Renal disease, abnormal glucose and lipid metabolism are sometimes associated. Some children have decreased levels of C3, a component of complement, which makes them prone to bacterial infections.

Generalized lipodystrophy, also known as Seip–Lawrence syndrome, is an autosomal recessive disorder. Total loss of body fat is associated with abnormal skin pigmentation; there is a freckled appearance of the axillae known as acanthosis nigricans. The condition is associated with hypothalamic abnormalities and similar metabolic abnormalities to those found in partial lipodystrophy. There is no specific treatment.

Mastocytosis

In this condition there is infiltration of skin and sometimes deeper tissues with mastocytes. The cause is unknown. The skin lesions are pigmented macules and papules with bullae. Release of histamine from the mastocytes may be caused by physical means (rubbing of the skin, heat or cold) or certain drugs. The symptoms of wheezing, diarrhoea, headache and flushing are produced.

The symptoms are controlled with H_1 and sometimes H_2 blockers. The problem tends to resolve spontaneously.

Pyogenic granuloma (Fig. 9.11)

Localized areas of granulation tissue occur in the skin. These require chemical or electrical cautery.

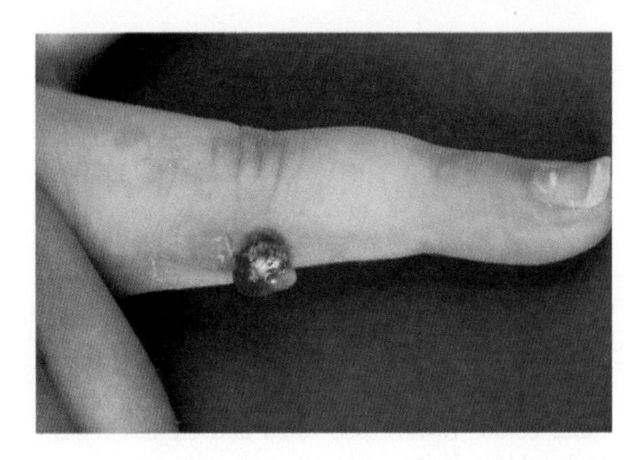

Fig 9.11
Pyogenic granuloma.

10 Endocrinology and growth disorders

Growth under the age of 1 year is largely determined by nutritional factors. Increasingly thyroid hormone and growth hormone determine growth rate after infancy. The pubertal growth spurt is determined by androgenic or oestrogenic hormones.

Some endocrine disorders (such as congenital adrenal hyperplasia) are rare and others (such as diabetes mellitus) are more common but they have potentially life-threatening complications and important long-term implications.

Adrenal disorders

Congenital adrenal hyperplasia (adrenogenital syndrome)

Clinical features
Important to think of congenital adrenal hyperplasia in a neonate who becomes shocked.

Prognosis
Over- and undertreatment both lead to short stature, due to excess exogenous or endogenous steroids.

This is a rare (1/10 000) congential dysfunction of the adrenal gland due to five inborn errors of steroid biosynthesis (Table 10.1). Deficiency of cortisol production stimulates ACTH production which in turn stimulates the adrenal to overproduce whichever steroid hormones the adrenal gland can synthesize. These are recessive disorders; the genes are on chromosome 6.

Table 10.1
Steroid biosynthetic enzymes which may be defective in congenital adrenal hyperplasia

Enzyme defect	Habitus	Salt loss	Salt retention
21-Hydroxylase	Virilized	+/−	−
11β-Hydroxylase	Virilized	−	+
3β-Hydroxysteroid dehydrogenase	Virilized (mild)	+	−
17α-Hydroxylase	Feminized	−	+
P_{450}SCC	Feminized	+	−

21-Hydroxylase deficiency accounts for 95% of occurrences of this disorder. A quarter of affected children are virilized; the remainder also lose salt. Males are described as 'infant Hercules' with enlargement of the penis, pubic hair, deep voice, acne and well developed muscles developing after 6 months. Early growth is rapid but adult height is reduced due to premature fusion of the epiphyses. Females show pseudohermaphroditism, with clitoral enlargement and labial fusion. Salt loss, due to defective mineralocorticoid production, causes hyponatraemia, hyperkalaemia, failure to thrive, vomiting and dehydration with eventual collapse and death without treatment.

The 11β-hydroxylase and 17α-hydroxylase deficiencies cause excess production of 11-deoxycorticosterone, which leads to salt retention, hypokalaemia and hypertension rather than salt loss. Urinary 17-ketosteroids are elevated in congenital adrenal hyperplasia. The levels are suppressed by hydrocortisone, unless the adrenal hyperfunction is due to a tumour.

Treatment consists of inhibiting excess adrenal steroid production with hydrocortisone and 9α-fluorocortisol if salt loss is present. The treatment is monitored by measuring growth progress and hormonal concentrations.

Phaeochromocytoma

This is a very rare tumour of chromaffin cells, which arises from the adrenal medulla or sympathetic ganglia. An autosomal dominant trait may be involved, and it is commoner in families with neurofibromatosis.

Secretion of adrenaline and noradrenaline (catecholamines) by this tumour produces hypertension, headache, sweating and vomiting. The diagnosis is made by demonstrating an elevated concentration of catecholamines in the urine, and the tumour is located by means of a CAT scan. It is removed under alpha- and beta-adrenergic blockade. Transient hypotension may occur postoperatively.

Pituitary disorders

Diabetes insipidus (see also septo-optic dysplasia)

> Nomenclature
> Diabetes means 'flowing through'; insipidus refers to the diluted urine.
>
> Diagnosis
> Needs to be differentiated from the much commoner psychogenic polydipsia.

Antidiuretic hormone (ADH) is produced in the posterior pituitary gland which may be damaged by tumours or their surgical removal, or by head injury. Damage to the posterior pituitary gland results in transient diabetes insipidus. An autoimmune form can occur, analogous to the islet cell destruction seen in diabetes mellitus. The diagnosis is suggested by a urine osmolality of 50–200 mOsm/kg which may rise to 300 during water deprivation. Water deprivation is potentially hazardous because of the obligatory water loss. In psychogenic polydipsia, urine osmolality becomes greater than plasma osmolality during water deprivation. Low plasma concentrations of ADH are confirmatory. This is treated with desmopressin, an analogue of ADH, by nasal spray or more recently tablets.

Nephrogenic diabetes insipidus

This is caused by a congenital inability of distal kidney tubule tissue to reabsorb urine formed in the proximal tubules, despite the presence of pituitary antidiuretic hormone (i.e. insensitivity to ADH). It is a rare cause of failure to thrive in infancy. Physical growth and mental development may be delayed. The diagnosis is often not made until it is noted that the infant is passing excessive quantities of urine. The condition is X-linked.

Surprisingly, diuretic drugs such as hydrochlorothiazide can help the kidney defect. Other drugs including indomethacin are sometimes useful. Supplementary potassium is often needed. It is vital that the child always has plenty of fluid available to drink and that intake is never restricted.

Pancreatic disorders

Diabetes mellitus: insulin-dependent (IDDM or type I diabetes)

> Nomenclature
> Mellitus or 'sweet with honey' refers to the sugar content of the urine.
>
> Prognosis
> The vascular, renal and ocular complications are usually delayed until adult life and are also delayed by good control.

INTRODUCTION

Virtually all children with diabetes are insulin-dependent (juvenile type).

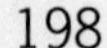

AETIOLOGY AND PATHOGENESIS

Insulin-dependent diabetes is thought to result from autoimmune-mediated damage to beta cells of the pancreatic islets. At presentation most diabetic children have antibodies including islet cell antibodies (ICA) and the recently recognized GAD and IA-2 antibodies. Pancreatic islets are infiltrated with T lymphocytes and islet cell-specific T cells may be present in the circulation. The antibodies may be detected in first-degree relatives; if they are strongly seropositive (occurring in approximately 3%), up to 85% might develop diabetes within 10 years. Genetic factors are present including the strong association of DR3 and DR4 HLA (tissue) types. An identical twin sibling has a 30–40% risk of developing diabetes. The remaining risk is believed to be 'environmental'. Non-twin siblings have a 7% risk. If one parent has IDDM, the risk to a child is 2%.

INCIDENCE

Approximately 1/13 000–25 000 children in the UK, according to region. The incidence is rising, for reasons unknown.

CLINICAL PRESENTATION

Occasionally diabetes presents in the neonate with profound ketoacidosis and fluid loss. Extremely small doses of insulin are needed. The disorder is nearly always transitory, presumably associated with some unidentified substance that has crossed the placenta. These children are the only group whose diabetes spontaneously remits. Otherwise the typical presentation of diabetes mellitus in a child is a history of thirst, excessive urination (often with a return of bedwetting), tachypnoea (Kussmaul breathing), tiredness and weight loss. The history is usually no more than 3 weeks at most. Delayed diagnosis leads to vomiting, abdominal pain, dehydration, ketoacidosis, drowsiness and coma. Diabetic ketoacidosis (DKA) has a 10% mortality. The sweet smell of ketotic breath is an important sign.

DIAGNOSIS

Fever suggests intercurrent infection. Abdominal tenderness may mimic surgical emergency. Common differential or mistaken diagnoses include enuresis, urinary tract infection, tonsillitis, pneumonia, asthma and gastroenteritis. Urine should be tested for glucose in all children with thirst or urinary symptoms. The oral glucose tolerance test is not used in childhood IDDM; the diagnostic test is an urgent random blood glucose (>11 mmol/L). Referral that day to the local diabetes unit is indicated. There must not be any delay. Children can become seriously ill overnight with untreated diabetes.

Transient hyperglycaemia occurs in acute illness (gastroenteritis, severe burns) or during treatment with steroids.

MANAGEMENT

Most children are not severely ill. Management is aimed at stabilizing control and starting an education programme at home if possible. Hospital admission is required in the case of diabetic ketoacidosis, dehydration or unavailability of a paediatric home care team. The management of diabetic ketoacidosis is summarized in Emergency box 10.1.

Insulin (see Information box 10.1) is given subcutaneously, or intravenously if parenteral fluids are required. Return to subcutaneous insulin when ketonuria clears. Many paediatricians prefer pre-mixed insulin for maintenance use (e.g. 30% soluble, 70% isophane), usually twice daily before breakfast and the evening meal. Optimal control may require a different ratio of insulins. Insulin requirement may fall shortly after diagnosis, due to partial recovery of insulin secretion. This period of easier diabetic control (the honeymoon period) may last a few weeks or up to a year, but is usually a few months, before pancreatic

Emergency Box 10.1

Diabetic ketoacidosis

- Intravenous normal saline and potassium
- Bicarbonate not routinely given
  - Increases risk of hypokalaemia
  - Acidosis corrects with adequate fluid and insulin replacement
- Intravenous insulin
- Watch out for
  - Hypoglycaemia
  - Hypokalaemia
  - Cerebral oedema, if present treat with mannitol and consult with neurosurgeons

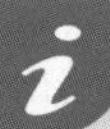

Information Box 10.1

Insulin treatment

- Synthetic human insulin is preferred. Beef and pork insulins are now seldom used because of possible development of antibodies.
- Soluble (unmodified) insulin acts within 30 minutes with peak effect at 1–4 hours, and duration of action 6–8 hours.
- Only soluble insulin should be given intravenously.
- Isophane is a modified insulin, with delayed absorption, acting after 1–2 hours, peak effect after 4–12 hours and duration of action 14–24 hours.

insulin reserve is further lost. Insulin dose increases with body size (0.7–1.0 IU/kg/day), and by an extra factor of 1.5–2-fold during puberty.

Diet

This is designed to provide normal nutritional requirements while regulating the pattern of carbohydrate intake during each day. Carbohydrate is spread across three main meals, with snacks between meals and before bed. Refined sugars are avoided where possible, with carbohydrate taken mainly in complex forms (starch, etc.) requiring digestion before absorption. This reduces the risks of hypo- and hyperglycaemia. Sweets are reserved for top-ups in relation to exercise, during illness or as an occasional treat (best at the end of a meal).

Education

Childhood diabetes requires initial parental responsibility and supervision with evolving patient understanding and responsibility. Age, growth, adolescence and family dynamics are changing factors and psychological and social worker support may be required. Parents must initially learn 'survival skills': how to draw up and inject insulin, test blood glucose and urine ketones, cope with hypoglycaemia, and organize diet. Education thereafter is a continual process, designed to shift responsibility to the child in keeping with age-related expectations.

Home blood glucose monitoring was introduced in the early 1980s and largely replaced urine glucose testing as a more precise means of assessing control. Patients are encouraged to do tests 1–4 times a day (before or after meals and when opportunities arise). Occasional bedtime tests are needed, and if glucose is below about 7 mmol/L an extra carbohydrate snack should be given.

Adjusting insulin dosage

A favoured approach is to assess insulin on 3–5-day blood glucose patterns. Adjustments are intended to prevent recurring abnormal (high or low) glucose levels (aim for 4–10 mmol/L). Virus infections may occur fairly frequently and these perturb the blood sugar levels (up with stress, down with anorexia). Children who exercise a lot may achieve better control than those who do little. Exercise increases insulin sensitivity and glucose demand. This may cause early or delayed (e.g. nocturnal) hypoglycaemia. If marked exercise is anticipated, extra carbohydrate can be taken beforehand, or the insulin dose reduced.

Hypoglycaemia ('hypos')

These episodes usually occur after vigorous exercise, when part or all of a meal is missed, when excess insulin has been given, or (in the older child) with alcohol. There is much variation in recognition and tolerance of hypoglycaemia. Factors include the rate of fall in blood glucose and the patient's habitual blood glucose level. Hypoglycaemia may cause sweating, pallor, shaking, irritability, crying, confusion, irrational behaviour, bad temper, headaches, abdominal pain and weakness, seizures or paralysis, before unconsciousness depending on the severity.

Mild to moderate hypoglycaemia can be treated with rapidly absorbed refined carbohydrate orally; this is inappropriate if a child is uncooperative or cannot swallow safely. Children are encouraged always to have a supply of glucose tablets, sweets or biscuits to hand (or in teacher's desk). Unconsciousness, seizures, or impaired airway protection require urgent treatment with glucagon (subcutaneously, intramuscularly or as hypostop gel) which can be given by relatives or friends with little training, whereas administration of intravenous dextrose requires a doctor. After glucagon injection (which stimulates hepatic glycogenolysis), the child should top up with oral carbohydrate on regaining consciousness.

Nocturnal hypoglycaemic episodes do not always waken the patient and may pass unnoticed, so parents should occasionally check their child's blood glucose at 2–3 a.m.

Intercurrent illness

Viral infections are frequent in childhood. The stress will usually increase insulin requirement. Sometimes there will be anorexia or nausea, reduced food intake and increased risk of hypoglycaemia. Systemic disturbance, especially vomiting, may be associated with hyperglycaemia and ketosis which could progress rapidly to ketoacidosis. With anorexia a small reduction in insulin dose may be needed to avoid hypoglycaemia, and glucose drinks should be encouraged. Blood glucose should be checked 3–4-hourly, and urine tested for ketones if glucose levels are greater than 5 mmol/L. A rising glucose level is treated by supplementary doses of soluble insulin. Medical attention should be sought, as the underlying cause of illness may need treatment. Repeated vomiting should be managed in hospital.

Long-term management

Glycosylated haemoglobin (HbA_1C) is a measure of glycaemic control over the previous 2–3 months. It is the best parameter to use in assessing long-term control. High HbA_1C levels are associated with increased risk of diabetes complications. In a large multicentre trial in North America (the DCCT) it was concluded recently that levels below 8% (normal range up to 6.5% approximately) were associated with slower progression of complications in adolescents and young adults. Patients are asked to aim for results below 8%, but no 'safe' level above normal is known. Levels persistently above 10% cause concern. Children should be managed by a specialist paediatric diabetes unit, with paediatrician, dietician, diabetes nurse specialist and access to adult diabetes care facilities. Reviews are generally at least 3-monthly (to adjust treatment according to HbA_1C). Families are encouraged to join the British Diabetic Association for support and education. Diabetes holiday camps may prove invaluable. Financial support is available as the Disability Living Allowance. A MedicAlert (or similar) bracelet is an advisable investment. Family planning advice, medical requirements for a driving licence, further education after school and transition to care by the adult diabetes team are important issues.

The needs of children with diabetes vary with development. Diabetes in infancy is rare but often difficult to manage because of the child's inability to communicate and inconsistent dietary intake. The major aim is to avoid hypoglycaemia and damage to the developing infant brain. Diabetes is often unstable in preschool children because of unpredictable physical activity and inability to keep to a planned regimen of meals and injections. School may offer a settled routine and acceptance of discipline with improved control. Adolescence may be a time of particular difficulty. Diabetes care may become the most neglected part of life just when insulin requirements are highest. Some require frequent hospitalization for acute care. Most recurrent admissions have an emotional, rather than physical, basis. Complex family and emotional issues need the involvement of a psychiatrist or psychologist experienced with diabetic children. Omission of insulin to cause ketoacidosis, or taking extra doses to cause hypoglycaemia are often practised as manipulative behaviour, particularly by girls, and should be viewed as cries for help.

Complications of diabetes

Growth failure and pubertal delay are uncommon, but may occur with poor diabetic control and there should be routine monitoring to detect these. Diabetes complications do occur in childhood; severe problems are rare. Early background retinopathy (up to 25%) is the commonest complication by the teenage years, compared with early nephropathy in about only 1–2%. Annual screening for complications is being widely introduced for children with diabetes of 5–10 years' duration and for adolescents.

Hyperinsulinaemia

> Clinical approach
> The maintenance of normoglycaemia in these children presents a formidable problem.

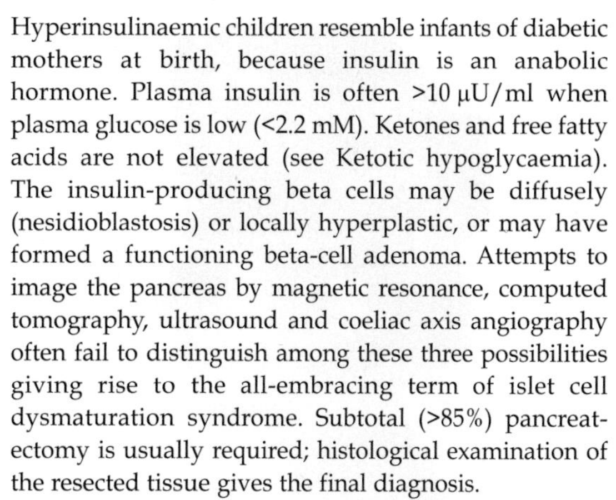

Hyperinsulinaemic children resemble infants of diabetic mothers at birth, because insulin is an anabolic hormone. Plasma insulin is often >10 μU/ml when plasma glucose is low (<2.2 mM). Ketones and free fatty acids are not elevated (see Ketotic hypoglycaemia). The insulin-producing beta cells may be diffusely (nesidioblastosis) or locally hyperplastic, or may have formed a functioning beta-cell adenoma. Attempts to image the pancreas by magnetic resonance, computed tomography, ultrasound and coeliac axis angiography often fail to distinguish among these three possibilities giving rise to the all-embracing term of islet cell dysmaturation syndrome. Subtotal (>85%) pancreatectomy is usually required; histological examination of the resected tissue gives the final diagnosis.

Blood glucose may be maintained preoperatively with the help of steroids, diazoxide and somatostatin; the latter, amongst many paracrine inhibitory actions, inhibits beta-cell activity. Leucine-sensitive hypoglycaemia is probably a variant of hyperinsulinaemia in which one of the triggers for insulin release is leucine, and hence dietary protein.

Other causes of hypoglycaemia

Ketotic hypoglycaemia

This is the commonest cause of hypoglycaemia in childhood. Fasting for >18 hours results in hypoglycaemia, ketonaemia and ketonuria, and insulin secretion is appropriately suppressed (<10 μU/ml). These features can occur in normal children after a fast of 36 hours.

A variety of metabolic defects may be involved, including protein catabolism, and amino acid metabolism (especially alanine, an important source of glucose during fasting).

The condition tends to remit at the end of the first decade.

Thyroid disorders

Goitre

> Nomenclature
> From the Latin *guttur*, meaning throat (Fig. 10.1).
>
> Epidemiology
> The most important worldwide cause of goitre is iodine deficiency which also causes developmental delay.

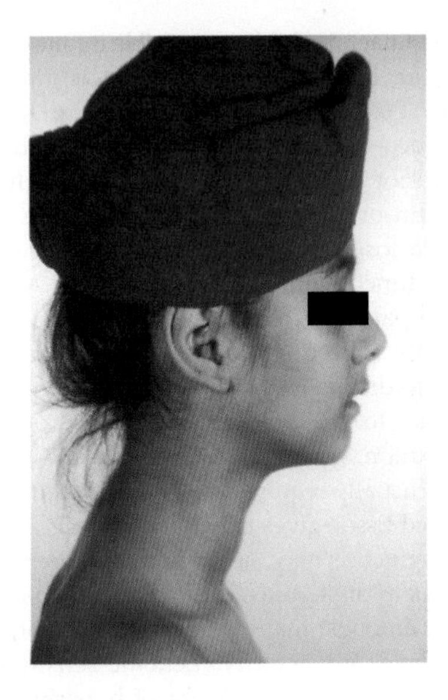

Fig 10.1
Goitre in thyrotoxicosis.

The causes of goitre in children are shown in Information box 10.2. Extreme degrees of congenital goitre may require partial thyroidectomy to relieve respiratory obstruction. Infants with congenital goitre and elevated TSH should receive thyroxine to enhance regression of the goitre and improve psychomotor development until thyroid hormone production improves. Infants with autosomal recessive inherited enzyme defects in thyroxine synthesis also require thyroxine. Iodine deficiency causes goitre in neonates, in adolescence and during pregnancy and lactation. If it is severe, brain damage and growth failure will result. Administration of injections of iodinated poppy seed oil to women is one way to prevent this problem during pregnancy. Large doses of iodine inhibit thyroxine synthesis in children with thyroid disorders.

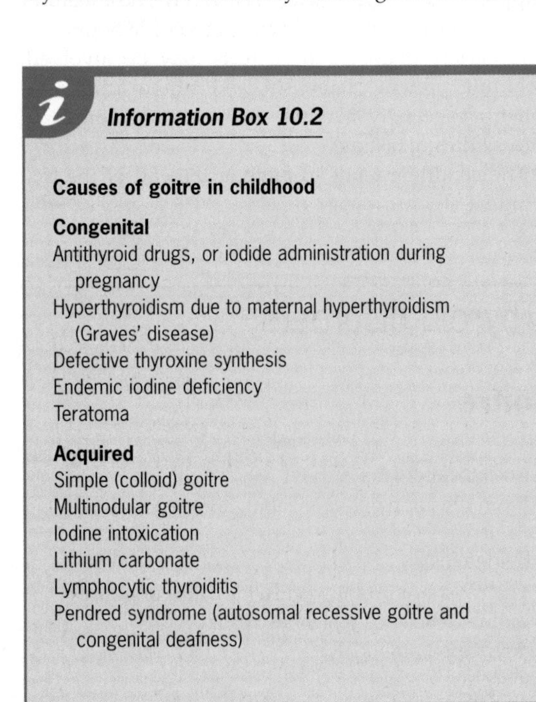

Information Box 10.2

Causes of goitre in childhood

Congenital
Antithyroid drugs, or iodide administration during pregnancy
Hyperthyroidism due to maternal hyperthyroidism (Graves' disease)
Defective thyroxine synthesis
Endemic iodine deficiency
Teratoma

Acquired
Simple (colloid) goitre
Multinodular goitre
Iodine intoxication
Lithium carbonate
Lymphocytic thyroiditis
Pendred syndrome (autosomal recessive goitre and congenital deafness)

Hypothyroidism

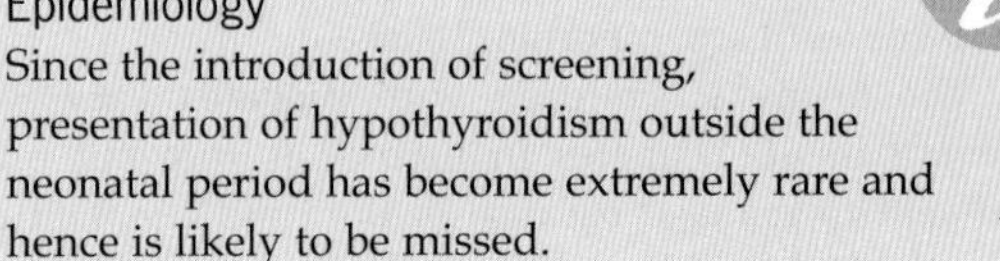

Epidemiology
Since the introduction of screening, presentation of hypothyroidism outside the neonatal period has become extremely rare and hence is likely to be missed.

Congenital hypothyroidism occurs in about 1 in 3500 infants; effective national screening programmes are in place. This means that to encounter the clinical appearance of congenital hypothyroidism (Information box 10.3; Fig. 10.2) is now virtually a thing of the past. An awareness of the condition is still important as laboratory errors can occur. Most affected infants have absence (aplasia) of the thyroid gland, or ectopic rudimentary thyroid tissue for instance at the base of the tongue (lingual thyroid). The condition is usually sporadic. Screening at birth is necessary because most infants are asymptomatic on account of the

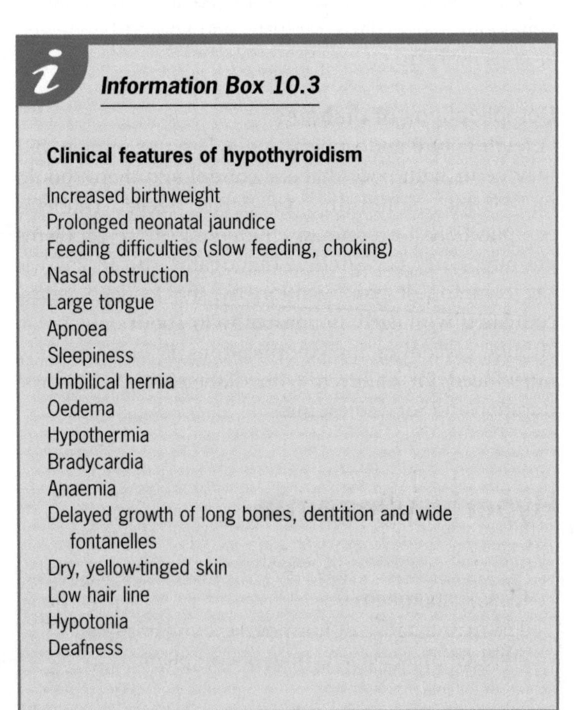

Information Box 10.3

Clinical features of hypothyroidism
Increased birthweight
Prolonged neonatal jaundice
Feeding difficulties (slow feeding, choking)
Nasal obstruction
Large tongue
Apnoea
Sleepiness
Umbilical hernia
Oedema
Hypothermia
Bradycardia
Anaemia
Delayed growth of long bones, dentition and wide fontanelles
Dry, yellow-tinged skin
Low hair line
Hypotonia
Deafness

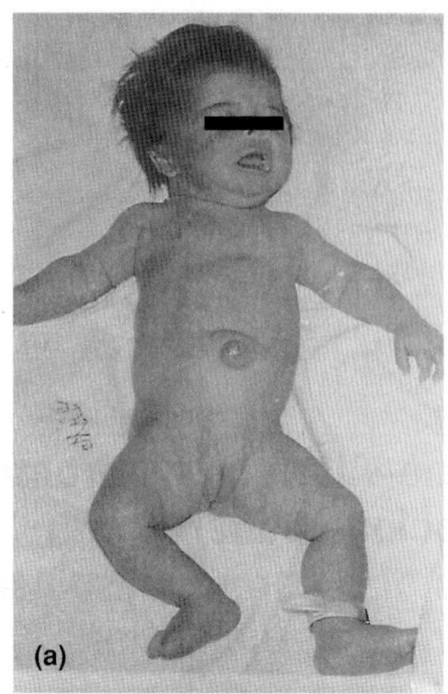

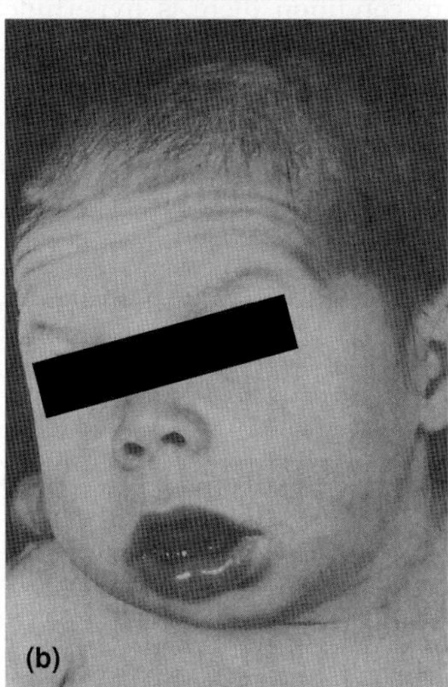

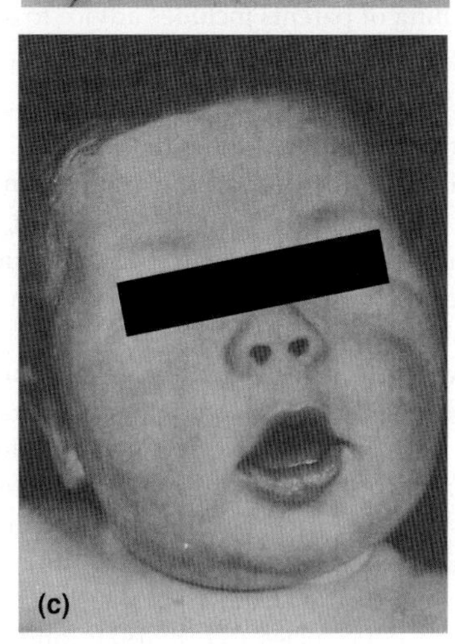

Fig 10.2
(a) Infant with hypothyroidism. Note the large tongue, umbilical hernia and hypotonic posture. (b) Hypothyroid child before treatment. (c) Same child after treatment.

transplacental passage of thyroxine (T_4). TSH is measured on the Guthrie card, an elevated concentration indicating hypothyroidism. Thyroxine must also be measured to diagnose hypothyroidism of hypothalamic origin which will be missed by the screening programme. Ectopic thyroid tissue may sustain normal development until later in childhood. Autosomal recessive disorders of thyroxine or thyroglobulin (thyroxine storage protein) production are rare, and cause a goitre due to stimulation of the thyroid by TSH.

The prognosis for affected infants has improved since the introduction of screening. Treatment with sodium-L-thyroxine is lifelong.

Hypothalamic and pituitary disorders

Growth hormone insufficiency

Causes

Congenital (e.g. aplasia, septo-optic dysplasia) and destructive (neoplastic, infection, trauma, radiation) lesions of the hypothalamus and pituitary may result in growth hormone deficiency.

Of interest are those in whom no structural lesion exists in whom there may be a deletion of the growth hormone, or growth hormone-releasing hormone gene or growth hormone receptor genes (Laron syndrome; growth hormone resistance). Secretion of an abnormal, biologically inactive growth hormone has also been described.

Children with lesions of the pituitary gland show features of other endocrine dysfunctions in addition to growth failure, including weight loss, cold sensitivity, impaired intellect, hypoglycaemia, and diabetes insipidus. Symptoms of raised intracranial pressure and visual field defects accompany expanding lesions. If the pituitary is normal, signs of growth failure occur during the second year of life. Growth hormone deficiency should be considered in any child who is failing to grow at the expected velocity. Those whose height is below the 3rd centile should be remeasured at least 6-monthly so that their growth velocity (cm/year) can be determined. Failure of growth hormone to increase above 7 ng/ml (15-20 iu) following 20 minutes of hard exercise or insulin-induced hypoglycaemia is strongly suggestive of growth hormone deficiency. Children with biologically inactive growth hormone may be missed if the hormone is measured by immunoassay but not by radioreceptor assay. Some normal short children growing at rates of less than 6 cm/year will grow faster with growth hormone although the effect on final height is not known. Subcutaneous injections of recombinant growth hormone are required.

Hypopituitarism (see also Growth hormone insufficiency)

Epidemiology
Rare and complex disorder.

Congenital defects resulting in hypopituitarism are rare and usually associated with other CNS defects such as anencephaly (see p. 309), optic nerve hypoplasia, or septo-optic dysplasia (see p. 326) when the septum pellucidum is also absent. A further example is the Hall–Pallister syndrome. Other midline defects such as cleft lip and palate or presence of a single midline tooth are intriguingly associated. The endocrine defect usually resides in the hypothalamus, with defective pituitary function being caused by lack of hypothalamic-releasing hormones. Any lesion such as craniopharyngioma which damages the pituitary or hypothalamus, will also be responsible. No anatomic lesion is demonstrable in most children with hypopituitarism, although traumatic birth has been cited as a factor. The condition is inherited in up to 10% of affected children and dominant, recessive and X-linked patterns of inheritance have been described.

Growth failure in the second year of life, as demonstrated by careful serial measurement, is the most striking clinical finding. Subsequent sexual and skeletal maturation are delayed. The latter is assessed by determining the state of maturation of epiphyses by X-ray of the hands. Hypoglycaemia (see p. 201) occurs readily during fasting. Destructive lesions of the pituitary cause secondary hypoadrenalism, hypogonadism (see p. 205), hypothyroidism (see p. 202) and diabetes insipidus (see p. 198) as well as symptoms of raised intracranial pressure (headache, vomiting, visual disturbance and drowsiness).

Replacement therapy includes growth hormone, thyroxine, hydrocortisone, sex hormones at puberty or vasopressin, according to which hormonal deficiencies are demonstrated by endocrinological investigation.

Kallmann syndrome

This is a luteinizing hormone-releasing hormone (LHRH) deficiency which causes hypogonadism. It is associated with agenesis of the olfactory lobes and hence the ability to smell. The inheritance pattern is variable. The X-linked variety may be associated with a number of X-linked conditions whose genes are adjacent on the X chromosome, including:

- Steroid sulphatase deficiency (X-linked ichthyosis, see p. 191)
- Chondrodysplasia punctata (Conradi syndrome, see p. 294)
- Others.

McCune–Albright syndrome (precocious puberty with polyostotic fibrous dysplasia and abnormal pigmentation)

In this rare condition there is hyperfunction of the endocrine glands. Precocious puberty occurs, mainly in girls. Hyperthyroidism, Cushing syndrome, café-au-lait spots, acromegaly and pathological fractures, due to fibrous lesions in the skeletal system, are all associated with this syndrome.

Gonadal disorders

Hermaphroditism (intersex)

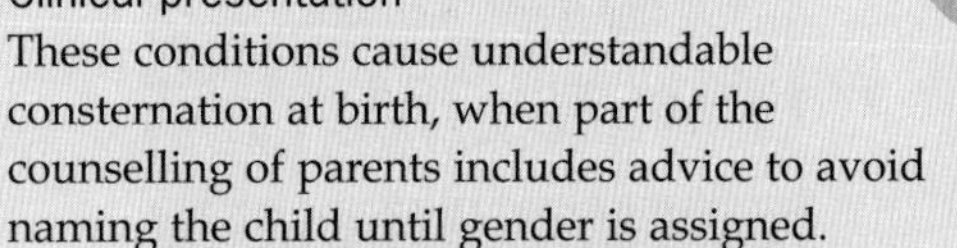

Clinical presentation
These conditions cause understandable consternation at birth, when part of the counselling of parents includes advice to avoid naming the child until gender is assigned.

True hermaphroditism can be caused when an individual has some cells with a female genotype (46, XX) and others with a male genotype (46, XY). The gonads contain ovarian and testicular tissue and the external genitalia are intermediate between male and female (ambiguous genitalia; Fig. 10.3). In others, all cells have the 46, XX genotype; the underlying mechanisms in this group are poorly understood. The testicular tissue is removed and the individual is raised as female; successful pregnancies have resulted. Female (46, XX) fetuses which become virilized are said to have female pseudohermaphroditism. Possible causes include congenital adrenal hyperplasia (21- and 11-hydroxylase deficiencies (see p. 197)), and androgen-producing adrenal or ovarian tumours in the mother. Male (46, XY) fetuses that are feminized may have XY gonadal agenesis syndrome (see below) or defects in testosterone synthesis by the testis which allow

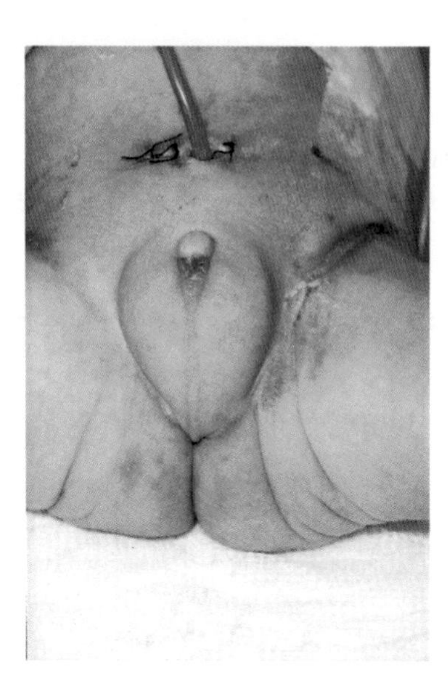

Fig 10.3
Ambiguous genitalia.

unopposed effects of maternal hormones on gonadal development during pregnancy.

Essential investigations include chromosome analysis and pelvic ultrasound to establish whether or not a uterus is present. Those with 5α-reductase deficiency are raised as males because virilization occurs at puberty. Otherwise infants with intersex are best reared as females because attempts at reconstructive surgery are likely to be more successful.

XY gonadal agenesis syndrome

When testicular degeneration occurs during the 8th to 12th week of gestation, the resulting male baby resembles a female. The absence of ovaries means that no secondary sexual characteristics develop at puberty. Degeneration after the 20th week of gestation produces a phenotypic male with no testes (anorchia). These conditions are familial.

Testicular feminization syndrome

This is an X-linked recessively inherited insensitivity to androgens. Affected males are indistinguishable from females, apart from a blind-ending vagina with absent uterus and the presence of intraabdominal testes. The boys should be reared as females. The testes should be removed because of the high risk of malignant change.

Hypogonadism

This damage to the testes can be caused by chemotherapy, radiotherapy, surgery, mumps, orchitis (which should be eradicated by MMR immunization), or Del Castillo syndrome, where the seminiferous tubules fail to develop, resulting in infertility.

Parathyroid disorders

Hypoparathyroidism (pseudohypoparathyroidism, pseudopseudohypoparathyroidism)

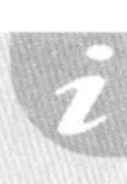

Epidemiology
Rare.

The various types of hypoparathyroidism are detailed in Table 10.2.

Coexistent hypomagnesaemia should be checked for and corrected if necessary. Excess intake of phosphate (e.g. from phosphate enemata) or release of phosphate from cell lysis (see Cancer, p. 333), also cause hypocalcaemia.

Hyperparathyoidism

This may be primary, associated with hyperplasia or functioning adenoma of the parathyroid glands. Secondary hyperparathyroidism may be linked to hypocalcaemia due to vitamin D-resistant rickets or malabsorption of calcium.

Growth disorders

Cerebral gigantism (Sotos overgrowth syndrome)

In this condition accelerated growth begins antenatally and continues until 5 years old. Clumsiness and low developmental quotients are associated. The aetiology is unknown; most cases are sporadic. Autosomal dominant and recessive forms occur.

Russell–Silver syndrome

This is named after the two doctors who described the same problem independently in the 1950s.

Table 10.2
Hypoparathyroidsim

Type	Causes	Symptoms	Treatment
Neonatal	Functional immaturity or hypoplasia of parathyroid glands, maternal hyperparathyroidsim or ^{131}I therapy	Hypocalcaemic convulsions	Calcium supplements. Breast milk is protective because of low phosphate concentration
Familial	X-linked recessive	Hypocalcaemic convulsions	Calcium and vitamin D supplements to maintain serum calcium
Traumatic	Surgery	Hypocalcaemic convulsions, cataracts	As above
Storage disorders	Iron (thalassaemia), or copper (Wilson disease)		Prevention by chelation
Autoimmune	Antiparathyroid antibodies	Presence of other autoimmune disorders	Calcium and vitamin D
Idiopathic			As above
Pseudohypoparathyroidism	Parathyroid hormone receptor defect	Tetany, soft tissue calcification, short stature, developmental delay, abnormal 4th and 5th metacarpophalangeal joints	
Pseudopseudo-hypoparathyroidism	Receptor defect but normal serum calcium		

Affected infants are undersized for their length of gestation; they grow poorly in infancy, and tend to be less than 5 ft tall. The fontanelle closes late. One side of the body tends to be larger than the other (hemihypertrophy). The face appears triangular with a small down-pointing mouth, but the head size is usually normal. The fifth finger often curves inwards (camptodactyly). Affected infants can develop hypoglycaemia. Intelligence is usually normal. This syndrome may be inherited, but is usually a 'one-off' or sporadic condition, of unknown cause.

Referral to a special growth clinic is advisable.

11 Gastroenterology

Until recently, the most common cause of death in childhood on a worldwide basis was dehydration due to acute diarrhoea. As a result of improved treatment of dehydration, respiratory infections are now the most common cause of death in childhood. Also, with improvement in the management of acute diarrhoea, chronic diarrhoea is becoming more prominent as a cause of death by malnutrition.

In developed countries, death from diarrhoea is almost unknown. Coeliac disease is also becoming less common, at least in childhood. However acute abdominal pain remains a frequent cause for admission, although appendicitis is becoming less common. Poorly understood gastrointestinal conditions such as chronic abdominal pain continue to cause considerable morbidity and loss of time at school. Childhood chronic inflammatory bowel disease also appears to be increasing.

Acute abdominal pain

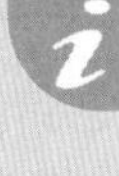

Epidemiology
Acute abdominal pain is a frequent cause of admission to hospital; 90% of children with acute abdominal pain do not require surgery.

INTRODUCTION

Assessment of abdominal pain is particularly difficult in young children. The history from the parents is often limited and physical signs may be minimal.

AETIOLOGY AND PATHOGENESIS

Common causes of the acute abdomen in adults (e.g. complications of peptic ulceration, biliary disease,

Information Box 11.1

Important causes of acute abdominal pain in childhood

Common causes
Mesenteric adenitis
Appendicitis
Trauma
Pyelonephritis
Henoch–Schönlein syndrome
Pneumonia
Acute intestinal obstruction (intussusception, incarcerated hernia, volvulus)
Gastroenteritis
Sickle cell crisis
Diabetic ketoacidosis
Renal colic

Less common causes
Peptic ulcer disease (NB: Meckel diverticulum)
Poison (lead, iron, corrosives)
Inflammatory bowel disease
Volvulus
Pancreatitis
Rheumatic fever
Torsion of ovarian cyst
Mittelschmerz
Porphyria
Neoplasia
Angioedema

gynaecological problems) rarely occur in children. Less common causes are included in Information box 11.1.

CLINICAL PRESENTATION

Infants with intra-abdominal emergencies are very difficult to assess because of the nonspecific presentation and limited history. The time of onset and severity of pain should be recorded. Associated symptoms such as site, radiation and character should be obtainable from older children. Enquiry should always be made about symptoms such as vomiting of gastric contents or bile-stained fluid, dysphagia, change in bowel habit, haematuria and dysuria.

DIAGNOSIS

Assessment should be unhurried and relaxed in a warm environment. Note should be taken of the general physical state, especially of the skin and respiratory tract. Because of the thin abdominal wall in infants, inspection may reveal local or generalized distension and peristalsis. General palpation is along the same principles as in adults, remembering to inspect the hernial orifices. Auscultation of the abdomen is rarely helpful (except in appendicitis, see below). A rectal examination, if warranted, is best performed once, and hence by a surgeon.

MANAGEMENT

A chest X-ray, erect and supine abdominal film, ultrasound, full blood count, urinalysis and culture, blood culture, urea and electrolytes should be requested. Nonsurgical, remedial causes (e.g. pneumonia, urinary tract infection, acute follicular tonsillitis) and real emergencies should be excluded by history and physical examination. A short period of observation (4–24 hours) before surgery is warranted.

Mesenteric adenitis

This common condition mimics acute appendicitis. It is rare in children under 3 years and in adults.

Symptoms and signs of viraemia are often associated. The child may complain of nausea, anorexia, vomiting, diarrhoea or sore throat. Pain is often intermittent and periumbilical or in the right iliac fossa. There is poorly localized tenderness and sometimes guarding.

If the child comes to surgery, the mesenteric nodes are found to be enlarged and fleshy.

Appendicitis

Epidemiology
Incidence is decreasing.
Remains the commonest abdominal emergency in childhood.

The diagnosis is easily missed at the extremes of life, hence the high mortality in these age groups. The classical features, of low grade fever, anorexia and/or vomiting, change in bowel habit (usually constipation), right iliac fossa and/or central abdominal pain, guarding and tenderness with rebound tenderness and rectal tenderness are often absent, especially in infants. An infected Meckel diverticulum (persistent vitello-intestinal duct present in 2% of the population) may mimic appendicitis. When peritonitis has occurred, the tenderness becomes generalized, bowel sounds are absent and the child is systemically unwell (unless receiving steroids or other immunosuppression).

Broad-spectrum antibiotics are required (including metronidazole for anaerobic cover) and surgery should follow correction of dehydration with intravenous fluids. If the signs of peritonitis are localized, and there is a mass palpable in the right iliac fossa, then an appendix abscess may have formed. If the history is over 48 hours and the child is not deteriorating, management can be conservative (as for generalized peritonitis) with 'interval' appendectomy after 2–3 months. If the history is less than 48 hours, immediate appendectomy is performed. Postoperative infections are common, even if the appendix was normal, in surgical wounds, in left and right iliac fossae, in the pelvis, or subdiaphragmatic. Drainage and antibiotics, which should include metronidazole, are required.

Intussusception

Epidemiology
Mainly seen from 3 months to 2 years (1–2/1000 live births).

The intussusception is due to invagination of one segment of bowel into another (Fig. 11.1). The commonest type is the invagination of terminal ileum into the caecum.

Infants present with distress, drawing up the legs; they are often initially thought to have colic, but the symptoms become increasingly intense. They may then subside inducing a false sense of security. There is abdominal distension on examination, with a sausage-shaped mass which is often curved and concave to the umbilicus. The swelling is painful and palpation may trigger colicky pain. Red-coloured, soft (redcurrant jelly) stool may be passed or seen on the glove on PR. Sometimes the head of the intussusceptum may be felt this way. Plain X-ray may show the obstruction as a radio-opaque mass with crescentic shadow, but it may be normal. Ultrasound may show a mass with characteristic echoes of multiple layers of intestine.

Early cases may be relieved by a diagnostic and therapeutic air enema under radiological control; if this does not bring immediate relief, operative reduction and possibly local resection is needed. The head of the intussusceptum can be examined for polyp, reduplication or presence of Meckel diverticulum which may have started the intussusception. Differential diagnosis includes dysentery, volvulus, appendicitis and Meckel diverticulitis.

Henoch–Schönlein syndrome

Definition
Acute inflammatory reaction of unknown cause occurring in small blood vessels.

Henoch–Schönlein purpura is due to bleeding from the damaged blood vessels and is most noticeable on the extensor surface of the limbs, particularly the lower limbs and buttocks (Fig. 11.2). Oedema is present in the face and extremities, and in the periarticular tissues of wrists, knees and ankles, where it may be painful.

Gut involvement produces abdominal pain, haematemesis and melaena. Haematoma of the gut wall can form the head of an intussusception. If abdominal pain is the first feature to appear then it may mimic an acute abdomen.

Renal involvement causes haematuria and

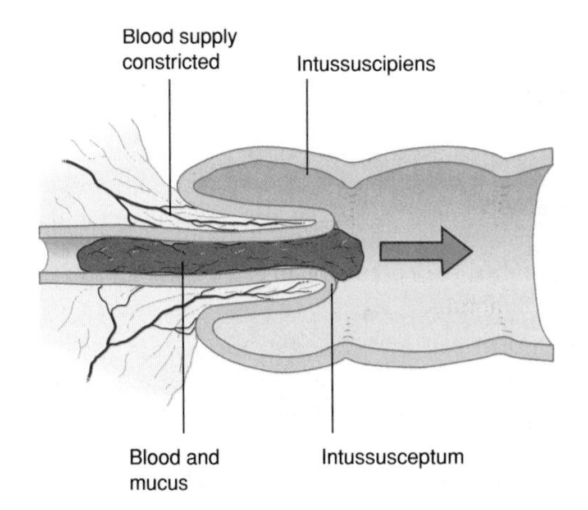

Fig 11.1
Pathology of intussusception.

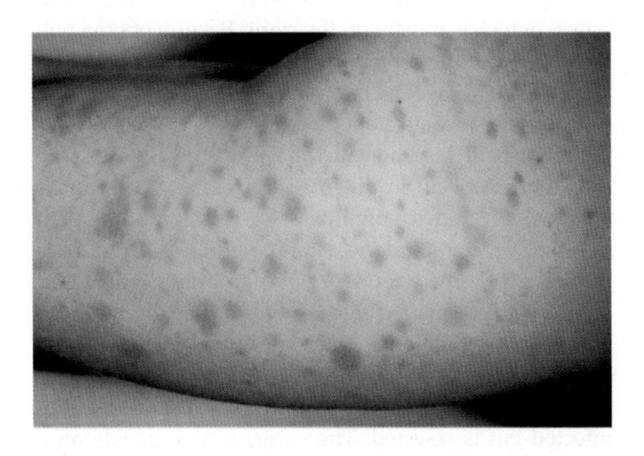

Fig 11.2
Skin rash in Henoch–Schönlein syndrome.

proteinuria. Occasionally renal failure may occur, with hypertensive encephalopathy, and progressing to chronic renal failure.

There is no specific therapy. High dose steroids, and transfusions for intestinal haemorrhage, may be given. The prognosis is usually excellent, although relapses can occur for up to 1 year.

Malrotation

> Clinical significance
> Essential to diagnose this before the occurrence of the life-threatening complication of volvulus.

Malrotation is a congenital malformation of the bowel occurring between the 6th and 16th weeks of gestation. There is failure of the caecum to rotate around the small intestine. The caecum remains mobile on account of the failure of the caecal mesentery to fuse with the parietal peritoneum. The blood supply to the caecum is conveyed in bands of Ladd, which sweep across the second part of the duodenum. The large bowel is on the left side of the abdomen and the small intestine on the right. The small intestine has a narrow pedicle and can rotate on this to produce a volvulus.

Malrotation can produce bile-stained vomiting from duodenal obstruction by Ladd bands. Volvulus produces partial, intermittent or complete duodenal or small intestinal obstruction with food refusal, bile-stained vomiting, abdominal distension, abdominal pain and passage of blood in the faeces. Complete duodenal obstruction produces a 'double bubble' on plain erect abdominal X-ray (Fig. 11.3) due to gaseous distension of the stomach and duodenum. Intermittent obstruction shows a characteristic S-shaped duodenum turning down or right at the third part to the small bowel, which is mostly on the right. Barium enema will show the caecum in the midline or left hypochondrium and the large bowel mostly on the left.

Volvulus is a surgical emergency because massive infarction and resection of the small intestine may be the result of delay in diagnosis or surgery. Surgery is always indicated if volvulus is suspected, although it may not need to be done as an emergency if there are no signs of obstruction or strangulation. The Ladd bands will be divided and attempts may be made to lengthen the small bowel mesentery and fixation of the bowel to the abdominal wall. Appendectomy may assist fixation. If strangulation is present, frankly infected gut is resected. The surgeon may decide on a 'second look' laparotomy after 24 hours, to check the viability of the gut.

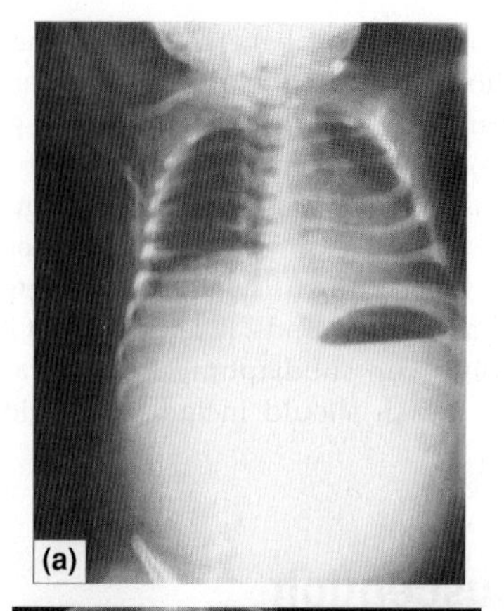

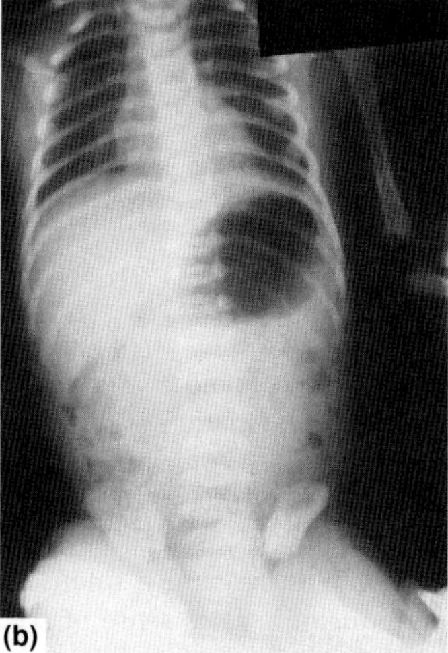

Fig 11.3
Erect X-rays of infant with duodenal obstruction due to malrotation. (a) Large gas bubble in stomach with no gas beyond. (b) Inflation of stomach with air produces gas in bowel, showing that the obstruction is incomplete.

Chronic recurrent abdominal pain

> Definition
> The occurrence of more than three attacks of abdominal pain occurring over a period greater than 3 months.

AETIOLOGY AND PATHOGENESIS

Important organic causes include recurrent subacute intestinal obstruction, e.g. intussusception, malrotation, and volvulus, urinary tract infection, pelviureteric obstruction, peptic ulcer, Crohn disease, tuberculosis and lead poisoning (Information box 11.2). It should be

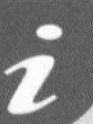

Information Box 11.2

Important organic causes of chronic recurrent abdominal pain

Recurrent, subacute intestinal obstruction
- Intussusception
- Malrotation
- Duplication
- Volvulus
- Internal herniae
- Stenosis

Aerophagy
Cholecystitis
Cholelithiasis
Urinary tract
- Infection
- Pelviureteric obstruction
- Stone

Splenic infarction
Ovarian tumours/cysts
Referred spinal pain
Tuberculosis
Crohn disease
Peptic ulcer
Pancreatitis
Lead poisoning
Porphyria

emphasized that in 95% of affected children, no cause is found.

Clinical features that may suggest the possibility of an organic and nonorganic diagnosis are shown in Information boxes 11.3 and 11.4.

DIAGNOSIS

At the initial consultation an organically orientated history is taken and a physical examination is performed. Minimum investigation should include urine microbiology, haemoglobin and ESR. Prominent organic symptoms e.g. vomiting, should be investigated appropriately (e.g. barium follow through). At this stage, the idea of a functional aetiology can be introduced. The offer to see the child during an attack will help to reassure the parents and child. During an acute attack, repeated physical examination, full blood count, urine culture and plain erect X-ray of abdomen should be performed. Stool microscopy and culture are also performed if the child has diarrhoea. The presence of nocturnal pain, vomiting and a family history of peptic ulceration suggest duodenal ulceration, which should be excluded radiologically or by endoscopy.

INCIDENCE

This affects 10% of children and as many as one in four 9-year-old girls. Episodes of 'abdominal pain' are an almost universal symptom.

MANAGEMENT

Management is directed towards excluding an organic cause and optimizing optimal therapy for a functional disorder. Because the main emphasis is rightly on a functional disorder, organic causes may be missed initially but will be diagnosed when 'functional' management fails or new features (e.g. weight loss) appear.

The aim of the initial consultation is to gain the confidence of parents and child, exclude obvious organic pathology and to sow the seeds of the idea of a possible functional cause. In addition to a full medical history, superficial exploration of likely causes of stress

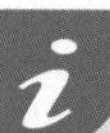

Information Box 11.3

Features associated with organic causes for abdominal pain

- Growth failure
  - Check longitudinal growth data
- Gross abdominal distension
  - May be due to air swallowing (aerophagy)
- Pain distant from umbilicus
- Occurrence in robust extrovert
- Failure to respond to simple tests and reassurance

Information Box 11.4

Features of inorganic abdominal pain

- Usually periumbilical
- Often severe
  - Transient
  - Rarely interferes with sleep, appetite or activities
- Prominent on schooldays and before bedtime
- Associated symptoms may reinforce concerns about organic disease
  - Nausea
  - Pallor
  - Lassitude
  - Low grade pyrexia
  - Abdominal distension
  - Headache
  - Limb pain
  - Constipation or diarrhoea

can begin. Potential areas might include family stress, change of house or school or death of close family friends, relatives or pets, and problems at school. Growth is assessed and a full physical examination is required to reassure both the doctor and the family. A successful consultation results in reassurance that a thorough examination has found nothing serious and provides hints that there may be a functional cause in many children with the problem.

When the child is seen again, growth velocity is measured, results of investigations reviewed with the family, and the opportunity is taken to enquire about the development of new symptoms and school attendance. The functional nature of the complaint is reinforced by comparisons with, for example, simple headache, for which a cause is rarely found. The likely functional aetiology is explored, perhaps separately at parental and child level. It is rarely profitable to attempt identification of the precipitating or maintenance factors responsible. Such identification is rarely accurate and is unnecessary for simple management. It may be helpful to point out the frequency of the symptom in normal children. Likewise it may be helpful to suggest that it occurs commonly in thoughtful, sensitive children. If precipitating factors can be identified then it may be possible to reduce them. Reassurance in itself may allow this. Indeed, the opportunity for the child to attend clinic for someone to take an interest in their problem, and to be reassured that they are not going to be rushed into hospital, or be subjected to distressing investigation, often improves the symptom. About 80% respond by disappearance or major reduction in symptoms. One way to increase the child's sense of security in the family is for one or other parent to give the child their undivided attention for a short period each day to do something of the child's choice.

At a further review, if there has been no improvement, the possible organic causes should be reviewed. If there are overt psychosocial problems, psychiatric referral should be suggested. Prolonged hospital follow up should be avoided, as this may reinforce the family's suspicions of an organic aetiology.

Onset of functional abdominal pain before 5 years old, positive family history of abdominal pain and a prolonged history are bad prognostic signs. About one-third resolve, one-third continue and one-third develop other psychosomatic symptoms such as headaches or limb pains. As adults, over 50% will develop some gastrointestinal symptom such as irritable bowel syndrome. Peptic ulceration is more common than in the general population, and their children are six times more likely to have recurrent abdominal pain compared with the rest of the population. Management of a specific cause of chronic abdominal pain, namely peptic ulceration, is described below.

Peptic ulceration

Epidemiology

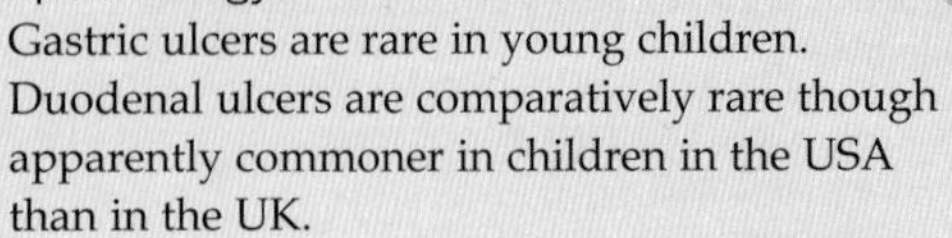

Gastric ulcers are rare in young children. Duodenal ulcers are comparatively rare though apparently commoner in children in the USA than in the UK.

Gastric ulcers occur in the neonatal period, in acute stress (e.g. caused by burns or raised intracranial pressure) and with salicylates and other drugs. Duodenal ulcers usually present with recurrent pain. Vomiting is a commoner presenting feature than in adults. The pain, which may be nocturnal, can be precisely located in the epigastrium. There may be a positive family history. When the diagnosis is made radiologically, it should be confirmed endoscopically. The child's *Helicobacter pylori* status should be ascertained. *H. pylori* infects the cells lining the gastric antrum, causing chronic gastritis. When duodenal enterocytes undergo metaplasia to gastric epithelium they are also susceptible to *H. pylori*-induced duodenitis. The infection is probably asymptomatic in childhood, but predisposes to duodenal ulceration and recurrence of ulceration after treatment. The organism can be demonstrated by histological examination of gastric biopsies, or on the basis of the organism's ability to produce urease, which converts urea into ammonia. Thus ammonia is released from infected gastric biopsies placed in culture medium containing urea. A breath test for detecting *H. pylori* is based on the release of ^{13}C from ingested ^{13}C-labelled urea into expired air. Antibody tests are also available but these do not necessarily detect current infection. Antibiotics such as amoxicillin and metronidazole and antibacterial agents such as bismuth are effective in eradicating the organism and should be included in the treatment of duodenal ulceration. Omeprazole or ranitidine are also given to assist ulcer healing. If frequent relapses occur, consideration is given to selective vagotomy and pyloroplasty. Peptic oesphagitis is relatively common in children, producing symptoms of regurgitation and/or dysphagia, especially in children with cerebral palsy.

Congenital disorders

Abetalipoproteinaemia

In this rare and recessively inherited disorder, absence of beta apoprotein results in failure of chylomicron formation and therefore in steatorrhoea and failure to thrive. Later, ataxia, neuropathy and pigmentary retinopathy develop, because of vitamin E deficiency. Acanthocytosis (irregular shaped erythrocytes, Fig. 11.4(a)), low plasma cholesterol and low or absent beta lipoprotein are present in the peripheral blood. Even after treatment vitamin E is undetectable, as it is transported in chylomicrons; vitamin E activity can be monitored with the erythrocyte peroxidase test. The mucosal cells of the jejunum are laden with fat (Fig. 11.4(b)).

Treatment is by low fat diet with vitamin E and essential fatty acid supplements. Growth is improved and neurological sequelae are prevented.

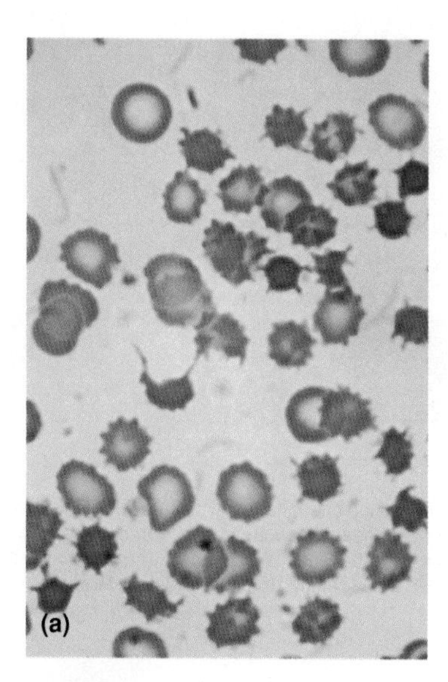

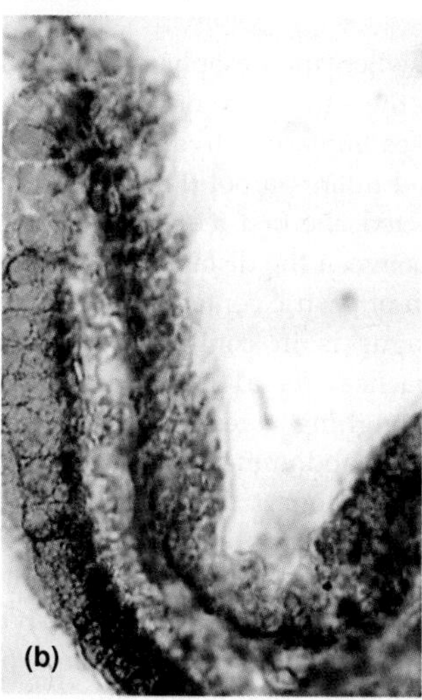

Fig 11.4
(a) Irregular erythrocytes from a child with abetalipoproteinaemia. The shape is due to an abnormal red cell membrane. (b) Frozen section of a jejunal biopsy from the same child with abetalipoproteinaemia. The fat in the enterocytes is stained orange. Virtually no fat is present in normal jejunal biopsies.

Cricopharyngeal incoordination

Babies who repeatedly choke and aspirate their feeds may show retention of contrast media in the pharynx on X-ray screening. The problem resolves spontaneously with age, and speech therapists can help with feeding difficulties.

Diaphragmatic hernia

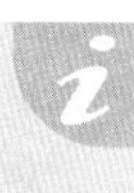

Treatment
Pioneering intrauterine surgery has been tried for this condition.

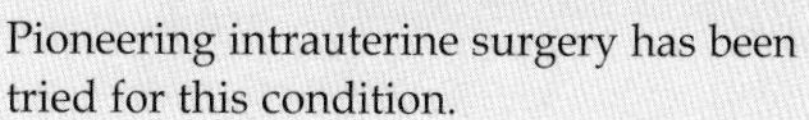

This is a rare (1 per 2000 births) but very important congenital defect due to failure of closure of the pleuroperitoneal canal. In fetal life there are connections between the abdominal and the thoracic cavities, called the foramen of Bockdalek, and the pericardial cavity called the foramen of Morgagni. When these fail to close, then herniation of abdominal viscera into the chest occurs. The lung on the affected side (most commonly the left) is compressed and hypoplastic (Fig. 11.5). As the gut fills with gas, severe, progressive respiratory distress occurs. Eventration of the diaphragm, due to weakness or absence of diaphragmatic muscle, produces an identical clinical picture. The earlier the presentation the more severe the lung hypoplasia and the worse the prognosis.

Presenting features include increasing respiratory distress, displacement of the heart (usually to the right), scaphoid (empty) abdomen and decreased air entry on the affected side. Alternative presentations include a subacute type, with vomiting, feeding difficulty and constipation, dyspnoea, or as a chance finding on chest X-ray ('cystic' appearance due to multiple loops of gas-filled bowel in the thorax).

The infant should be nursed in an erect posture, with a nasogastric tube to aspirate the stomach. If ventilatory support is required this may have to be given by a high frequency ventilator or heart–lung bypass (extra-corporeal membrane oxygenation) until surgical correction. The immediate prognosis depends on prompt diagnosis and management. The mortality rate is high for those infants who present in the first 3 days of life, but following successful corrective surgery the prognosis is good. The long-term prognosis is determined by the degree of lung hypoplasia.

Epigastric hernia

When the contents of a body cavity protrude through the wall of the cavity, this is described as a hernia. A

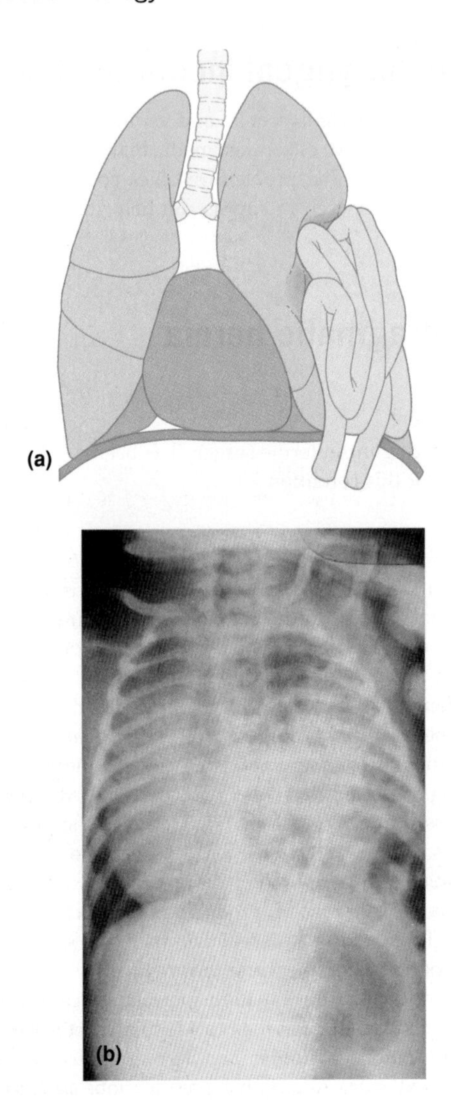

Fig 11.5
(a) Diaphragmatic hernia. (b) X-ray appearance. Courtesy of Milupa.

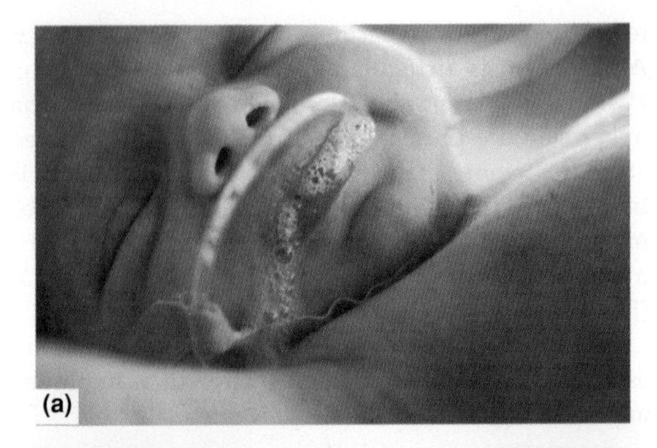

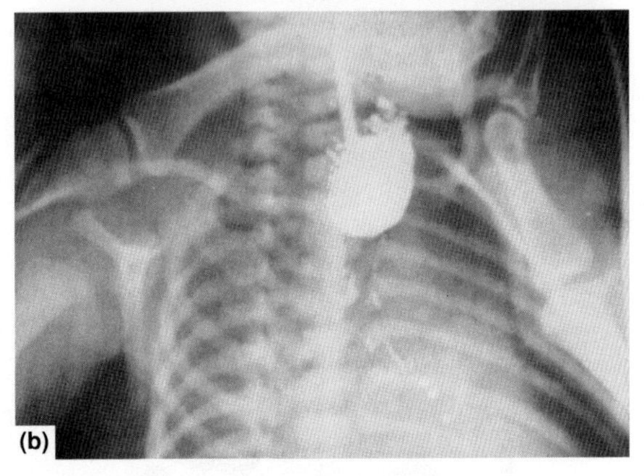

Fig 11.6
(a) Infant with tracheo-oesophageal fistula unable to swallow saliva.
(b) Proximal oesophageal pouch outlined with contrast media. Contrast should not be used because of aspiration. The pouch can be outlined by injecting air via a feeding tube. (Courtesy of Milupa.)

protrusion through the linea alba between the umbilicus and xiphisternum is called an epigastric hernia. A hernia may become painful if the contents become incarcerated; surgery is required if this occurs. The hernia must be marked with a skin pencil preoperatively as they are difficult to locate under anaesthesia.

Tracheo-oesophageal fistula

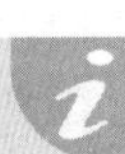

Epidemiology
One in 3000 births.

This occurs when the oesophagus and trachea fail to separate in the 4th week of gestation. Oesophageal atresia causes maternal hydramnios in 25%. After birth, affected infants drool (Fig. 11.6). If the diagnosis is not suspected, the first feed causes choking. If there is a fistula between the distal oesophagus and trachea, regurgitation of gastric contents causes pneumonitis. If the oesophagus is in continuity but communicates with the trachea via a fistula ('H'-type), recurrent choking, coughing, respiratory distress, chest infections and abdominal distension occur. Ideally a large bore nasogastric tube is passed into the oesophagus. If it 'arrests' before reaching the stomach, a little air is injected which may outline the blind-ending oesophagus on chest X-ray. H-type fistula is more difficult to diagnose, often requiring repeated expert paediatric radiology and endoscopy to demonstrate it.

The immediate management is directed towards prevention of aspiration and pneumonia by nursing upright and aspirating the proximal oesophageal pouch by continuous suction. The tracheal aspirate is cultured and broad-spectrum antibiotics are given if aspiration has occurred.

Three-quarters can be treated by primary closure of the fistula and oesophageal anastomosis. Feeding can be commenced from 5 days postoperatively via a transanastomotic tube, providing the Lipiodol swallow is normal. If primary anastomosis is impossible, the fistula is divided and a feeding gastrostomy performed. The proximal pouch may be formed into an oesophagostomy to allow drainage of saliva and sham feeding. When the child is older, secondary anastomosis or alternative surgery such as restoring continuity of the oesophagus with a length of colon may be performed. Early postoperative complications include breakdown of the anastomosis, erosion of the posterior wall of the trachea to form an acquired H-type fistula, mediastinitis, pneumothorax and pyothorax. Late complications include swallowing difficulties, obstruction of the oesophagus with solid foods and recurrent aspiration.

Tracheo-oesophageal fistula can occur as part of the VATER association (vertebral anomalies, ventricular septal defects, anal atresia, tracheo-oesophageal fistula, radial dysplasia and renal anomaly).

Cleft lip and palate (Fig. 11.7)

> **Treatment**
> Operative correction is being carried out at an increasingly early stage to improve speech and feeding development, prevent recurrent otitis media and improve maternal bonding.

INTRODUCTION

Cleft lip is the failure of the medial nasal and maxillary processes to fuse. Cleft palate is failure of the palatal shelves to fuse.

AETIOLOGY AND PATHOGENESIS

Genetic factors are more important in cleft lip with or without cleft palate, than in cleft palate alone. Both can be sporadic. Clefts may be unilateral or bilateral.

INCIDENCE

Cleft lip with or without cleft palate occurs in 1:1000 births and is commoner in males. Isolated cleft palate occurs in 1:2500 births. The incidence is higher in people from Asia and lower amongst the negroid race. The risks of cleft lip and palate to a sibling and offspring are approximately 3–6% and 40% in an identical twin. There is an increased risk of cleft palate in children with chromosomal disorders.

CLINICAL PRESENTATION

The severity of cleft lip varies from a small indentation in the vermilion border of the lip to a full-thickness cleft reaching to the floor of the nose. Unilateral clefts are commoner on the left side. Isolated cleft palates are midline. When associated with cleft lip, the cleft palate begins in the midline of the soft palate then may become bilateral, connecting one or both nasal cavities with the mouth.

MANAGEMENT

Immediate treatment of cleft palate is to place a plastic dental plate to temporarily close the defect. A new plate will be required every few weeks to allow for growth. Surgical repair, especially of cleft lip, is being performed earlier, with palate closure before 1 year allowing normal speech development. If the cleft palate crosses the alveolar ridge, the child will need expert dental surgery to move adjacent teeth and replace missing teeth. Careful nursing will be required in the immediate postoperative period to prevent aspiration of secretions. Complications include otitis media, hearing loss, defective speech, malposition of teeth, dental decay and feeding problems.

Defective speech may persist even after anatomically correct closure of palate. Particular difficulty is experienced with b, d, t, h, y, s, sh and ch. If speech therapy is unsuccessful, a plastic operation is required to raise a flap of mucosa from the posterior pharyngeal wall against which the palate may successfully separate the mouth and nose.

Gastroschisis

This is a congenital defect in the abdominal wall, usually to the right of the midline (not at the umbilicus). The abdominal viscera protrude through the defect without a covering of amnion.

Management is as described for exomphalos (see Fig. 12.3, p. 246).

Inguinal hernia

> **Practice point**
> Inguinal herniae should be repaired as soon as possible because the risk of incarceration is high in infancy.

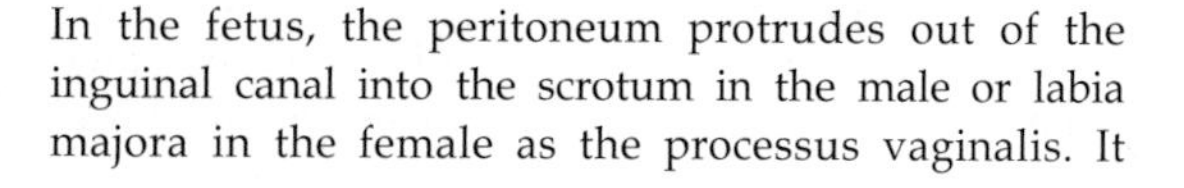

In the fetus, the peritoneum protrudes out of the inguinal canal into the scrotum in the male or labia majora in the female as the processus vaginalis. It

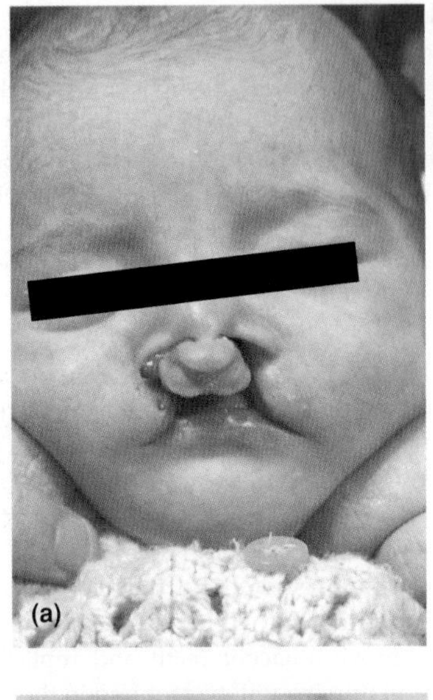

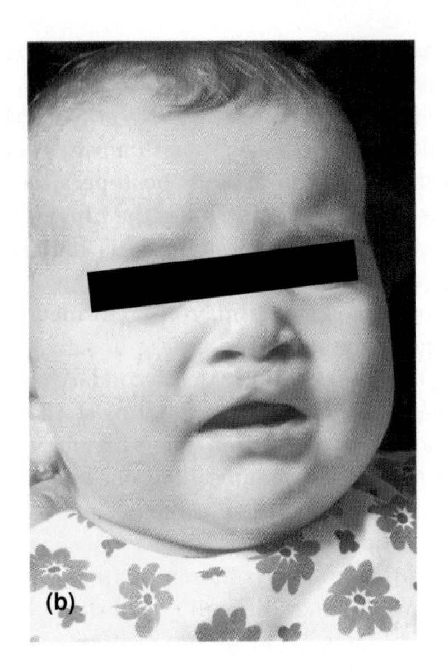

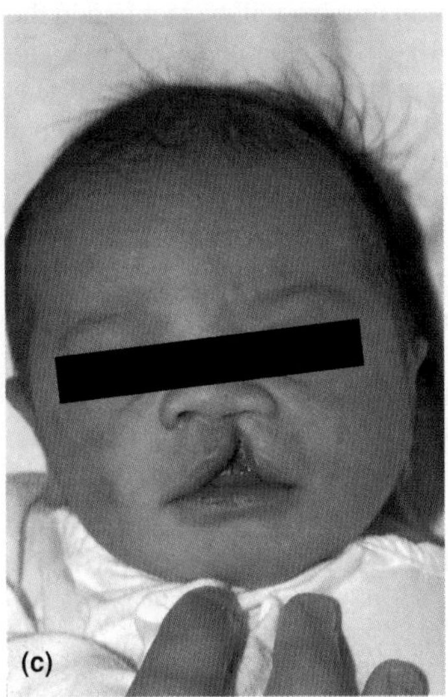

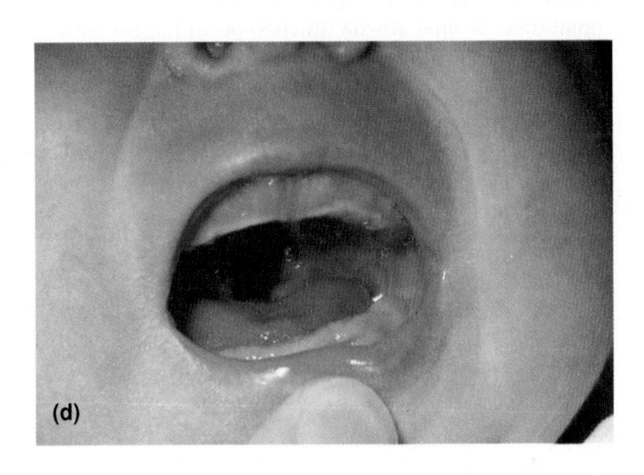

Fig 11.7
Bilateral cleft lip and palate: (a) before repair, and (b) after repair. (c) Cleft lip. (d) Cleft soft palate.

obliterates at birth, except for the portion in the scrotum that envelops the testis as the tunica vaginalis. Failure of obliteration gives rise to an indirect inguinal hernia. Accumulation of fluid in the tunica vaginalis is called hydrocele. The characteristic sign is an inguinal mass that disappears when the hernia is reduced. Incarcerated herniae should be treated by sedation and elevation of the legs using skin traction. If the hernia does not reduce rapidly it should be explored for infarcted intestine.

A Richter hernia is a rare form of incarcerated inguinal hernia in which only part of the intestinal wall is present in the hernia, so that necrosis of the intestine can occur without intestinal obstruction.

Intestinal atresias

Presentation

Suspect in any neonate who vomits green bile.

Atresia can involve the oesophagus, duodenum, jejunum, colon and anus. The higher the obstruction the earlier symptoms occur in the newborn period. Hydramnios is another feature of high obstruction, attributed to the failure of the infant to swallow amniotic fluid.

Duodenal atresia occurs in 1 : 5000 live births, and in 30% of instances it is associated with Down syndrome. Vomiting of bile-stained fluid usually occurs in the first 24 hours as the lesion is at the second part of the duodenum or beyond. Injecting 5–10 ml of air down a nasogastric tube assists with the diagnosis by emphasizing the 'double bubble' appearance on erect abdominal X-ray, caused by air in the stomach and duodenal cap (Fig. 11.8). The rest of the abdomen resembles 'ground glass' on X-ray because the gut contains no gas.

Jejunal and ileal atresias occur in 1 : 6000 births and may be multiple. Abdominal distension may be severe in distal lesions. Erect abdominal X-ray shows fluid levels in the centre of the abdomen and no gas in the rectum.

Colonic atresia is 20 times less common than small intestinal atresia and presentation is delayed.

Anal atresia is categorized as low, middle and high (Fig. 11.9). A low atresia ('covered anus') terminates below the pelvic floor and is treated by uncovering and dilatation. A high atresia terminates above the pelvic floor, either blind or with a fistula. A transverse colostomy is required followed by a 'pull through', at 6–12 months. Faecal continence depends on the length of the effective internal anal sphincter zone, function of the puborectalis sling and avoidance of constipation with overflow incontinence.

At surgery, it is important to determine the residual length of small bowel; whether or not the ileocaecal valve is present is a determinant of outcome. Provided the ileocaecal valve is intact, then a few centimetres of ileum will allow survival. If the terminal ileum is resected, B_{12} supplements may be required.

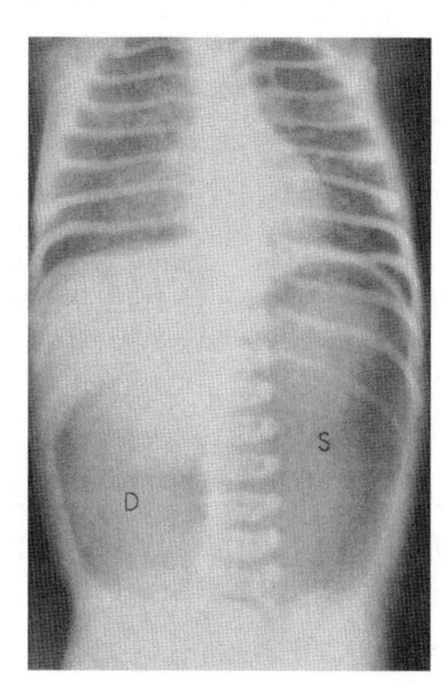

Fig 11.8
X-ray showing 'double bubble'. D, duodenum; S, stomach. (Courtesy of Milupa.)

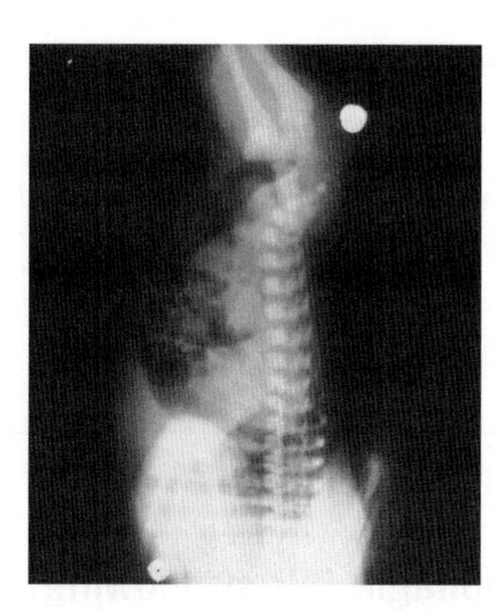

Fig 11.9
High anal atresia. The length of the atresia is demonstrated by X-ray of the baby upside-down, with a radio-opaque marker at the site of the anus.

Intestinal duplication cyst

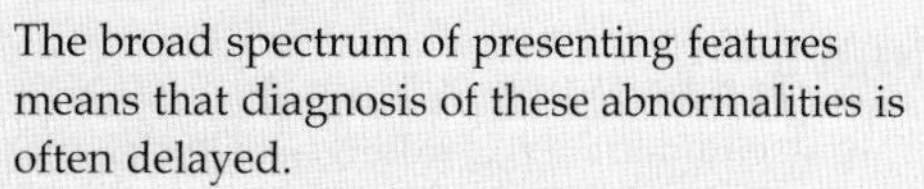

Presentation
The broad spectrum of presenting features means that diagnosis of these abnormalities is often delayed.

These occur on the mesenteric border of normal gut. Duplications often share the same outer muscle layer and can be cystic or tubular. They may be entirely separate and blind-ending, or communicate at both ends with the normal gut. Thoracic duplications are associated with anterior spina bifida as the split notochord syndrome. They may track down through the diaphragm and communicate with abdominal viscera. Presenting features include neonatal respiratory distress, or cyst or space-occupying lesion on chest X-ray, meningitis from anterior spina bifida, intestinal obstruction, volvulus, abdominal distension or mass, bleeding from heterotopic gastric mucosa and small intestinal bacterial overgrowth (p. 230). Contrast studies show stretching of the intestine over the lesion and possible filling of communicating lesions.

Small or cystic duplications are excised with the adjacent normal gut, because of the shared blood supply. Tubular duplications are managed by stripping the mucosa from inside the duplication, leaving the serosa and muscle in situ to avoid lengthy resections of normal intestine.

Umbilical hernia

An umbilical hernia is a protrusion through an incompletely closed umbilical ring. Most resolve spontaneously, and surgery is reserved for those still present after 5 years of age.

(For neonatal surgery, see also Ch. 2 and Ch. 17 (Nephrology and Urology)).

Functional disorders

Aerophagia (air swallowing)

Air swallowing is the commonest cause of abdominal distension. The child's abdomen is flat in the morning and becomes increasingly distended during the day; it deflates at night as the child passes flatus. Other causes of abdominal distension such as malabsorption, or surgical problems do not show this diurnal variation.

The abdomen of toddlers often looks distended because of their posture when standing.

Bezoars

These are accumulations of foreign material in the stomach. They are classified according to their composition as trichobezoars (hair), phytobezoars (vegetable matter), lactobezoars (milk curd) or polybezoars (mixed). They present with abdominal pain, vomiting and mobile epigastric mass, and are best visualized by endoscopy.

Lactobezoars can be broken up with the endoscope. Other types are removed surgically, but there is a considerable hazard of contamination of the peritoneal cavity.

Food refusal

Aetiological factors include a resistance to weaning by the infant; a failure of parental persistence allowing the infant to gain control; and an overestimation of the nutritional requirements of infants causing parents to offer attractive alternatives when food is refused.

Management includes reassurance, which may increase the child's food intake; the avoidance of snacks; eating with parents; attendance at therapeutic play groups; and appropriate rewards.

The prognosis is usually, but not invariably excellent. Occasionally children continue to have a very low intake and fail to thrive, and psychological intervention may be required.

Disordered swallowing

This may be caused by immaturity. Mechanisms of swallowing begin to develop at 16 weeks' gestation and are mature by 34 weeks. Anatomical causes include micrognathia (Pierre Robin anomaly), macroglossia or cleft palate, or the cause may be neurological, i.e. cerebral palsy.

The diagnosis is made by observation, nasal endoscopy or cine video swallow. Treatment is by tube feeding, attention to the child's posture, facial and oral desensitization or the use of palatal appliances.

Disordered oesophageal transit

When there is no stricture, disorders of oesophageal transit may be caused by post-tracheo-oesophageal fistula surgery or by neuropathy, as in familial dysautonomia. If a stricture is present the disorder may be due to post-tracheo-oesophageal fistula surgery, achalasia, peptic oesophagitis, corrosives, compression, duplications, mediastinal mass or vascular rings.

Infantile colic

This is found in more than 1 in 10 infants. There is periodic irritability with drawing up of legs, flatus and borborygmi. It is usually related to the latter half of the feed, and characteristically occurs in the afternoon or evening. It may remit by 3 months but not always. It is found in bottle- and breastfed infants. Maternal anxiety may be a secondary cause. Management should include consideration of other causes of crying, such as underfeeding, learnt behaviour, or infection of the urinary tract or otitis. Reassurance should be given in the hope of a natural remission. A cow's milk-free diet for the mother if the infant is breastfed may also be effective; calcium, vitamin A and vitamin D supplements are then required for the mother.

Disorders of unknown aetiology

Achalasia

In this condition, swallowed food which fails to pass through the cardiac sphincter accumulates in the dilated oesophagus. Aspiration into the trachea is frequent. The disorder may present as anorexia nervosa. Treatment is to dilate the cardiac sphincter of the oesophagus.

Aphthous stomatitis/ulcers

Many children suffer from repeated episodes of small (<1 cm), superficial, often multiple ulcers of the buccal and gingival mucous membrane. The aetiology is unknown, but predisposed individuals appear to react in this way to minor trauma to the oral mucosa. Aphthous ulcers are linked with iron deficiency, coeliac disease and Crohn disease. However, they are so common that it is difficult to ascertain the significance of these ulcerations

Topical corticosteroid pellets (Corlan) are recommended, but the lesions are generally too painful to allow topical medication.

Constipation, soiling and encopresis

> **Lifestyle**
> Constipation is often attributed to poor intake of fibre but children with or without constipation both eat little fibre.
>
> **Genetics**
> If one identical twin is constipated, the other is much more likely to be affected than in nonidentical twins.
> A family history on the mother's side is common.

INTRODUCTION

Constipation is difficulty or delay in the passage of stool. As a result the lower rectum, which is normally empty, is full of stool; the latter is often hard but may be of normal consistency. Soiling is the inappropriate passage of stool that may occur in chronic constipation. Soiling occurs involuntarily. The leakage of soft stools and fluid past large, impacted faeces or 'scybala' is referred to as spurious diarrhoea. By contrast encopresis is the inappropriate passage (e.g. into pants or behind furniture) of normal stools in a child with normal anorectal function. Bowel control is normally present in the majority of children older than 2 years. Encopresis occurring in school-age children is part of an emotional disturbance.

AETIOLOGY AND PATHOGENESIS

Acute constipation occurring, for example, during an acute illness may result in difficult and painful defecation. The passage of large, hard faeces may even tear the lining of the anus, resulting in an intensely painful acute anal fissure. The child will avoid defecating, thus compounding the problem. Inappropriate toilet training or lack of suitable facilities at nursery or school will make matters worse. The final result may be chronic constipation.

When faeces enter the rectum, this produces the desire to defecate. This process occurs after a meal, as the 'gastrocolic reflex'. If the rectum is chronically distended, this sensation is no longer produced and spontaneous 'overflow' of faeces (soiling) results.

Organic causes are rare but important (Information box 11.5).

Neurological problems such as cerebral palsy, paraplegia and spina bifida may be associated with severe constipation because the abdominal wall muscles cannot play their normal part in defecation.

INCIDENCE

Acute constipation will occur in most children, in response to events such as hospitalization or illness. As many as 5–10% of school age children have chronic constipation.

CLINICAL PRESENTATION

Although most children present in the toddler age group, the history may date from birth. Constipation from birth is an important feature as it may indicate an organic cause. Those with soiling or 'spurious' diarrhoea may have been treated with repeated courses of antidiarrhoeal therapy.

DIAGNOSIS

The history will help distinguish between encopresis and constipation with soiling. Consider an organic cause (Information box 11.5) if the onset is from birth with delayed passage of meconium, severe constipation in the first year of life, alternating constipation and diarrhoea,

> **Information Box 11.5**
>
> **Specific causes of chronic constipation**
>
> - Hirschsprung disease
> - Hypercalcaemia
> - Hypothyroidism
> - Chronic dehydration
>   - Diabetes
>   - Chronic renal failure
>   - Renal tubular disorders
> - Anal stenosis
> - Intestinal pseudo-obstruction
> - Drugs (e.g. opiates)

and failure to thrive. Confirmation of the degree of constipation by abdominal and rectal examination is mandatory. Rectal examination will also identify anal stenosis. Anal stenosis is a rare cause of constipation present from birth. The stenosis responds to repeated digital or instrumental dilatation. Gross abdominal distension, with a 'squirt' of faeces on withdrawing the finger from the rectum, suggests Hirschsprung disease.

Clinical examination underestimates faecal loading. A plain X-ray of the abdomen is useful in distinguishing encopresis without faecal loading and constipation (Fig. 11.10). An X-ray can also help distinguish between spurious diarrhoea secondary to constipation and actual diarrhoea.

MANAGEMENT

Management of children with idiopathic constipation begins with reassuring the family that it is a common problem albeit one which families are loath to discuss. Although the ultimate prognosis is good, the parents need to understand that it may take as long to solve the problem as it took to develop in the first place. It is helpful to explain the loss of normal rectal sensation, such that children who soil are not aware of the problem and do not experience a call to defecate.

The aim should be a regular, painless bowel action and regaining continence. To achieve continence, the rectum must first be emptied, by regular suppositories (say daily for 2–10 days), or one or two phosphate enemas, or the use of a powerful laxative such as Movicol®. At some centres the anus is stretched under general anaesthesia. This approach may be helpful if there is a history of anal fissuring. Once the rectum is empty, lactulose 5–15 ml twice daily will soften the stool and Senokot 2.5–10 ml daily will encourage a more regular bowel action by stimulating peristalsis. The parents should know not to change the dose more frequently than weekly in order to assess the effect of change. They should increase the lactulose to produce a softer stool and the Senokot to produce a more frequent stool. A good fibre and fluid intake are encouraged but are unlikely to succeed without medication. Many parents will have already tried this approach. The laxatives do need to be reinforced by behaviour modification. The child should spend at least 5 minutes on the toilet after each meal. If no bowel action results, then this is 'made light of' but if a stool is produced then the child is praised to excess! Success can be reinforced by a reward system using a star chart in the early stages. A star may be awarded for the lowest level of cooperation required, i.e. sitting on the toilet. An extra star is given for a day without soiling and a further star for three clean days. When this reward system starts to wane, then the use of extra treats can be given after a week of success.

This approach needs frequent reinforcement from the paediatrician initially, and continued follow up at 4–6-week intervals until the child is weaned off laxatives (after 6 months or longer). If this approach fails, occasionally it may be necessary to admit a child for more detailed assessment.

Children with encopresis should have formal psychological assessment to explore what precipitating, exacerbating environmental factors are present. Behavioural, analytical and family therapies are all potentially successful approaches.

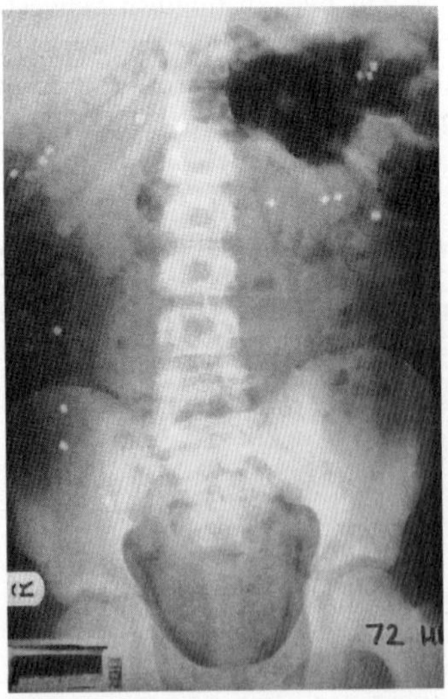

Fig 11.10
X-ray of abdomen of child with constipation. The entire colon and rectum are loaded with faeces outlined by small gas bubbles. The white dots are radioopaque markers used to measure transit time. After 72 hours none have reached the rectum.

Hirschsprung disease

Definition

Absence of nerve ganglion cells (aganglionosis) in the intramuscular and submucous plexuses of the bowel. A variable length of gut is affected but aganglionosis always involves the anus and extends proximally.

This disease usually involves the sigmoid colon but can extend proximally into the small bowel. Ultra-long segment may be familial or genetic. The illness may present in the newborn period with failure to pass meconium. (NB: 10% of normal infants do not pass meconium in the first 24 h and 2% do not pass meconium in the first 48 h.) The rectum is empty and withdrawal of the examining finger may induce a 'spurt' of meconium. There may be signs of large bowel obstruction with gross abdominal distension and late vomiting which may be faeculent. An important differential diagnosis of delayed passage of meconium is meconium ileus (see cystic fibrosis, p. 352). A later presentation is with chronic constipation from birth with abdominal distension and failure to thrive.

The diagnosis is made by taking suction rectal biopsies which show absent ganglion cells in Hirschsprung disease. Nerve fibres in the biopsy show increased staining for cholinesterase. Anal pressures may be measured during rectal distension with a fluid-filled balloon. Normal relaxation of the anal sphincter does not occur in Hirschsprung disease. Barium enema shows a characteristic 'funnel' or 'cone' of dilated normal bowel leading to the affected segment. This test may be useful for estimating the length of affected segment but false-positive and false-negative results can occur. For example the normal bowel may force faeces into the aganglionic segment, thereby dilating the aganglionic segment and shortening the distance between the 'cone' and the anus.

The treatment is surgical. The subacute obstruction is relieved by an enterostomy, using frozen sections of gut examined for ganglion cells to establish the site. At 1 year a bypass operation is performed. The Soave operation is popular, in which the aganglionic bowel is resected, the anal mucosa is removed and the normal gut is pulled through the anus and anastomosed. In older children a single stage operation is usual.

The illness may be complicated by acute or subacute enterocolitis (Fig. 11.11). Acute enterocolitis may occur before or after neonatal surgery for Hirschsprung disease and carries a high mortality. The management includes relief of the obstruction if this has not already been done. The illness is managed along the lines of necrotizing enterocolitis. The subacute form presents in infancy with diarrhoea. Continence is achieved after surgery in 70–90% although this may be delayed until after adolescence. A permanent colostomy may be required in those who do not achieve continence.

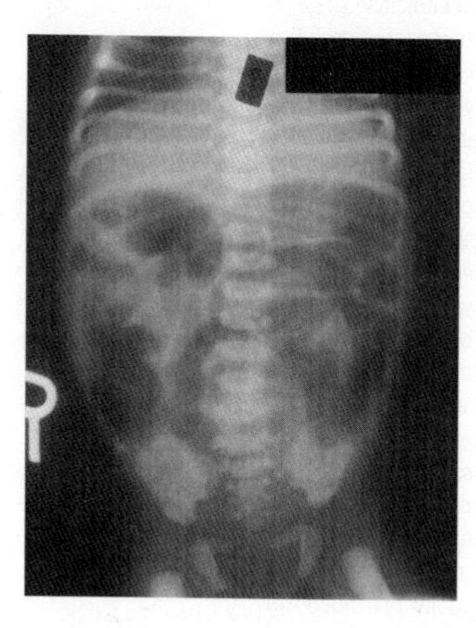

Fig 11.11
Supine X-ray of infant with Hirschsprung enterocolitis. Note the degree of distension of bowel loops proximal to the aganglionic segment.

Diarrhoea

Acute diarrhoea

Epidemiology
One of the most important public health problems on a worldwide scale.

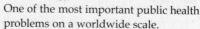

Lifestyle
Breastfeeding confers a strong protective advantage.

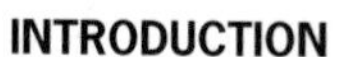

INTRODUCTION

The causes of acute diarrhoea and vomiting are acute gastrointestinal infections and other causes, listed in Information box 11.6. Any systemic infection may be associated with acute diarrhoea and vomiting, but these symptoms are usually a manifestation of a gastrointestinal infection. The term 'acute diarrhoea and vomiting' or 'acute intestinal infection' is preferred to 'gastroenteritis' as there is little evidence for gastric involvement in this acute infectious disease. Furthermore 'enteritis' or inflammation of the gut is not prominent in acute watery diarrhoea from many specific causes.

AETIOLOGY AND PATHOGENESIS

The commonest pathogen in infants is rotavirus, especially during the colder months of the year. The virus infects the absorptive cells of the villi of the small intestine. These cells are shed, resulting in shortening of villi, and loss of surface area, digestive enzymes and transport proteins that are normally found in the brush borders of these cells. The cells that migrate from the crypts are better equipped to secrete fluid than absorb it; this adds to the diarrhoea.

The commonest bacterial pathogen in the developed countries is *Campylobacter jejuni*, which causes fever, severe abdominal pain and diarrhoea, which may be bloody as this bacterium invades the mucosa of the distal gut. Infection with the protozoan *Giardia lamblia* is usually acquired from infected food or water, and cryptosporidia are acquired from contact with farm animals or drinking contaminated water, and then to other children. They cause acute or persistent diarrhoea especially in immunocompromised individuals. Other causes are listed in Information box 11.6.

Information Box 11.6

Intestinal pathogens associated with acute diarrhoea

Viruses
Rotavirus
Picornavirus (Norwalk, Hawaii, etc.)
Small round viruses (astro, calici)
Corona-like virus
Adenovirus

Bacteria
Campylobacter jejuni
Nontyphoid salmonellae
Shigellae
Yersiniae
Staphylococci
Bacillus cereus
Clostridia
Vibrio parahaemolyticus
Vibrio cholerae
Escherichia coli
- Enterotoxigenic
- Enteroinvasive
- Enteropathogenic
- Enterohaemorrhagic

Bacteroides fragilis
Aeromonas sp.
Plesiomonas sp.

Protozoa
Entamoeba histolytica
Giardia lamblia
Cryptosporidium parvum

INCIDENCE

Surveys and other sources carried out in 1988 revealed that over 1.3 thousand million episodes of diarrhoea occurred each year in children under 5 years of age in Asia (excluding China), Africa and Latin America. Four million children in this age group died annually from diarrhoea. Since then the mortality rate has fallen, due to the increased availability of simple, effective treatment (see below). A very different picture emerges in developed countries, where mortality rates are low. Some European countries now report annual mortality rates of zero. In England and Wales there has been a marked decrease from approximately 700 deaths per year in the late 1970s to around 25 in the late 1980s. The statistics should be compared with mortality rates for England and Wales at the beginning of the 20th century when 30 000–50 000 children died each year. Nonetheless acute diarrhoea continues to be a significant cause of morbidity in children from developed countries.

CLINICAL PRESENTATION

Depending on the causative agent and severity of the infection, the child may present with watery or bloody diarrhoea, with or without vomiting. The most important clinical signs are those of dehydration that include thirst, restlessness or irritability, decreased skin turgor (assessed by lifting and releasing the skin of the abdomen and observing the rate of flattening), sunken eyes, sunken fontanelle (in infants) and suppression of tear and saliva formation. These signs become more pronounced in severe dehydration and are accompanied by hypovolaemic shock (absence of peripheral pulses, peripheral cyanosis and drowsiness). The child with some signs of dehydration has a fluid deficit of 50–100 ml/kg; severe dehydration is associated with a deficit of greater than 100 ml/kg.

DIAGNOSIS

The differential diagnosis of acute diarrhoea and/or vomiting is shown in Information box 11.7.

While children commonly develop diarrhoea while receiving antibiotics, antibiotic-associated diarrhoea due to *Clostridium difficile* is rare in childhood. Neonates

Information Box 11.7

Causes of acute diarrhoea and/or vomiting

- Gastrointestinal infections (see Information box 11.6)
- Systemic infections
  - Urinary tract infection
  - Septicaemia
  - Meningitis
  - Respiratory tract infections
- Surgical conditions
  - Appendicitis
  - Intussusception
  - Hirschsprung disease
  - Pyloric stenosis
- Metabolic conditions
  - Diabetic ketoacidosis
  - Congenital adrenal insufficiency
- Miscellaneous
  - Antibiotic-associated diarrhoea
  - Cystic fibrosis
  - Coeliac disease
  - Chronic inflammatory bowel disease
  - Immunodeficiency
  - Kawasaki disease
  - Laxatives
  - Cow's milk protein intolerance
  - Enterocolitis
  - Poisoning
  - Toddler diarrhoea
  - Toxic shock syndrome

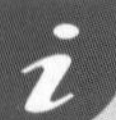

Information Box 11.8

Indications for stool examination during diarrhoea

- During an epidemic
- Immunodeficient patients
- Severely ill children
- Bloody diarrhoea
- Overseas travel
- Chronic diarrhoea >14 days

can carry toxigenic strains of *C. difficile* without symptoms.

Indications for stool examination to determine specific causes of gastrointestinal infection are shown in Information box 11.8.

MANAGEMENT

Patients with some dehydration require 50–100 ml/kg of oral rehydration therapy with solutions containing sodium (60 mM), potassium (20 mM) and glucose (100 mM), over 4–6 hours, followed by a return to the usual diet. Further oral rehydration therapy is administered if diarrhoea continues (50–100 ml oral rehydration therapy following each loose stool in children under 2 years of age, 100–200 ml if older than 2 years). Intravenous rehydration is required for severe dehydration, and for patients with coma or ileus, or if other intra-abdominal pathology is suspected. Excess vomiting or stool output (>10 ml/kg/h) can be managed by administration of oral rehydration therapy via a nasogastric tube. If hydration has not improved after 4–6 hours intravenous fluids should be administered.

If there is blood in the stool, the diarrhoea is likely to be due to an invasive organism such as campylobacter, shigella, or salmonella. If the child is systemically unwell, antibiotic therapy should be considered. If the bloody diarrhoea is due to enterohaemorrhagic *E. coli* then antibiotics are not advised.

Giardiasis is treated with a single dose of tinidazole 50 mg/kg. Persistent cryptosporidiosis has been shown to respond to clarithromycin. In the immunocompromised it may be improved but not cured.

Hyponatraemia (serum Na^+ <130 mmol/l), which is associated with lethargy and convulsions, also responds to oral rehydration therapy. Hypokalaemia (serum K^+ <3 mmol/l) may be associated with weakness, ileus, impairment of renal concentrating ability and cardiac arrhythmias, but in practice it is almost invariably asymptomatic. The amount of K^+ in oral rehydration solutions (ORS) (usually 20 mmol/l) is often inadequate to replace K^+ deficits during rehydration. Hypernatraemic dehydration (serum Na^+ >150 mmol/l) is one of the most feared complications of acute diarrhoea, because of the association with cerebral haemorrhage, cerebral oedema during therapy, death, and brain damage in survivors. While this complication has virtually disappeared in developed countries, it is still a cause for serious concern in developing countries. Risk factors for hypernatraemic dehydration include severe dehydration, age less than 1 year, consumption of excessively concentrated ORS, the prescription of antibiotics and antidiarrhoeal drugs with consequent delay in starting oral rehydration therapy, and the use of traditional drinks containing sucrose. Once the circulation has been restored, oral rehydration therapy is the treatment of choice. Extending the rehydration phase from 6–8 hours to 12–16 hours, is recommended to allow slower re-equilibration of hyperosmolar dehydration.

Severe enteritis may lead to transient lactose intolerance. Lactose intolerance complicating acute diarrhoea appears to be a declining problem. This has allowed the abandonment of slow reintroduction of milk into the diets of children recovering from gastroenteritis. Lactose in breast milk is well tolerated during acute diarrhoea. Rapid reintroduction of full strength milk is recommended. Breastfeeding should not be stopped.

If diarrhoea with or without blood lasts 14 days or more, the diarrhoea is said to be persistent. After 14 days, mortality rates begin to rise. Investigations should include stool microscopy to detect pathogens such as *Entamoeba histolytica*, *Giardia lamblia* and *Cryptosporidium parvum*. Intravenous fluid and electrolytes may be required to maintain hydration if monosaccharide intolerance is present. The most essential intervention in such infants is to maintain nutrition. This is best achieved with a protein source such as comminuted (ground up) chicken to which are added starch, vegetable oil, vitamins and minerals. In developed countries a lactose-free milk containing extensively hydrolysed protein is used.

Important strategies for preventing diarrhoea exist, including promotion of hygiene and breastfeeding, nutritional supplementation and improving water supplies. Nevertheless the results of vaccine trials in which cholera and noncholera deaths were prevented by the expedient of administering cholera vaccine orally, rather than by injection, demonstrated the utility of immunization. In addition to cholera, development of vaccines against shigella dysentery, enterotoxigenic *E. coli* and rotavirus is a priority with the prospect of reducing attendances at hospitals with diarrhoea by more than 20%. Unfortunately, the prospects of a rotavirus vaccine have been set back by experiences in the USA where the introduction of a rotavirus vaccine was associated with an increased incidence of intussusception. The vaccine has now been withdrawn.

Chronic diarrhoea

> Lifestyle
> Breastfeeding protects against chronic as well as acute diarrhoea.

INTRODUCTION

Diarrhoea is defined as a change in stool consistency towards looseness or increased frequency. If the symptom lasts more than 14 days it is called chronic. Chronic diarrhoea can occur in the presence or absence of failure to thrive.

AETIOLOGY AND PATHOGENESIS

Chronic diarrhoea without failure to thrive can occur in breastfed babies. Other important causes of chronic diarrhoea are listed in Information box 11.9. Specific causes are dealt with below.

Information Box 11.9

Causes of chronic diarrhoea

Causes	Examples
Food protein intolerance	Coeliac disease Eosinophilic gastroenteropathy Food allergy
Carbohydrate intolerance	Primary and secondary sucrose and lactose intolerance
Surgical	Malrotation Hirschsprung disease Stenosis Bacterial overgrowth
Intestinal infection	*Giardia lamblia* Cryptosporidia Dysentery
Antibiotics	Pseudomembranous colitis
Pancreatic insufficiency	Cystic fibrosis Schwachman syndrome
Immunodeficiency	AIDS Severe combined immunodeficiency Hypogammaglobulinaemia
Tumours	Ganglioneuroma Langerhans cell histiocytosis Lymphoma
Chronic inflammatory bowel disease	Ulcerative colitis Crohn disease
Other	Necrotizing enterocolitis Lymphangiectasia Toddler diarrhoea Chloride- or sodium-losing diarrhoea

Coeliac disease (gluten enteropathy)

> Lifestyle
> The cereals which form the staple part of our diet are capable of immunologically mediated damage to the small intestinal mucosa in susceptible individuals.
>
> Aetiology
> The protein fraction that causes the damage is called 'gluten' hence the alternative name 'gluten-sensitive enteropathy'.

The fraction of gluten that is toxic to the small intestinal mucosa is called 'alpha gliadin'. Gliadin from wheat is the most toxic, followed by rye, oats and barley. Rice and maize cereal are nontoxic to children with coeliac disease. The damage is probably caused by a delayed hypersensitivity reaction to gliadin, occurring in the small intestinal mucosa. People of tissue type HLA-B8 are predisposed.

Although the whole length of the small intestine is sensitive to gluten, the proximal small intestine is most severely affected because the distal intestine is not exposed to intact gluten. The histopathological appearance is described as 'subtotal villous atrophy' (Fig. 11.12). There is loss of villi and hypertrophy of crypts. The surface epithelium changes from columnar to cuboidal and increased numbers of lymphocytes are seen within the epithelium. The lamina propria is infiltrated with plasma cells. The crypts of the small intestinal mucosa are hypertrophied and increased numbers of the lining cells undergo mitosis. As a result of damage and loss to the mature enterocytes of the villi, the upper small intestinal mucosa is turning over faster. The cells that line the small intestine are immature, with poorly developed enzyme systems for digesting disaccharides such as lactose and sucrose or absorbing monosaccharides such as glucose, galactose and fructose.

In the mid-1970s the prevalence was 1 in 2000 in the UK, and as high as 1 in 300 in the west of Ireland. The risk to first-degree relatives is about 10%. The incidence in childhood has been falling in recent years, possibly as a result of the delayed introduction of gluten in infancy. It will probably present later in life, because of the genetic factors involved in the disease.

The 'classical' presentation of coeliac disease is failure to thrive occurring after the introduction of cereals into the diet. Weight gain slows first, followed by a slowing of the rate of height increase and then of head growth (Fig. 11.13). The stools are frequent, soft and pale. The child becomes irritable and the appetite is

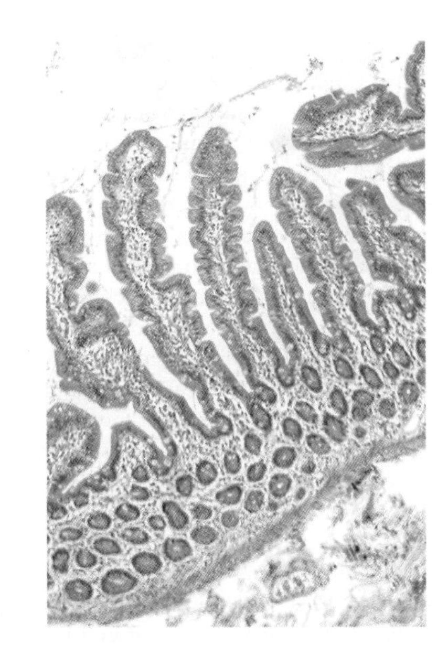

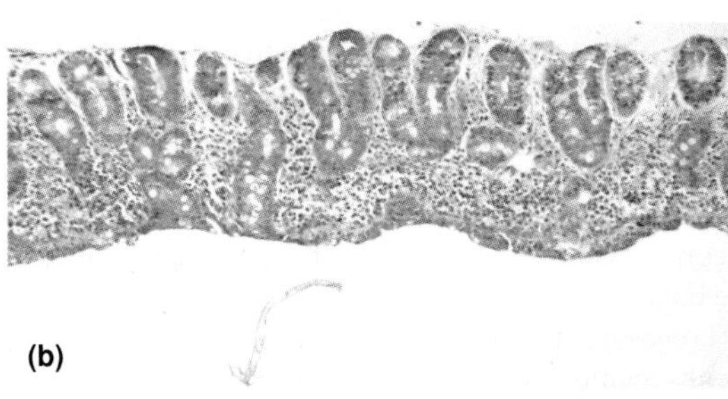

Fig 11.12
(a) Normal small intestine showing finger-shaped villi. (b) Subtotal villous atrophy; villi virtually absent.

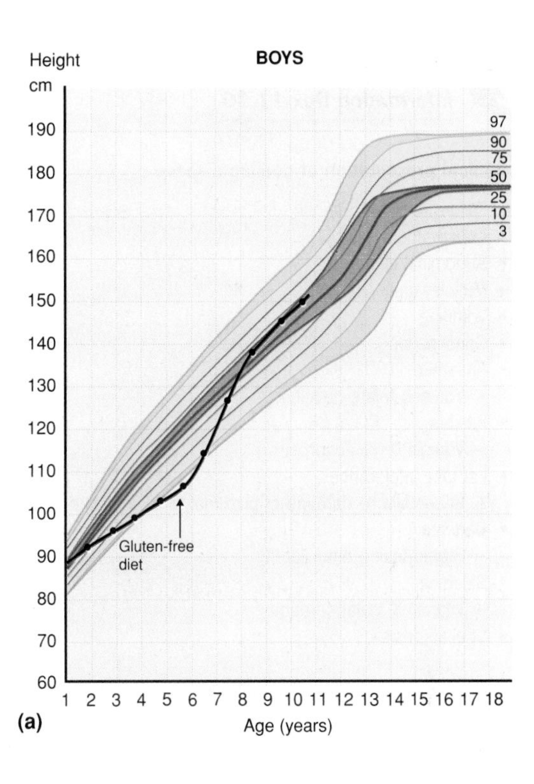

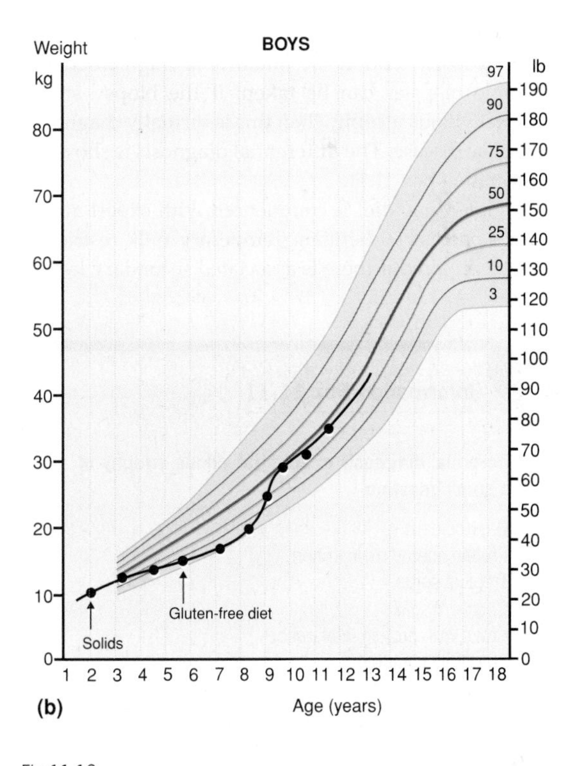

Fig 11.13
Typical growth charts for a boy with coeliac disease. (a) Height. (b) Weight – notice how weight is gained after the commencement of a gluten-free diet. The classic presentation is failure to thrive after the introduction of cereals to the diet. Weight gain slows, followed by a slowing of height increase.

poor. The abdomen becomes distended and muscle wasting is most obvious clinically in the proximal limb muscles, especially the gluteal muscle. In practice alternative presentations occur (see Information box 11.10).

Screening tests such as serum and red cell folate, serum iron, plasma calcium, phosphate and alkaline phosphatase and xylose loading tests are not recommended. False-positives and false-negatives occur and they add to the distress of the experience. The newer generation of tests involving, for example, serum IgA alpha-gliadin and antiendomysial antibodies and differential absorption of oligosaccharides such as lactulose and mannitol, show more specificity and sensitivity and are useful for checking compliance with the diet. The initial diagnosis is made by peroral jejunal biopsy with subsequent confirmation by gluten challenge.

The jejunal biopsy is now obtained under general

Information Box 11.10

Clinical presentation of coeliac disease

- Failure to thrive
- Loose stools
- Abdominal distension
- Muscle wasting
- Vomiting
- Constipation
- Anaemia
  - Iron and folate deficiency
- Rickets
  - Vitamin D malabsorption
- Lactose intolerance
  - Secondary to damage of proximal small intestine
- Oedema
  - Protein-losing enteropathy
- Bleeding
  - Vitamin K malabsorption
- Coeliac crisis
  - Dehydration
- Growth failure without gastrointestinal symptoms

anaesthetic with biopsy forceps passed down an endoscope. The biopsy samples obtained directly with an endoscope tend to be small and fragmented but multiple biopsies can be taken. If the biopsy shows subtotal villous atrophy then this is virtually diagnostic of coeliac disease. The differential diagnosis is shown in Information box 11.11.

A gluten-free diet is commenced with expert advice from a paediatric dietitian. Temporary milk restriction may be required if there is associated secondary lactose intolerance. The handbook published by the Coeliac Society (The Coeliac Society, PO Box 181, London NW2 2QY) is helpful and up-to-date. If the child responds with decrease in symptoms (mood is first to improve) and weight gain accelerates, then the diagnosis is confirmed by gluten challenge. A repeat biopsy on a gluten-free diet shows normal histology, with a return to abnormal following gluten challenge. This is delayed for 2–4 years if catch-up growth is occurring. It is best carried out before starting school when the child will be eating more often outside the home and also the procedure can be explained to the child. If the diagnosis was made after the second year of life, then the challenge can be monitored by measuring titres of pre- and post-gluten challenge serum anti-endomyseal antibodies rather than by biopsies. If the diagnosis was made under the age of 2, when other causes of subtotal villous atrophy are possible (see Information box 11.11) or if no diagnostic biopsy was obtained, then the challenge is monitored by pre- and post-challenge jejunal biopsies. The pre-challenge biopsy must be morphologically normal for comparison with the post-challenge specimen.

The gluten challenge is administered as either gluten powder added to the diet (10–15 g/day) or the equivalent in gluten-containing foods (e.g. at least four slices of bread per day). The post-challenge biopsy is performed after 3–4 months unless marked symptoms occur. A deterioration in the histological appearance in the biopsy confirms the diagnosis.

Long-term follow up is required to monitor growth, and to maintain contact with a dietitian. The need for a lifelong diet is re-emphasized, even though symptoms may not occur when the diet is broken. There is increasing evidence that good compliance prevents the development of small bowel malignancy, which is increased 20-fold in adults with coeliac disease. Disorders associated with coeliac disease are listed in Information box 11.12.

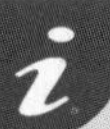

Information Box 11.11

Differential diagnosis of subtotal villous atrophy of the small intestine

- Gastroenteritis
- Protein energy malnutrition
- Tropical sprue
- Coeliac disease
- Cow's milk protein intolerance
- Soy protein intolerance
- Temporary gluten intolerance
- Antineoplastic therapy
- Severe combined immunodeficiency
- Autoimmune enteropathy
- Protracted diarrhoea of unknown cause
- Bacterial overgrowth of the small intestine

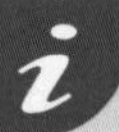

Information Box 11.12

Disorders associated with coeliac disease

- Dermatitis herpetiformis (Fig. 11.14)
- HLA-B8 tissue type associated diseases
  - Diabetes mellitus
  - Autoimmune thyroiditis
  - Pernicious anaemia
- IgA deficiency
- Small bowel malignancy (especially lymphoma)

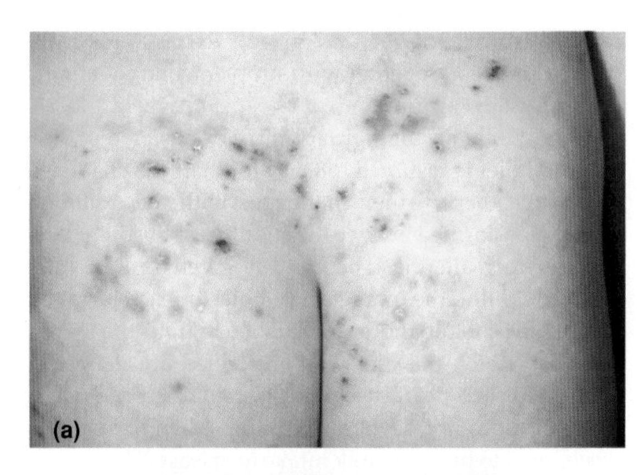

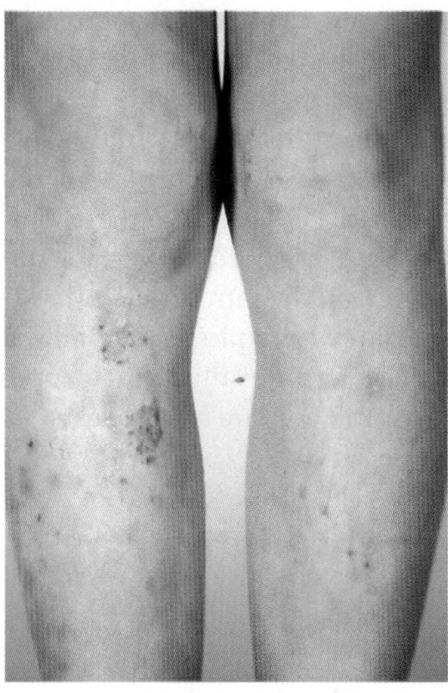

Fig 11.14
Dermatitis herpetiformis (a) on the buttocks and (b) on the legs.

Eosinophilic gastroenteropathy

Allergic children may have eosinophilic infiltration of their gastrointestinal tracts, associated with vomiting, chronic diarrhoea and protein-losing enteropathy.

Food allergy

> Epidemiology
> At least 5% and as many as 30% of infants may show immunologically mediated reactions to the ingestion of food, most notably to cow's milk.

Reactions to food are due either to intolerances (e.g. intolerance to lactose) or to allergies mediated by immune mechanisms. Such reactions are commoner in the first year of life. Hypersensitivity to dietary protein is more common in atopic individuals with a personal and/or family history of eczema, hayfever and asthma.

Apart from cow's milk, many other foods have been implicated. Gluten, soy, rice, fish and chicken proteins have been shown to cause damage to the small intestine (enteropathy). Wheat protein (gluten) is the only protein known to cause lifelong sensitivity.

Detectable amounts of whole protein are absorbed across the gut mucosa in humans. The amounts absorbed are increased in young infants (particularly if preterm). The amount is further increased in IgA-deficient individuals. The presence of IgA is one factor which prevents food intolerance. In lactating mothers, detectable amounts of food protein are excreted in the breast milk and this may be sufficient to precipitate dietary food intolerance in their infants.

The entry of whole protein across the gut mucosa of certain infants predisposes them to develop hypersensitivity reactions. These may be immediate, usually in association with raised IgE, or delayed, mediated by lymphocytes. The soluble milk proteins (lactalbumin and lactoglobulin) are more potent allergens than insoluble milk protein (casein). A high proportion of the cow's milk protein in infant formulae is in the soluble form.

The symptoms which may occur as a result of ingestion of a food to which a child is allergic are listed in Information box 11.13.

Diagnosis is based on remission of symptoms on withdrawal of the suspect food from the diet. The symptoms should return on reintroduction and remit again on withdrawal. If the initial response is dramatic then challenge with the suspect food is delayed for

> ***Information Box 11.13***
>
> **Symptoms which may be precipitated by food allergy**
>
> - Acute anaphylaxis
> - Urticaria
> - Eczema
> - Wheezing
> - Vomiting
>   - Occasionally as only manifestation
> - Acute diarrhoea
>   - Usually with vomiting
> - Chronic diarrhoea
> - Acute colitis
> - Occult gastrointestinal blood loss
>   - Iron-deficiency anaemia
> - Colic
> - Migraine
> - Constipation

6–12 months and until after 12–18 months of age. Supportive laboratory tests include:

- A positive intradermal skin prick test with a negative control
- A positive radioallergosorbent test (RAST) indicating the presence of a specific IgE
- Total plasma IgE raised for age
- High eosinophil count.

The management of dietary protein intolerances may be modelled on that of cow's milk protein intolerance. When the diagnosis is suspected, the exclusion diet should be supervised by a paediatric dietitian. Fully milk-fed infants may be fed on a variety of milk substitutes which are available for treatment of cow's milk protein intolerance. Soy protein-based formulae are the simplest, cheapest and most widely available cow's milk protein-free diet. Unfortunately it is said that as many as 30% of children with cow's milk protein intolerance have soy protein intolerance. In order to avoid prolonging the symptoms, many clinicians use milks in which the protein part is hydrolysed to peptides that are not recognized as milk protein by the allergic child's immune system. Some children appear not to respond until they receive a milk in which the peptides are replaced by free amino acids. Those few children who fail to respond to the amino acid-based diet can be tried on a diet based on comminuted (ground up) chicken with added carbohydrate, fat, electrolytes, trace metals, and vitamins. This diet is exceedingly complex to prepare (Fig. 11.15). Such feeds have unusual smells and tastes. It is essential to explain that in spite of this, the food intolerant infant may enjoy and thrive on them.

If the infant is breastfed then the mother has to be placed on a cow's milk protein-free diet in order that her breast milk becomes cow's milk protein-free. This is usually best accomplished by removing cow's milk protein from her diet and giving extra cow's milk protein-free food together with supplementary vitamins A and D with calcium.

If the child fails to improve on the exclusion diet then a normal diet is resumed after 1 month. If the challenge is positive then further challenges with the excluded food are performed every 6–12 months, in hospital if the child is very allergic. The child is given 1 ml of milk orally, doubling the intake every hour to reach 32 ml by 5 hours. Do not abandon the challenge until the symptoms for which the diet was prescribed are definitely confirmed (except in case of suspected anaphylaxis). If the child does not develop symptoms then the child is discharged to increase milk intake to at least 250 ml/day. Follow up is required because symptoms may not be immediate and may take days to develop.

The diet must be strict for the trial period. After this, partially denatured cow's milk protein may be introduced as in cheese, yoghurt and chocolate. Many children do not react adversely to these. They should be introduced when the condition is stable on diet. Only one new food should be introduced every 2 weeks with careful monitoring of symptoms. The clinical symptoms related to the gastrointestinal tract appear to remit spontanteously and are rare after 6 years of age.

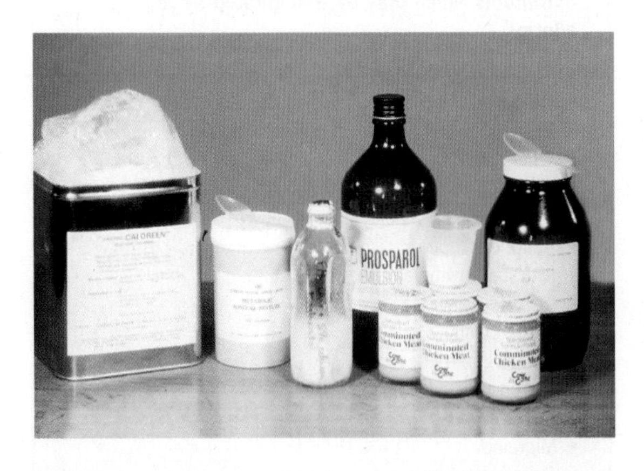

Fig 11.15
Constituents of comminuted chicken feed used with children who fail to respond to amino-acid based diet.

Carbohydrate intolerance

> Lifestyle
> In parts of the world where few cattle are kept for milking, non-caucasian lactose intolerance is common.

In early infancy, lactose is the only carbohydrate ingested, to which are added starch and sucrose (see Information box 11.14). Some carbohydrate is

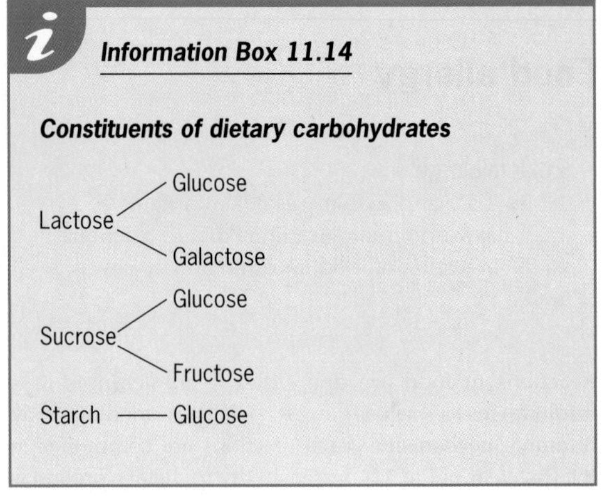

obligatory to provide glucose for metabolism by erythrocytes, otherwise protein must be degraded to form glucose. Carbohydrate is stored as glycogen and excess is converted into fat; fat cannot be converted by humans to carbohydrate. Carbohydrate intolerance results in malabsorption, then loose, watery, frothy stools and anal excoriation occur. Glucose and galactose are malabsorbed in a rare autosomal recessive disorder, presenting in the neonatal period, because of a defective small intestinal carrier protein that transports glucose and galactose. Lactose sucrose and glucose must be avoided, with carbohydrate supplied as fructose. Lactose intolerance is described as congenital, non-caucasian or secondary. The congenital variety is a rare autosomal recessive disorder with absent lactase activity. Sucrose and glucose are tolerated normally. Low or absent small intestinal lactase activity is normal in non-caucasian individuals over 5 years of age. Persistence of lactase activity is dominantly inherited. Milk is avoided by older children and adults with lactose intolerance since drinking large amounts causes colicky abdominal pain and/or diarrhoea. Lactase is the most vulnerable of small intestinal brush border enzymes, and any disease process that damages the small bowel (such as gastroenteritis, gastrointestinal surgery or coeliac disease in relapse) can cause secondary lactose intolerance. Treatment of secondary lactose intolerance is with lactose-free milks and regular challenges with lactose or cow's milk.

Sucrose intolerance can also be primary or secondary and is invariably associated with a degree of starch intolerance because the sucrase enzyme complex contains isomaltase and both are involved in starch digestion. The primary disorder is autosomal recessive and commoner than congenital lactase deficiency. Secondary intolerance is rarer than secondary lactase deficiency. Malabsorption of carbohydrates can be detected by stool and breath hydrogen testing (Practical box 11.1).

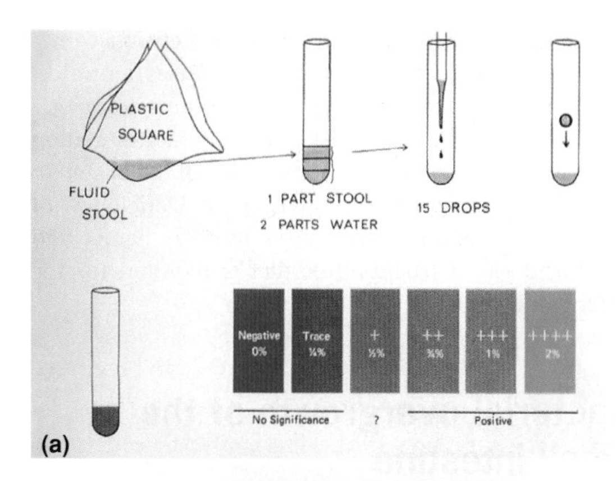

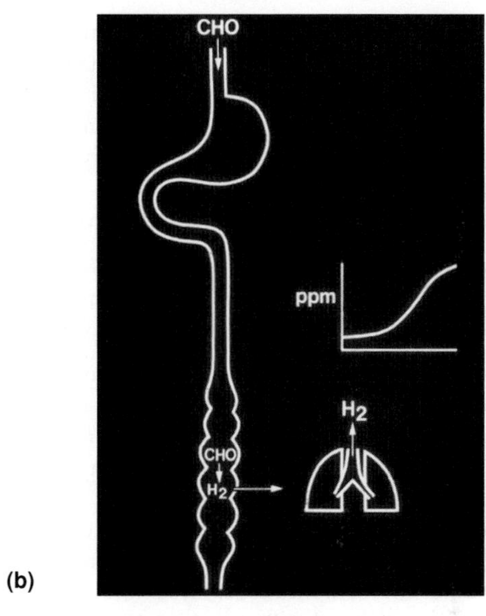

Fig 11.16
(a) Testing stool for malabsorbed reducing sugars (lactose, glucose, fructose and sucrose after hydrolysis; see Practical box 11.1). From Anderson CM, Burke V, Gracey G. Paediatric Gastroenterology 2nd Ed. Blackwell Publications, Melbourne, 1987. (b) Breath hydrogen test. Hydrogen (H_2) is released from malabsorbed carbohydrate (CHO) absorbed and excreted in the breath. Monitors are commercially available which give an instant reading of H_2 concentration in the breath.

Practical Box 11.1

Testing for carbohydrate intolerance

Malabsorbed carbohydrates can be detected in the watery phase of stool by testing with Clinitest tablets (Ames). Sucrose is not a reducing sugar, and hence the stool has to be boiled with hydrochloric acid (5 volumes of stool to 10 volumes of HCl) to hydrolyse the sucrose to fructose and glucose which will reduce the Clinitest.

Carbohydrate intolerance can also be diagnosed by challenging with the suspect carbohydrate and measuring hydrogen concentration in expired air (Fig. 11.16).

The monosaccharide fructose, which is found in the disaccharide sucrose, is absorbed from the intestine by a specific carrier by a process termed facilitated diffusion. In contrast to glucose, the process is independent of absorption of sodium and is not energy-dependent. The resulting process is less efficient than glucose absorption and subject to variation between individuals. Some children who ingest large volumes of fruit juice can exceed their absorptive capacity for fructose and develop diarrhoea. Other specific deficiencies of enzymes involved in the metabolism of fructose have been described. Deficiency of fructokinase (1 in 120 000) results in failure to metabolize fructose that is excreted in the urine. This autosomal recessive condition is not associated with clinical abnormalities and hence is termed benign fructosuria. Deficiency of 1-phosphofructaldolase (1 in 40 000) causes jaundice, hepatomegaly, vomiting and CNS symptoms, following fructose ingestion. Fructose-1-phosphate accumulation competitively inhibits the conversion of glycogen to glucose, resulting in hypoglycaemia. Deficiency of fructose-1,6-diphosphatase causes hypoglycaemia and lactic acidosis. A fructose-free diet is required for the latter two conditions.

Bacterial overgrowth of the small intestine

This is defined as the presence of $>10^4$/ml viable bacteria in the jejunal fluid. The sample is obtained by intubation of the jejunum. Anaerobic and aerobic culture of the fluid is required. Causes include blind loops, strictures, abnormal motility, surgery of the intestine and short gut syndrome.

The bacteria may damage the intestinal mucosa.

Amoebiasis

Infection with *Entamoeba histolytica* is a worldwide problem, commoner in developing countries. It results from the ingestion of cysts in contaminated food and water. The cysts are digested in the stomach and the resulting trophozooites colonize the colon.

There is intermittent diarrhoea with blood and mucus (amoebic dysentery), and peritoneal and liver abscesses are rare complications. Cysts and amoebae containing ingested red cells are seen in fresh stool samples; elevated antibody titres occur with abscesses.

Metronidazole is effective. Occasionally drainage of abscesses is required.

Toddler diarrhoea (chronic nonspecific diarrhoea of infancy, irritable bowel syndrome of infancy)

> **Nomenclature**
> Sometimes known as the 'peas and carrots' syndrome because of the contents of the stool.
>
> **Epidemiology**
> The majority of young children presenting with chronic diarrhoea will have toddler diarrhoea.

This begins between 6 months and 2 years of age. The stool pattern and frequency are variable, in that diarrhoea may alternate with constipation. The first stool of the day may be formed. A high fibre diet makes the diarrhoea worse, and the stools contain undigested vegetable lumps, e.g. peas and carrots, as well as mucus. Meanwhile the child remains well and thrives. The 'disorder' tends to decrease with age and rarely persists beyond 6 years.

The diagnosis is made by recognizing the clinical features, checking the growth velocity and excluding giardiasis (p. 223) and carbohydrate intolerance (p. 228). Clinical skill is then required to reassure the parents that they have a healthy child albeit with loose stools. Suggesting that toddler diarrhoea represents a delay in the maturation of normal bowel motility may help. The presence of normal growth is reassuring. If the symptom is causing family distress, the occasional use of loperamide may help but this may reinforce the parents' suspicion of bowel disease.

Chloride-losing diarrhoea

This is an inborn error of chloride absorption, caused by defective Cl^-–HCO_3^- exchange in the terminal ileum and colon. A defect in Na^+ – H^+ exchange can also occur. They presents with watery diarrhoea from birth. Treatment is with intravenous and eventually oral rehydration.

Gastrointestinal haemorrhage

> **Prognosis**
> Gastrointestinal haemorrhage in childhood may be life-threatening (e.g. bleeding oesophageal varices). Generally speaking it is less serious than in adult life.
>
> **Investigation**
> A cause is frequently not found.

INTRODUCTION

Rectal bleeding may be massive with circulatory collapse, intermittent with a history of melaena, chronic (occult) presenting with anaemia or subclinical and causing no symptoms. The site is often difficult to ascertain at presentation. 'Coffee grounds' (denatured blood) or fresh haematemesis indicates upper gastrointestinal bleeding. Small amounts of fresh blood per rectum indicate lower gastrointestinal bleeding. Streaking of stools indicates rectal or anal bleeding.

AETIOLOGY AND PATHOGENESIS

Neonatal rectal bleeding is usually swallowed maternal blood (use Apt test to distinguish, the infant's blood is mainly fetal haemoglobin which is more resistant to alkali than adult). Causes of rectal bleeding are shown in Information box 11.15 (see also Bleeding disorders in the newborn, p. 55).

CLINICAL PRESENTATION

The investigation is undertaken jointly with a paediatric radiologist and surgeon. The nose and nasal cavity are inspected for bleeding; the presence of blood in the nose suggests that the blood was swallowed. A history of previous occurrences suggests a vascular lesion, and epigastric pain, a peptic lesion. Vomiting suggests a Mallory–Weiss lesion, a tear of the mucosa of the distal oesophagus. Examine for signs of portal hypertension/cirrhosis (hepatosplenomegaly, jaundice, enlarged abdominal veins, haemorrhoids, ascites and oedema, spider naevi, liver palms and nails), bleeding diathesis (bleeding from other sites including venepuncture), and skin manifestations of an underlying disorder (Peutz–Jegher syndrome, hereditary telangiectasia, Ehlers–Danlos syndrome), and abdominal signs suggesting ruptured viscus or enterocolitis. Passage of a nasogastric tube and gastric washout may confirm that the bleeding is gastric or oesophageal rather than postpyloric.

MANAGEMENT

Following a large bleed, resuscitation precedes investigation. Use whole blood, plasma, plasma expanders or normal saline (10–30 ml/kg rapidly) in a shocked patient, monitoring central venous pressure. A rising pulse or falling blood pressure gives late confirmation of transfusion requirement, especially in children who are able to maintain their systemic blood pressure in the face of extensive blood loss. Over-transfusion results in an increased risk of continuing bleeding or re-bleeding, as well as risks of pulmonary oedema.

Initial investigations include coagulation studies and platelets which should be repeated after a massive transfusion. Plain X-rays may demonstrate a mass, foreign body, perforation, intestinal obstruction or enterocolitis. Special techniques may enable confirmation of the site of bleeding prior to laparotomy. Barium contrast studies are of limited value since they may demonstrate abnormalities (e.g. varices) which are not bleeding. Upper and lower GI endoscopy (and even pan-endoscopy) are more informative, at least in adults. Angiography during an acute bleed is occasionally the only helpful test but success depends on a brisk bleeding rate. Meckel diverticulum (or duplication) with ectopic gastric mucosa is demonstrated with a [^{99}Tc]-pertechnate scan.

Information Box 11.15

Causes of gastrointestinal bleeding in children

Upper and/or lower tract bleeding
- Blood disorders
  - Idiopathic thrombocytopenic purpura
  - Blood dyscrasia
  - Disseminated intravascular coagulation
  - Congenital bleeding disorder (may have local bleeding lesion)
    - E.g. Factor VIII deficiency
    - Vascular disorders
- Haemorrhagic disease of the newborn (early and late)
- Haemangioma
  - Hereditary telangiectasia
  - Vasculitis (e.g. collagen disorder)
  - Ehlers–Danlos syndrome
- Anomalies
  - Duplications
- Neoplasm
  - Polyps
    - Single
    - Multiple
    - Peutz–Jegher
- Mechanical
  - Foreign body

Upper tract bleeding
- Pseudo
  - Swallowed blood
- Peptic
  - Oesophagitis
  - Acute gastritis
- Mechanical
  - Mallory–Weiss
- Vascular
  - Varices
  - Malformations

Lower tract bleeding
- Inflammatory
  - Ulcerative colitis
  - Crohn disease
  - Allergy
    - Cow's milk
    - Soya
  - Enterocolitis
    - Necrotizing (Fig. 11.17)
    - Hirschsprung
    - Bacterial
    - Pseudomembranous
    - Radiation
- Anomalies
  - Meckel diverticulum
- Vascular
  - Haemorrhoids
  - Varices
- Mechanical
  - Volvulus
  - Intussusception
  - Anal fissure
  - Rectal prolapse

Note: massive bleeds usually originate in the upper GI tract. Enterocolitis may produce massive bleeding as a late manifestation.

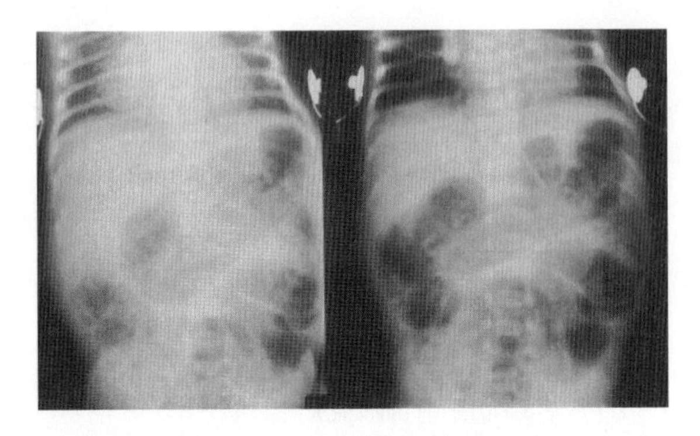

Fig 11.17
Necrotizing enterocolitis in twins.

Meckel diverticulum

This is a persistent vitellointestinal duct, present in 2% of the population. It may connect with the umbilicus as an enterocutaneous fistula (persistent omphalomesenteric duct). Ectopic gastric mucosa may cause bleeding by peptic ulceration of the distal ileum; the mucosa takes up [^{99}Tc]-pertechnate which can be demonstrated by scanning.

If symptoms are caused, surgical excision is performed.

Bleeding from a peptic lesion

Massive bleeding from a peptic ulcer is rare in children, but acute gastritis may cause severe haemorrhage.

Management is usually medical with nasogastric suction, antacids and H_2 blockers. There is no evidence that bleeding is less with this treatment, but it may hasten healing. Surgery may be required if the exact diagnosis is obtained or bleeding is uncontrollable.

Polyposis

Prognosis
Colonic polyps either predispose to malignancy (juvenile polyposis, Peutz–Jegher syndrome) or are premalignant (familial adenomatous polyposis coli).

Generalized juvenile polyposis, familial polyposis coli or Peutz–Jegher syndrome may all present with episodes of gastrointestinal bleeding. Juvenile polyps are the commonest. They are nonmalignant, isolated, pedunculated, hamartomatous, and rarely familial. The polyps contain mucin retention cysts. Gastrointestinal malignancy risk is increased. Offending lesions can be removed but they are usually too numerous to be completely excised. Therefore management is expectant, reserving surgery for removal of polyps causing excessive bleeding or intussusception.

Intestinal polyposis (familial adenomatous polyposis coli) is a dominantly inherited syndrome where there are multiple adenomatous polyps of the colon. It occurs in 1 in 6000 people, due to a gene on chromosome 5. The polyps cause rectal bleeding and abdominal pain. Pancolectomy is required to prevent malignant change. Unaffected relatives should have a yearly colonoscopy with surgery if lesions are recognized.

Peutz–Jegher syndrome is dominantly inherited and is characterized by freckle-like pigmentation of the lips and buccal mucosa with benign tumours of the stomach and small bowel. These are classified as hamartomas, that is, excessive outgrowths of normal tissue. They produce bleeding and intussusception. Management is as for juvenile polyps.

Lower tract bleeding

In children this is less common than upper tract bleeding, and usually denotes a serious condition such as enterocolitis. Occasionally it is due to a vascular malformation.

The general management is as for an upper GI tract bleed, with the following provisos:

- Contrast studies are contraindicated in acute colitis
- Endoscopy is the best investigation
- Angiography is occasionally useful.

Rectal bleeding

Small quantities of frank blood can be passed per rectum, either with or without faeces. The cause may be seen on proctoscopy, and is usually associated with rectal polyp, rectal prolapse, anal fissure or haemorrhoids. These conditions characteristically cause bleeding at the end of defecation and not mixed in with the stool. All of these are managed conservatively.

There may occasionally be signs of ulcerative colitis or Crohn disease.

Hereditary haemorrhagic telangiectasia (Osler–Weber–Rendu disease)

This dominantly inherited condition may present in childhood as recurrent epistaxis.

Telangiectasia develops at puberty, involving nose, mouth, lips, and tongue.

Life-threatening bleeding may occur from nose,

mouth, lungs, urinary tract, or gut. Surgery may be required to control the bleeding.

Management of occult gastrointestinal blood loss

Occult gastrointestinal blood loss presents with anaemia, and other gastrointestinal symptoms. Commoner causes include:

- Reflux oesophagitis
- Anatomical abnormalities (e.g. duplication)
- Inflammatory bowel disease
- Amoebiasis (on a worldwide scale; rare in the UK)
- Gastrointestinal allergy (e.g. cow's milk protein intolerance)
- Ileocolic anastomoses
- Meat-based diet.

Kits are available which distinguish human haemoglobin from that of animals. The amidopyrine test is the most reliable for confirming the presence of faecal occult blood in childhood. Weak positive results (only positive with 20% amidopyrine) are not usually clinically significant.

If a cause is established then this may be treated. If none is found, a cow's milk-free diet can be tried in infancy. Iron supplements are given with follow up after iron therapy.

Management of problem bleeding

Problem bleeding is the occurrence of more than one severe bleed for which no cause can be found.

Investigations should be repeated, with:

- Contrast studies such as a small bowel 'enema'
  - Direct introduction of barium into the duodenum
- Double contrast barium enema, using a mixture of air and contrast
- Upper and lower endoscopy
- [^{99}Tc]-pertechnate gamma scan
  - May detect a 'flush' in an arteriovenous malformation in an early picture
  - Standard timed pictures may detect ectopic gastric mucosa in a Meckel diverticulum
- Gamma scan using [^{99}Tc]-labelled red cells
  - May demonstrate a site of blood loss while still bleeding
  - Investigation is less invasive than angiography.

If these techniques fail to suggest a site, then selective angiography, and ultimately laparotomy, may be performed. At operation, panendoscopy can be performed by threading the small bowel over the endoscope.

Management after recovery

Most bleeds resolve with medical management. After recovery, contrast radiography has a greater role than in the acute phase. Endoscopy remains important, but angiography is usually unrewarding.

If no cause is found with the above investigations, then await events, as many bleeds do not recur.

Chronic inflammatory bowel disease

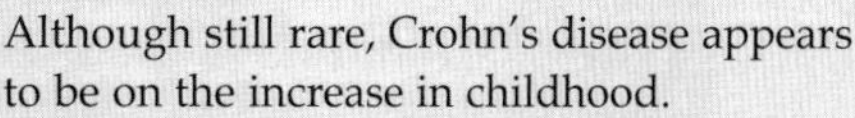

Epidemiology
Although still rare, Crohn's disease appears to be on the increase in childhood.

Aetiology
The cause may lie in an abnormal intestinal immune response to the bowel flora.

History
Burrill Crohn, a North American gastroenterologist, described the disease in the 1930s; hence it may be a relatively new disease.

Chronic inflammatory bowel disease is a general term encompassing Crohn's disease and ulcerative colitis. Although the two types are thought to be variations of the same disease, their clinical features are dissimilar. Crohn disease occurs in about 5–8/100 000 people per year often beginning in the second decade. The presenting features of abdominal pain, diarrhoea, and weight loss are similar in childhood and adult life. Presentation with growth failure occurs in childhood and the associated anorexia may be wrongly labelled anorexia nervosa. The diagnosis is suggested by demonstration of ulceration in the terminal ileum on barium follow through (Fig. 11.18(b)). Colonoscopy is used to confirm the extent of ulceration and obtain biopsies (Fig. 11.18(a)).

Ulcerative colitis is commoner than Crohn's disease generally, but is less common than Crohn's disease in childhood because the illness usually presents in later life with bloody diarrhoea and abdominal pain. The diagnostic work-up is the same as for Crohn's disease (Fig. 11.18). However the colonic ulceration is continuous and the small bowel is not involved. It is important to exclude an infective cause for the bloody diarrhoea when the child first presents. In view of the rarity of these conditions, they are best managed by a

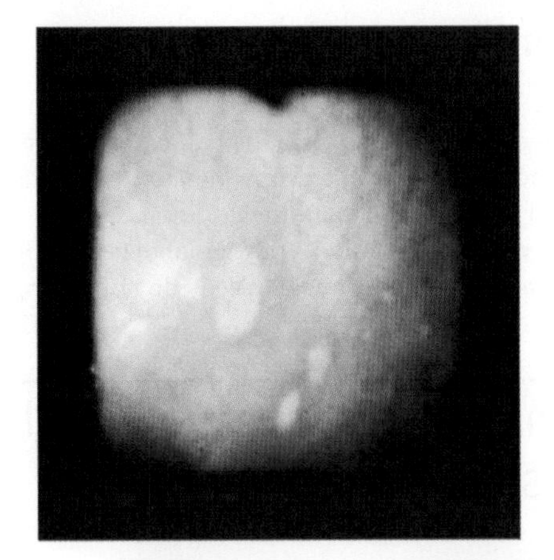

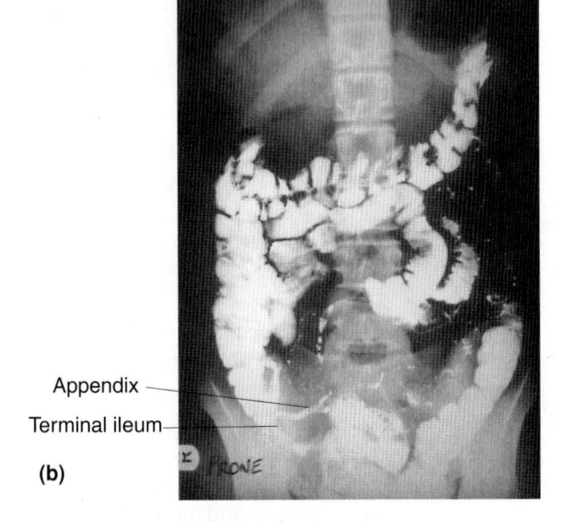

Fig 11.18
(a) Characteristic ulceration of colon in Crohn's disease. The ulcers resemble aphthous ulcers commonly seen in the mouth. (b) Barium follow through in teenager with Crohn's disease. In the right iliac fossa the appendix can be seen, and below, the abnormal terminal ileum.

paediatric gastroenterologist in consultation with a paediatric surgeon. Steroids are used in high doses to obtain a remission of symptoms in both conditions. Elemental diets can also induce a remission in Crohn's disease without the side-effects of steroids. In both conditions, relapse occurs and lifelong follow up is required.

Protein-losing enteropathy

Any gut disease can cause loss of protein into the lumen of the gastrointestinal tract, and when the rate of loss exceeds the synthesis rate, hypoproteinaemic oedema results. The condition can be screened for by measuring alpha-1-antitrypsin in stool. Coeliac disease is a common cause.

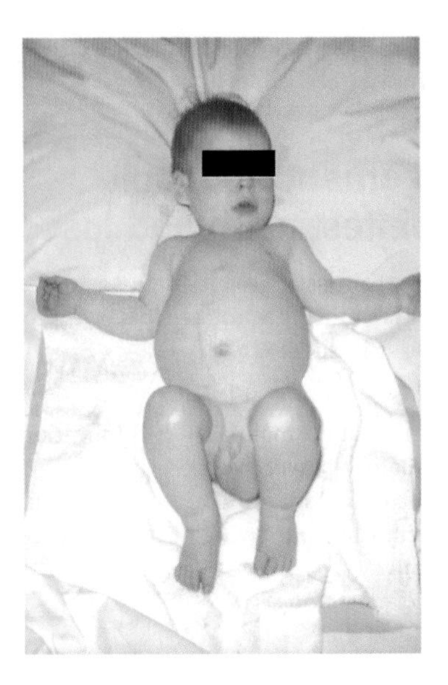

Fig 11.19
Generalized oedema in child with protein-losing enteropathy due to lymphangiectasia.

Primary intestinal lymphangiectasia presents in this way (Fig. 11.19). Protein and lymphocytes are lost from dilated lymphatics which cause coarse mucosal folds on barium follow through. Intestinal lymphangiectasia is treated with a low fat diet supplemented with medium chain triglycerides (MCT). The latter are absorbed by the portal vein rather than via lymphatics.

Vomiting

Gastro-oesophageal reflux

Aetiology
Immaturity of lower oesophageal sphincter.

Lifestyle
Symptom is better tolerated by mothers who breastfeed.

Presentation
Broad spectrum of symptoms from failure to thrive to wheezing.

Varying degrees of gastro-oesophageal reflux are common in infancy. There is often an associated sliding hiatus hernia present, but severe reflux may occur in the

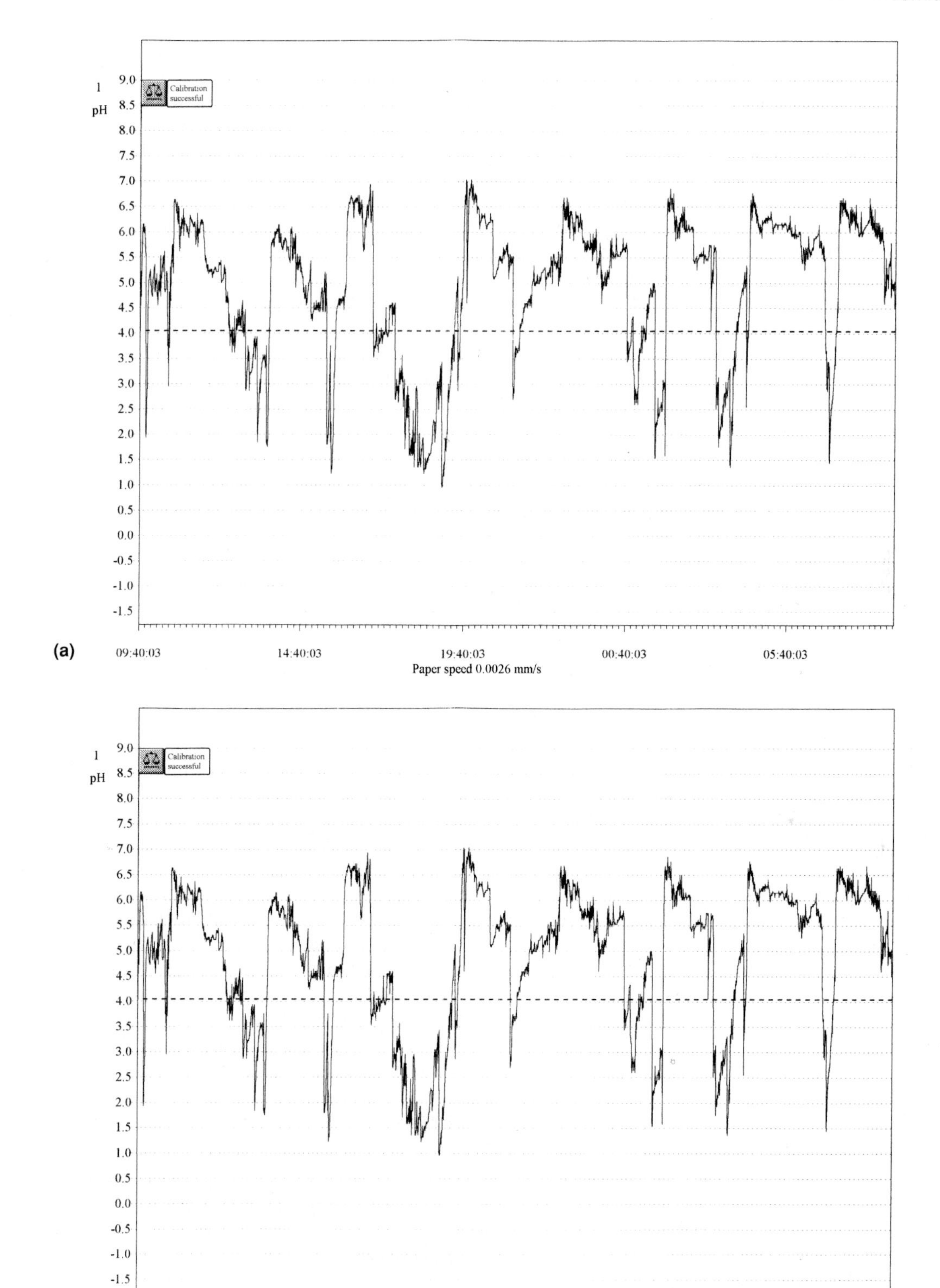

Fig 11.20
Oesophageal pH monitoring. A pH less than 4 is abnormal. (a) Tracing from a neonate with recurrent apnoea. Note pH less than 4 for almost 2 hours on one occasion. Apnoea responded to antireflux treatment. (b) Tracing from neonate whose apnoeic attacks ceased at start of study. Note pH greater than 4 almost throughout study.

absence of a hernia. Vomiting of curdled milk, with occasional haematemesis begins in the first week of life. The differential diagnosis includes vomiting secondary to infection, a feeding problem and pyloric stenosis. Recurrent aspiration of gastric contents can masquerade as asthma. Severe reflux may be complicated by failure to thrive, with secondary feeding problems, anaemia secondary to blood loss, and stricture of the oesophagus. Infants with failure to thrive, severe vomiting, recurrent aspiration and dysphagia should be investigated. A barium swallow is usually performed, and demonstrates the mechanism of swallowing, presence of spasm or stricture of the oesophagus, and anatomy and motility of the stomach, pylorus and duodenum. Detection of fluid reflux by ultrasound examination is a complementary technique, which has the advantage that prolonged examinations are possible without X-ray exposure. The technique does not demonstrate anatomy and function to the same degree as radiological examination. Endoscopy is of value in the assessment of stricture and oesophagitis. Prolonged monitoring of lower oesophageal pH is useful for objectively assessing the severity of reflux and therapy (Fig. 11.20). An alternative approach is to detect the presence of reflux in technetium-labelled milk, but access to a gamma camera is required. Mild reflux generally responds to thickening milk feeds with 0.5–1.5% Nestargel or Carobel. Prone or left-side posture, with 30° head-up tilt is also beneficial (Fig. 11.21). More severe symptoms respond to continuous nasogastric feeding for 2 or 3 weeks. Other adjuncts include prokinetic drugs (e.g. domperidone), H_2 receptor blockade (e.g. ranitidine) or proton pump inhibitor (e.g. omeprazole) for peptic oesophagitis. If there is no response to intensive medical treatment, the infant should be referred for the operation of fundoplication.

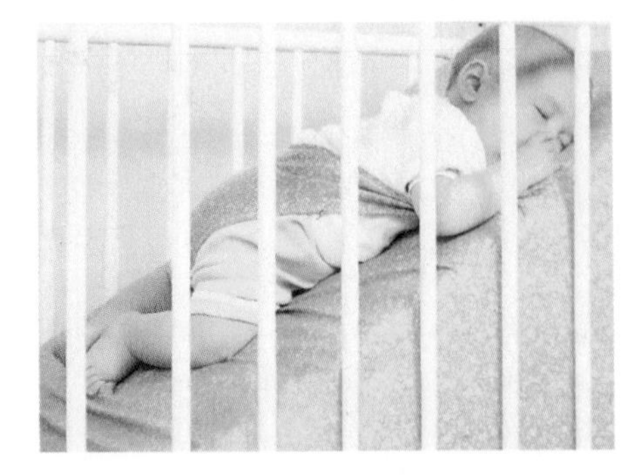

Fig 11.21
Optimal posture for prevention of reflux is prone or on the left side with 30° elevation of the head.

Sandifer syndrome is a variant of gastro-oesophageal reflux in which an abnormal head posture of extension is adopted during episodes of gastro-oesophageal reflux. The head positioning is thought to reduce to some extent the severity of the reflux. It is commoner in children with cerebral palsy. The condition was described by a paediatric neurologist who originally thought it was a movement disorder.

Pyloric stenosis

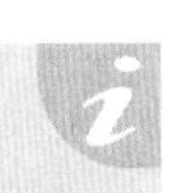

Clinical features
An uncommon and readily correctable cause of vomiting.

Hypertrophic pyloric stenosis affects 3/1000 liveborn infants with a male to female ratio of 4:1. It is much commoner in firstborns, especially caucasian boys and also when there is a family history (especially maternal). Vomiting usually begins between the 3rd and 8th weeks and gradually increases in severity, developing a characteristic projectile nature. Examination during a feed shows visible waves of peristalsis (Fig. 11.22(a)) moving from left to right and downwards in the left hypochondrium. An ovoid swelling (like an olive) can be felt between the liver and rectus muscle in the right hypochondrium. The swelling varies in size and consistency as the pyloric muscle contracts and relaxes. Persistent severe vomiting results in constipation, hyponatraemia, hypokalaemia, hypochloraemia, alkalosis and eventually dehydration. The hypertrophied pylorus (Fig. 11.22(b)) can be demonstrated by ultrasound examination or contrast studies showing gastric outlet obstruction and an elongated, narrow pyloric canal.

The electrolyte disturbances are corrected with intravenous saline with added potassium. When the alkalosis has been corrected, a pyloromyotomy (Ramstedt operation) is carried out. Breast- or bottle-feeding can be resumed soon after recovery from anaesthesia.

Short bowel (short gut) syndrome

This follows massive intestinal resections on account of:

- Volvulus
- Multiple atresias
- Necrotizing enterocolitis
- Gastroschisis.

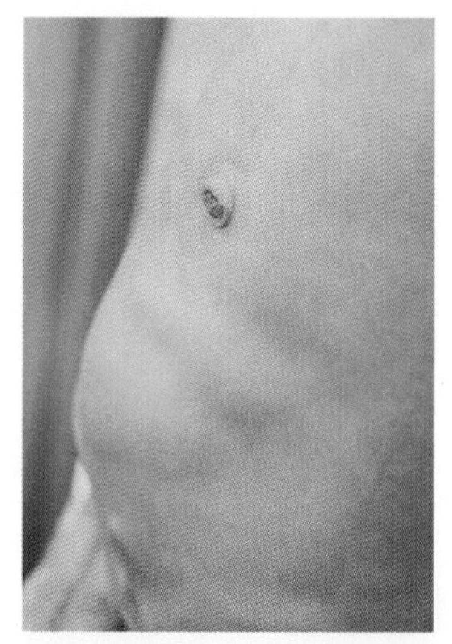
(a)

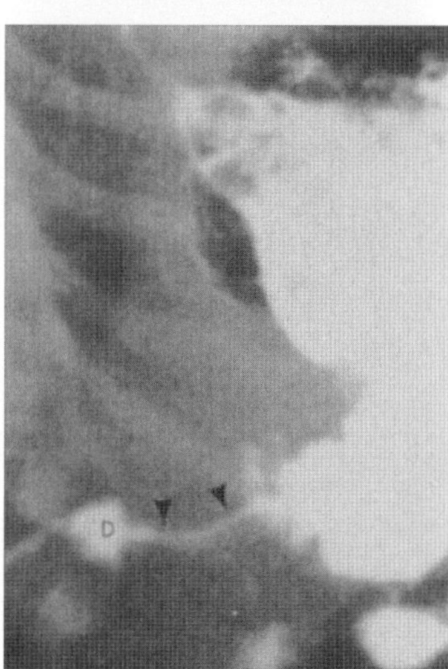

(b)

Fig 11.22
(a) Visible gastric peristalsis. (b) Barium meal appearance of pyloric stenosis. Hypertrophied pylorus shown by arrows. D, duodenum.

Prolonged parenteral nutrition is required and the slow introduction of an elemental or modular diet.

Bile salt malabsorption complicates terminal ileal resection and the resulting diarrhoea can be helped with cholestyramine.

Pancreatic disorders (see also Cystic fibrosis)

Schwachman syndrome (Schwachman–Diamond syndrome)

This is the other autosomal recessive cause of pancreatic insufficiency, albeit much rarer than cystic fibrosis. It is differentiated by the presence of normal concentrations of electrolyte in sweat in this condition. Chest infections occur because of the associated intermittent, or cyclical neutropenia which can be fatal. The pancreas is replaced with adipose tissue, and growth tends to be poor even if pancreatic supplements are given.

Pancreatitis

Acute pancreatitis can complicate mumps and other viral infections and abdominal trauma. Chronic pancreatitis is associated with congential abnormalities of the biliary tree or pancreatic ducts, hypercalcaemia and hyperlipidaemia (p. 291).

12 Genetics and dysmorphology

Genetics is one of the most rapidly advancing areas of medicine, and especially paediatrics, paving the way to new understanding of the cause of congenital diseases. As the human genome is being sequenced, new genetic probes are becoming available for the diagnosis of dysmorphic children. Once a gene is identified, the gene product can be synthesized and the precise mechanism of genetic disorders elucidated. This means that this is a rapidly expanding field, from which we have chosen some illustrative examples. There are enormous technical difficulties to be overcome, but families with children with genetic disorders such as cystic fibrosis live in hope of the arrival of gene therapy.

Chromosome abnormalities

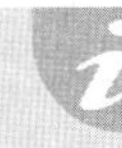

Historical
Chromosomal abnormalities were the first genetic disorders to be described because the morphology of whole chromosomes could be observed directly under the microscope.

INTRODUCTION

Every human cell contains 46 chromosomes (in pairs of 23) which were formed from half the chromosomes of each parent. Each chromosome carries the genes encoding proteins which order the behaviour of the cell. In the past 25 years it has become increasingly possible to examine the chromosomes and look at the genetic factors carried on them (Table 12.1). Occasionally a chromosome may become abnormal through a variety of mechanisms including radiation, and ageing of the parental gametes. Other anomalies are inherited although the majority of parents with chromosomally abnormal children are normal themselves. Although most conceptuses with chromosome abnormalities abort early in pregnancy, a few survive to deliver. Down syndrome is the commonest example but there are a host of other chromosomal conditions. These can be divided into those that affect the X and Y chromosomes, giving rise to conditions such as Turner XO and Klinefelter XYY and fragile X syndromes, and those disorders involving the remaining 22 pairs of chromosomes, the autosomes. Examples include Down and other more severe conditions, such as Edward and

Table 12.1
Detection of chromosomal abnormalities

Chromosomal abnormality	Method of detection
Gross abnormality of number, e.g. trisomy (p. 241)	Standard cytogenetics or fluorescent in situ hybridization (FISH)
Translocations (part of one chromosome displaced onto another). May cause a number of disorders	Standard cytogenetics
Small deletions or duplications	Standard cytogenetics with banding
Single-gene defects where the gene has been identified, and in the particular family:	
(a) the precise mutation is known	Mutation analysis: several techniques including single-strand conformational polymorphism analysis (SSCP), direct sequencing, restriction enzyme digestion
(b) the precise mutation has not been identified	Linkage analysis: family linkage studies using restriction fragment length polymorphism (RFLP) analysis with closely linked polymorphic markers
Single-gene defects where the chromosomal location is known but the gene has not been identified	Linkage analysis

Patau syndromes which are rarely compatible with survival. These conditions will be described in this section. Rare chromosome abnormality syndromes are still being described and clarified. These often involve abnormalities of chromosomal regions, e.g. a deletion of a small part of a chromosome, such as the cri-du-chat syndrome (depletions of short arm of chromosome 5) so named because affected infant's cry sounds like that of kittens.

X chromosome abnormalities

Fragile X

Nomenclature
X stands for the X or female chromosome.

Epidemiology
Up to 30% of boys with otherwise unexplained mild to moderate learning difficulties are found to have an abnormality of their X chromosome when studied using special techniques.

Girls are affected more often than boys but, as the retardation is usually milder, fewer girls are diagnosed. 'Fragile' means that the stained chromosome examined under a very high powered microscope has an apparent break or fracture across the end of the long arm of the X chromosome. Postpubertal boys have enlarged testes though no other sexual abnormality. There is a risk of recurrence. The inheritance pattern is X-linked. The carrier mother will donate either a normal or an abnormal sex chromosome to her offspring. This means that one-half of male offspring will be affected and one-half of female offspring will be carriers. The girls will be protected from full expression of the disease by the normal X chromosome inherited from their fathers.

Gonadal dysgenesis syndrome (Turner XO syndrome)

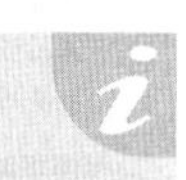

Epidemiology
1 : 3000 births.

The condition is explained by abnormality of the sex chromosomes. Normal females have two XX chromosomes in every body cell while in Turner syndrome there is only one. The chromosomal basis of this syndrome was described as long ago as 1959. This has a profound effect on the whole body, starting from intrauterine life.

At birth infants tend to be underweight and have characteristic puffy feet. Close examination reveals a number of abnormal features that include webbing of the neck, hypoplastic and widely spaced nipples and an inability to fully straighten out the arm at the elbow. Growth in height is restricted and sexual changes at the time of expected puberty do not occur. There is no possibility of spontaneous pregnancy, because of failure of ovarian development, unless the affected girl has a mosaic chromosomal configuration. Many females with Turner syndrome have configurations of 45,X/46,XX and these patients may be fertile. When different chromosomal configurations occur in the same individual, this is referred to as mosaicism and the proportion of those with mosaicism (25%) is higher for Turner syndrome than any other chromosomal disorder. Another related mosaic is 45,X/46,XY in which the phenotype can vary between Turner syndrome and normal male.

The child should be given growth hormone from the time of diagnosis, and oestrogenic hormonal therapy starting at puberty to give her breast development and an adult female shape. In general intelligence is normal or slightly reduced and probably not as high as that expected in the particular family. Heart defects, particularly coarctation of the aorta, are common and should be sought. The girl and her family will need much counselling. It is difficult to break the news to a girl that she will be infertile. When to do this requires a joint decision by the professional advisers and family. It should not be left to late teens. Many girls with Turner syndrome marry. They need to be advised about adoption and early contact with adoption agencies in view of the shortage of available babies. Ovum donation and in vitro fertilization is another possibility.

Noonan syndrome has a superficial resemblance to Turner syndrome. The essential difference is that both boys and girls can be affected, unlike Turner, which only affects girls, and no chromosomal abnormality has been described so far. Children with Noonan syndrome have learning difficulties and are very small. The heart is often abnormal with defects such as pulmonary stenosis. As in Turner syndrome, the neck is webbed, there are facial abnormalities, particularly affecting the appearance of the eyes and external ears. Mild forms are less likely to be diagnosed and textbook descriptions tend to dwell on the severe cases. There is no specific diagnostic test. In general it is recognized by a paediatrician who has seen the condition before. There is no specific treatment, though a variety of specialists may be needed to help minimize the handicaps such as kyphoscoliosis, which are associated with the condition.

Klinefelter syndrome (XXY syndrome)

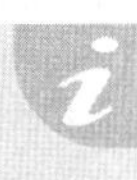

Epidemiology
1 : 750 boys.

Typically, the boy looks normal in childhood. Intelligence tends to be lower than average for the family but there is a wide scatter of ability. Puberty may be delayed or never fully completed. The body tends to be tall and thin and the genitalia relatively underdeveloped. Infertility is usual. The diagnosis is confirmed by chromosome analysis. The basic problem is that there is an extra X chromosome in every cell giving the format XXY. In the majority of cases the presence of the condition will not come to light in childhood unless routine chromosome studies are being undertaken for research purposes. Considerable ethical problems occur if a symptom-free boy is discovered to have this anomaly. Some come to light at infertility clinics. It is likely that many cases are never diagnosed. There is no convincing explanation for the occurrence of Klinefelter syndrome; it is a sporadic disorder that will be revealed if antenatal fetal chromosome analysis is undertaken.

Trisomic autosomal chromosome abnormalities

Down syndrome

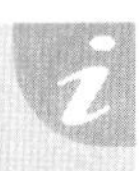

Epidemiology
1 : 600 births.
The commonest of the trisomic conditions.

In 90% of instances, Down syndrome is associated with 'regular' 21 trisomy giving a total 47 chromosomes (Fig. 12.1). The other 10% are due to balanced translocation involving chromosome 21. Part of an extra chromosome is attached to another, usually 13, 14, 15, 21 or 22, but there is a total chromosome count of 46. The parents of these children are devoid of the condition but 20–40% have a balanced translocation in their cell lines. Since this group has a one-in-two risk of having more affected infants it is essential that all parents with a Down's infant are offered chromosome testing so that they know their future risks. The risk rises sharply with maternal age. For mothers over 40 the risk is 1 in 100 pregnancies and for those over 45, 1 in 30 pregnancies. There is a lower order of association with older fathers, particularly with those over 60.

Measurement of alpha fetoprotein, human chorionic gonadotrophin and unconjugated oestriols on maternal blood at 16 weeks' gestation predicts 60% of pregnancies complicated by Down syndrome, and helps select which pregnancies should be investigated by amniocentesis. Ultrasound examination of the affected fetus often shows thickened folds of tissue at the nape of the neck (Fig. 1.10).

Birthweight tends to be low. Main neonatal features include poor muscle tone, poor feeding and mild jaundice. Close observation reveals the features listed in Information box 12.1.

Associated congenital heart disease may be a tetralogy of Fallot, but is most commonly a simple ventricular septal defect or an atrioventricular canal defect. These children have a much higher risk of developing irreversible pulmonary hypertension (some have already done so by the time of birth), and the decision to close the defect must be implemented within the first year. Until recent years there was a reluctance to operate on these children, partly because of their other handicaps, but in particular because of the high mortality associated with cardiac surgery (up to 50%). Although the mortality rate remains very high compared with children without Down syndrome, surgery should always be offered when technically

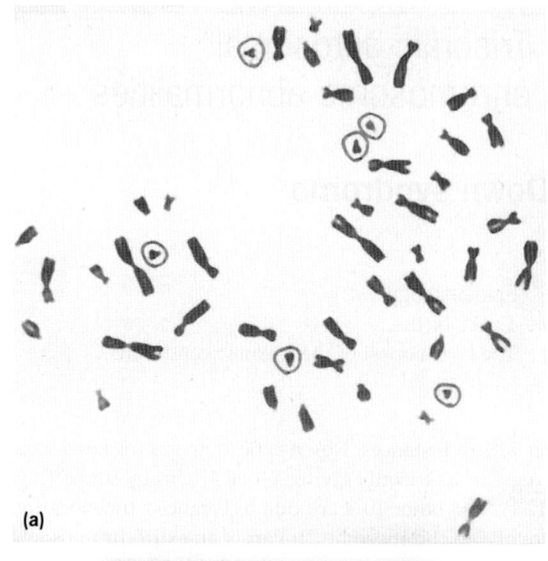

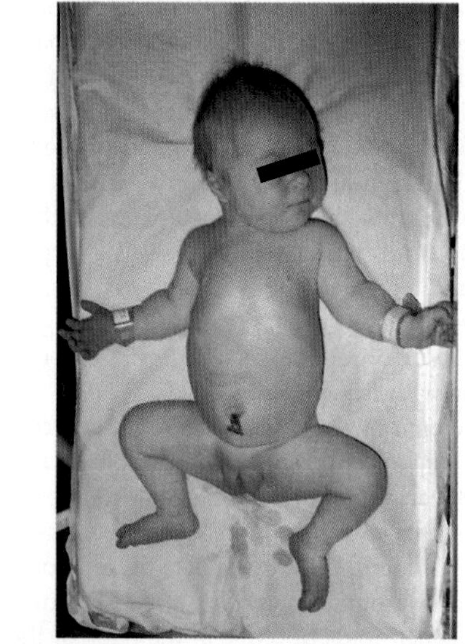

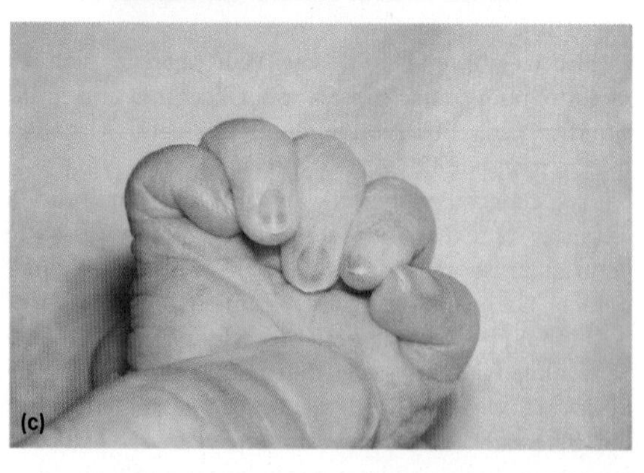

Fig 12.1
(a) Trisomy 21. The chromosomes circled are the morphologically similar X chromosome (this child is male), two 22 chromosomes and three 21 chromosomes. (b) A neonate with Down syndrome. (c) Single palmar crease and incurving little finger in Down syndrome.

Information Box 12.1

Features of Down syndrome (see also Fig. 12.1)

- Typical eyelids
  - Narrow palpebral fissures
  - Almond-shaped eyes
- Brushfield spots
  - Small streaks on the iris
- Ears
  - Simple
  - Small lobes
- Hands and feet
  - Small hands
  - Single palmar crease on hands and feet
  - Incurving fifth fingers
  - Widely spaced first and second toes
- Increased risk of duodenal atresia and Hirschsprung disease
- In later life, much increase in
  - Profound myopia
  - Deafness
  - Leukaemia
  - Premature senility
  - Moderate to severe learning difficulties
- 75% have congenital heart disease
  - Severe in 20–40%

feasible, to prevent them from dying prematurely and unpleasantly from pulmonary hypertension.

Occasionally a child of typical Down appearance has a mosaic chromosome pattern and proves to have abilities in the normal range. This is rare, but it is important that it should be detected so that a better prognosis can be given to the parents.

In any case the most important early step is full appropriate counselling undertaken by those who are very experienced with the condition. This needs to be started when the condition is suspected – not left until the diagnosis is confirmed. In practice chromosome testing is needed to confirm the diagnosis. It is important that parents know what is wrong with their infant so that fantasies can be replaced by fact. It is best that the paediatrician involved with the child organizes this, so that information can be shared.

Parents have to be helped to appreciate the nature of the condition, that the prospects for their child will be limited, but that in infancy the precise extent of limitation cannot be predicted. A programme for helping the child to make maximum progress is needed right from the start. Visual and hearing problems need to be anticipated; suitable schooling should be organized at an early stage. Parents may be greatly helped by joining a parents' organization; in the UK the Down's Parents' Association is very effective.

It is also vital that everything possible is learnt about the patterns of abnormality found in a community so that the possible influence of environmental factors can be researched. Although chromosome abnormalities are common in the newly conceived embryo, most lead to spontaneous abortion. Down syndrome is particularly common because the affected fetus is more viable than those with other trisomies. So far little is known about the process whereby the abnormal fetus has a high chance of spontaneous abortion.

Down syndrome raises serious ethical issues, for example concerning the rightness of antenatal screening: is it a laudable aim to abort all Down's fetuses? Should the characteristic features of Down syndrome be altered by surgery? What should be done if a potentially lethal but treatable condition presents, such as duodenal atresia or congenital heart disease, and the parents do not want surgery?

Edward syndrome

This is the second commonest autosomal chromosomal defect, occurring in 1 : 8000 births, and is due to trisomy of chromosome 18. Physical features include:

- Low birthweight
- Stiffness (hypertonia)
- Severe flexion of the fingers and toes (producing overlapping fingers and 'rocker bottom' feet (Fig. 12.2)
- Prominent occiput
- Low set ears
- Mental retardation
- Failure to thrive
- Congenital heart disease (ventricular septal defect and patent ductus arteriosus).

Most affected children die in early infancy. As with Down syndrome, translocation and mosaicism do occur, and advanced maternal age is a factor.

Patau syndrome

The incidence of this condition is 1 : 20 000 births. The 13th chromosome is trisomic. Features of an affected infant include:

- Failure to thrive
- Underdevelopment of the brain often with convulsions
- Deafness
- Underdevelopment of the eyes (microphthalmia)
- Cleft lip and often palate

(a)

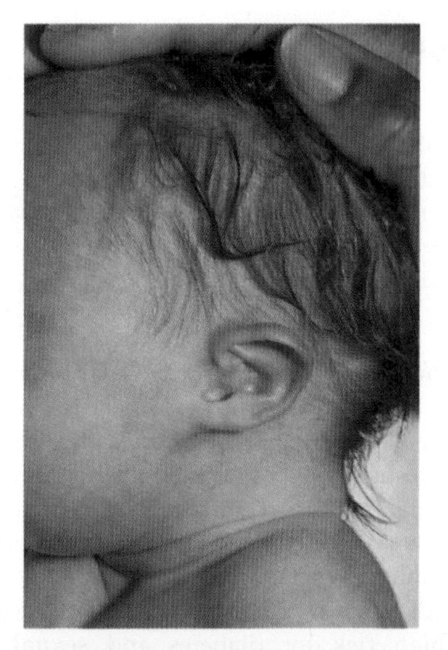

(b)

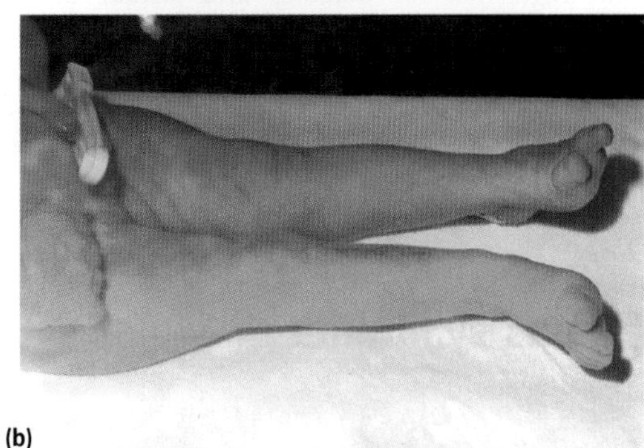

Fig 12.2
(a) Low set ears in Edward syndrome. (b) Dorsiflexed toes producing 'rocker-bottom' feet, in Edward syndrome.

- Congenital heart defect (especially septal defects and patent ductus arteriosus)
- Absent testes in males
- Herniae
- Flexion deformity of the fingers.

The cause is unknown, although the condition is found more commonly in babies born to older mothers. Prolonged survival is most unlikely, and one hardly need stress the plight of parents who are caring for a very severely handicapped child with a minimal chance of survival.

Some inherited syndromes

Some syndromes are not associated with chromosomal abnormalitites. Ever increasing numbers are being recognized.

Prader–Willi syndrome

> Diagnosis
> Suspect in short, obese, poorly coordinated children with developmental delay, small hands and feet and cryptorchidism.
> The diagnosis is often missed.

This syndrome was named after the Swiss paediatricians who described it in 1956. The typical features may not be present at birth though it is an important cause of hypotonia and feeding difficulty in the neonatal period, resulting in failure to thrive. Obesity usually presents in older children. Some have strange eating habits and food intake may need to be reduced; dietary advice is often needed. These children are at high risk for diabetes and sexual under-development. Teenage boys may not develop pubertal changes without replacement male hormone. The cause is unknown. Some have deletions of chromosome 15. Recurrence in the same family is unusual but is not unknown. The diagnosis is made by clinical observation.

Williams syndrome (see also Hypercalcaemia)

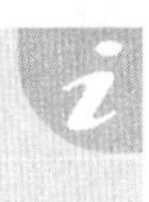

> Developmental profile
> Motor and perceptual delay with good speech development and sociability.

This condition, first described in 1961, includes several very serious problems including stenosis above the aortic heart valve and other congenital heart abnormalities; an abnormal facial appearance with very blue eyes and large lips; teeth that decay readily, small stature and slow growth rate, and a relatively low intelligence. Whilst both sexes can have this rare syndrome, the clue in boys is an extremely small penis; testes may be undescended but not invariably. In girls the labia are underdeveloped. Normal pubertal changes can occur. The skull is large and the eyes wide-spaced with underdevelopment of the lower face. Arms, particularly forearms, are short. A wide variety of other features can be present including epilepsy.

Both autosomal dominant and recessive inheritance patterns have been reported. The cause of this syndrome is unknown. It is not expected to recur in further children. Parents of affected children need a great deal of counselling about this puzzling disorder that poses many unsolved questions. Some of its features are similar to those seen in idiopathic hypercalcaemia syndrome, which is due to the effect of an excess absorption of calcium in early infancy in a minority of infants who are excessively sensitive to large amounts of vitamin D. Williams syndrome however is not caused by excessive intake of calcium. Diagnosis depends on the child being seen by a doctor who is sensitive to the existence of the condition. Diagnosing rare syndromes requires a great deal of experience because many affected children do not have all the recorded features of the condition. Williams syndrome should be remembered where there is a congenital heart disorder, failure to grow and low intelligence. There is no specific treatment though heart surgery may be needed. The defect has recently been mapped to chromosome 7.

There are other chromosomal disorders that are individually very rare. They usually cause severe deficits including mental retardation.

Aarskog syndrome

Those affected by this very rare condition have very short stature but normal growth hormone output. Behaviour is rather simple though engaging; IQ is low. The eyes are wide-spaced (hypertelorism) and the lower face is under-developed. Second teeth are delayed and irregular. In males, the testes are undescended and there is an unusually flat round (shawl) scrotum. Only males have the full features; carrier females may have lesser manifestations.

Alport syndrome

Chronic renal failure characterizes Alport syndrome, with mesangial proliferation, glomerulosclerosis and atrophy of renal tubules. Renal transplantation may be required.

The syndrome may be associated with sensorineural deafness and eye abnormalities such as cataract. X-linked and autosomal recessive varieties have been described.

Autosomal dominant disorders

Achondroplasia

This autosomal dominant trait is found in 1:25 000 births. There is no family history in about 70–80% of instances, indicating new mutations. The condition presents at birth with:

- Large head
- Prominent frontal bone ('bossing')
- Depressed nasal bridge
- Prominent jaw ('prognathism')
- Short limbs (especially proximal)
- Short, broad hands.

Older children have marked lumbar lordosis, and are at risk of atlantoaxial instability.

Early hypotonia and joint laxity results in delayed motor development, which improves in later childhood. Mental development and life expectancy are normal.

Holt–Oram syndrome

In this autosomal dominant disorder there is an atrial septal defect associated with an abnormal or absent thumb. The thumb may have three phalangeal bones (triphalangeal).

Marfan syndrome

The incidence of Marfan syndrome is 1:66 000. It may be present in a child who is exceptionally tall, yet the span of the arms exceeds the height. Affected children have long fingers and toes, and a long thin face with a high arch palate. Lax connective tissue is associated with herniae and 'double jointedness'. Hazards of this syndrome include severe myopia, dislocation of the lens, aneurysms (which may be fatal) in early middle age and other cardiac defects. This worrying diagnosis should not be made mistakenly in perfectly normal tall, thin children.

The cause of this unfortunate condition is not known. In most cases it is dominantly inherited, but a minority are due to new mutations. Both sexes can be affected, with varying severity. The nature of the defect is not understood nor are the reasons why it occurs.

Robinow syndrome (mesomelic dysplasia)

Both sexes can have this rare syndrome. Affected boys have an extremely small penis, and the testes may be undescended but not invariably. In girls the labia are underdeveloped. Normal pubertal changes can occur. Affected individuals tend to be short. The skull is large and the eyes wide-spaced with underdevelopment of the lower face, and the arms, particularly the forearms, are short. A wide variety of other features can be present, including epilepsy. Intelligence varies but may be normal.

Both autosomal dominant and recessive inheritance patterns have been reported.

Treacher Collins syndrome

This is an autosomal dominant condition presenting with downward sloping (antimongoloid) facial abnormality. Features include clefts (colobomata) of the lower eyelids, ear deformity, growth of hair on the cheeks, and receding chin.

Laurence–Moon–Biedl syndrome

This unexplained recessive disorder was described in 1865. Features include obesity, mental retardation, extra or joined fingers, and degeneration of the retina which eventually leads to blindness in a high proportion of cases. It is often associated with deafness, short stature and glomerulonephritis. Not all affected children have all the above features.

There is no specific treatment for the various features, but excessive weight gain must be avoided.

Polycystic disease

In this autosomal recessive disorder kidney cysts are associated with cysts of the liver (congenital hepatic fibrosis). The common presentation is with bilateral masses due to gross kidney enlargement. If kidney function is grossly impaired there may be resulting oligohydramnios, and Potter syndrome, characterized by:

- Low set ears
- Recessed chin
- Flat nose
- Pulmonary hypoplasia
- Limb abnormalities.

Renal transplantation may be required in later life, and hepatic cysts may lead to portal hypertension and cirrhosis.

Adult polycystic disease is an autosomal dominant condition. Polycystic disease inherited in this way rarely presents in childhood.

Sporadic disorders

Beckwith (Beckwith–Wiedemann) syndrome

Affected newborn babies with this condition are large. The following features are found:

- Hypoglycaemia
- Macroglossia

- Omphalocele (Fig. 12.3)
- Creased earlobes
- Renal medullary dysplasia
- Increased risk of neoplasia (Wilms' tumour).

Occurrence is usually sporadic, and the prognosis is good if hypoglycaemia (due to pancreatic beta islet-cell hyperplasia) is avoided.

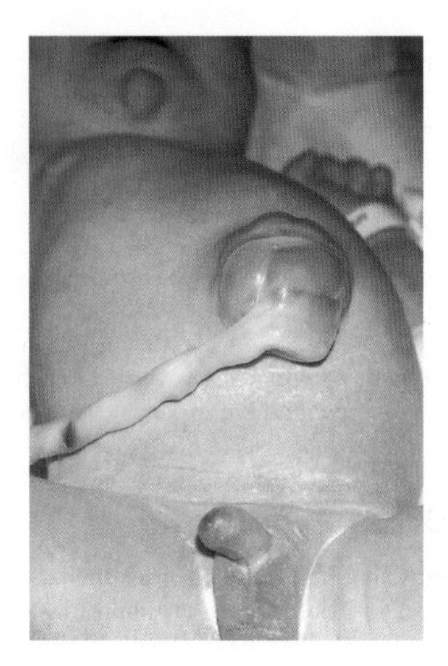

Fig 12.3
Omphalocele in Beckwith–Wiedemann syndrome.

Exomphalos (see Fig. 12.3)

This is any protrusion at the umbilicus. It occurs in 1 : 10 000 births. Associated problems include:

- Meckel diverticulum (p. 232)
- Intestinal atresias (p. 216)
- Malrotation (p. 210)
- Beckwith–Wiedemann syndrome (p. 245).

Hernia into the cord is a persistence of the normal fetal umbilical hernia, without an abdominal wall defect. Surgical repair is straightforward (see Practical box 12.1).

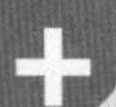

Practical Box 12.1

Surgery for exomphalos

Surgical repair of small defects is straightforward, unless the hernia has been trapped in the cord clamp, leading to perforation.

Omphalocele is a cord hernia with a muscular defect in the abdominal wall at the umbilicus.

Small defects can be closed with skin flaps. Large defects, which cannot be closed without splinting the diaphragm and compromising respiration, are covered with a sac (e.g. Silastic or Prolene) which is sutured around the edge of the lesion. The sac is then gradually reduced over a period of weeks. The gut will not function well while outside the abdominal cavity and prolonged parenteral nutrition may be required.

Cornelia de Lange syndrome

This occurs in about 1 in 10 000 births. Affected children have extreme short stature, a low hair line, long eyelashes and eyebrows that meet in the midline (synophrys).

Small hands and feet (micromelia) are characteristic. There is severe retardation and a tendency to self-mutilate.

Ellis–van Creveld syndrome (chondroectodermal dysplasia)

This is one of several syndromes featuring short ribs which restrict breathing. It presents with short limbs, polydactyly and congenital heart disease with atrial septal defects. Epispadias is also present and the nails are hypoplastic. There are multiple frenulae of the upper lip, a cleft palate, and teeth present at birth.

Poland anomaly

Dr Poland of Guy's Hospital, London described the syndrome in 1841. Affected children have a disorder of the muscles which run from the front of the chest to the clavicle. The pectoralis minor is missing, and the extent to which the pectoralis major is present is variable. This is possibly the result of interruption of local blood supply in the uterus.

The condition is variable in its extent and is usually unilateral, with the right side being affected in most cases. Three times as many boys as girls are affected.

Often the fingers are webbed together (syndactyly), and surgery may be required. Some have very underdeveloped fingers which add to their difficulties. There is underdevelopment of the breast and nipple. Intelligence is in the normal range.

The cause is unknown, but the disorder can be familial.

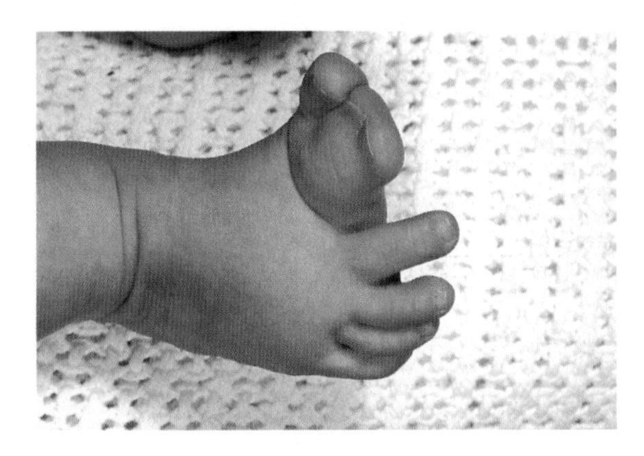

Fig 12.4
Polydactyly and syndactyly.

Polydactyly

Extra fingers may be sporadic. Polydactyly may be associated with:

- Cleft palate
- Spinal abnormalities
- Absent tibiae (as is toe polydactyly)
- Imperforate anus
- Fanconi anaemia
- Radial aplasia–thrombocytopenia syndrome
- Down syndrome
- Laurence–Moon–Biedl syndrome
- Holt–Oram syndrome.

Syndactyly

Fusion or webbing of digits is usually sporadic, occurring in 1/2000 births. The long and ring fingers are most often involved, and early surgery is required.

Syndactyly of the toes generally involves the second and third toes (Fig. 12.4). Surgery is usually not required.

Syndactyly is found in the following disorders:

- Apert
- de Lange
- Holt–Oram
- Laurence–Moon–Biedl
- Radial aplasia–thrombocytopenia syndrome
- Trisomies 13, 18 and 21.

Thyroglossal cyst/fistula

A midline thyroglossal cyst of the neck may extend to the base of the tongue and contain ectopic thyroid tissue. It may form a fistula and discharge mucus.

If excision is contemplated, it is important to ensure that there is sufficient thyroid tissue remaining after surgery.

13 Haematology

Inherited haematological disorders are commoner in children who live in parts of the world where malaria is found. These include conditions such as thalassaemia and other haemoglobinopathies, sickle cell anaemia and glucose-6-phosphate dehydrogenase deficiency. With increasing migration these disorders are being seen in non malarial regions.

Haematological malignancies, i.e. leukaemia, are the commonest form of neoplasia in children and, even though treatment has improved, acute lymphatic leukaemia is the cause of a substantial proportion of deaths in childhood.

Anaemias

> Epidemiology
> Iron deficiency anaemia is the commonest haematological disorder in disadvantaged children throughout the world, with important implications for their development.

INTRODUCTION

Anaemia can be defined as a circulating haemoglobin level that is below the normal age-related range. A more physiological definition would be a haemoglobin level below that necessary to meet the tissues' demand for oxygen delivery. This might mean that in certain conditions, such as heart and lung disease, anaemia could be present at a haemoglobin level within the normal range. The normal haemoglobin concentration changes at different ages. The values for the first 6 months of life are shown in Table 3.3, p. 89.

AETIOLOGY AND PATHOGENESIS

There are a large number of causes of anaemia, which are summarized in Information box 13.1. Notes on the most important of the individual conditions are given below.

CLINICAL PRESENTATION

The clinical features of anaemia are secondary to the failure of oxygen delivery to the tissues and the physiological compensatory mechanisms which the body employs. Children may present with pallor,

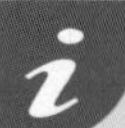

Information Box 13.1

Causes of anaemia in childhood

Failure of red cell production
Congenital disorders
- Pure red cell aplasia (Diamond–Blackfan) anaemia
- Fanconi anaemia

Transient erythoblastopenia
Parvovirus infection
Aplastic anaemia:
- Idiopathic
- Secondary, e.g. drug reactions, direct or indirect effect of antimetabolites

Marrow replacement by malignant disease
Leukaemia, lymphoma
Storage disorders, e.g. Gaucher disease
Marrow depression due to chronic disease
Deficiency states
- Iron deficiency
- Folic acid deficiency
- Vitamin B_{12} deficiency
- Vitamin B_6 deficiency
- Vitamin E deficiency

Haemoglobinopathies
- Thalassaemias
- Sickle cell disorders

Excessive red cell destruction states
Red cell membrane disorders
- Hereditary spherocytosis
- Ellipsocytosis
- Stomatocytosis

Enzyme deficiencies
- Glucose-6-phosphate dehydrogenase (G6PD) deficiency
- Pyruvate kinase deficiency

Autoimmune haemolytic anaemia
Disseminated intravascular coagulation

Blood loss
Acute
- Trauma, surgery

Chronic
- Usually from the gastrointestinal tract in children

lethargy, irritability, headache, failure to thrive, or being nonspecifically unwell. In sickle cell anaemia, a history of painful crisis and infective episodes (salmonella, pneumococci) may be obtained.

On examination, in addition to pallor, there may be signs of cardiovascular changes with tachycardia, and hyperdynamic circulation with cardiac flow murmurs. Children with preexisting heart or lung disorders may present in heart failure. Children with specific disorders may present in different ways. For instance, in leukaemia, there may be bruising and infection from depression of the other haematological components. In haemolytic states, jaundice may be apparent. In thalassaemia, splenomegaly occurs and bone marrow overgrowth causes facial and other skeletal changes.

DIAGNOSIS

A blood count confirms the presence of low haemoglobin and often provides clues to the underlying diagnosis. Measurement of mean corpuscular volume (MCV) and mean corpuscular haemoglobin concentration (MCHC) give further clues. If the MCV is small (microcytic) and the MCHC low (hypochromic) the anaemia is likely to be due to iron deficiency, or iron loss from chronic gastrointestinal (GI) bleeding, or due to haemoglobinopathy. If the MCV is large (macrocytic) possible causes include folic acid deficiency due to malabsorption. If MCV and MCHC are normal (normocytic and normochromic) the anaemia may be caused by a chronic illness such as juvenile arthritis.

Further evidence may be obtained from a family history of inherited red cell disorders such as thalassaemia, sickle cell disease, etc. Dietary history and/or evidence of malabsorption will be needed to identify possible deficiency states. Inquiry should also be made about exposure to drugs or toxins. On examination the signs of jaundice and presence or absence of splenomegaly may be helpful. The presence of skeletal abnormalities (acquired as in thalassaemia, or congenital as in Fanconi anaemia) should be noted. Further tests may include:

- Measurement of haematinics
  - Iron and ferritin
  - Serum and red cell folate
  - B_{12} (deficiency very rare in childhood: see below)
- Haemoglobin electrophoresis
- Coombs' test
- Red cell enzyme measurement
- Red cell fragility test (for membrane disorders)
- Bone marrow aspirate and/or trephine.

MANAGEMENT

The management of anaemia will depend on the underlying condition.

Iron deficiency anaemia

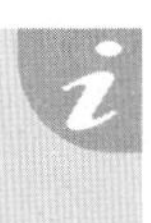

Epidemiology
Commonest form of anaemia in childhood (up to 40% in inner cities).

Deficiency of iron may be due to inadequate dietary intake, chronic blood loss as in GI bleeding, or malabsorption states. The commonest of these will be inadequate dietary intake and it is usually associated with delayed weaning and with prolonged and excessive milk intake in toddlers. Children from the Indian subcontinent seem to be particularly at risk in the UK. Commonly there is a secondary loss of appetite that aggravates the problem, and other symptoms may include pica (dirt eating) as well as lethargy and slowing in development. Physical signs include nail deformity, having a slightly concave profile, (koilonychia) or angular cheilitis. Confirmation of the diagnosis is made by measuring iron and ferritin concentrations. The typical picture is low iron and ferritin.

Treatment is with an iron medicine (preferably one of the more palatable and better tolerated preparations), while the possibility of malabsorption or chronic blood loss should be borne in mind. Darkening of the stools with iron medicine is a good sign of compliance. Where dietary causes are present, input from a paediatric dietician is helpful to prevent recurrence. Iron therapy should normally continue for 1–2 months. If there is failure to respond one should consider again the possibility of other haematological conditions, such as thalassaemia minor or malabsorption.

Folic acid deficiency

Epidemiology
Much less common than iron deficiency.

Folic acid deficiency is often associated with malabsorption due to disorders of the small intestine. Children with other haematological conditions leading to increased red cell turnover are more prone to develop this problem. In addition children on long-term phenytoin treatment or long-term cotrimoxazole occasionally develop folic acid deficiency. The blood film typically shows a macrocytic anaemia and the bone marrow may be megaloblastic. Measurement of red cell folate is an indicator of body stores and is more useful than serum folate levels. Treatment with folic acid supplements is required. In some conditions with a high rate of red cell turnover such as sickle cell anaemia folic acid may be used prophylactically.

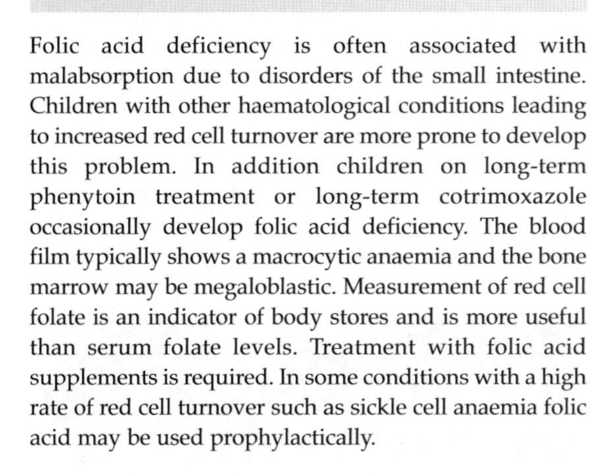

Vitamin B_{12} deficiency

Epidemiology
Very rare in childhood.

This is most commonly caused by congenital absence of intrinsic factor and other defects in vitamin B_{12} transport. Because transplacental B_{12} stores last in the infant for several years, B_{12} deficiency will usually present in mid-childhood. Acquired B_{12} deficiency may be due to pernicious anaemia or may follow resection of the terminal ileum. Treatment is with vitamin B_{12} injections.

β-Thalassaemia

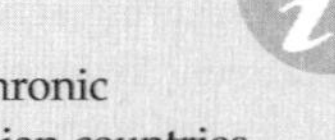

Epidemiology
One of the commonest forms of chronic anaemia in Mediterranean and Asian countries.

This arises from a defect in the genes controlling beta globin synthesis. Heterozygotes have thalassaemia minor which results in a mild asymptomatic low haemoglobin and microcytosis (which can be confused with iron deficiency). In thalassaemia major, inherited as an autosomal and recessive condition, there is failure to produce beta globin chains and therefore haemoglobin A is absent from the blood. Without beta chains, the haemoglobin produced is unstable and this results in ineffective erythropoiesis with many red cells failing to leave the bone marrow. The bone marrow will hypertrophy to compensate and this leads to the characteristic facial and other skeletal changes. Children usually present in infancy when fetal haemoglobin levels have declined and will have a sallow appearance (Fig. 13.1) with splenomegaly.

Treatment involves long-term transfusion therapy with the aim of maintaining the haemoglobin at such a

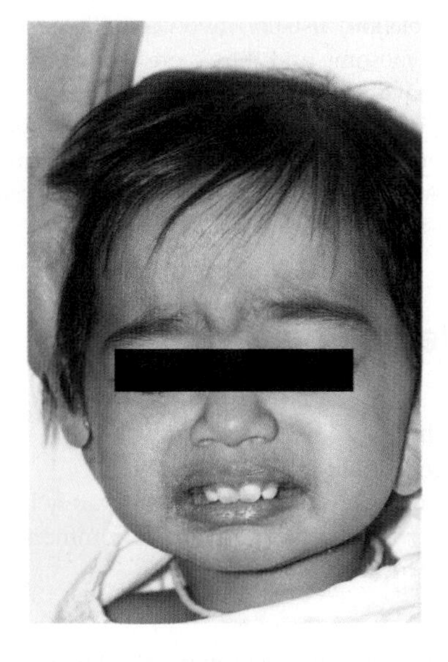

Fig 13.1
Child with β-thalassaemia major.

level as to switch off erythropoiesis. Most children need transfusion on a monthly basis approximately. Unfortunately the consequence of frequent transfusions is that iron overload develops and if unchecked this will lead to cardiomyopathy, endocrinopathy, and liver disease. If the cardiomyopathy is allowed to progress, it will eventually prove fatal. To remove iron from the body, children have to start on iron chelation therapy which involves subcutaneous infusions of desferrioxamine (Desferal) usually given into the abdominal wall at night. The effectiveness of this can be monitored by measuring serum ferritin levels. Adherence to this treatment regimen may be poor, particularly during adolescent years. It is hoped that in the next few years an oral iron-chelating agent will become available.

α-Thalassaemia

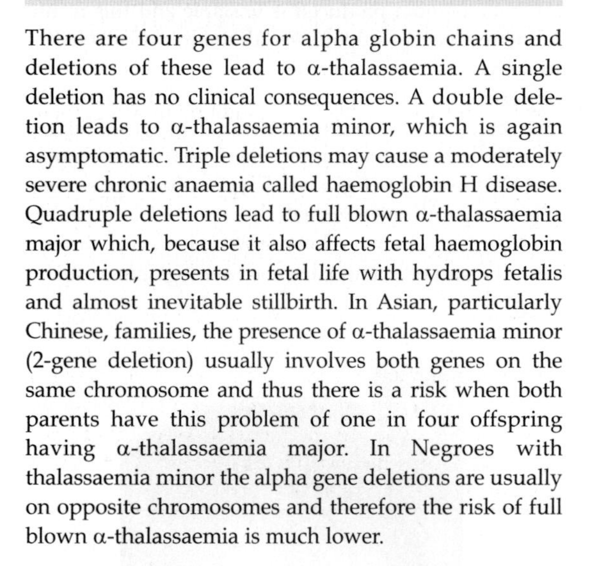

Epidemiology
Prevalent in Africa, Asia and Mediterranean countries.

There are four genes for alpha globin chains and deletions of these lead to α-thalassaemia. A single deletion has no clinical consequences. A double deletion leads to α-thalassaemia minor, which is again asymptomatic. Triple deletions may cause a moderately severe chronic anaemia called haemoglobin H disease. Quadruple deletions lead to full blown α-thalassaemia major which, because it also affects fetal haemoglobin production, presents in fetal life with hydrops fetalis and almost inevitable stillbirth. In Asian, particularly Chinese, families, the presence of α-thalassaemia minor (2-gene deletion) usually involves both genes on the same chromosome and thus there is a risk when both parents have this problem of one in four offspring having α-thalassaemia major. In Negroes with thalassaemia minor the alpha gene deletions are usually on opposite chromosomes and therefore the risk of full blown α-thalassaemia is much lower.

Sickle cell disease

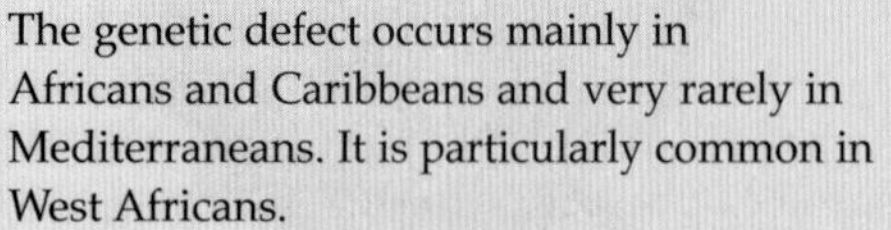

Epidemiology
The genetic defect occurs mainly in Africans and Caribbeans and very rarely in Mediterraneans. It is particularly common in West Africans.

A single amino-acid substitution of valine for glutamine at position six in the beta globin chain is responsible for sickle cell anaemia. The heterozygous state with haemoglobin AS is asymptomatic and usually associated with a mildly depressed haemoglobin level. Homozygous SS disease results in the full blown syndrome. In these individuals the abnormal beta globin chains under certain circumstances (hypoxia, acidosis) polymerize in red cells causing distortion of the cells into a sickle shape (hence the name; Fig. 13.2). Because of their shape and abnormal rigidity these sickle cells will not pass normally through capillaries, resulting in ischaemia in tissues leading to tissue damage and necrosis. Most commonly this occurs in bones leading to painful sickle crisis, but it can occur in any organ of the body. The spleen is a particularly common site for sickling and initially children have a large compensatory enlargement of the spleen. One unusual but devastating complication usually triggered by infection and sickle crisis is splenic sequestration. In this syndrome sickling leads to massive pooling of red cells in the spleen, which becomes grossly enlarged. The child becomes profoundly pale and unwell.

Gradually by a process of piecemeal necrosis the spleen shrinks and disappears by a process of autosplenectomy. The resultant splenic dysfunction combined with other ill defined effects on the immune system leads to the second major complication of sickle cell disease, which is susceptibility to infection with encapsulated bacteria, particularly *Streptococcus pneumoniae*. This organism causes pneumonia, septicaemia and meningitis. Another common infection in sickle cell patients is osteomyelitis that may be caused by unusual organisms such as salmonella. The abnormal red cells in these patients show shortened survival and therefore the marrow is hyperactive. For this reason folic acid supplements are usually given. Exposure to parvovirus infection which causes transient red cell aplasia can result in a profound aplastic crisis.

Prophylactic treatment involves pneumococcal vaccination, long-term treatment with penicillin (because vaccination is not fully protective and in any

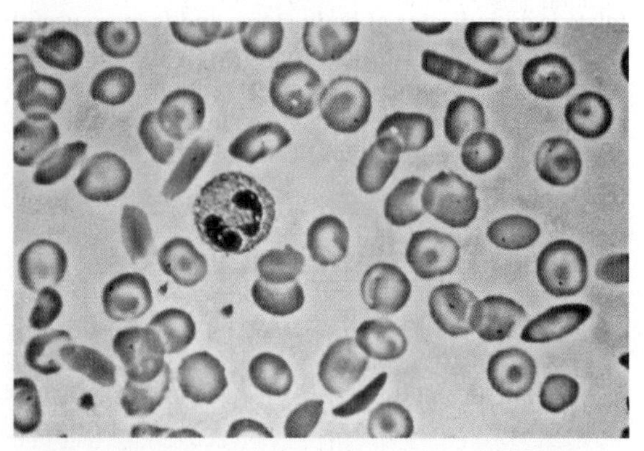

Fig 13.2
Sickle cells.

case does not cover all pneumococcal serotypes) and long-term folic acid. The frequency of crises can be reduced by avoiding exposure to cold, dehydration and acidosis. Supportive management during painful crisis consists of analgesia which may involve infusion of morphine, copious fluid intake, and treating any underlying infections. Exchange transfusion is sometimes required.

Haemoglobins (sickle) C disease behaves as a milder version of homozygous sickle cell anaemia. This is due to the co-inheritance of the haemoglobin C gene and the haemoglobin S gene (C is the result of another variant mutation on the beta globin chain). Crises are less common than in SS disease and though there is an increase in the risk of infection this is also less. Management is along the same lines as sickle cell anaemia.

Another variant in haemoglobinopathy is the co-inheritance of the sickle gene and the beta-thalassaemia gene, resulting in sickle β-thalassaemia. This disorder may behave more like thalassaemia major, like homozygous sickle cell disease or with a mixture of symptoms. If thalassaemia major symptoms pre-dominate, the patient will need to go on to long-term transfusions.

Glucose-6-phosphate dehydrogenase (G6PD) deficiency

> Epidemiology
> Found predominantly in Mediterranean, Asian and African families in slightly different forms.

This is an X-linked condition. Glucose-6-dehydrogenase is needed to keep glutathione in a reduced state necessary to keep the red cell membrane intact. In affected individuals this enzyme is unstable. Deficiency may present in the neonatal period with prolonged hyperbilirubinaemia. Alternatively it presents later with haemolytic episodes which may be precipitated by intercurrent infections or by drugs which act as oxidizing agents. Precipitants include certain antimalarial drugs (e.g. primaquine) antipyretics, sulphonamides, vitamin K or ingestion of fava beans, *Vicia faba* (favism). The prognosis is generally good provided these precipitating agents can be avoided.

Hereditary spherocytosis

> Epidemiology
> Commonest congenital haemolytic disorder after G6PD deficiency.

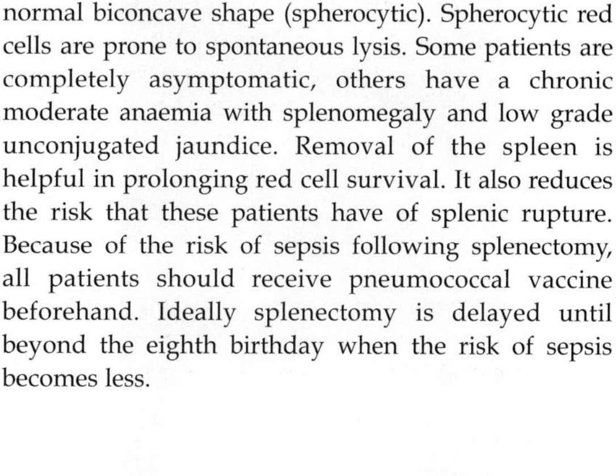

This is an autosomal dominantly inherited condition where there is an abnormality of the red cell membrane resulting in formation of red cells which have lost the normal biconcave shape (spherocytic). Spherocytic red cells are prone to spontaneous lysis. Some patients are completely asymptomatic, others have a chronic moderate anaemia with splenomegaly and low grade unconjugated jaundice. Removal of the spleen is helpful in prolonging red cell survival. It also reduces the risk that these patients have of splenic rupture. Because of the risk of sepsis following splenectomy, all patients should receive pneumococcal vaccine beforehand. Ideally splenectomy is delayed until beyond the eighth birthday when the risk of sepsis becomes less.

Fanconi anaemia (pancytopenia)

> Associations
> Absence of the radius may be associated with pancytopenia (Fanconi) or thrombocytopenia (thrombocytopenia with absent radius (TAR) syndrome (Fig. 13.3)).

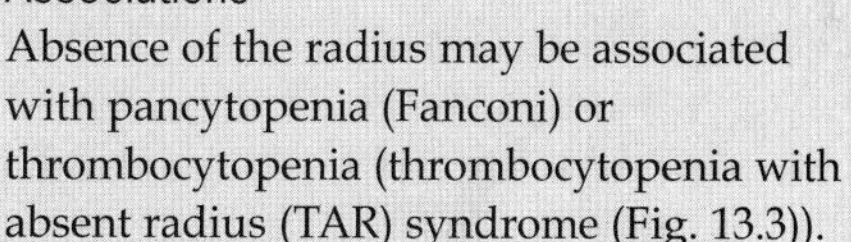

This is an autosomal recessive condition in which there is an abnormality of DNA repair. The children develop a progressive bone marrow failure, usually starting in the early years of life with the development of pancytopenia. Androgens may produce temporary improvement but without bone marrow transplantation the children will ultimately die. There is a high incidence of leukaemia in these children and other congenital abnormalities may include aplasia of the radius, abnormalities of the thumb (Fig. 13.3), changes in skin pigmentation, renal defects and growth failure. Note that Fanconi anaemia must not be confused with Fanconi syndrome, which was described by the same paediatrician.

Diamond–Blackfan red cell aplasia

> Epidemiology
> Rare.

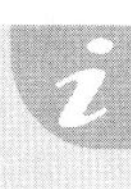

This is an autosomal recessive condition causing failure of red cell production by the bone marrow, starting in the early months of life. Other abnormalities such as short stature, abnormal thumbs, cleft lip and palate may be present but less commonly than in Fanconi anaemia.

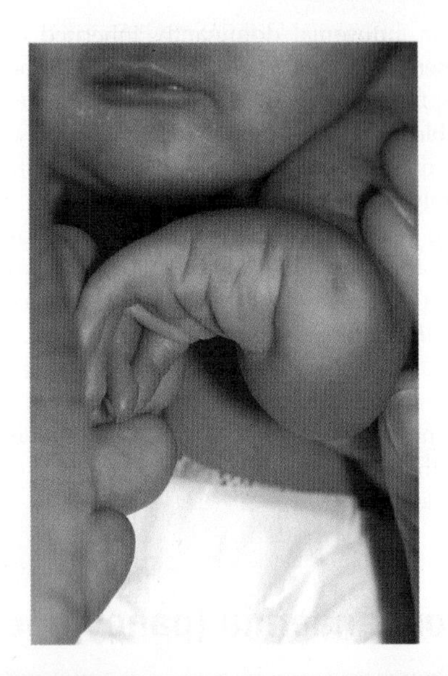
(a)

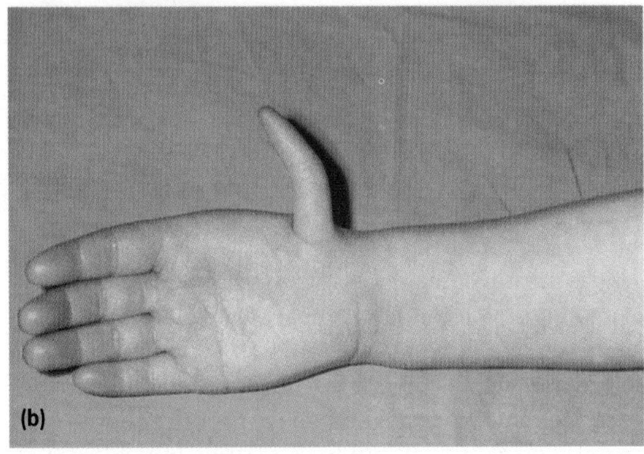

Fig 13.3
(a) Radial aplasia. The infant also had thrombocytopenia.
(b) Abnormal position and shape of thumb in Fanconi anaemia.

Some of these patients respond to prednisolone treatment but others do not and require long-term transfusion therapy. Treatment with erythropoietin has not been found helpful. Bone marrow transplantation is being evaluated.

Transient erythroblastopenia

Aetiology
Increasingly recognized disorder of the red blood cell precursors, probably immune-mediated.

In this condition a transient, pure red cell aplasia develops possibly following a viral infection. Differentiation from Diamond–Blackfan red cell aplasia can usually be made by means of age of presentation and by other tests. Children may often become so profoundly anaemic that they need transfusion, but the prognosis is usually good with spontaneous recovery in a matter of months.

Immune haemolytic anaemias

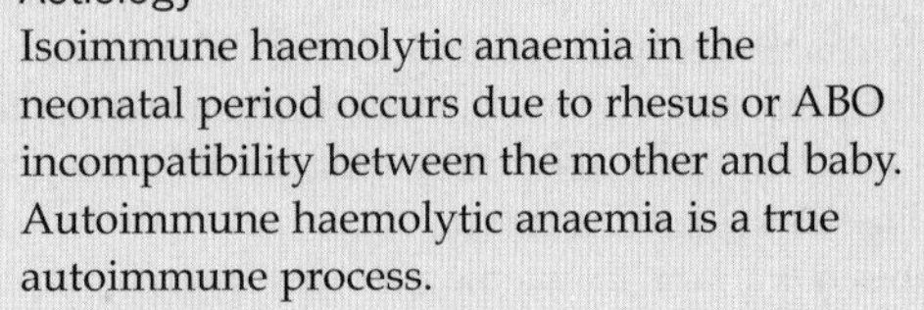
Aetiology
Isoimmune haemolytic anaemia in the neonatal period occurs due to rhesus or ABO incompatibility between the mother and baby. Autoimmune haemolytic anaemia is a true autoimmune process.

In full blown rhesus disease there will be gross oedema of the fetus (fetal hydrops) and usually this can be diagnosed antenatally by ultrasound. Intrauterine blood transfusions have been successful in helping these babies to survive until they can be delivered. The use of anti-D prophylaxis to prevent rhesus sensitization has greatly reduced the incidence of the problem of rhesus disease in recent years.

Less severe disease due to rhesus and ABO incompatibility usually presents in the neonatal period with the early development of jaundice that may rapidly rise to levels requiring exchange transfusion (see Ch. 2). Treatment is by exchange transfusion (Fig. 13.4) with the appropriate blood type to treat anaemia and prevent brain damage (kernicterus). Nowadays ABO incompatibility is a more common cause of this problem than rhesus incompatibility.

Autoimmune haemolytic anaemia is rare in childhood. It may occur as an isolated phenomenon most commonly following a virus infection in which case the prognosis for recovery is good. It may be part of an autoimmune disorder such as systemic lupus

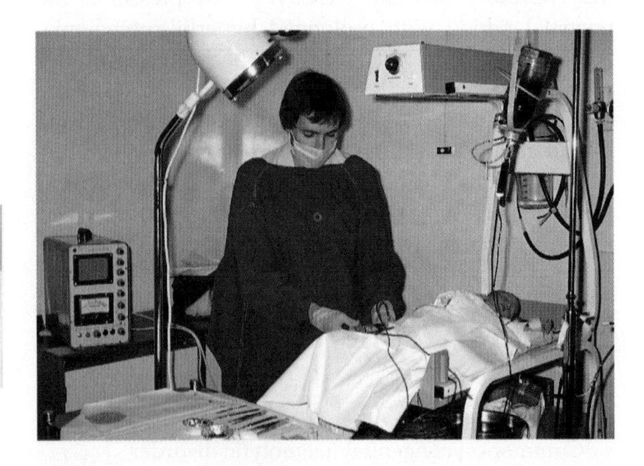

Fig 13.4
Infant with immune haemolytic anaemia receiving exchange transfusion.

erythematosus. Diagnosis is confirmed by the finding of a positive Coombs' test. Sometimes drug-induced haemolytic anaemias have an autoimmune basis and again a positive Coombs' test is usually found.

Platelet disorders

Idiopathic thrombocytopenic purpura (Fig. 13.5)

This disease commonly follows a viral infection. The megakaryocytes cease platelet production, and profound thrombocytopenia leads to bruising and a generalized purpuric rash, especially in the first 3 weeks of the illness. Intracranial haemorrhage is an occasional complication. Platelets are extremely scanty and large on peripheral blood smear. Bone marrow is normal except that megakaryocytes may be increased.

Most patients recover spontaneously within 3 months. When a decision is made to treat, high dose intravenous immunoglobulin for 4 days, or high dose steroids for 3 weeks may be given. A second course may be given if remission has not been obtained by 6 months. Splenectomy may be considered if a response is not obtained.

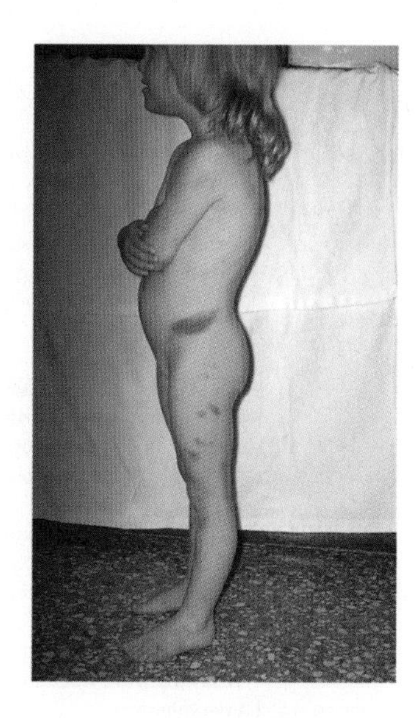

Fig 13.5
Idiopathic thrombocytopenic purpura.

Other causes of thrombocytopenia

These include:

- Bone marrow suppression, e.g. after chemotherapy
- Drug-induced, which may either be due to bone marrow suppression or the induction of immune-mediated platelet destruction
- Consumption of platelets which can occur in severe infection or vasculitis (as in haemolytic uraemic syndrome, see p. 302)
- Genetic disorders, e.g. Wiskott–Aldrich syndrome (see Chapter 15, p. 265) or thrombocytopenia with absent radius (TAR) syndrome (p. 344 (Fig 13.3))
- Neonatal thrombocytopenia due to transplacental (p. 253) maternal antibodies or allo-antibodies (most frequently involving a platelet antigen called PLA-1).

Thrombocytosis

This may occur as part of a chronic inflammatory or infective process. It is a frequent occurrence in the convalescent phase of Kawasaki disease. Very high platelet counts may occur transiently after splenectomy.

If the child is considered to be at risk of thrombotic disease, very low dose aspirin may be used to reduce platelet adhesiveness.

White cell disorders

Functional deficits of white cells are covered in Chapter 15, Immunology and infectious diseases. Leukaemia is discussed in Chapter 20, Oncology.

Deficiency of neutrophils (neutropenia)

Neutropenia leads to an increased susceptibility to infection with bacteria and fungi. In severe neutropenia (< 200/mm^3) translocation of colonizing bacteria in the gastrointestinal tract, nasopharynx or from skin wounds may occur, causing septicaemia which may lead rapidly to shock and death. Most cases of neutropenia are secondary, often iatrogenic due to myelosuppresive treatments. However, there are also rare but important primary causes. Table 13.1 lists the causes of neutropenia.

Investigation of neutropenia involves full clinical assessment and careful examination of the blood film. A bone marrow examination may help distinguish deficiency of production from excessive destruction, but in cases of severe marrow hypoplasia a trephine biopsy will be required as well as a simple aspirate. For

Table 13.1
Causes of neutropenia

Lack of production	Primary marrow disorders – Congenital agranulocytosis – Cyclic neutropenia – Primary myelodysplasia – Part of a syndrome, e.g. Schwachmann syndrome (see p. 237) – Fanconi anaemia – Idiopathic aplastic anaemia Secondary marrow disorders – Infiltration, e.g. leukaemia – Metabolic storage disorders, e.g. Gaucher disease – Drug effect, e.g. chemotherapy (dose-dependent), or idiosyncratic side-effect (non dose-dependent) – Secondary myelodysplasia resulting from infection
Excessive destruction	Hypersplenism Overwhelming infection (especially in neonates) Autoimmune neutropenia Alloimmune neutropenia (in neonates)

immune-mediated neutropenia, measurement of neutrophil antibodies may be helpful.

Management of the neutropenic child will involve minimizing the risk of infection by avoidance of contamination of wounds and vascular lines. Prophylactic antifungal drugs are often used and, in some cases, prophylactic antibacterials may be considered, though infection with resistant organisms may be a problem. Antiseptic mouth washes and soaps are often used.

Treatment of the underlying disorder depends on the cause. In secondary neutropenia treatment is aimed at the underlying disorder, e.g. leukaemia. Recombinant haemopoetic growth factors such as granulocyte colony stimulating factor (GCSF) may be useful in both primary and secondary lack of production of neutrophils. Since permanent severe neutropenia carries a poor prognosis, bone marrow transplantation may be required.

Coagulopathies

Haemophilia

Haemophilia A is the commonest genetic coagulation defect. It is due to an X-linked deficiency in Factor VIII production. Residual levels of Factor VIII determine the severity of the disorder (<1% = severe; 1–5% = moderate; 6–30% = mild). Levels are usually consistent within the same affected family.

Spontaneous deep bleeds, particularly affecting the muscles and joints, are the most frequent clinical problems. Intracranial bleeding can also occur, and bleeding after even minor surgery such as circumcision or dental extraction.

Treatment is aimed at avoidance of trauma and early and vigorous treatment of bleeds with purified Factor VIII infusions. This treatment, together with physiotherapy to maintain mobility of joints affected by bleeds, is important in preventing the disabling joint problems that were previously common in these boys. When bleeds are very frequent prophylactic Factor VIII infusions can be given and these are also used prior to surgery.

Immunization against hepatitis A and B is required because the child will frequently receive blood products.

Factor IX deficiency (Christmas disease, haemophilia B) is identical clinically to factor VIII deficiency. It is also X-linked. Factor IX concentrates are required.

Factor XI deficiency (haemophilia C) is autosomal recessive and milder. Fresh frozen plasma is required.

von Willebrand disease

This autosomal dominant (rarely recessive) defect predisposes to abnormal bleeding. The missing factor (von Willebrand protein) binds platelets and factor VIII. Excessive bleeding occurs from epistaxes, menorrhagia and after trauma. Bleeding time is prolonged and platelets show decreased adhesiveness. The severity of the disease is very variable.

Replacement therapy with fresh frozen plasma or cryoprecipitate is sometimes necessary, particularly to cover surgical procedures.

14 Hepatology

Liver disorders in childhood are relatively rare but important. They are therefore best managed in special centres. Hence it is important to be able to recognize paediatric liver disease early so that appropriate referral can be made.

Paediatric hepatology includes hepatitis B, which is one of the most frequent causes of cancer in the world.

Congenital disorders

α_1-antitrypsin deficiency

The glycoprotein α_1-antitrypsin inhibits other proteolytic enzymes. It exists in more than 20 different forms encoded by the same gene (alleles). The commonest allele is called M and the normal phenotype is protease inhibitor (Pi) MM.

The Z allele is defective, and 20% of people with the phenotype PiZZ (1 in 3000) have neonatal cholestatic jaundice, and serum α_1-antitrypsin concentrations are 10–20% of normal. Granules of α_1-antitrypsin are present in hepatocytes. The jaundice may resolve completely or become chronic with cirrhosis, requiring transplantation.

Other phenotypes (e.g. PiMZ) are not associated with liver disease. PiZZ and PiSZ are associated with early onset of emphysema; this is presumably related to an inability to neutralize the proteolytic activity of leukocytes.

Enzyme replacement therapy is being tried.

Crigler–Najjar syndrome

This deficiency of the enzyme UDP glucuronyl transferase causes severe unconjugated hyperbilirubinaemia and kernicterus.

Serum bilirubin is maintained at <340 μmol/l (less in preterm infants) by means of phototherapy and repeated exchange transfusions. Liver transplantation is curative and prevents the development of kernicterus. The latter can still occur in adult life if bilirubin is >680 μmol/l.

Type I is autosomal recessive. Type II is a less severe autosomal dominant condition and the prognosis is much better.

Gilbert syndrome

About 5% of the population have low activities of UDP glucuronyl transferase, resulting in slight elevation of serum bilirubin (<100 μmol/l). The condition is entirely harmless unless the patient is investigated unnecessarily for liver disease.

Dubin–Johnson syndrome

In this condition an autosomal recessive defect of bilirubin excretion results in chronic, mild conjugated hyperbilirubinaemia. Liver function remains normal.

Biliary atresia

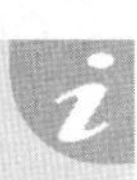

Epidemiology
1 : 4000 live births with males outnumbering females by 2 to 1.

One-third of infants with cholestasis have biliary atresia. The aetiology is unknown but a progressive, fibrosing obliteration of the intra- and extrahepatic bile ducts occurs. Associated congenital anomalies occur in about one-quarter, such as vascular anomalies, malrotation and polysplenia. The affected infant is usually full term; physiological jaundice fails to fade and pale stools are the leading symptom. Haemorrhagic disease of the newborn is an alternative presentation.

Liver function tests are of limited value in distinguishing from neonatal hepatitis and such children should be referred to a special centre. If no cause is found for neonatal hepatitis and the DISIDA (^{99m}Tc-diisopropyliminodiacetic acid) scan shows no excretion then a laparotomy and operative cholangiogram is performed. If biliary atresia is confirmed then a loop of intestine is anastomosed to the porta hepatis (Kasai procedure). Cholangitis occurs in one-half postoperatively in the first year, and adversely affects the prognosis in 50% of those affected. Portal hypertension and varices are also common. The results are much worse following late referral, hence the decision to refer should be made in the first month of life. If the operation fails, and liver function deteriorates a liver transplant is the next option.

Choledochal cyst

This congenital abnormality of the biliary tree presents with pain, mass and obstructive jaundice. The cyst should be excised rather than drained because of a risk of malignant change.

Alagille syndrome (syndrome of paucity of the intrahepatic bile ducts)

Epidemiology
Very rare.

The typical features are severe failure to thrive in infancy coupled with persistent neonatal jaundice caused by conjugated hyperbilirubinaemia and pruritus, due to underdevelopment of the hepatic bile ducts. Other abnormalities include unusual facies (broad forehead, hypertelorism, long straight nose and small mandible), ocular abnormalities (posterior embryotoxon), pulmonary stenosis and failure of anterior vertebral arch fusion (butterfly vertebrae). It is important that the child is seen at a unit with specialized knowledge of liver disorders (Department of Child Health, King's College Hospital, London, or The Children's Hospital, Birmingham, in the UK).

Acquired disorders

Cholelithiasis

Cholelithiasis is rare in childhood, except in haemolytic diseases such as sickle cell anaemia and red cell enzyme defects. Pigment stones may develop.

Cholestasis

Definition
Serum conjugated bilirubin >25 μmol/l.

The leading sign is decreased stool pigment; dark urine also results. Urgent investigation is required in infants to exclude sepsis, coagulopathy (vitamin K deficiency), galactosaemia (RBC galactose-1-phosphate or galactose-1-phosphate uridyl transferase deficiency) and biliary atresia. Other causes include neonatal hepatitis following perinatal or intrauterine infection (hepatitis B, cytomegalovirus (CMV), syphilis, toxoplasmosis). Other metabolic causes of neonatal hepatitis include α_1-antitrypsin deficiency (check phenotype) cystic fibrosis, fructose intolerance (fructose in urine) and tyrosinaemia I.

Examination should be carried out for specific syndromes (Alagille, see above, Zellweger, see p. 294) and intrauterine infection (small for dates, purpura, congenital heart disease). Hepatosplenomegaly occurs both in obstructive lesions of the bile ducts and in intrahepatic cholestasis. The child should be referred to a paediatric hepatology centre for diagnosis by ultrasound, liver biopsy and DISIDA scan, proceeding to laparotomy if results suggest biliary obstruction.

Cirrhosis

Definition
Development of fibrosis within the liver.

The causes of cirrhosis are listed in Information box 14.1.

Malnutrition is a major complication of cirrhosis that may require overnight tube feeding with a special feed. These children can also develop portal hypertension. Obstruction of venous return causes back pressure, resulting in splenomegaly, ascites, and oesophageal varices. The varices are a major problem when they bleed. A Sengstaken–Blakemore tube may be required to compress the varices from the oesophageal lumen and stop the bleeding. Injection of the varices with a sclerosing agent by endoscopy is increasingly used to prevent bleeding. Hepatocellular carcinoma (Ch. 20) may complicate advanced cirrhosis.

Information Box 14.1

Causes of cirrhosis

Metabolic
Galactosaemia
Glycogen storage disease type IV
Tyrosinaemia
Niemann–Pick C
α_1-antitrypsin
Wilson disease
Indian childhood cirrhosis
Haemochromatosis
Haemosiderosis

Biliary obstruction

Infection
Hepatitis B (+ delta)
Hepatitis C
Non-A non-B hepatitis

Cystic fibrosis

Autoimmune
Chronic active hepatitis
Primary sclerosing cholangitis

Toxic
Chronic veno-occlusive disease

Hepatitis

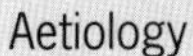

Epidemiology
A serious worldwide health problem.

Aetiology
There are five types of hepatitis viruses, and many other types of viruses, bacteria, fungi and protozoa which can cause hepatitis.

The hepatitis viruses A–E, the adenoviruses, coxsackieviruses, cytomegalovirus, Epstein–Barr virus, echoviruses, herpes, measles, mumps, rubella, varicella and human immunodeficiency viruses can all cause hepatitis. Nonviral causes include brucellosis, leptospirosis and malaria.

Hepatitis A (infectious hepatitis) is spread by direct contact and contaminated food and water and only rarely by blood products. The infection is usually asymptomatic in young children. After an incubation period of about a month, older children and adolescents with hepatitis A develop fever, malaise, anorexia, nausea and epigastric pain and tenderness. Jaundice is due to obstruction of bile canaliculi by swollen hepatocytes and hepatocyte damage. Urobilinogen, which is synthesized in the intestine from bilirubin and reabsorbed, appears in the urine because the damaged liver cannot excrete it in bile. The urine becomes dark and the stools pale. Enzymes are released into the blood from the obstructed bile ducts (alkaline phosphatase, 5′-nucleotidase and γ-glutamyl transpeptidase) and damaged hepatocytes (alanine aminotransferase and lactic dehydrogenase). Convalescence lasts several weeks.

Hepatitis B (serum hepatitis), C and D are acquired from direct contact, infected blood products and needles. Transmission of hepatitis B to infants also occurs antenatally and from maternal blood and faeces at birth but not by breastfeeding. The incubation period of hepatitis B is 2–6 months and is usually asymptomatic in infants and children although they are at risk for hepatocellular carcinoma as in adult life. Immunization against hepatitis B decreases the risk. The onset of hepatitis B is more insidious than that of hepatitis A and is associated with skin rashes. The illness lasts longer than hepatitis A but is otherwise similar.

Hepatitis C is milder than A or B but, like hepatitis B, may result in chronic active hepatitis leading to cirrhosis and hepatocellular carcinoma. The hepatitis D virus is an incomplete RNA virus, which can only replicate in the presence of hepatitis B virus, a DNA virus. Hepatitis D may be very severe (fulminant) hepatitis. Hepatitis E is waterborne and causes an acute hepatitis with joint pain in adults. It also causes fetal loss in pregnant women. Vaccines are available for hepatitis A and B.

Liver failure

Hepatic encephalopathy

Acute or chronic liver failure can produce disturbances of consciousness. This has been ascribed to accumulation of ammonia, γ-aminobutyric acid and other neurotransmitters.

These and other substances (such as mercaptans and phenols) may be produced by the colonic bacteria, not metabolized by the diseased liver and can cross the blood–brain barrier. Treatment of hepatic encephalopathy is described in Information box 14.2. Mortality is high.

Information Box 14.2

Treatment of hepatic encephalopathy

- Mannitol and dexamethasone for raised intracranial pressure
- Treatment of the underlying liver failure
- Supporting the patient until liver function returns or the liver is transplanted
- Avoidance of sedatives, diuretics and antiemetics
- Administration of neomycin and lactulose
- Prevention of hypoglycaemia, electrolyte and acid–base imbalance
- Correction of clotting abnormalities with vitamin K and fresh frozen plasma
- Treatment of sepsis

Reye syndrome

Reye syndrome is an acute encephalopathy accompanied by microvesicular fatty changes in the liver. It may be precipitated by influenza, varicella, or respiratory or gastrointestinal infections, especially when treated with aspirin. With the banning of the administration of aspirin to children the condition has become less common. Inborn errors of metabolism such as urea cycle defects can present in a similar fashion to Reye syndrome.

The disease produces:

- Vomiting
- Depressed conscious state
- Hepatomegaly
- Hyperammonaemia (serum ammonia >100 μmol/l)
- Raised transaminase (AAT >100 IU/l)
- Prolonged prothrombin (>4 seconds prolonged)
- Hypoglycaemia.

Treatment is as for liver failure. The treatment of raised intracranial pressure requires direct monitoring, with ventilation to maintain $P\text{CO}_2$ between 3.5 and 4.0 kPa, and administration of mannitol.

The mortality rate is high.

15 Immunology and infectious diseases

The brunt of infectious disease falls on children because of their immature immune systems. The greatest worldwide killers of the under-5s are pneumonia, acute diarrhoea (generally of infectious cause), measles, malaria and tuberculosis. Poliomyelitis, which tends to maim rather than kill, is at the point of probable global eradication as a result of vigorously conducted vaccine initiatives. In developed countries, better nutrition, immunization and availability of treatment has reduced mortality. Nevertheless toddlers will suffer an infectious disease (most commonly upper respiratory) every 6 weeks, and the majority of acute hospital admissions are either directly or indirectly infection-associated (for example by precipitation of asthma symptoms or febrile convulsions).

Advances in the treatment of malignant diseases and immunopathological disorders in children, as well as the HIV epidemic, have led to an increase in the number of children with secondary immunodeficiency. Taken together with children with primary (genetic) disorders of the immune system, paediatricians are having to deal increasingly with complex infections in immunocompromised children.

Immunology

A knowledge of immunology is important to the understanding of many disease processes including the very common allergic disorders. Deficiency of the immune response, either primary or secondary, leads to problems with infection which may be complex and atypical in presentation. Newborn babies and young children have a 'physiological' immune deficiency, partly compensated by passive transfer of immunoglobulin across the placenta and through breast milk.

Some forms of primary immunodeficiency, such as IgA deficiency, are relatively common while other more major deficiencies are rare. It is important to recognize the latter, as treatments such as immunoglobulin replacement or bone marrow transplantation may be lifesaving.

The discipline of immunology also encompasses autoimmunity and allergy. Autoimmune disorders are discussed in the organ specialty chapters and in the Rheumatology chapter (p. 361). Allergic diseases are also covered in the organ specialty chapters, mainly

Respirology and Dermatology. Important immunodeficiency disorders are listed below.

Antibody deficiency disorders

The most common infections associated with these disorders are caused by pyogenic bacteria, particularly the polysaccharide-encapsulated organisms such as pneumococcus. In severe antibody deficiency states there are also problems handling the enteroviruses, which include ECHO, coxsackie and polio viruses. Opportunistic infections are rare and their presence usually indicates a cell-mediated deficiency component to the disorder.

Agammaglobulinaemia (Bruton disease)

This panhypogammaglobulinaemia affects all immunoglobulin classes. Inheritance is X-linked, with an incidence of 1 in 100 000. The disorder is caused by a defect in an intracellular enzyme, Bruton tyrosine kinase (btk), necessary for the development of B lymphocytes, which are therefore usually absent or very low in the blood.

Repeated bacterial infections start from around 4 months of age, as maternal antibodies are waning.

Treatment comprises:

- Lifelong immunoglobulin replacement therapy
- Frequent use of antibiotics for respiratory infections.

Common variable immunodeficiency (CVID)

This variable hypogammaglobulinaemia affects IgA and IgG, with or without IgM. Some patients have a degree of T-cell deficiency. The condition may be present from birth or develop later (late-onset hypogammaglobulinaemia).

It is familial, with complex genetics linked to selective IgA deficiency and autoimmune disease. The incidence is 1 : 20 000, and both sexes are affected. B lymphocytes are usually present in the blood.

CVID may present with:

- Repeated respiratory tract infections
- Gastrointestinal problems (infective or inflammatory)
- Autoimmune phenomena
- Opportunistic infections (if there is a significant T-cell deficiency component).

Treatment comprises:

- Lifelong immunoglobulin replacement therapy
- Frequent use of antibiotics for respiratory infections
- Monitoring and treating associated complications.

Selective IgA deficiency

Selective IgA deficiency has two forms:

- Complete IgA deficiency, with absence of IgA in blood and secretions
- Partial IgA deficiency, with detectable but low levels of IgA.

The complete form, usually permanent, has an incidence of 1 in 500. The partial form occurs in early childhood and often resolves (transient). The disorder may be linked with disturbed IgG subclass levels.

It is associated with recurrent respiratory tract (including ear) and gastrointestinal infections, and increased incidence of coeliac disease and autoimmune disorders. The susceptibility to infections improves with age, even if the deficiency persists.

Treatment comprises:

- Prophylactic antibiotics, especially during winter months
- Monitoring and treating associated complications.

Immunoglobulin replacement therapy is not indicated. Some patients develop antibodies to IgA in blood products, which potentially may cause severe reactions.

Immunoglobulin G subclass deficiencies

These are a relatively common finding in children with recurrent infections. The deficiencies are usually caused by an immunoregulatory problem, and rarely, due to deletions in the relevant Ig heavy chain genes.

IgG2 deficiency, which may be partial or complete, is the most common. It is often transient in early childhood, and may be associated with IgA deficiency. It can be associated with recurrent respiratory infections, although not always.

IgG1 and IgG3 deficiencies are also associated with infections, but are less well characterized. IgG4 deficiency is of doubtful clinical significance.

Management may be expectant or involve prophylactic antibiotics. Immunoglobulin replacement is rarely required, and is restricted to children with persistent chest problems and/or a failure of antibody response to vaccines.

Antibody deficiency with normal immunoglobulins

This condition is poorly understood; it may occur as part of a combined immunodeficiency or as an isolated problem. It is diagnosed by finding absence of specific antibody responses to vaccine antigens following booster doses. Immunoglobulin replacement therapy may be required, depending on clinical status.

Defective anti-polysaccharide responsiveness is a form of this problem in which response to protein or conjugate protein–polysaccharide antigens is normal, but there is failure of response to pure polysaccharide (such as pneumococcal) vaccine. This problem cannot be diagnosed in the first 2 years of life when polysaccharide responses are inherently poor. Prophylactic antibiotic therapy or immunoglobulin replacement may be required, depending on clinical status.

Transient hypogammaglobulinaemia of infancy

In this poorly defined condition there are low levels of one or more immunoglobulin classes. It is often an incidental finding or associated with relatively minor infections, and usually resolves by 36 months of age.

Differential diagnoses include Bruton disease and CVID (see p. 262). B cells are present in blood, and specific antibody responses to vaccines are present.

Management is expectant. Antibiotic prophylaxis is sometimes used.

Combined immunodeficiency disorders

Nearly all defects of T cells (cell-mediated immune defects) result in at least a degree of failure of antibody production. They are therefore called combined (T-cell and antibody) defects. Affected children suffer a wide range of infections including bacterial, fungal, viral and protozoal types. Many of these are called opportunistic infections, meaning that the organism does not normally cause the problem in immunocompetent children but is acting opportunistically. Examples include the fungus *Pneumocystis carinii* and cytomegalovirus. Although the latter may be responsible for mild illness in normal children, it can cause severe life-threatening illness in immunodeficient children.

Severe combined immunodeficiency (SCID)

This is a group of disorders, with an overall incidence of around 1 in 50 000, which result in profound deficiency of cell-mediated and humoral immunity. Several different molecular defects have been identified as causes. Inheritance is autosomal recessive in some cases or X-linked in others.

The disorder presents in infancy with:

- Pneumonitis
- Diarrhoea
- Failure to thrive
- Candidiasis.

Lymphopenia is present in most cases, compared with age-related levels; this provides a clue for early diagnosis. The T cells are invariably absent (or very low). B cells and NK cells are present or absent depending on the molecular type of SCID.

Supportive treatment includes prophylactic cotrimoxazole and immunoglobulin. Blood products should be CMV-negative and irradiated to prevent transfusion-acquired graft versus host disease. Bone marrow transplantation is curative if performed early before excessive morbidity develops, and somatic gene therapy is being explored.

Antenatal diagnosis is available; in the first trimester if the molecular defect is known, otherwise in the second trimester, by fetal blood analysis of T cell numbers.

Combined immunodeficiency

This is similar to SCID but slightly less severe with some T cells present. Some have the same molecular defect as SCID but with incomplete expression; others have different or as yet unidentified defects. It presents with similar problems to SCID, particularly diarrhoea, often due to a noninfective, presumed autoimmune enteropathy.

Management is on the same lines as for SCID. Antenatal diagnosis is only available where the molecular defect in the family is known.

Hyper-IgM syndrome

This condition, usually inherited in an X-linked fashion but occasionally in an autosomal recessive fashion, results in failure to produce IgG and IgA. The IgM level is high or normal. In the X-linked variety the defect is due to a failure to express the molecule CD40 ligand on activated T cells.

This molecule is important in enabling B cells to switch immunoglobulin isotype production. The molecule is also important in signalling to macrophages to facilitate killing of intracellular organisms. Affected individuals suffer recurrent bacterial infections, but are also susceptible to *Pneumocystis carinii*, mycobacterial and cryptosporidial infections.

Management involves immunoglobulin replacement and *Pneumocystis carinii* prophylaxis. Bone marrow transplantation is under evaluation.

In the long term liver problems (sclerosing cholangitis) may occur, often due to chronic infection with *Cryptosporidium parvum*.

X-linked lymphoproliferative disease

Affected boys remain well with normal immune function until they encounter the Epstein–Barr virus. They then develop serious life-threatening illness. Severe chronic infectious mononucleosis with secondary immune depression leads to susceptibility to a wide range of other pathogens, including:

- Hypogammaglobulinaemia
- Lymphoproliferative disease
- Aplastic anaemia.

Mortality is very high, being greater than 80%.

Management involves:

- Supportive care
- Immunoglobulin replacement
- Bone marrow transplantation.

Recent identification of the gene will allow the diagnosis to be made (and possibly corrected by bone marrow transplantation) in at-risk boys before the disease develops.

Disorders associated with syndromes

Di George anomalad

In 90% of cases this is associated with a microdeletion on chromosome 22q which can be detected using a fluorescent in situ hybridization (FISH) technique. It forms part of a wider developmental problem causing velofacial cardiac (Shprintzen) syndrome involving structures derived from the 3rd and 4th pharyngeal arches.

Affected children have an unusual face with:

- Fish-mouth deformity
- Hypertelorism
- Anti-mongoloid (downward sloping) slanting eyes
- Low set ears
- Bifid uvula.

The condition is also associated with congenital heart disease (usually aortic arch anomalies), hypoparathyroidism and thymic hypoplasia.

Early assessment of immune function is required. Significant immunodeficiency occurs in the minority of cases and comprises:

- Low T-cell numbers and defective T-cell responses
- Defective antibody responses (usually with normal immunoglobulin levels).

There is a tendency for the immune deficiency to improve with time. In those with severe immunodeficiency, avoidance of live vaccines, *Pneumocystis carinii* pneumonia prophylaxis, immunoglobulin therapy and sometimes bone marrow transplantation are required.

Ataxia telangiectasia (see also Neurology, Ch. 18)

This is caused by a defect in a cell cycle control protein ATM. Immunodeficiency of variable severity is found in 80% of cases. In order of frequency: IgA deficiency, defective polysaccharide responses, low IgG, T-cell lymphopenia and defective T-cell responses may occur.

There may be recurrent respiratory infections leading to bronchiectasis, and there is a high incidence of malignancy, mainly of the lymphoid system.

Treatment comprises prophylactic antibiotics and, in some cases, immunoglobulin.

Hyper immunoglobulin E syndrome (Job syndrome)

In this condition, there is extreme elevation of serum IgE, associated with deep-seated bacterial and fungal infections. Inheritance is autosomal dominant with incomplete penetrance.

The syndrome is associated with dermatitis (not true eczema), abnormal (coarse) facies, delayed dentition and osteopenia with increased risk of fractures. Staphylococcal lung infections typically lead to pneumatoceles which often require surgical removal to prevent secondary fungal infection. There is defective neutrophil chemotaxis and sometimes poor polysaccharide antibody responses.

Treatment is with:

- Prophylactic antistaphylococcal antibiotics
- Immunoglobulin replacement if there is a demonstrated deficiency of antibody response.

(Job was a red-headed, fair-skinned Biblical character who was afflicted with a plague of boils, and the condition was first described in fair red-headed children.)

Wiskott–Aldrich syndrome

This X-linked recessive condition is caused by a mutation in the gene encoding a protein (Wiskott–Aldrich syndrome protein, WASP) involved in cytoskeletal functioning of haemopoeitic cells. Features include:

- Eczema
- Thrombocytopenia with abnormally small platelets
- Recurrent bacterial infections
- Risk of opportunistic infections
- Low serum IgM and high IgE and IgA
- Progressive lymphopenia
- Risk of developing autoimmune and vasculitic disorders
- High incidence of lymphoid malignancy.

Treatment includes immunoglobulin replacement, prophylaxis against *Pneumocystis carinii*, splenectomy (to control bleeding), and bone marrow transplantation if a suitable donor can be found.

Chronic mucocutaneous candidiasis

This probably represents a heterogenous group of genetic disorders with susceptibility to candida infection. Inheritance is variable but often autosomal dominant.

Patients suffer recurrent or persistent candidal infections of skin, nails and mucous membranes. They can also suffer an excess of other (mainly bacterial) infections. In some pedigrees the disorder is associated with autoimmune endocrinopathy, as the APECED syndrome (autoimmune poly-endocrinopathy, candidiasis and ectodermal dystrophy), inherited as a single gene defect. Hypoparathyroidism, hypothyroidism, diabetes mellitus, pernicious anaemia, Addison disease and gonadal failure may all occur in this condition. (Cancer of the mouth and oesophagus may occur in adults.)

Treatment is with systemic imidazole class antifungals (such as itraconazole) but resistance may be a problem.

Neutrophil disorders

Lack of neutrophils (neutropenia) is covered in the Haematology chapter (p. 255). Neutrophil function disorders result in problems handling bacterial (especially staphylococcal) and fungal infections.

Chronic granulomatous disease

This may be X-linked (in two-thirds) or autosomal recessive (in one-third). It represents a group of defects of neutrophil NADPH oxidase, which prevents generation of hydrogen peroxide and hydroxyl radicals in the neutrophil phagolysosome, resulting in a failure of microbial killing.

Clinical features include:

- Recurrent bacterial and fungal infections affecting skin, lymph nodes, bone, lung and gastrointestinal tract
- Hepatosplenomegaly
- Recurrent noninfective granuloma formation particularly in the gastrointestinal and urinary tracts.

Stimulated neutrophils fail to reduce the dye nitroblue tetrazolium; this is used as a diagnostic test.

Continuous prophylaxis is required with:

- Cotrimoxazole, as an antibacterial agent which penetrates well into neutrophils
- Itraconazole; a broad-spectrum antifungal agent.

Steroid therapy may be required to combat the noninfective granulomatous problems. Bone marrow transplantation is being evaluated, and the possibility of somatic gene therapy is being explored.

Antenatal diagnosis is possible using umbilical cord blood obtained by fetoscopy or mutation analysis or a chorionic villous sample if the gene defect is known.

Leukocyte adhesion deficiency

In this disorder there is a defect of a leukocyte surface molecule used in helping cells adhere to other cells by receptor–ligand interaction. Such interaction is essential to permit neutrophils to egress from the circulation. Inheritance is autosomal recessive.

Affected children show:

- Delayed separation of the umbilical cord (which depends on migration of neutrophils)
- Recurrent bacterial infections with poor pus formation
- Severe periodontitis
- Necrotizing skin lesions
- Poor wound healing
- High circulating neutrophil count (cells can't get out).

Partial forms are described, with less severe problems. The full blown form is usually fatal in early life.

Bone marrow transplantation is indicated.

Complement disorders

Primary deficiencies of complement factors are rare, but secondary consumption of C3 and C4 may occur in sepsis, certain autoimmune diseases and in nephritis. Deficiency of any one factor breaks the complement cascade, but the alternative complement pathway can bypass C1, C4 and C2 to activate C3 which is the main factor involved in opsonization of bacteria. Deficiency of one of the terminal components (C6–9), relatively common in some Middle Eastern and Japanese populations, affects complement-mediated bacterial lysis.

C1, C4 and C2 predispose to autoimmune diseases such as systemic lupus erythematosus (SLE), rather than to infections.

C3 deficiency (nearly always secondary to consumption) leads to a high susceptibility to pyogenic infections, whereas C5 deficiency is associated with a mild excess of infections.

C6–9 deficiencies lead to specific problems only with neisserial species (meningococcus and gonococcus).

Management involves monitoring for autoimmune disease, use of prophylactic antibiotics and immunization against meningococcus.

Hereditary angioedema

This is a deficiency of C1 esterase inhibitor, a protein which inhibits early complement activation. Inheritance is autosomal dominant.

Patients develop inappropriate complement activation leading to localized areas of increased vascular permeability and angioedema. This occurs spontaneously or is induced by physical trauma, including surgery and dental treatment. Attacks affecting the airway are life-threatening. Gastrointestinal involvement may produce a picture mimicking appendicitis or other acute abdomen.

Attacks are self-limiting, but if they are life-threatening they can be limited by infusing the purified inhibitor. Infusions of C1 inhibitor concentrate can be used prophylactically prior to surgery or dental work. Frequency of attacks is reduced by prophylaxis with tranexamic acid or anabolic steroids such as danazol. Use of the latter is best avoided before puberty.

Asplenia

Absence of the spleen is associated with:

- Midline liver
- Right-sided stomach
- Dextrocardia
- Complex cyanotic congenital heart disease
- Increased risk of sepsis
- Howell–Jolly and Heinz bodies in pitted erythrocytes.
- Both lungs have three lobes.

When multiple spleens are present (polysplenia) both lungs have two lobes. The manifestations of asplenia occur except for sepsis and red cell changes.

Secondary immunodeficiencies

Many disease states as well as treatments may cause immune suppression. Table 15.1 gives some of the more common examples and their consequences. The list is not exhaustive and many other disease processes, including malignancy, diabetes and uraemia, all cause ill-defined depression of immunity. Recognition of some of the susceptibilities allows appropriate prophylactic measures to be taken such as penicillin prophylaxis and pneumococcal immunization in hyposplenic patients. The list of prophylactic drugs that some children have to take can get very long, for example after bone marrow transplantation. It should be borne in mind that no prophylaxis is 100% effective.

Bacterial infections

Congenital bacterial infections are covered in Chapter 1.

Group A beta-haemolytic streptococcal pharyngitis

Pharyngitis presents with fever, sore throat and enlarged cervical (tonsillar) glands. There is usually but not always a purulent pharyngeal exudate or a follicular appearance (Fig. 15.3) though similar appearances may be seen with viral pharyngitis. A positive throat swab in the presence of symptoms confirms the diagnosis. Treatment is with penicillin for a full 10 days or a macrolide antibiotic if the child is penicillin-allergic.

Complications include peritonsillar abscess (quinsy (see Fig. 15.3)), suppurative cervical lymphadenopathy, scarlet fever or, rarely, streptococcal toxic shock syndrome. Poststreptococcal glomerulonephritis can occur after infection with particular nephritogenic strains. Raised levels of antistreptococcal antibodies (antistreptolysin O or anti DNA-ase) may help confirm this diagnosis. Rheumatic fever (see p. 180) following streptococcal infection is nowadays a rare event which is preventable by antibiotic treatment of the initial infection.

Table 15.1
Secondary immunodeficiency states

Cause	System affected	Clinical problems
Acute infection, e.g. measles, varicella, overwhelming sepsis	Immune responses, neutrophil function	Secondary infections, mainly bacterial or fungal
Chronic infection, e.g. viral, malaria, TB See also HIV, p. 274	Immune responses	Secondary infections, all types
Major trauma, burns, surgery and anaesthesia	Immune responses and neutrophil function	Bacterial and fungal infections
Drugs		
Corticosteroids*	Immune responses and inflammation	Bacterial infections Fungal, especially candida Viral – varicella
Chemotherapy, acute	Myelosuppression	Bacterial/fungal sepsis
Chemotherapy, longer term	Immune responses	Opportunistic infections, e.g. *Pneumocystis carinii* pneumonia
Immunosuppressives, e.g. cyclosporin A	Specifically depressed immune responses	Opportunistic infections Epstein–Barr virus-driven lymphoproliferative disease
Bone marrow transplant with chemo- and/or radiotherapy	Early myelosuppression and prolonged depression of immune responses	Early: bacterial/fungal sepsis Late: opportunistic infections
Splenectomy/hyposplenism	Handling of capsulated bacteria	Pneumococcal sepsis
Protein-losing states (nephrotic syndrome, gastrointestinal disease	Loss of IgG antibody	Bacterial infections especially pneumococcal

* The immunosuppressive dose of steroids in children is not well established. A dose of 2 mg/kg for >1 week or 1 mg/kg for 2 weeks is often taken as being significant.

Scarlet fever (scarlatina)

This group A streptococcal infection has an incubation period of 2–5 days.

Clinical manifestations include pharyngitis and a strawberry tongue. There is a generalized erythematous rash (day 2), and desquamation with healing (Fig. 15.1). The syndrome can be prevented with early penicillin treatment.

Rare complications include rheumatic fever, acute glomerulonephritis and other poststreptococcal syndromes. Streptococcal toxic shock may also occur.

Group B β-haemolytic Streptococcus

S. agalactiae causes serious invasive infection (pneumonia, septicaemia and meningitis) in newborn infants (see Ch. 1, p. 18).

α-haemolytic streptococcal infection: endocarditis

See Chapter 7, Cardiology, page 179.

Streptococcus pneumoniae (pneumococcus) infection

See Pneumonia (p. 359), Otitis media (p. 119) and Meningitis (p. 280).

Impetigo and furunculosis

See Chapter 9, Dermatology, page 194.

Deep-seated staphylococcal infections

See relevant organ specialty section.

Toxic epidermal necrolysis (scalded skin syndrome)

This is caused by toxin (epidermolysin)-producing *Staphylococcus aureus*. It is commonest in neonates.

Clinical manifestations include extensive superficial fragile blistering, which desquamates to leave raw

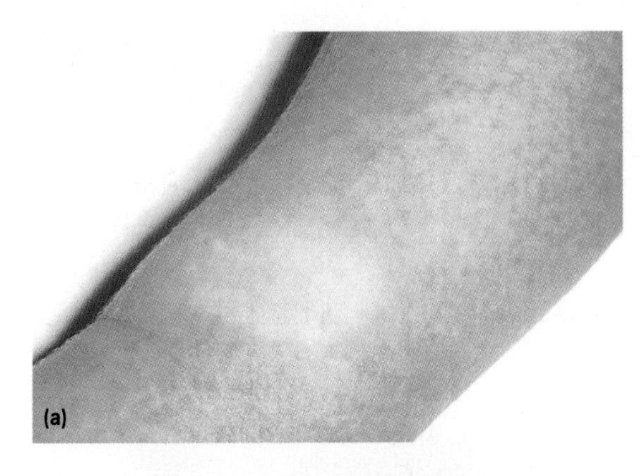

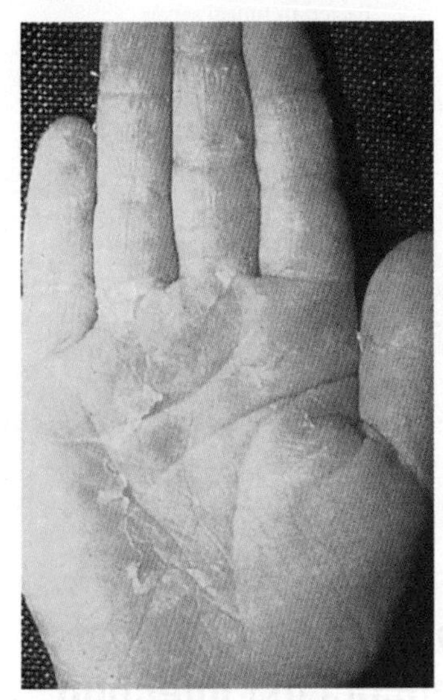

Fig 15.1
Scarlet fever: (a) rash showing sign of prolonged blanching after pressure; (b) desquamation during convalescence (Courtesy of Milupa).

areas. The skin can come off on the examiner's hands (Nikolski sign). Toxic shock may be associated. In older children the disease is often localized. It may complicate chickenpox.

Complications include hypovolaemia, because of oozing from raw skin areas, and shock.

Toxic shock syndrome

This is caused by toxin-producing *Staphylococcus aureus*, or occasionally by group A Streptococcus.

It presents with fever, vomiting with or without diarrhoea, impaired consciousness and a generalized erythematous rash. Nonpurulent conjunctivitis may or may not be found. There is a focus of staphylococcal infection, which is often minor, and shock.

Complications of shock may occur.

Meningococcal infections

See Meningitis (p. 280) and Septicaemia (p. 280).

Haemophilus infections

Haemophilus influenzae may be capsulated in serotypes a–g. Type b causes the vast majority of invasive disease: bacteraemia, meningitis and epiglottitis. The introduction of conjugate vaccine against the type b capsulated organism (Hib vaccine) has virtually eliminated invasive disease due to this serotype. Non-encapsulated (or nontypable) strains are important causes of bronchitis, pneumonia and otitis media. The vaccination programme has not reduced the incidence of these problems.

Treatment of serious *H. influenzae* infections is with a third-generation cephalosporin such as cefotaxime. Amoxycillin can be used in the first instance for less serious infections, such as otitis media, but there is an antibiotic resistance rate of around 15%.

Enteric fever (typhoid fever)

Epidemiology
Common in low income countries. Occurs only in humans.

This is infection with *Salmonella typhi*, *S. paratyphi* A, *S. schottmuelleri* (previously *S. paratyphi* B) and *S. hirschfield* (previously *S. paratyphi* C). After ingestion of contaminated water or food, the salmonellae reach the bloodstream via Peyer patches of the small intestine. They collect in reticuloendothelial cells and re-seed the blood stream.

Symptoms commence on average 14 days after exposure and can vary from an apparently mild febrile illness to severe septicaemia. Typically there is constipation in the early phases, though young children tend to suffer diarrhoea. A dry cough is a common symptom. A sparse maculopapular rash may occur over the chest and abdomen ('rose spots') (Fig. 15.2). There is lymphocytosis and a relative bradycardia in the face of fever. The illness can be complicated by intestinal haemorrhage and perforation. The organisms can be isolated from blood cultures and later in the illness from urine and stool.

Treatment with chloramphenicol or cotrimoxazole is required. Two vaccines are available, an injectable killed preparation based on the carbohydrate 'Vi' antigen of *S. typhi* and a live oral vaccine based on an attenuated strain of *S. typhi* called Ty21a.

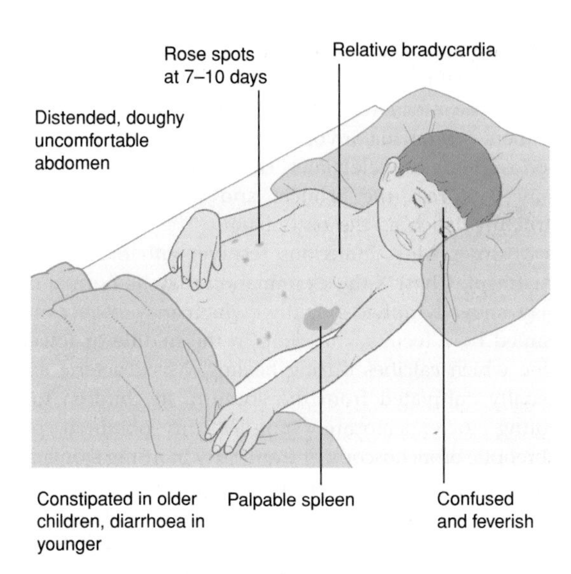

Fig 15.2
Typhoid.

Diphtheria

Epidemiology
Rare in the UK, but it can return when immunization programmes fail, as in Russia.

Diphtheria is prevented by immunization with a toxoid derived from the toxin of *Corynebacterium diphtheriae*.

The organism infects the upper respiratory tract and, after an incubation period of 1–6 days, the released toxin damages first the local tissues, and then the heart, kidneys and nervous system by inhibiting protein synthesis. A firmly adherent greyish-white pseudo-membrane of fibrin, erythrocytes, epithelial and inflammatory cells is seen on the nasal septum or pharynx (Fig. 15.3). Nasal diphtheria may be less easy to diagnose and produces a serosanguinous discharge. Oedema of the neck results in the so-called 'bull neck' appearance. Heart failure, coma and death may occur after 1 week due to systemic effects of the toxin. Extension of the local infection to the larynx causes severe obstruction. Diagnosis is confirmed by culturing the organism from nasal or throat swabs and demonstrating toxin production.

Antitoxin (antiserum raised in horses) must be administered immediately after first excluding sensitivity to horse serum (administration of a small dose intradermally). Anaphylactic reactions are treated with adrenaline. Sensitivity is an indication for

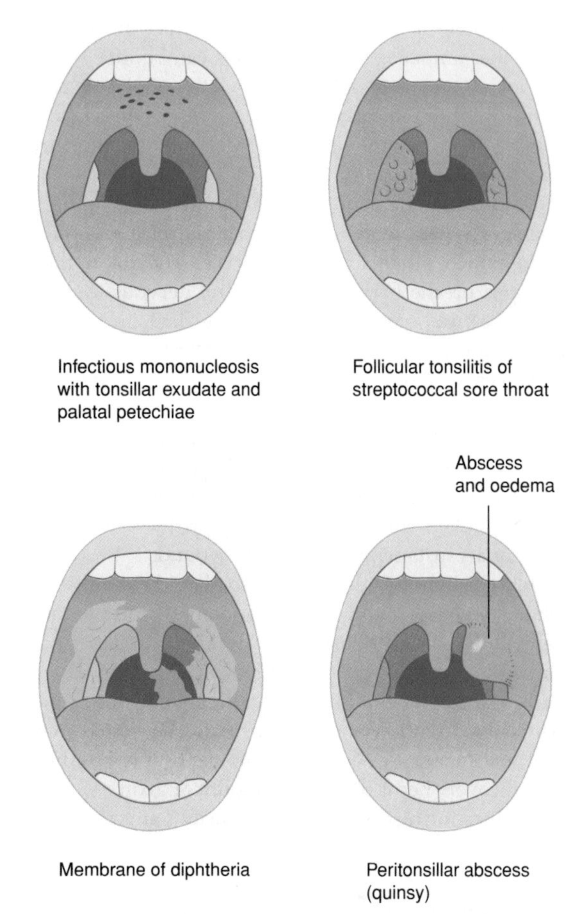

Fig 15.3
The appearance of the pharynx in different illnesses. In diphtheria, a firmly adherent greyish pseudomembrane is seen.

desensitization with progressively increasing doses. Penicillin (or erythromycin) is also given. Contacts should be immunized if they have not received a booster for 5 years. Unimmunized close contacts should receive antibiotics, although the efficacy of chemo-prophylaxis has not been established.

Tetanus

Epidemiology
Rare in countries with a high immunization rate.

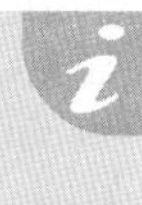

Tetanus is caused by the toxin of *Clostridium tetani*. Spores of the organism are widespread in the environment, including the intestinal tract of humans and other animals. Newborn babies can be infected in low income countries if there is a practice of placing cow dung on the umbilical cord stump. In many areas health education programmes and maternal immunization are reducing this problem.

More usually a wound is contaminated by spores. The spores germinate and the bacteria release tetanus toxin which binds to motor nerves. The toxin then migrates up the nerves to the central nervous system. Prolonged and painful muscle spasms develop, usually within 2 weeks of injury. Spasm of the facial muscles produces a fixed sardonic grin (*risus sardonicus*). Consciousness is not affected.

The disease can be prevented by immunization with tetanus toxoid. Maternal immunization prevents neonatal tetanus. Wounds should be carefully debrided and human tetanus immune globulin given to nonimmune individuals sustaining deep or dirty wounds.

Tetanus immune globulin is also given in established tetanus together with wound debridement. Intravenous penicillin G is administered. The affected patient is nursed in a darkened room. Muscle spasms are treated with diazepam. Paralysis with pancuronium and artificial ventilation may be required. The illness may continue for up to 6 weeks. Immunization is required after recovery because the tiny amount of toxin required to produce the disease is not necessarily immunogenic.

Tuberculosis

> Epidemiology
> The global burden of infection with this disease is enormous. It has been estimated that 35% of the world population is infected. Most of the burden is in low income countries, where low standards of living and in some cases HIV infection are contributory factors. In the UK the incidence of tuberculosis fell dramatically through the 20th century until the 1990s when there was a rise in the number of cases reported.

Most tuberculous infections are caused by *Mycobacterium tuberculosis*. Prior to the introduction of tuberculin testing of cattle *M. bovis* was another cause but this is now very rare. The main route of infection is by inhalation of infected droplets produced by coughing and sneezing. Two months after infection the patient will respond to the intradermal injection of *Mycobacterium tuberculosis* antigen (purified protein derivative; PPD) by development of induration after 2–3 days at the site of injection. The induration is produced by activated lymphocytes accumulating at the site of antigen injection (Mantoux test, Fig. 5.20, p. 147).

In primary pulmonary infection, bacilli infect the periphery of the lungs and draining lymph nodes at the hilum. The infection is asymptomatic initially but cough (if there is bronchial involvement), fever, and erythema nodosum may develop later. The enlarged lymph nodes may compress the bronchi and other mediastinal structures such as the oesophagus. The Mantoux test is positive. Most infections resolve with or without treatment. Chest X-ray examination may be normal or may show lymphadenopathy which may be accompanied by a focus of infection in the middle or lower lobe which calcifies during healing. Mycobacteria are usually cultivated from the sputum. In children too young to expectorate, samples are obtained by fibreoptic bronchoscopy or from early morning stomach washings via a nasogastric tube.

Rarely the primary pulmonary infection may spread to involve a whole lobe of the lung, causing cough, fever and anorexia. The primary infection may reactivate in adult life in the apices of the lungs. The infection causes fever and night sweats. Cough with haemoptysis begins when the infected lung cavitates.

Primary infections can disseminate throughout the body. This form is called miliary tuberculosis because of the resemblance of the tuberculous granulomata to millet seeds. Symptoms include fever, anorexia and cough. TB meningitis may be present (see Meningitis, p. 280).

M. tuberculosis can cause cervical lymphadenopathy which is managed with antituberculous chemotherapy. If a biopsy is required this should ideally be a full excision in case the cause turns out to be a nontuberculous mycobacterium (see below).

Commonly used antituberculous drugs are rifampicin, which is hepatoxic and colours urine, sweat, tears (and contact lenses) orange. Ethambutol can rarely cause visual disturbance including colour blindness. Pyrazinamide can cause hepatotoxicity. Isoniazid, which can cause hepatotoxicity and peripheral neuropathy, is given as prophylaxis for 6 months to children who are Mantoux positive but well, to prevent reactivation and potential development of miliary TB. Established tuberculosis is treated with isoniazid, rifampicin and pyrizinamide for 6 months.

Prevention involves contact tracing, chemoprophylaxis and BCG vaccination.

Nontuberculous mycobacterial infection

> Epidemiology
> Unlike *M. tuberculosis* and *M. bovis* these organisms are widely distributed in soil and water. Person-to-person spread does not occur.

The organisms mainly responsible are *M. avium, M. intracellulare, M. scrofulaceum, M. kansasii, M. fortuitum, M. marinum* and *M. chelonae*. In young children they cause cervical lymphadenitis or occasionally pulmonary infection. The last three organisms listed can cause localized cutaneous granulomas. Disseminated disease only occurs in the profoundly immunocompromised. The natural history of these infections is to resolve spontaneously but this may take many months or even years.

The differential diagnosis of cervical lymphadenitis due to one of these organisms includes tuberculosis, cat scratch disease and lymphoma. Biopsy of the lesions is therefore often undertaken. This should ideally be a complete excision biopsy otherwise a chronically discharging sinus may result. If complete excision can be achieved this is usually curative.

The organisms are mostly inherently resistant to standard antituberculous drugs, but other antibiotics such as ciprofloxacin, clarithromycin and cotrimoxazole may be of some benefit in difficult cases.

Children affected by these infections are not seriously ill but a lot of anxiety can be generated because of the chronicity of the symptoms and the disfigurement which can occur with discharging sinuses.

Fungal infections

Candida infections

These are most commonly caused by *Candida albicans* but others, for example *C. tropicalis*, also occur.

Oral and napkin candidiasis are common in newborn infants (see Ch. 2). Candidal infections are less common in other age groups, but risk factors include general debility, treatment with antibiotics, steroids or other immunosuppressives. They usually respond to topical therapy such as nystatin or miconazole.

In immunosuppressed children there may be recurrent superficial infection, resistant to treatment or involving unusual sites such as the oesophagus. Deep (invasive) infection, for example pneumonia or septicaemia, occurs in the immunosuppressed, particularly in those with prolonged periods of neutropenia.

Invasive disease is treated with amphotericin B which can be administered in a liposomal form to reduce its toxicity. Azole drugs such as fluconazole are also used, but resistance may be a problem.

Aspergillus infections

Aspergillus fumigatus, A. flavus and other species are ubiquitous in the environment. Transmission is by inhalation of spores.

Allergic bronchopulmonary aspergillosis occurs in atopic patients, especially those with asthma, causing wheezing with flitting perihilar opacities seen on the chest radiograph. In immunocompetent individuals, sinus and external ear infections can occur. Aspergilloma is a fungal ball which develops in pre-existing lung cavities/cysts.

Serious invasive aspergillosis, causing pneumonia, fungaemia and widespread fungal abscess formation, occurs in immunocompromised patients particularly those undergoing prolonged myelosuppressive treatment and those with neutrophil function disorders. Mortality is high.

Treatment is with amphotericin B. Newer imidazole drugs, such as itraconazole, may be useful prophylactically in high risk patients.

Dermatophytoses

These superficial fungal infections are caused by Trichophyton and Microsporidium species, and are commonly known as ringworm, affecting the scalp (tinea capitis), body (tinea corporis), feet (tinea pedis or athlete's foot) and nails (tinea unguum). Transmission is by direct or indirect contact with affected humans, animals or fomites.

Tinea pedis can be treated with topical antifungal agents such as clotrimazole or miconazole. Other forms of the infection require systemic treatment with griseofulvin (taken for a prolonged period in the case of nail infections), which can be combined with topical preparations.

Other fungal infections

For cryptococcosis, see below; for *Pneumocystis carinii* pneumonia, see Chapter 23, Respirology, page 360.

Viral infections

Exanthems

(Congenital viral infections are covered in Chapter 1)

Definition
Exanthem means a rash produced by an infection, either viral or bacterial.

Epidemiology
Exanthemata such as rubella and measles are becoming rare since the introduction of vaccines. Others such as varicella are almost universal in childhood, although often subclinical.

Measles (rubeola) (Fig. 15.4)

The incubation period is 8–14 days. Measles presents with coryza, cough, fever and Koplik spots which resemble grains of sugar on the buccal membranes (days 1–2). The rash, which appears on days 3–4, is florid and maculopapular. It starts at the hairline and spreads down. It is nonpruritic and leaves brown staining.

Complications of measles include secondary bacterial infection, which may cause conjunctivitis, otitis media or pneumonia. Post infectious encephalitis occurs in 1–2 per 1000 cases. Subacute sclerosing panencephalitis, a chronic, degenerative brain disease due to measles, is late and very rare.

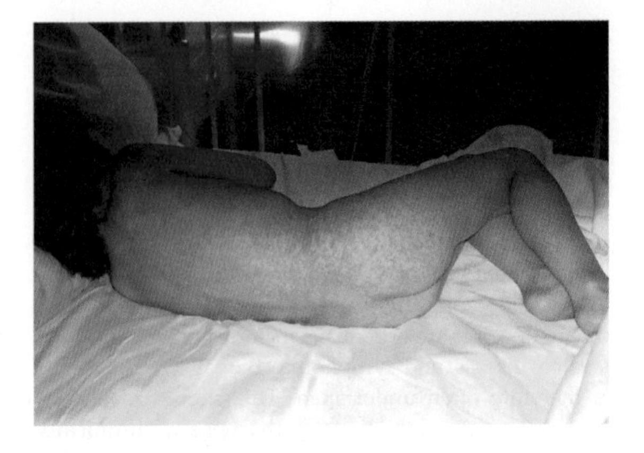

Fig 15.4
Measles.

Mumps

The incubation period is 12–25 days. The illness may be subclinical. Clinical presentation includes fever, parotitis (Fig. 15.5) or other salivary gland inflammation, and aseptic meningitis. Mumps may be complicated by epididymo-orchitis, postinfectious encephalitis, pancreatitis, deafness or facial nerve paralysis.

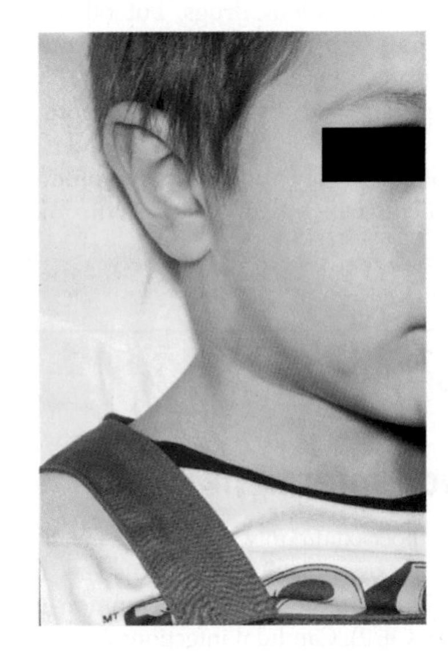

Fig 15.5
Parotid gland enlargement caused by mumps. Note filling in of the angle of the jaw.

Rubella

The incubation period is 14–21 days. Rubella presents as a mild, often asymptomatic, illness. There is lymphadenopathy, especially post-auricular, and low grade fever. The rash, which usually appears on day 1 of the illness, is transient and less florid than that of measles (Fig. 15.6). Complications include polyarthritis, especially of the hands; this is more common in adults. Other complications are post-infectious encephalitis and congenital rubella syndrome.

Erythema infectiosum (fifth disease, slapped cheek disease)

This is a parvovirus infection with an incubation period of 4–14 days. Clinical manifestations include a rubella-like rash with or without a 'slapped cheek' appearance, which can persist or recur for several weeks. There is fever, coryza and pharyngitis with cervical lymphadenopathy. Polyarthritis may occur as a complication, usually in adults. The virus transiently switches off red cell production. This may cause an aplastic crisis in disorders with increased red blood cell turnover, such as sickle cell anaemia, G6PD deficiency or spherocytosis. Hydrops fetalis may occur as a result of in utero infection.

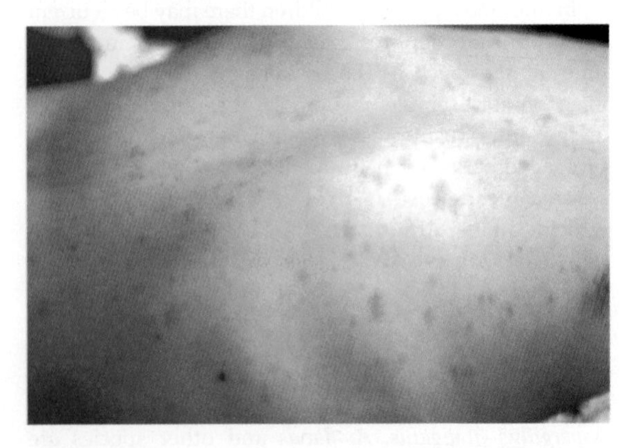

Fig 15.6
Rubella. (Courtesy of Milupa.)

Roseola infantum (erythema subitum)

This is caused by human herpes viruses 6 or 7. The incubation period is 7–15 days. The illness presents with high fever and irritability which lasts 3 days. As the fever resolves, a faint macular rash is seen on the trunk (Fig. 15.7). Febrile convulsions are a common complication.

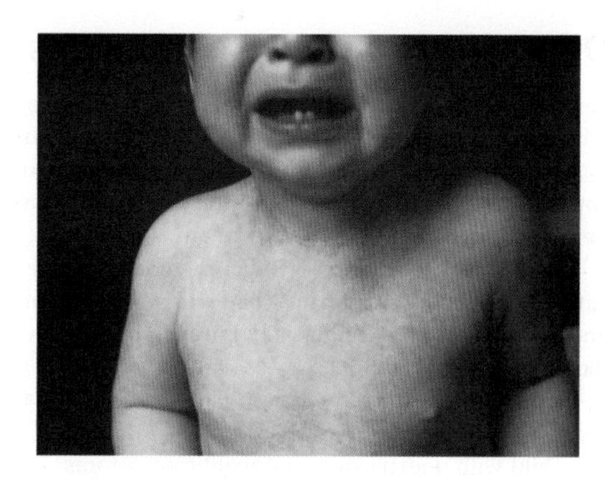

Fig 15.7
Rash of roseola infantum. (Courtesy of Milupa.)

Varicella (chickenpox)

The incubation period is 10–21 days. Chickenpox presents with coryza, fever, and a rash developing after 24–48 hours (Fig. 15.8) which evolves through papular, vesicular, and pustular phases. Once the lesions are dry the patient is non-infectious. Permanent scarring may occur, particularly after secondary bacterial infection.

Chickenpox may be complicated by encephalitis which is often cerebellar. Other complications are secondary bacterial infection or VZV pneumonia, the latter occurring especially in adults and smokers. Shingles may be a late complication, occasionally occurring in childhood.

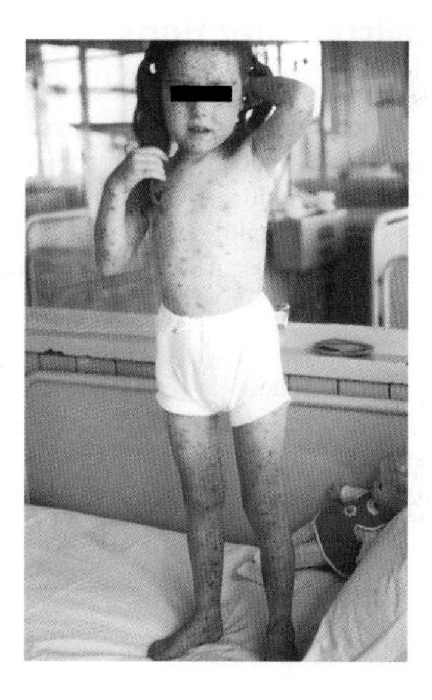

Fig 15.8
Varicella. Courtesy of Milupa.

Herpes simplex infections

Gingivostomatitis

The first contact with *Herpes simplex* virus can induce multiple small ulcers in the mouth. These are intensely painful, often preventing eating and sometimes drinking.

Aciclovir is probably of no benefit. Antifungal (nystatin) and antibiotic (flucloxacillin) treatment may be needed for secondary infection. Some children require hospital admission for nasogastric or intravenous fluid therapy.

The lesions heal in 7–10 days, but recurrence is likely as a localized lesion on the lip (herpes labialis or 'cold sore') which will respond to topical aciclovir if given early.

Neonatal herpes infections

Most of these are caused by type II (genital) *Herpes simplex*, acquired from the maternal genital tract at delivery. Primary infection in the mother carries the highest risk.

The localized form affects the skin, mouth and eyes as a vesicular eruption or keratoconjunctivitis. It can progress to more invasive forms. The encephalitic type presents with altered consciousness level and convulsions. The generalized systemic form presents with pneumonitis, hepatitis and sometimes septic shock-like illness.

Disease which is recognized early (at the localized stage) responds well to treatment with aciclovir, while late disease carries a high morbidity and mortality.

Infants of mothers with active genital disease should be delivered by caesarean section, if this can be done within 4 hours of rupture of the amniotic membranes. Any carers of newborns who have cold sores should wear masks, use topical aciclovir to shorten the period of their infectivity and wash their hands thoroughly.

Other *Herpes simplex* infections

Herpetic whitlows are localized lesions on the fingers whose main significance is that they are highly infectious.

Ocular herpes infections involve the conjunctiva and cornea. Dendritic ulcers affecting the latter can cause permanent scarring; specialist treatment is required.

Eczema herpeticum (Fig. 9.8 p. 192) is a serious extensive cutaneous herpetic eruption in a child with atopic eczema, and requires hospitalization and intravenous aciclovir therapy.

Herpes encephalitis in children is rare but devastating. It should be considered as a possible diagnosis in any child with unexplained encephalitic symptoms.

Other viral infections

Enterovirus infections

These may be caused by coxsackie A, B or ECHO viruses. The incubation period is 3–6 days.

Clinical features include those of a nonspecific febrile illness, with pharyngitis, myalgia and headache. A nonspecific rash and mild gastro-intestinal symptoms may or may not be present. With specific agents there may be:

- Herpangina (coxsackie A)
- Pharyngeal ulceration
- Hand, foot and mouth disease (coxsackie A16)
- Anterior mouth ulcers
- Pleurodynia (Bornholm disease; coxsackie B group).

Possible complications include the following:

- Conjunctivitis
- Myositis
- Pneumonia
- Myocarditis
- Encephalitis
- Aseptic meningitis
- ?Postviral fatigue syndrome
- Fulminant septic shock-like illness in neonates, with or without hepatic necrosis.

Infectious mononucleosis

The incubation period is 14–21 days.

The illness presents with fever, pharyngitis (Fig. 15.3) (cervical adenopathy), a maculopapular rash (in 15%) and anicteric hepatitis with splenomegaly. A florid rash follows ampicillin or amoxycillin treatment almost invariably.

Complications include:

- Upper airway obstruction
- Myocarditis (pericarditis)
- Ruptured spleen
- Chronic infectious mononucleosis
- Encephalitis (mainly in the immunocompromised)
- Postviral fatigue.

Cytomegalovirus infections

This is caused by a herpes virus which becomes latent after primary infection, and is the commonest cause of congenital infection (see Ch. 1, p. 16).

Postnatal primary infection usually results in an asymptomatic or mild illness. Cytomegalovirus can cause an infectious mononucleosis type illness. Serious life-threatening illness occurs in the immunocompromised as a result of the realighting of latent infection. After bone marrow transplantation severe pneumonitis and viraemia may occur. HIV-infected children suffer focal infections including retinitis, encephalitis, colitis. Gauciclovir and foscarnet are active against the virus.

Adenovirus infections

Adenovirus is a DNA virus with nearly 50 different types, most of which cause respiratory disease.

Upper respiratory illness usually manifests as pharyngitis or laryngitis (croup) with cervical lymphadenopathy. Conjunctivitis may occur (kerato-conjunctival fever). In very young children (<2 years), lower respiratory illness may occur including bronchiolitis or pneumonia. The latter may result in severe lung damage.

Types 40 and 41 are associated with gastrointestinal infection (see p. 221).

Adenoviruses are a particular problem in severely immunocompromised patients.

Respiratory viral infections

See Respirology, Chapter 23, page 357.

Gastrointestinal viral infections

See Gastroenterology, Chapter 11, page 221.

Hepatitis viruses

See Hepatology, Chapter 14, page 259.

HIV/AIDS (Fig. 15.9)

INTRODUCTION

HIV infection is caused by one of the two known human immunodeficiency viruses, HIV1 and HIV2. Affected

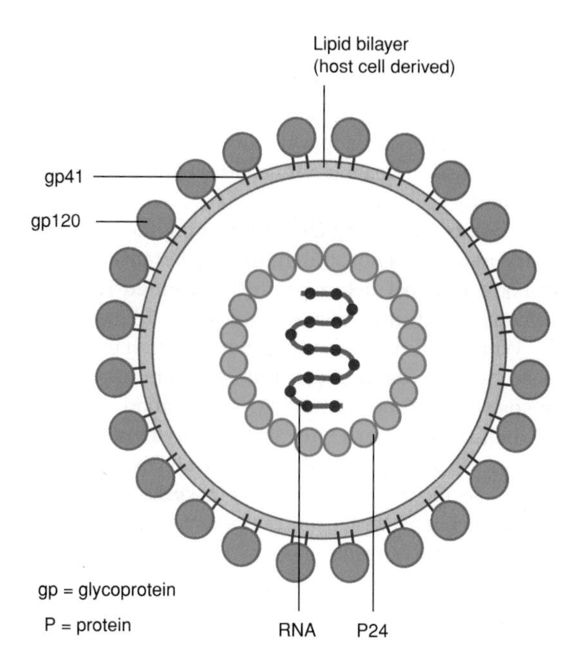

Fig 15.9
Schematic representation of the HIV virus.

individuals may be symptomatic or asymptomatic. In the immune system the virus infects the helper (CD4-positive) cells which gradually decline in number, leading to a weakening of the immune system and secondary susceptibility to infections including those caused by opportunist agents. The virus may also directly infect other organs leading to encephalopathy, cardiac disease, renal disease, etc. Acquired immunodeficiency syndrome (AIDS) is the end stage of symptomatic HIV infection when the patient develops certain AIDS indicator diseases (see below).

EPIDEMIOLOGY AND INCIDENCE

Since the onset of the HIV/AIDS epidemic, the virus has infected more than 45 million people in the world. With more than 2.2 million deaths in 1998, HIV/AIDS has become the fourth leading cause of mortality and it is going to increase. Over 95% of all cases occur in the developing world, mainly among young adults.

Infection in children occurs mainly by vertical transmission from an infected mother, in utero, during delivery or possibly postnatally through breast milk. The rate of transmission from an infected mother in the absence of breastfeeding varies from 15–25% in developed countries to 39% in Africa. Transmission can also occur through use of infected blood products, from intravenous drug abuse (in adolescence) and by sexual transmission, which in children usually means sexual abuse. Fortunately this mode of transmission is uncommon. Horizontal transmission by other means is extremely rare, and when reported has involved potential mixing of blood or other body fluids.

Blood product transfusion has produced a sizeable cohort of infected children in the UK (mainly boys with haemophilia) and a larger and even more tragic problem in Romanian orphans who were given repeated blood transfusions. Now that the problem has been identified, the numbers of children in Europe who have acquired infection by this route will slowly dwindle. However, this mode of transmission remains a major concern in low income countries.

The main concern for paediatricians is the epidemic of HIV infection in the heterosexual population and the resultant increase in children who have been vertically infected. In Africa the number of children infected by this route is vast. In certain East African countries the seroprevalence of HIV in the general population is approximately one in five. There is also a large and rapidly increasing problem of heterosexual HIV transmission in the Indian subcontinent. In the United Kingdom and Europe the numbers are still relatively small and largely restricted to high risk groups. Unlinked anonymous testing of neonatal dried blood spots (see Neonatal screening Ch. 2) facilitates good epidemiological monitoring in the UK.

In recent years it has become evident that certain interventions such as the avoidance of breastfeeding and the use of antiretroviral therapy in pregnancy and labour can greatly reduce the risk of vertical transmission from HIV-positive mothers. The implementation of these measures has significantly reduced the number of new paediatric cases in the USA and continental European countries. This is only just being achieved in the UK, because until recently there were very low levels of uptake of antenatal testing and therefore identification of women at risk. Recent evidence suggests that even a single dose of a relatively cheap antiviral agent given in labour can halve the risk of transmission and this offers hope for controlling the problem in low income countries.

AETIOLOGY AND PATHOGENESIS

When infection occurs, DNA proviral copies of the viral genome are made and integrated into the host cell DNA. Latent infection is therefore set up and, as for other viruses that exhibit latency, there is no known way of eliminating this proviral DNA from the body. The virus has a predilection for three major cell types; the CD4-positive helper T lymphocyte, the macrophage, and the cells of the central nervous system. In young children many of the manifestations of HIV infection can be attributed to infection in these cell types and involve development of immunodeficiency and neurological disorders.

CLINICAL PRESENTATION

In older children who acquire the virus from blood transfusions or sexually, the disease behaves much as it does in adults. The reader is referred to textbooks of adult medicine for details. There are certain differences however from adults, in that opportunist infection with reactivated infections such as toxoplasma is less common in children, simply because those in this age group are less likely to have previously encountered these agents and to have established latent infection. Possibly for the same reason, Kaposi sarcoma is relatively unusual in children.

The spectrum of the disease in infants who have acquired the virus from their mothers is often quite different from that in older individuals. Clinical presentation may occur in the following ways:

- The mother is identified as having HIV infection and the child is then screened (see below for problems in confirming infection in infants)
- The infant presents within the first 6 months of life with an AIDS-defining illness (see Information box 15.1), most commonly *Pneumocystis carinii* pneumonia
- An infant or young child develops symptoms suggestive of HIV infection which include:
  - Recurrent respiratory infections
  - Tachypnoea with chest radiological appearances of lymphoid interstitial pneumonitis
  - Diarrhoea
  - Candidiasis, persistent or recurrent
  - Lympadenopathy
  - Hepatosplenomegaly
  - Parotid enlargement
  - Neurological symptoms: motor disorder, e.g. spastic diplegia, developmental regression

Not all of these are AIDS-defining; see Information box 15.1.

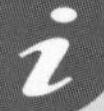

Information Box 15.1

AIDS-defining illness in childhood

- Opportunistic infections
  - *Pneumocystis carinii*
  - Cytomegalovirus
  - Disseminated TB or atypical mycobacterial infection
  - Candidiasis affecting oesophagus or respiratory tract
  - Other opportunistic infections
- Two or more serious bacterial infections, e.g.
  - Septicaemia, meningitis
- Chronic severe respiratory disease (due to lymphoid interstitial pneumonitis (LIP) and/or infections)
- Severe failure to thrive
- Encephalopathy (Fig. 15.10)
- Malignancy, mainly lymphoma + Kaposi sarcoma

DIAGNOSIS

In the older child the diagnosis when suspected is easily confirmed with an HIV antibody test. Pre-test counselling and post-test support from a counsellor specifically trained in dealing with children and adolescents is mandatory.

In infants and young children making the diagnosis of HIV infection is not straightforward because the HIV antibody test will detect passively acquired maternal antibody which may persist until up to 18 months of age. While viral culture and antigen detection tests have been used to circumvent this problem, these are expensive and time-consuming. The method of choice for diagnosis in early life is the polymerase chain reaction (PCR) test to detect proviral DNA. This is highly specific and sensitive after 2 weeks of age and should be infants tested on two separate occasions to confirm a positive result.

MANAGEMENT

Follow up is best conducted in a family clinic because the mother, father and siblings are often affected.

In older children the management of HIV and AIDS is similar to that in adults with the disease. Prophylaxis against *P. carinii* and bacterial infections is along standard lines, being related to the circulating CD4 cell count. Early identification and treatment of opportunist infections are required and antiretroviral treatment is useful in slowing down the progress of the disease (see below). The paediatrician's role will include tackling specific problems which may occur in relation to schooling and in helping the child and family cope with this life-threatening and stigmatizing disease. Counselling and support should be provided by persons experienced with dealing with children and adolescents suffering chronic and fatal disorders.

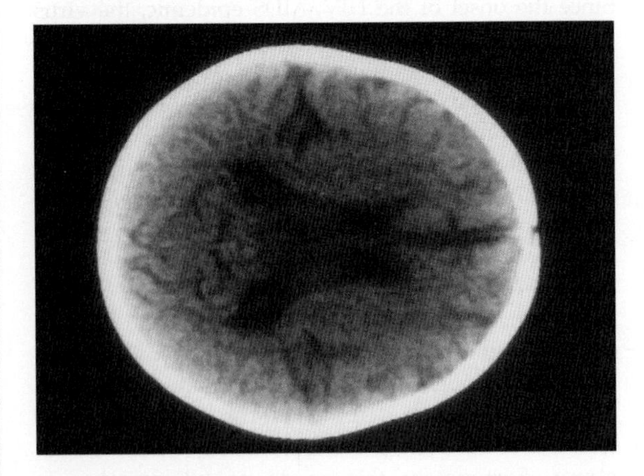

Fig 15.10
HIV encephalopathy showing cerebral atrophy (enlarged ventricles and sulci).

In infants born to known HIV-positive mothers, initial management will be aimed at trying to establish whether or not the infant is infected. In high income countries, breastfeeding is discouraged to decrease the risk of HIV transmission. In low income countries the benefits of breastfeeding outweigh the risks of viral transmission, although very prolonged breastfeeding may unnecessarily increase the risks; this is an issue currently under study.

Monitoring of growth development and susceptibility to infection will form part of clinical assessment.

Infection prophylaxis involves immunizations, which should all be given except for BCG. The last is omitted (because of the risk of disseminated BCGosis) in this country, though it is given in low income countries where the risks of tuberculosis outweigh the risks of vaccine-related problems. The killed injectable polio vaccine is preferred to the standard live oral vaccine because of the risk of vaccine-associated poliomyelitis in the recipient or in family contacts who may also be immunodeficient. All other vaccines including the live MMR vaccine are safe and are indicated.

Drug prophylaxis includes the use of cotrimoxazole against *P. carinii* pneumonia, and this also provides some protection against bacterial infections. The use of intravenous immunoglobulin has also been suggested in those with recurrent bacterial infections occurring despite antibiotic prophylaxis, but is not employed generally. Other types of secondary antimicrobial prophylaxis, for example antifungal agents, antivirals against cytomegalovirus and antimycobacterial drugs, also need to be employed in some cases.

There have been considerable advances in the use of antiretroviral drugs in the last 5 years. A number of different agents, including nucleoside and non-nucleoside reverse transcriptase inhibitors and viral protease inhibitors, are used in combinations of three or four drugs, known as highly active antiretroviral therapy (HAART). Such treatments have been shown to arrest the progress of the disease and can reverse the immune incompetence that has developed. There has been a significant fall in hospitalization rates for complications of HIV in both adults and children since the introduction of this treatment. There is concern that the development of viral resistance will reverse this trend and this is being monitored. It has not yet been fully established in which children and at what stage of the illness this treatment should be started, but it depends on clinical parameters, HIV viral load and CD4 count. There is no doubt that treatment should be commenced when AIDS-defining illnesses develop. Marked improvement, at least on a temporary basis, can be seen in neurological manifestations when drug regimens which include zidovudine are used.

The overall outcomes for children who prove to be infected from their mothers are shown in Information box 15.2.

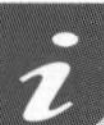

Information Box 15.2

Outcomes for children infected with HIV from their mothers

- Up to 20% will develop AIDS within 6 months of birth
  - These are so-called rapid progressors
  - There is a high mortality, though some will respond to treatment
- The remainder (slow progressors) have a delayed onset of severe disease
  - Most have some symptoms which are usually responsive to treatment
  - Some remain completely asymptomatic
  - If symptoms are mainly lymphoid interstitial pneumonitis (LIP)-related, prolonged survival can be expected
  - Many of these children have a relatively long life expectancy
- A number of vertically infected children are still alive in teenage years
  - Prevention of transmission of the disease as these youngsters become sexually active is an important public health objective

Protozoal diseases

Gastrointestinal protozoa

See Gastroenterology, Chapter 11 (Amoebiasis, Giardiasis and Cryptosporidiosis).

Malaria

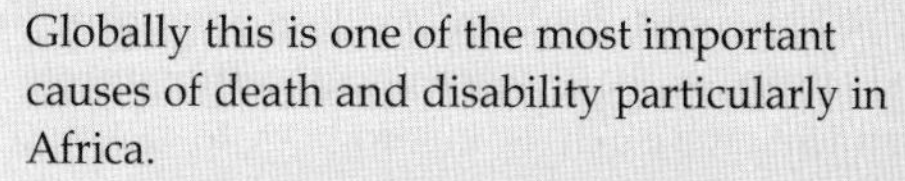

Epidemiology

Globally this is one of the most important causes of death and disability particularly in Africa.

Because of increased world travel, it is a possible cause of fever in any country.

In the UK there are 200–300 imported cases each year in children.

A small number of individuals die in the UK each year, nearly all due to falciparum malaria and usually associated with delayed diagnosis and treatment.

Malaria is an infection due to *Plasmodium falciparum* (most severe), *P. ovale*, *P. vivax* and *P. ovale*, acquired from the bite of the female anopheline mosquito. The disease occurs in the tropics but is commonly imported into temperate climates. The diagnosis should be considered in children returned from the tropics who develop fever.

The parasites develop in red cells causing haemolysis. Symptoms include malaise, very high fever, headache, myalgia, abdominal pain, diarrhoea, vomiting and jaundice. *P. falciparum* produces convulsions and coma (cerebral malaria) and haemoglobinuria (blackwater fever).

The diagnosis is made by detecting the parasites in thick and thin blood films. Repeated examinations may be required and the most useful samples are taken just as the fever is rising. The differential diagnosis will include other diseases acquired in the tropics, including typhoid fever, and it should be remembered that in returning travellers it is not unusual for more than one disease to be present.

The infection is prevented by avoidance of mosquito bites (using insect repellents and mosquito nets impregnated with insecticide) and chemoprophylaxis. The choice of chemoprophylactic agents is determined by local parasite sensitivity but examples include a combination of proguanil and chloroquine or mefloquine.

Malaria caused by *P. falciparum* is treated with quinine because of the possibility of chloroquine resistance. A 5-day course of this treatment is followed up with a single dose of Fansidar (pyrimethamine and sulfadoxine) unless the child is glucose-6-phosphate dehydrogenase (G6PD)-deficient. In the UK all cases of malaria are tested for G6PD deficiency since its presence will influence subsequent treatment (see p. 253). The deficiency is particularly common in certain populations in West Africa, probably because it confers a degree of protection against severe malaria.

In other (more benign) forms of malaria oral chloroquine is used. Since these forms have an exoerythrocytic phase, patients who will not be returning to endemic areas should also be treated with primaquine unless they are G6PD-deficient.

Severe falciparum malaria (high parasite load with or without coma) should be treated with intravenous quinine in a specialist centre, with close monitoring for both the effects of the disease and the side-effects of the treatment. Research is in progress to develop a vaccine.

Helminthic infections

Epidemiology
Virtually all higher life forms and the surface of the earth are colonized by helminths.

Nematodes (roundworms)

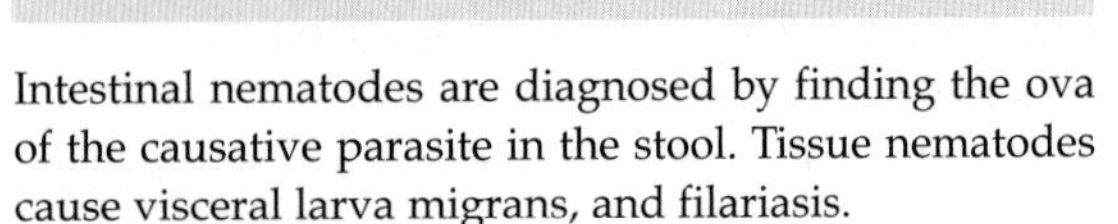
Illnesses caused
Ancylostomiasis, ascariasis, strongyloidiasis, enterobiasis and trichuriasis.

Intestinal nematodes are diagnosed by finding the ova of the causative parasite in the stool. Tissue nematodes cause visceral larva migrans, and filariasis.

Ancylostomiasis is caused by hookworm (*Ancylostoma duodenale, Ancylostoma ceylanicum* or *Necator americanus*) in the tropics. Hookworm larvae living in damp, warm soil can infect the human host by direct penetration through the skin. Children living in farming communities in tropical countries are particularly at risk. The larvae travel in the circulation to the lungs where they enter and travel up the bronchial tree to the larynx, then pharynx, where they are swallowed and pass to the small intestine. After a month the mature worms develop. They are about 1 cm long and attach to the mucosa of the small intestine by specialized mouth parts through which they suck blood. Worm eggs are passed in the faeces and hatch to produce larvae capable of infecting the next host. The main manifestations of infection are anaemia due to iron loss and protein-losing enteropathy. The diagnosis is made by finding ova in fresh faecal smears. Mebendazole eradicates the parasite.

Ascariasis is acquired by ingesting eggs of the roundworm *Ascaris lumbricoides*, which hatch in the small intestine. The larvae gain access to the circulation by penetrating the intestinal wall. They enter in the lungs, penetrate the alveoli, then ascend the bronchial tree and are swallowed. The adult worm (15–35 cm) develops in the small intestine, the female shedding eggs in the stool of the host. The transit of larvae through the lungs may produce the Lœffler syndrome of pulmonary infiltration and eosinophilia (see p. 359). Watery diarrhoea is induced with heavy infestations causing intestinal obstruction. Mebendazole is an effective treatment.

Strongyloidiasis is acquired in the same way as ancylostomiasis. Ova from mature *Strongyloides stercoralis* can hatch in the intestinal lumen, allowing the larvae to penetrate the colonic or perianal skin and establish an overwhelming infection. Disseminated strongyloidiasis is more likely in immunodeficient states, as occur in severe malnutrition or AIDS. The symptoms are those of malabsorption, with disseminated strongyloidiasis sometimes producing shock. The treatment is thiabendazole.

Enterobiasis is caused worldwide by *Enterobius vermicularis* (pinworm or threadworm) which is acquired by ingesting eggs from clothing or bedding. The eggs hatch in the stomach and the larvae travel to the caecum to mature. Mature female worms (1 cm long) deposit eggs on perianal skin. Scratching the irritated skin results in dissemination of the infection under fingernails. The pinworm eggs are more easily seen if a piece of clear adhesive tape is pressed against the perianal skin first thing in the morning, rather than in faeces. Mebendazole is given to all members of the family. Repeated treatment may be required.

Trichuriasis, caused by *Trichuris trichiura* (whipworm) is acquired in the same way as enterobiasis. As the worm attaches to the colon and sucks blood, heavy infections are associated with iron deficiency and bloody diarrhoea (dysentery). Once again mebendazole reduces the worm burden.

Visceral larva migrans (toxocariasis) is caused by the dog and cat parasites *Toxocara canis, T. cati* and *T. leonina*. Ingestion of eggs from animal faeces by children results in dissemination from the gastrointestinal tract to lung, liver, eye, brain, kidney and heart. Migration of the parasites produces fever, myalgia, cough and wheeze and convulsions. Eye involvement produces decreased visual acuity. Granulomata, which have been mistaken for retinoblastoma, can be seen on the retina. The blood shows a marked eosinophilia, and measurement of antibodies against the eggs of toxocara confirms the diagnosis. The treatment is diethylcarbamazine.

Infection of lymphatic vessels with minute worms called filariae results in filariasis, lymphoedema (hydrocele and elephantiasis) 10–20 years after infection, caused by lymphatic obliteration by scarring. People may be infected by mosquitoes bearing larval forms of the worm. The diagnosis is made by demonstrating larval forms (microfilariae) in blood samples. Treatment with diethylcarbamazine or ivermectin must be given early in the disease when there is lymphangitis; there is no therapy for elephantiasis. Other forms of filiariasis infect the eye (onchocerciasis, river blindness). The vector is the blackfly (simulium). Microfiliariae can be seen by slit lamp in the anterior chamber of the eye. Tabanid flies transmit a form of filariasis called loa loa, which causes conjunctivitis and subcutaneous swellings. The presence of microfilariae in the blood can cause Lœffler syndrome (p. 359).

Trematodes (flukes) – schistosomiasis

Aetiology

Schistosomiasis is caused by blood flukes *Schistosoma haematobium, S. intercalatum, S. japonicum, S. mansoni,* and *S. mekongi* which infect children.

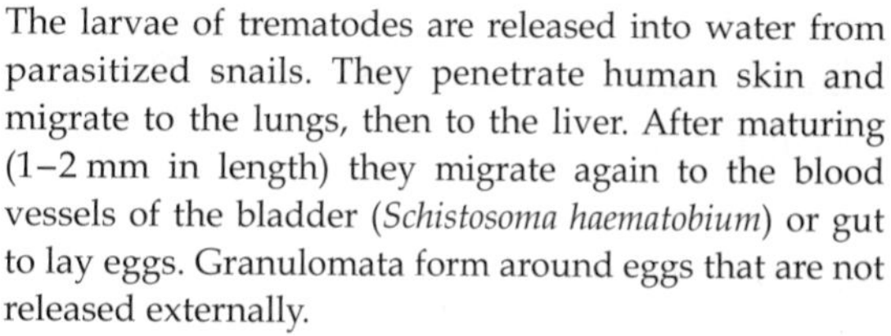

The larvae of trematodes are released into water from parasitized snails. They penetrate human skin and migrate to the lungs, then to the liver. After maturing (1–2 mm in length) they migrate again to the blood vessels of the bladder (*Schistosoma haematobium*) or gut to lay eggs. Granulomata form around eggs that are not released externally.

Acute schistosomiasis occurs shortly after infection, with fever, lymphadenopathy, hepatosplenomegaly and eosinophilia. Chronic schistosomiasis due to *S. haematobium* causes frequency, dysuria and haematuria leading to chronic kidney failure and bladder cancer. The other species of schistosomas produce bloody diarrhoea and portal hypertension.

Schistosomiasis is diagnosed by finding the eggs in the urine (best in the terminal part of the urinary stream) or stool. There are also serological tests.

The treatment is praziquantel.

Cestodes (tapeworms)

Aetiology

Taeniasis is caused by ingesting the larvae of *Taenia saginata* (beef tapeworm) or *Taenia solium* (pig tapeworm).

Echinococcosis (hydatid disease) is caused by *Echinococcus granulosus.*

The larvae of *T. saginata* and *T. solium* are found in undercooked meat. The tapeworms mature in the intestine to lengths of up to 10 metres. Infection is usually asymptomatic. Infection with *T. solium* may cause dissemination of larvae in the tissues (cysticercosis) which can cause seizures if localized in the brain. Treatment is niclosamide, or prizaquantel for cysticercosis.

The eggs of *Echinococcus granulosus* are acquired by contact with faeces of dogs that have become infected by ingestion of the viscera of parasitized sheep and cattle. The eggs hatch in the duodenum, penetrate the intestinal wall and travel to the liver, where the hydatid cyst forms. The cyst may grow to 20 cm in diameter. Cysts are also found in the lungs, bone and brain. Surgical removal is hazardous, since spillage of the cyst contents can result not only in disease dissemination but also in an overwhelming anaphylactoid reaction. The need for surgery may be avoided with the use of albendazole.

Some specific infections in children

Septicaemia

Epidemiology

The commonest cause of septicaemia is meningococcus. This causes septicaemia and/or meningitis. About two-thirds of meningococcal disease involves both processes with the remainder divided between a pure meningitis and a pure septicaemia without meningitis. The prognosis is worst for the last variety. Overall 4000 cases of meningococcal disease are reported per annum in the UK, of which 10% are fatal. Prior to the introduction of the conjugated meningococcal C vaccine, around 60% of these are caused by Group B organisms, one-third by Group C organisms and a small number by other groups. In developing countries, including the 'meningitis belt' in sub-Saharan Africa, Group A disease predominates.

Bacteraemia is defined as the presence of bacteria in the blood as identified on blood culture. This may be a primary process following invasion of organisms, for example from the nasopharynx, or it may be secondary and associated with a focal infection such as pneumonia or osteomyelitis. In septicaemia, bacteria are not only present in the blood but are actively multiplying. This leads to a profound illness with circulatory disturbance leading to shock in its most severe form. Damage to the endothelial lining of blood vessels, metabolic disturbance and coagulopathy all contribute to the development of multiorgan dysfunction and damage, thus compounding the problem. Both bacteraemia and septicaemia may be primary or secondary to bloodstream invasion from a site of focal infection.

Causative organisms in newborn infants include group B Streptococcus, *Escherichia coli*, and rarely *Listeria monocytogenes* (see Ch. 2).

In post-neonatal childhood the commonest and most devastating cause of septicaemia is *Neisseria meningitidis* (meningococcus). Other causes include *E. coli*, salmonella species including *S. typhi*, other Gram-negative bacilli, *S. aureus* and *S. pneumoniae*. *H. influenzae* type b is now a very rare cause.

The clinical presentation of sepsis in children will include fever and a number of nonspecific signs of being unwell which are described in Chapters 2–5. Meningococcal septicaemia usually but not invariably causes a haemorrhagic petechial or purpuric rash. In about one-third of cases this characteristic rash is preceded by a nonspecific maculopapular rash which can be mistaken for a nonspecific viral exanthem or the early stages of chickenpox. Petechial spots may coexist with this rash and should be looked for very carefully. Unlike most other childhood rashes the spots do not blanch on pressure and this is the basis of the tumbler test in which a glass tumbler is pressed to the skin over the spots and blanching or nonblanching observed. Purpuric spots are larger areas of haemorrhage in the skin secondary to the blood vessel damage which occurs in meningococcal sepsis.

Treatment of septicaemia is a medical emergency. From the first appearance of the rash to the stage of irreversible shock may take a matter of a few hours. Doctors seeing children with rashes suspected of being due to meningococcal infection must administer intravenous or intramuscular penicillin without delay and before transfer to hospital. Once in hospital treatment in an intensive care setting is usually required and involves treatment of shock and multiorgan dysfunction.

Prevention of meningococcal disease is a major research goal. A polysaccharide vaccine against group A and C organisms has been available for some time but is poorly effective in very young children (<2 years). It is recommended for travellers to developing countries with a high incidence of group A disease. Recently a conjugate group C vaccine has been licensed in the UK; this is immunogenic in young infants and should greatly reduce the proportion of disease due to this serogroup. Unfortunately a group B vaccine is not yet available. This is because the group B polysaccharide cross-reacts with a human antigen and is therefore non-immunogenic. Attempts at vaccine development are therefore aimed at using a meningococcal protein antigen rather than the polysaccharide.

Meningitis

INTRODUCTION

Two main forms of meningitis are viral (or aseptic) meningitis, and bacterial. A subtype of bacterial meningitis, often considered as a separate entity because it behaves differently, is tuberculous meningitis. In immunocompromised individuals, such as those with HIV and AIDS, fungal meningitis may also occur.

In viral meningitis there is usually an accompanying encephalitis to produce the clinical picture of meningoencephalitis. Sometimes there is a pure aseptic meningitis and in other cases a pure encephalitis without any meningeal inflammation. The range of possible viruses causing aseptic meningitis and meningoencephalitis is large. Some causes, particularly the insect-borne viruses (arboviruses), are only found in certain parts of the world. The main viral causes of aseptic meningitis in the UK are: enteroviruses

(ECHO and coxsackie viruses) and mumps. A variety of other common viral illnesses may occasionally be complicated by meningoencephalitis including infection with influenza, parainfluenza, RSV, measles, rubella and Epstein–Barr virus. Lymphocytic choriomeningitis virus is a rare but much vaunted cause of aseptic meningitis contracted from rodents.

The normal course of events is that there is a systemic illness with the virus then homing in on the central nervous system.

PATHOGENESIS AND AETIOLOGY OF BACTERIAL MENINGITIS

In bacterial meningitis the organisms gain access to the central nervous system via the bloodstream. A very small proportion of cases is associated with direct invasion of the central nervous system, either through defects in the dura, often in the region of the cribriform plate or from pericranial sepsis such as middle ear, sinus or dental sepsis. In those spread by the haematogenous route the three commonest organisms are *Neisseria meningitidis*, *Streptococcus pneumoniae* and *Haemophilus influenzae* type b (Hib). The proliferation of the bacteria in meninges produces a purulent response that gives rise to the symptoms and signs of the illness. Occasionally the cerebral tissue itself may become involved causing cerebritis. In neonates, the range of organisms causing meningitis is much greater and includes those derived from the maternal genital tract at birth such as group B Streptococcus and *Escherichia coli*. *Listeria monocytogenes* is also an important cause of meningitis in this age group. In the immunocompromised child, and in those with ventriculoperitoneal shunts in situ, the range of potential causative organisms is also much greater.

Tuberculous meningitis, caused by *Mycobacterium tuberculosis*, usually occurs following haematogenous spread from a primary focus elsewhere; most commonly the lungs. Multiple tubercles are produced throughout the meninges. There may also be larger foci of infection in the brain tissue itself, called tuberculomas.

INCIDENCE

There are approximately 4000 cases of bacterial meningitis reported annually in the UK. The greatest incidence occurs in infants and young children. There is a seasonal variation with an excess of cases occurring during the winter months. *H. influenzae* and *N. meningitidis* (meningococcus) were previously the two commonest varieties with *Streptococcus pneumoniae* (pneumococcus) in third place. We have now seen a marked fall in the incidence of *H. influenzae* meningitis, due to the introduction of a vaccine.

CLINICAL PRESENTATION

Inflammation of the meninges produces characteristic clinical findings. There will be fever, headache, bulging fontanelle (if patent), photophobia, pallor, vomiting, and signs of cerebral irritation such as high-pitched cry in young infants. The inflammation of the meninges produces reflex spasm of the neck muscles (neck stiffness) and pain on stretching the meninges, for instance in straight leg raising. These latter specific signs may be absent in children under 2 years of age. At that age the child often presents with a nonspecific febrile illness without specific signs. Most children will show an impaired conscious level that may range from mild drowsiness to coma. Seizures may be a presenting feature and occasionally focal neurological deficits. In meningococcal meningitis, the accompanying septicaemic component may produce a vasculitis leading to shock. In this condition there is usually but not inevitably a typical rash (Fig. 15.11) that is purpuric/petechial in appearance (this is caused by small haemorrhages due to leaky capillaries). The rash does not blanch on pressure in contrast to most other rashes that children get. In viral meningitis the signs and symptoms may be accompanied by evidence of a systemic viral infection and if these are specific as in mumps this may make the diagnosis easy.

In tuberculous meningitis the onset of symptoms is more insidious than with the other forms, with the features of drowsiness, headache, neck stiffness and vomiting often developing over several days to weeks. Mood changes, anorexia and vomiting progress to neck stiffness and cranial nerve palsies followed by coma. Focal neurological deficits such as squint or ophthalmoplegia are more likely to be present in this form of the disease. Disease elsewhere in the body may not be evident.

DIAGNOSIS

In some cases the diagnosis may be made on clinical grounds, e.g. a meningitic illness associated with the

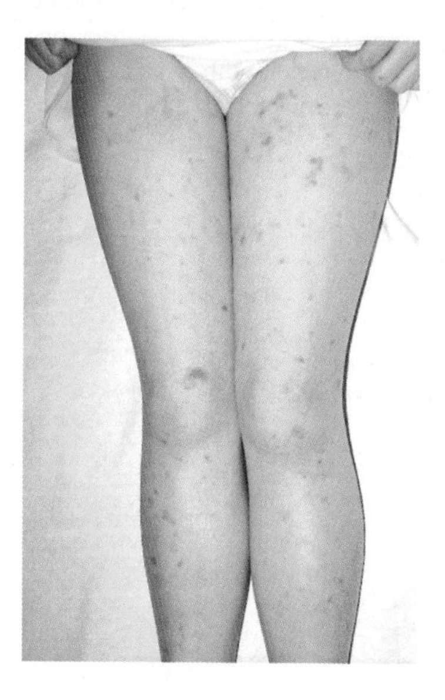

Fig 15.11
Rash of meningococcal septicaemia.

typical features of mumps or, more seriously, meningitis associated with the typical meningococcal rash. In most other cases the establishment of the diagnosis depends on the cerebrospinal fluid (CSF) appearances at lumbar puncture (Fig. 15.12). Performing the lumbar puncture carries some risks since there is usually raised intracranial pressure. As a rule if the symptoms are prolonged, the child is drowsy or if there have been focal seizures or a focal neurological deficit it is advisable to obtain a CT scan of the head before proceeding to lumbar puncture. However, even with a normal CT scan, if there are clinical signs of raised intracranial pressure a lumbar puncture may be contraindicated. Table 15.2 presents the typical findings in the main forms of meningitis.

In most cases the main forms of meningitis can be readily determined from the CSF findings but particular difficulties may occur in children who have received antibiotics and who therefore have a partially treated meningitis. Rapid bacterial antigen detection may be helpful in these cases. Polymerase chain reaction (PCR) techniques for detection of specific bacterial nucleic acid sequences allows precise diagnosis and is available for meningococcal disease.

Poliomyelitis is dealt with on page 319.

MANAGEMENT

Treatment of meningitis should be initiated as quickly as possible. In meningococcal disease with septicaemic rash, penicillin should be given immediately without waiting for a lumbar puncture. When a lumbar puncture is to be performed this should be done without delay. If there is inevitable delay, for instance in obtaining a CT scan, and bacterial meningitis is suspected then empirical antibiotics should be given. The antibiotic of choice is systemic penicillin for meningococcal infection with a rash. For other types of meningitis, where bacteriological confirmation may take some time, the antibiotic of choice is a third-generation cephalosporin such as ceftriaxone. In children under 3 months of age, ampicillin is added to cover the possibility of listeria meningitis.

Rifampicin is given to eliminate nasal carriage of *N. meningitidis* and *H. influenzae*. A 2- or 4-day course, respectively, is also given to household contacts (but only if there are members of the household who are less than school age in the case of *H. influenzae* meningitis).

In tuberculous meningitis, bacteriological culture may take several weeks. Once clinical diagnosis is made the patient should be started on antituberculous chemotherapy. Mortality may be as high as 50% if treatment is delayed, with permanent handicap in most of the survivors.

In viral meningitis there is usually a benign self-limiting course which does not require specific therapy. Antibiotics or antituberculous drugs are sometimes given if there is uncertainty about the possibility of bacterial or tuberculous meningitis. In suspected *Herpes simplex* encephalitis, aciclovir treatment is given.

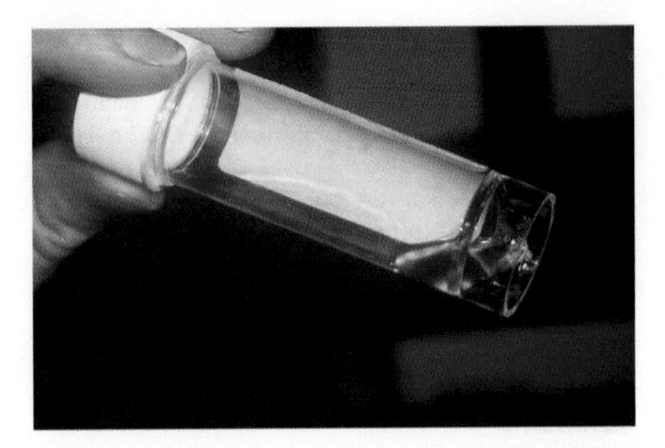

Fig 15.12
Cloudy CSF obtained by lumbar puncture of a child with meningococcal septicaemia.

Table 15.2
Cerebrospinal fluid (CSF) findings in meningitis

Cause	Cell count	Protein	Glucose	Microbiology
Bacterial	↑ Mainly neutrophils	Mildly ↑	↓	Positive Gram stain and culture
Partially treated bacterial	↑ Mixed mononuclear/ neutrophil	Normal or slightly ↑	Normal or ↓	Gram stain and culture often negative Antigens helpful PCR*
Viral	↑ Or occasionally normal, predominantly mononuclear	Normal or ↑	Normal	Negative bacterial culture Viral culture or PCR* may be positive
Tuberculosis	↑ Mononuclear cells	↑ May be very high	↓	Positive Ziehl–Nielsen stain Culture takes 6 weeks

* Polymerase chain reaction for detection of specific nucleic acid fragments of the bacteria or viruses

In addition to antibiotic treatment, it has recently been shown that with *H. influenzae* meningitis the use of corticosteroids reduces the likelihood of hearing loss and other damage after the infection. There is evidence that it may also help in cases of tuberculous meningitis. The antibiotic regimes used are now so powerful that the use of these immunosuppressive agents does not compromise the treatment.

In addition to the specific antimicrobial therapy, supportive care for the child is very important. In particular the management of the child's fluid balance may make all the difference to the outcome. Meningitis tends to cause inappropriate ADH secretion with water retention and a risk of developing cerebral oedema. On the other hand the severely ill child who has been vomiting and who may have septicaemic shock may need large volumes of fluid therapy. A great deal of experience is needed in judging how much and which fluid to give, and the child's fluid status and electrolytes should be carefully monitored throughout treatment. Analgesics are often underemployed in meningitis particularly if the child is too young to specifically complain of headache. Regular paracetamol should be given until improvement occurs.

Meningitis may be complicated by brain abscess which can also follow sinusitis, otitis, facial cellulitis and penetrating head injuries. Children with cyanotic congenital heart disease are predisposed to this. Infections may result from mixed aerobic and anaerobic bacteria. Early symptoms of headache, lethargy and fever proceed to hemiparesis with papilloedema. CSF examination shows a few leukocytes and increased protein. After demonstration of an abscess on CT, drainage and/or prolonged antibiotic therapy are required. Mortality is high, especially if the abscess ruptures, and permanent neurological deficits are common.

PREVENTION

Prevention of some types of meningitis is possible. Hib vaccination has virtually eliminated this type of meningitis over the last few years. Vaccines are also present against types A and C meningococcus, including the recently introduced type C conjugate vaccine, which is already having an impact in the UK. Unfortunately type B, the predominant cause of disease in the UK, cannot be vaccinated against at the present time. When families travel to certain parts of the world, particularly East Africa and the Middle East, they should receive immunization. In tuberculous meningitis, contact tracing and BCG immunization where appropriate should help reduce the risk. Mumps immunization has virtually eliminated what was the commonest cause of viral meningitis.

Bone and joint infections (See also p 346)

> **Epidemiology**
>
> Up to 80% of osteomyelitis and septic arthritis in children is caused by *S. aureus*. Other causes include streptococcal species, Gram-negative bacilli including salmonella species and *Haemophilus influenzae* type b.
>
> Tuberculosis should always be borne in mind as a possible cause of these infections.
>
> In sickle cell diseases and in immunocompromised individuals, osteomyelitis is more common and more likely to be caused by an unusual organism such as salmonella.

The organism usually finds its way to the skeleton via the bloodstream following a usually subclinical bacteraemia (haematogenous spread). The metaphyseal region of a long bone is most commonly affected in osteomyelitis or a single large joint in septic arthritis. In a small number of cases infection is caused by a penetrating injury or direct spread from an infected adjacent focus.

In acute infection the child will be febrile and ill. There will be failure to move the affected part of the body or failure to weight bear on an affected limb. The joint or bone will be swollen and tender. In chronic infections, such as those due to tuberculosis, the acute inflammatory signs are less and fever may not be present. Radiographic changes of osteomyelitis (areas of rarefaction and periosteal reaction) take at least 10 days though soft tissue swelling may be evident earlier. Isotope bone scan is much more sensitive from early in the illness except in very young infants (less than 3 months of age). Magnetic resonance imaging (MRI) may be useful, particularly in chronic or complicated cases. In septic arthritis joint aspiration is both diagnostically and therapeutically useful. The causative organism may be grown directly from aspirates or from blood cultures where it is found in approximately 60% of osteomyelitis and 40% of septic arthritis cases.

Treatment is with intravenous antibiotics in high dose to achieve good bone penetration. If the organism is not isolated then a broad-spectrum combination such as flucloxacillin and cefotaxime (or ampicillin) is used in previously healthy children. Wider Gram-negative antibiotic cover is needed in children with underlying disorders. After initial clinical response antibiotics are switched to the oral route and then must be continued for 4 weeks in septic arthritis and 6 weeks in osteomyelitis. Failure to respond suggests a resistant organism or abscess formation, and surgical exploration may be required. Serial measurement of inflammatory markers such as C-reactive protein or sedimentation rate may be useful for monitoring treatment progress.

Less common but important infections

The following infectious diseases are important on a global basis but are uncommon in the UK.

Brucellosis

Infected dairy products are the usual source of this disease (zoonoses, diseases of animals which can be transmitted to man). Organisms involved may be:

- *Brucella abortus* (cows)
- *B. melitensis* (goats)
- *B. suis* (pigs)
- *B. canis* (dogs)
- *B. ovis* (sheep)
- *B. neotomae* (desert rats).

The disease presents as an influenza-like illness. Diagnosis is by means of:

- Agglutinating and complement-fixing antibodies
- ELISA assay
- Blood assay and bone marrow cultures, the latter being most likely to be positive.

Treatment is with tetracycline or cotrimoxazole with or without streptomycin for 4 weeks.

Cat-scratch disease

The organism causing this disease, acquired as the name suggests, is *Rochalimea henselae*. A papule appears 10 days after the scratch or bite and there is massive enlargement of regional lymph nodes. The disease resolves spontaneously after 2 months.

Diagnosis is by means of lymph node biopsy, and antibiotics such as azithromycin may hasten spontaneous resolution.

Cryptococcosis

This is caused by *Cryptococcus neoformans*. The yeast spores are inhaled, usually by an immunocompromised host. From the lungs there is spread to the meninges, and the commonest form of presentation in children is as a subacute meningitis. Diagnosis is by microscopy of CSF.

Treatment is with antifungals including amphotericin B and flucytosine. Long-term prophylaxis with fluconazole may be required in immunocompromised children to prevent relapse.

Dengue fever

Dengue fever is a viral infection, the source being mosquitoes in tropical countries.

The disease presents with fever, headache and transient macular rash. There is myalgia and a second, morbilliform rash after the fever resolves. A second attack may be more severe with a haemorrhagic illness and shock. Diagnosis is by means of serological testing. Mosquito control helps prevention.

Histoplasmosis

This is a mycosis (fungal infection), caused by *Histoplasma capsulatum*, when fungal spores shed by birds and bats are inhaled. It presents as an influenza-like illness, becoming disseminated in immuno-compromised patients.

Diagnosis is by means of culture of blood, bone marrow, urine, CSF and sputum, if the disease is disseminated. Treatment is with amphotericin B.

Leishmaniasis (kala-azar)

This protozoal infection is caused by *Leishmania donovanii*, and the source is the sandfly, found in all continents except Australia.

Incubation may be up to 10 years. Nonspecific symptoms include fever, and malaise. These are accompanied by abdominal pain from a hugely enlarged spleen. The cutaneous form produces ulcerating erythematous macules. The illness may progress to involve the respiratory tract (mucocutaneous leishmaniasis).

Diagnosis is by means of serology, examination of biopsies of the lesion and specialized culture techniques.

Pentavalent antimony compounds, such as sodium stibogluconate and meglumine antimonate are standard treatments, but liposomal amphotericin is also effective and less toxic. Amphotericin is given for cutaneous leishmaniasis. Splenectomy may be required.

Prevention is by sandfly control.

Leptospirosis (Weil disease)

This illness is caused by *Leptospira interrogans*, the source being contamination of water and soil near rivers by rat urine.

The clinical features are:

- 1 week of fever, rigors, headache, vomiting and myalgia

- 1 month of aseptic meningitis
- 1 month of hepatic and renal dysfunction.

Diagnosis is made by prolonged culture for the organism from blood, CSF or urine, and the slide agglutination test for serological diagnosis.

Treatment is with penicillin (tetracycline in children over 12-years-old), but there is doubt about its effectiveness. There is no proven method of prevention except avoidance of exposure.

Lyme disease

This illness, named after a town in Connecticut, is caused by *Borrelia burgdorferi*, the source being the bite of a tick of genus Ixodes, which is parasitic on deer.

Clinical features include:

- An expanding annular rash (erythema chronicum migrans) beginning at the site of the tick bite
- Lymphadenopathy
- Fever
- After 1 month, may become latent for several months
- Then neurological symptoms (meningitis, facial nerve palsy, peripheral neuropathy) can occur
- Cardiac involvement, with heart block and myocarditis occurs in this secondary phase
- Arthritis is a late occurrence.

Diagnosis is from the clinical history.

Amoxicillin, or tetracycline in older children, is effective. Those with meningitis are given ceftriaxone.

Prevention is by means of insect repellent, protective clothing and frequent inspection of limbs for ticks when walking near deer.

Toxoplasmosis (Fig. 15.13)

This is caused by *Toxoplasma gondii*, an obligate intracellular protozoan. Toxoplasma oocysts are found in the faeces of cats infected by ingesting infected meat.

The disease presents as a glandular fever-like illness with lymphadenopathy. Congenital infection causes infection of the retina (chorioretinitis), calcification of the brain and hydrocephalus.

Diagnosis is by culture of the organism or PCR, or by serological diagnosis using the Sabin–Feldman dye test.

Infants with congenital toxoplasmosis are treated for 1 year with pyrimethamine and sulphadiazine. Pregnant women should be advised to avoid raw and rare meat, and cat faeces.

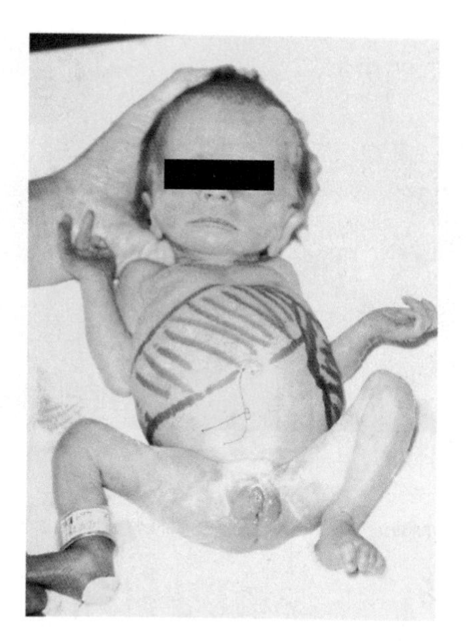

Fig 15.13
Neonate with congenital toxoplasmosis. Skin markings show the size of the liver and spleen. The child also has microphthalmia.

Kawasaki disease (Fig. 15.14)

The causative agent of this illness is not known.

This illness presents with fever (>5 days), irritability

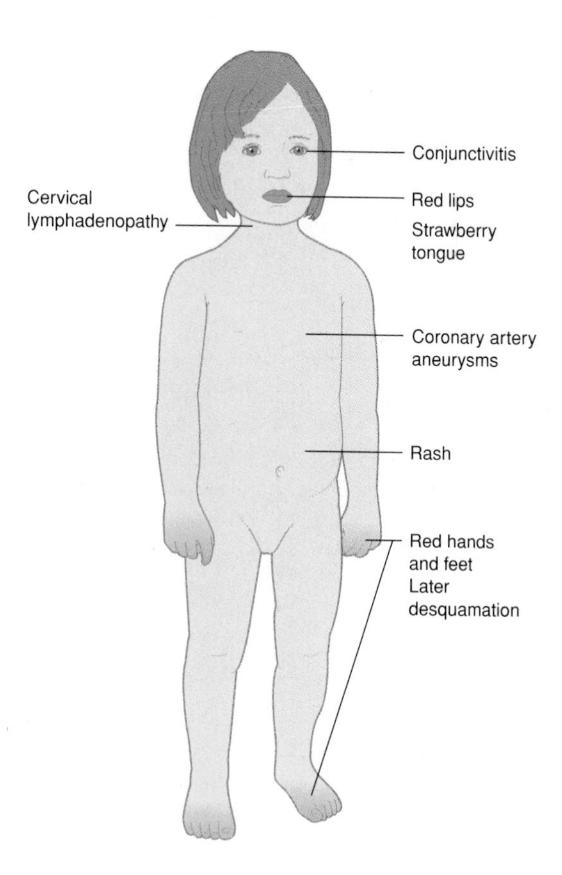

Fig 15.14
Features of Kawasaki disease.

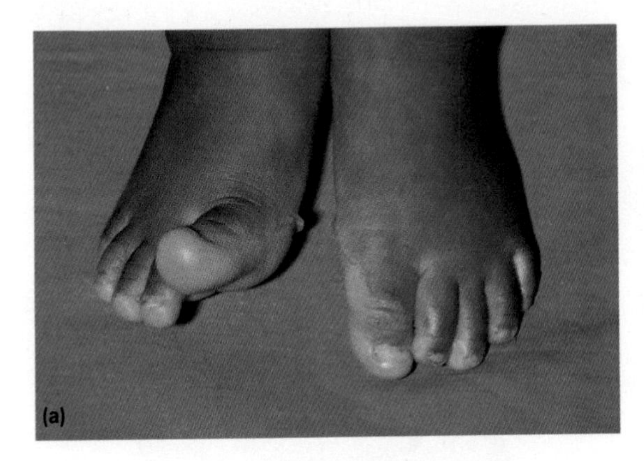

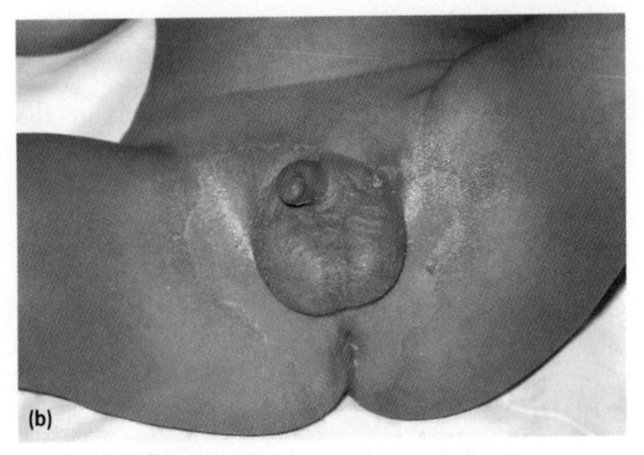

Fig 15.15
(a) and (b) Kawasaki disease. Desquamation often starts in the napkin area but classically affects the hands and feet.

and lymphadenopathy, before the macular rash appears. There is oedema, redness of hands and feet (Fig. 15.15) and nonpurulent conjunctivitis. There is late desquamation, especially fingers and toes.

Acute complications include:

- Myocarditis
- Myositis
- Arthritis
- Renal failure
- Aseptic meningitis.

Late complications include coronary artery aneurysms and myocardial infarctions, which may be prevented by the use of intravenous immunoglobulin during the acute illness.

16 Metabolism

Further examples of rare but important disorders are included in this section. At present all babies are screened for phenylketonuria, and there is growing pressure to screen for other metabolic disorders in which early treatment can improve prognosis.

Amino acid metabolism

Cystinosis (Fanconi syndrome with cystinosis, Lignac syndrome)

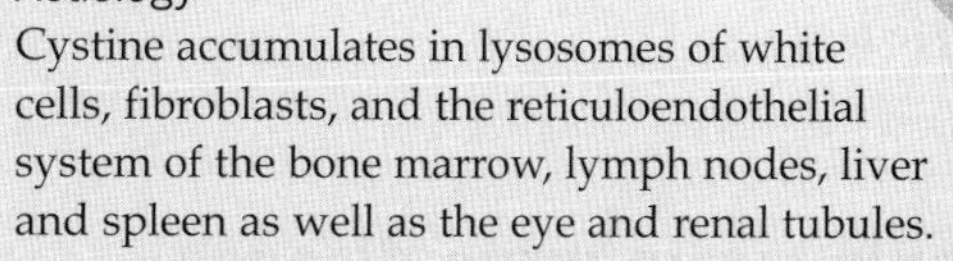

Aetiology

Cystine accumulates in lysosomes of white cells, fibroblasts, and the reticuloendothelial system of the bone marrow, lymph nodes, liver and spleen as well as the eye and renal tubules.

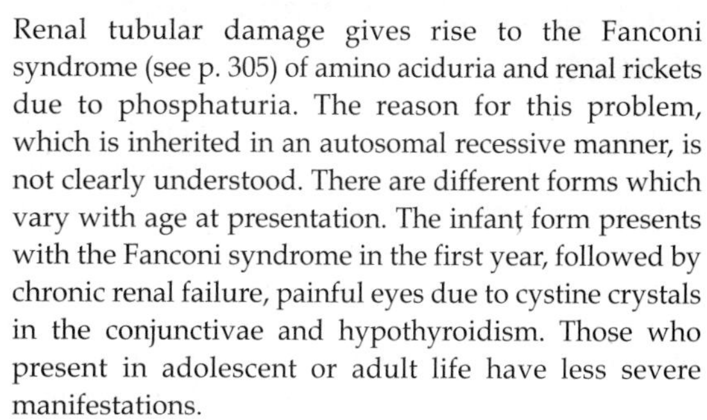

Renal tubular damage gives rise to the Fanconi syndrome (see p. 305) of amino aciduria and renal rickets due to phosphaturia. The reason for this problem, which is inherited in an autosomal recessive manner, is not clearly understood. There are different forms which vary with age at presentation. The infant form presents with the Fanconi syndrome in the first year, followed by chronic renal failure, painful eyes due to cystine crystals in the conjunctivae and hypothyroidism. Those who present in adolescent or adult life have less severe manifestations.

The condition is diagnosed by measuring cystine concentrations in white cells and blood and finding cystine crystals in the cornea on slit lamp examination. Treatment is directed towards the renal failure, and kidney transplantation may be needed. Cysteamine relieves some of the symptoms.

Do not confuse this condition with cystinuria or homocystinuria (see pp. 288, 289), which are different disorders despite their similar names, and remember that Fanconi described several syndromes that bear his name (e.g. see Congenital absence of radius).

Homocystinuria (methionine metabolic defect)

Homocystinuria is an autosomal recessive disorder of methionine metabolism due to deficiency of cystathione synthase (type I or classic), vitamin B_{12} (type II), or folic acid (type III). Type I is commonest (1 : 200 000 births).

The manifestations resemble those of Marfan syndrome, with tall stature, long fingers (arachnodactyly), lens subluxation, and atherosclerosis. Recurrent thromboses are another prominent feature. After birth, the diagnosis is suggested by the presence of methionine and homocystine in urine, and confirmed by assay of the enzyme in a liver biopsy or cultured fibroblasts. It may be diagnosed antenatally in biopsied chorionic villi or cultured amniotic cells.

A low methionine diet with high doses of vitamin B_6 and folic acid may be tried. Trimethylglycine supplements also help by converting homocysteine back to methionine.

Defects in vitamin B_{12} and folic acid metabolism cause elevation of homocystine because they are cofactors in the conversion of this amino acid to methionine. Types II and III both cause developmental delay and respond to B_{12} and folic acid supplements.

Maple syrup urine disease (branched-chain amino acid defect)

In this condition the activity of the branched-chain α-ketoacid dehydrogenase enzyme is defective. This normally catalyses the decarboxylation of by-products of metabolism of the branched-chain amino acids leucine, isoleucine and valine.

The urine and plasma contain high concentrations of these amino acids, and their presence with their associated ketoacids gives the urine and body secretions their characteristic sweet odour. Affected infants develop vomiting in early life, rapidly progressing to coma with hypoglycaemia and increased muscle tone. Untreated, the condition is rapidly fatal.

Emergency treatment includes peritoneal dialysis, and intravenous glucose. Synthetic formulae, free from leucine, isoleucine and valine, are available for long-term management. Some children respond to high doses of thiamine, a cofactor for the defective enzyme.

Phenylketonuria (aromatic amino acid defect)

Aetiology

Deficiency of phenylalanine hydroxylase results in accumulation of the essential amino acid phenylalanine, and breakdown products phenylpyruvic acid and phenylethylamine.

Development of mental retardation is delayed for several months, by which time the affected child will have been diagnosed by the neonatal screening programme. Blood from a heel prick on the 6th day of life is spotted onto a card for phenylalanine assay.

Treatment consists of feeding a synthetic breast milk substitute with no phenylalanine. Frequent estimates of phenylalanine are required to check for successful controls of levels. Under- and overtreatment should be avoided; the latter because phenylalanine is an essential amino acid. The diet is relaxed when the age of the child reaches double figures. Recent evidence has shown that relaxation of the diet in adolescence is associated with changes in brain myelin on MRI scan in adult life. Obsessive control is reinstituted in mothers with phenylketonuria whose babies otherwise develop microcephaly and congenital heart disease.

Albinism (aromatic amino acid defect)

This autosomal recessive condition has an incidence of 1 : 20 000. There is defective formation and distribution of melanin, normally synthesized from tyrosine by melanocytes. The depigmentation of the skin, iris and retina results in high risk for skin cancer and impaired vision, and a prominent red reflex in the eye. The defect may be confined to the eye (ocular albinism). When the skin defect is partial, the term 'piebaldism' has been used.

The genetic basis of the variants of albinism is not well understood; dominant and X-linked inheritance has been described.

Alkaptonuria (ochronosis; aromatic amino acid defect)

In this autosomal recessive disorder there is a deficiency of homogentisic acid oxidase, leading to an accumulation of excess homogentisic acid (a metabolite of tyrosine). Homogentisic acid is excreted in the urine which turns dark on standing, with oxidation and polymerization of the acid.

Deposition of the pigment in tissues causes spots in the sclera and ears (ochronosis), and arthritis. There is no treatment.

Amino acid transport disorders

Cystinuria

Cystinuria is an inborn error of dibasic amino acid transport which causes increased urinary excretion of ornithine, arginine, lysine and cystine. The relative insolubility of the latter can result in renal calculi.

Hartnup disease

This autosomal recessive condition was first reported in a family of the same name. There is a defect in the transport by the small intestine and kidney, of the neutral amino acids alanine, serine, threonine, valine, leucine, isoleucine, phenylalanine, tyrosine, tryptophan and histidine. Most of the 1 in 30 000 affected individuals are asymptomatic; some affected infants have a light-sensitive dermatitis resembling pellagra (see p. 329). The condition responds to a high protein diet and nicotinamide.

Carbohydrate metabolism disorders

Galactosaemia

This includes autosomal recessive deficiencies of galactokinase, galactose-1-phosphate uridyl transferase or uridyl diphosphogalactose-4-epimerase.

Galactokinase deficiency (1 in 40 000) causes galactosuria and cataract formation on ingestion of galactose. The latter is found in lactose, the disaccharide in milk; a galactose-free diet prevents progression of the cataracts.

Galactose-1-phosphate uridyl transferase deficiency (1 in 50 000) causes cataracts, jaundice, hepatomegaly and ascites. Accumulation of galactose-1-phosphate competitively inhibits the conversion of glycogen to glucose, resulting in hypoglycaemia.

Uridyl diphosphogalactose-4-epimerase deficiency can be asymptomatic or can produce the same symptoms as galactose-1-phosphate uridyl transferase deficiency, depending on the distribution of the enzyme deficiency in the body. A galactose-free diet is required if the condition is symptomatic.

Glycogen storage diseases (glycogenoses)

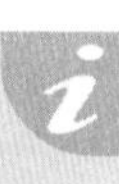

Classification

The 12 types and 8 subtypes are summarized in Table 16.1.

Blood tests show low glucose, and high urate, lactate, triglycerides and cholesterol. The treatment of glycogen storage diseases complicated by hypo glycaemia (types 0 and I) is to give high glucose and starch meals every 2 hours round the clock (by nasogastric infusion overnight).

Mucopolysaccharidoses

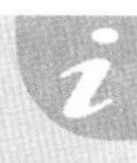

Classification

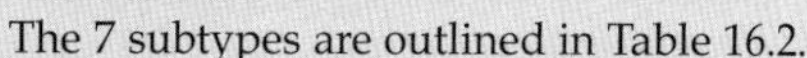

The 7 subtypes are outlined in Table 16.2.

These are a group of inborn errors of metabolism of mucopolysaccharides (glycosaminoglycans) which are constituents of the intercellular substance of connective tissue. The Hunter syndrome is X-linked recessive; the others are autosomal recessive. The defective enzyme activity can be detected in white blood cells or cultured fibroblasts from skin biopsies. All can be diagnosed antenatally.

Spondyloepiphyseal dysplasia may show similar X-ray appearances, and other defects of enzymes normally found in lysozymes (including GM_1 gangliosidosis, mannosidosis, fucosidosis, aspartylglucosaminuria, mucolipidoses, and multiple sulphatase deficiency) have similar clinical and biochemical findings. Bone marrow transplantation is being tried, to replace the deficient enzymes.

Lipid storage

Gaucher disease

Gaucher disease is an autosomal recessive condition common amongst Ashkenazi Jews. Deficiency of β-galactosidase results in accumulation of glucosylceramide, a specialized lipid.

The infantile and juvenile forms involve the central nervous system. Accumulation in the reticulo-endothelial system causes massive splenomegaly and

Table 16.1
The glycogenoses: disorders of glycogen structure or the ability to release glucose from glycogen (Fig 16.1)

Type	Enzyme defect	Tissues involved	Features
0 (Aglycogenosis)	Glycogen synthetase	Liver	Hypoglycaemia
Ia (von Gierke disease)	Glucose-6-phosphatase	Liver, kidney, gut	Hypoglycaemia, hepatomegaly, enlarged kidneys, 'doll-like' face
Ib	Glucose-6-phosphate translocase	As for Ia	As for Ia
Ic	Phosphate transport	Liver	Hepatomegaly, hypoglycaemia, brittle diabetes
IIa, b (Pompe disease, generalized glycogenosis)	Lysosomal acid α-glucosidase	All (IIa), heart spared in IIb	Hypotonia, cardiomegaly (IIa), death in infancy (IIa); IIb late onset
III (Limit dextrinosis, debrancher glycogenosis, Cori disease, Forbes disease	Amylo-1,6-glucosidase	Depends on subtype	Hepatomegaly
IV (amylopectinosis, brancher glycogenosis, Andersen disease)	Amylo-1,4→1,6-transglucosidase	All	Hepatosplenomegaly, liver failure and death
V (McArdle syndrome)	Muscle phosphorylase	Skeletal muscle	Weakness
VI	Liver phosphorylase	Liver	Hepatomegaly
VII	Phosphofructokinase	Skeletal muscle, erythrocytes	Minimal weakness
VIII	Liver phosphorylase inactivation	Liver, brain	Hepatomegaly, brain degeneration
IXa (autosomal recessive), b (X-linked recessive), c (autosomal recessive)	Liver phosphorylase kinase	Liver (muscle in type c)	Hepatomegaly
X	Cyclic AMP-dependent kinase	Liver	Hepatomegaly, muscle pain
XI	None	Liver, kidney	Fanconi syndrome (see p. 287/305)

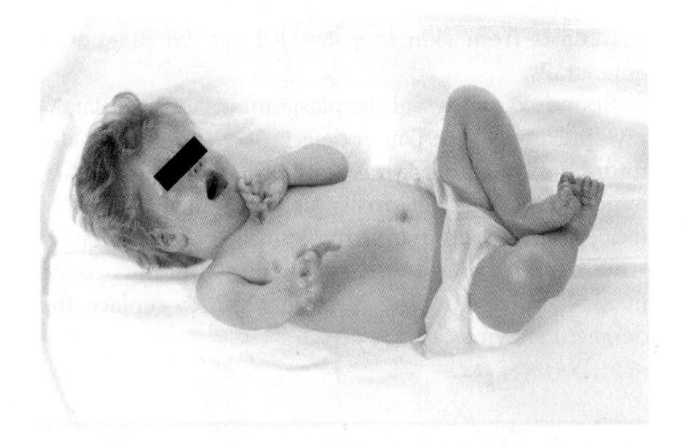

Fig 16.1
Glycogen storage disease. Note the large abdomen due to hepatomegaly, 'doll-like face' and hypotonic posture.

cells aspirated from the bone marrow are loaded with glucosylceramide.

Detection of carriers and antenatal diagnosis are available. Treatments by means of infusions of the missing enzyme and bone marrow transplantation are being tried.

Niemann–Pick disease

This is an autosomal recessive lipid storage disorder. The defective enzyme, sphingomyelinase, normally degrades the complex lipid sphingomyelin which is stored in lysosomes with cholesterol. The disorder is commoner amongst Ashkenazi Jewish children.

Development is delayed, with eventual regression. Hepatosplenomegaly and failure to thrive are also found. These features begin by 4 months of age. A characteristic but not invariable finding is a cherry red spot at the macula of the retina.

Antenatal diagnosis is possible.

Tay–Sachs disease

Here there is a deficiency of the lysosomal enzyme β-hexosamidase. The autosomal recessive trait is commonest in children of Ashkenazi Jewish descent.

Affected children begin to regress from 5 months, with the accumulation of GM_2 ganglioside in the central nervous system. A specific feature is an abnormal startle response to noise, called hyperacusis. The macula of the optic fundus may develop a cherry red spot.

Death occurs in early adult life. There is no treatment, hence prenatal diagnosis is vital.

Table 16.2
The mucopolysaccharidoses (MPS) (Fig 16.2)

Syndrome	Enzyme	Abnormal urinary metabolites	Clinical features
Hurler (MPS IH)	α-L-Iduronidase	Dermatan and heparan sulphates	• Begins in 2nd year • Progressive developmental delay • Coarsening of the features • Clouding of the corneas • Kyphoscoliosis: lumbar spine X-rays show beak-like projections of the lower anterior margins of vertebral bodies • Joint contractures • Herniae • Hepatosplenomegaly • Death in the second decade
Hunter (MPS II)	Iduronosulphate sulphatase	Dermatan and heparan sulphates	• Similar to Hurler syndrome • Less severe • No clouding of the cornea
Scheie (MPS IS)	Dermatan-specific α-L-iduronidase	Dermatan sulphate	• Similar to Hurler syndrome • Much less severe • Onset after 5th year of life • Normal life expectancy, IQ and height
Sanfilippo (MPS IV)	Sulphamidase, α-*N*-acetylhexosaminidase, acteyl CoA:α-glucosaminide *N*-acetyltransferase, or *N*-acetylglucosamine-6-sulphatase	Heparan sulphate	• Similar to Hurler syndrome • Much less severe • Severe neurological deterioration leading to death in the second decade
Morquio (MPS IV)	*N*-acetyl galactosamine-6-sulphate sulphatase or β-galactosidase	Keratan sulphate	• Onset in 2nd year • Corneal clouding • Short stature; flattened vertebral bodies • Joint laxity: atlantoaxial instability (see p. 344) • Normal IQ • Death in fourth decade from cardiorespiratory problems, secondary to vertebral deformities
Maroteaux–Lamy (MPS VI)	*N*-acetylglucosamine-4-sulphate-sulphatase	Dermatan sulphate	• Similar to Hurler syndrome • Normal IQ
β-Glucuronidase deficiency (MPS VII)	β-Glucuronidase	Chondroitin 4/6	Similar to Hurler syndrome but manifestations variable

Hyperlipidaemia and hypercholesterolaemia

Clinical importance
Screening may prevent premature arteriosclerosis.

The features of the most important primary genetic defects resulting in hyperlipidaemia are summarized in Table 16.3.

Hyperlipidaemia may be secondary to obesity, hypothyroidism, nephrotic syndrome, cholestasis, anorexia nervosa, steroid therapy, diabetes mellitus and, in adolescents, excess alcohol intake.

Children with moderately raised plasma cholesterol concentrations are at increased risk for premature coronary artery disease. Elevation occurs in primary genetic defects such as hyper-apobetalipoproteinaemia and diet can contribute. Screening of all children over

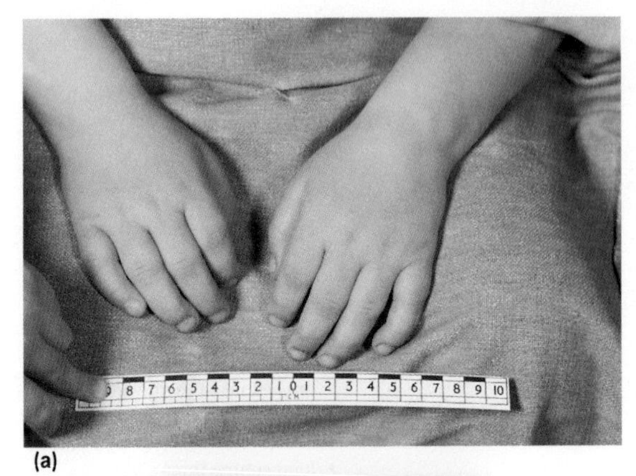

(a)

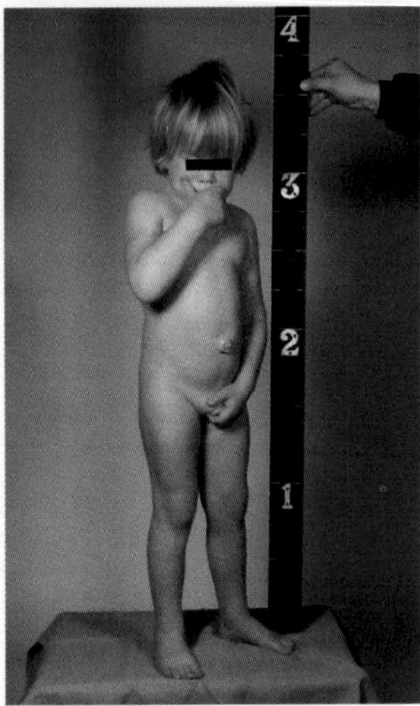

(b)

Fig 16.2
(a) and (b) Child with Hunter syndrome. Note the coarse features and umbilical hernia.

2 years of age has been suggested. Cholesterol or apobetalipoprotein may be measured.

Other metabolic disorders

Hyperuricaemia

Gout rarely occurs in childhood. Hyperuricaemia is a feature of the Lesch–Nyhan syndrome, a sex-linked deficiency of the enzyme hypoxanthine guanine phosphoribosyl transferase. It is characterized by spasticity, choreoathetosis, self-mutilation, and gout in later life.

The responsible gene has been isolated; gene therapy will be the next step.

Secondary hyperuricaemia occurs whenever cells are breaking down, for example due to malignancy (especially during treatment), or renal failure.

Leigh encephalopathy (subacute necrotizing encephalomyelopathy)

The severe CNS symptoms include convulsions, delayed development, optic atrophy and abnormal movements. Vomiting and lactic acidosis also occur. Pyruvate dehydrogenase, or pyruvate decarboxylase is defective. Defects in the respiratory chain in mitochondria lead to the same syndrome.

Some respond to supplementation with thiamine (as with Wernicke encephalopathy); most die within 6 months of presentation.

Orotic aciduria

Orotic acid is a precursor of pyrimidines, used in DNA and RNA synthesis. Deficiencies in the activities of the enzymes orotidylic acid pyrophosphorylase and decarboxylase result in excretion of orotic acid in urine and megaloblastic anaemia which responds to the administration of pyrimidines. The anaemia results from insufficient RNA and DNA production to support red cell production (erythropoiesis).

Trace element disorders

Acrodermatitis enteropathica

This zinc deficiency disorder (Fig. 16.3) is characterized by perineal and perioral dermatitis, diarrhoea, alopecia and paronychia. There is irritability and depression, anorexia and immunodeficiency. The disorder may be due to a primary inborn error of zinc absorption or secondary to malabsorption.

Menkes kinky hair syndrome

This very rare X-linked recessive disorder was named after a paediatric neurologist in California.

Infants usually appear normal at birth. However, as the weeks go by intellectual progress deteriorates, the infants feed poorly and seizures are likely to occur by 6 months of age. This condition is one of the causes of epilepsy in young infants. The most noticeable characteristic is the hair, which appears normal at birth but gradually depigments and becomes twisted and brittle.

Table 16.3
Features of primary hyperlipidaemias

Disorder	Inheritance	Prevalence	Defect	Clinical manifestations	Treatment
Familial hypercholesterolaemia (FH), heterozygous	Dominant	1:500	Low density lipoprotein (LDL) receptor impairs uptake of LDL from circulation	• Premature coronary atherosclerosis • Tendon xanthomata* • Xanthelasmas* • Arcus corneae* • Elevated total cholesterol and LDL cholesterol	• 'Prudent' diet† • Cholestyramine • Colestipol • Nicotinic acid
FH, homozygous	Dominant	1:100 000	Two genes encoding defective LDL receptor	• Markedly more severe than heterozygous FH	• Plasmapheresis to remove LDL • Liver transplantation
Familial combined hyperlipidaemia (FCHL)	Dominant	1:100	Overproduction of very low density lipoprotein (VLDL)	• Obesity • High risk of early myocardial infarction • Cholesterol or triglycerides or both elevated in adult life	• As for FH

* Xanthomata are nodules containing cholesteryl esters in macrophages. Xanthelasmas are similar lesions occurring in the eyelids. Arcus corneae refers to deposition around the rim of the cornea.
† The details of a 'prudent' diet are as follows: dietary fat 30% of total calories (saturated, monounsaturated and polyunsaturated) and <100 mg cholesterol/1000 calories.

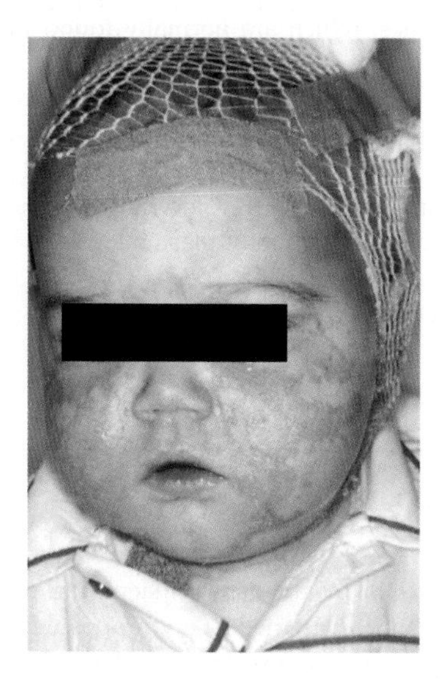
(a)

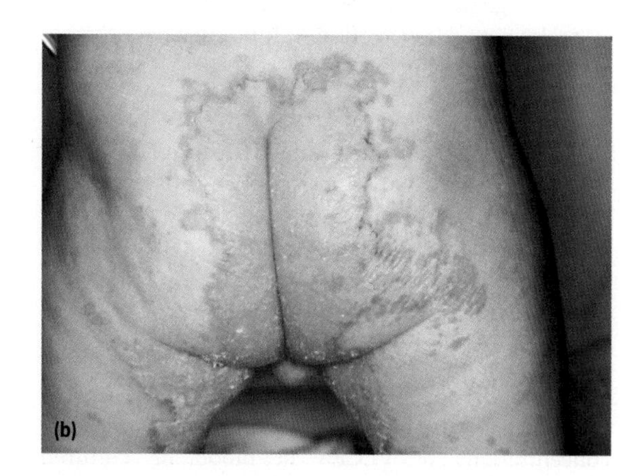
(b)

Fig 16.3
(a) and (b) Acquired acrodermatitis enteropathica, due to chronic diarrhoea. Note the symmetrical eczema-like rash on face and perineum.

The underlying problem is an inability to absorb the copper from the diet which is needed for correct function of enzymes. This leads to abnormalities of blood vessels, skin and hair. Other problems include fractures due to abnormal collagen synthesis, and poor feeding. The serum copper and caeruloplasmin are very low.

Unfortunately it is not possible to treat this condition with supplementary copper, and the outlook is bleak. Prenatal diagnosis is possible through amniocentesis.

Wilson disease (hepatolenticular degeneration)

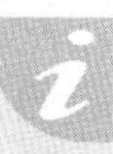

Epidemiology
5 per million people.

This is an autosomal recessive disorder of copper metabolism. Approximately one-half present before 15 years of age, with insidious onset of lethargy, malaise, anorexia, abdominal pain and hepatosplenomegaly. Alternative presentations include acute hepatitis, fulminant hepatic failure with haemolysis, haemolysis alone, portal hypertension and cirrhosis. Choreoathetosis and Fanconi syndrome are other associated features.

Slit lamp examination fails to show the characteristic Kaiser–Fleischer rings in the cornea in the first decade. Serum caeruloplasmin is low unless hepatic inflammation is present. Urine copper is high; serum copper is variable.

Treatment is by copper chelation with penicillamine. Side-effects (rash, fever, lymphadenopathy, lupus-like reaction, proteinuria) may necessitate a change to trientine or zinc sulphate.

Wilson disease presenting with fulminant liver failure has a poor prognosis without transplantation.

Peroxisomal disorders

Adrenoleukodystrophy, X-linked

Epidemiology

Although extremely rare, up to one-half of males with adrenocortical insufficiency have this biochemical defect.

This is a genetically determined disorder in which saturated, very long chain fatty acids (VLCFA) accumulate due to failure of degradation by intracellular organelles called peroxisomes using the enzyme lignoceroyl-CoA ligase. The adrenal cortex becomes distended with lipid. The white matter of the central nervous system undergoes demyelination. Steroid replacement therapy is required and restriction of VLCFA and bone marrow transplantation are being tried. Female carriers can be identified by measuring concentrations of VLCFA in blood or cultured fibroblasts, coupled with a DNA probe. Prenatal diagnosis of affected male fetuses is possible by measuring VLCFA on cells from amniotic fluid or chorionic villous biopsy.

Chondrodysplasia punctata (Conradi syndrome)

Nomenclature

'Chondro' means cartilage; 'dysplasia' means disorder of growth; 'punctata' describes the pinpoints of calcification seen on X-ray.

Taken together chondrodysplasia punctata implies that the child has one of a number of growth-restricting conditions. The epiphyses form abnormally resulting in a growth-retarded child who may have the characteristic collection of abnormalities seen in a specific syndrome. The severest type of condition, with very short limbs, is autosomal recessive. These children also have a defect of peroxisomes resembling Zellweger syndrome in which punctate cartilages are also found. An autosomal dominant form is known as Conradi–Hünermann syndrome. Specific features include short stature, cataracts, joint contractures and skin abnormality, with large pores giving the appearance of orange peel. Some affected infants fail to thrive in infancy. Affected children have associated problems, including mental retardation, which vary in severity from relatively mild to severe. A milder X-linked form also exists.

Zellweger syndrome

Peroxisomes are subcellular organelles, containing many enzymes, which are normally found in all cells except erythrocytes.

This autosomal recessive disorder, caused by defective peroxisomes, is characterized by high forehead, eye abnormalities, hypotonia and seizures. Death occurs within a few months. Absence of the enzymes causes elevation of plasma levels of very long chain fatty acids.

Antenatal diagnosis is possible.

Porphyrias

These defects in metabolism of haem, the pigment of haemoglobin, are classified as erythropoietic or hepatic depending on which system is involved. The enzyme defects are generally dominantly inherited and present in childhood to adulthood.

The chronic type produces photosensitivity. The acute type presents with colicky abdominal pain, psychiatric (neurovisceral) symptoms, peripheral neuropathy, tachycardia and hypertension.

When the diagnosis is made, family studies are important, to prevent unnecessary mortality from incorrect therapy. Treatment involves correction of fluid and electrolyte disturbances, and avoidance of alcohol, barbiturates, griseofulvin, and synthetic oestrogens and valproate and other antiepilepsy drugs.

Urea cycle defects

Epidemiology
1 : 30 000 live births (total of all defects)

The body detoxifies ammonia, produced by metabolism of amino acids, by converting it to urea. Five enzymes are required (carbamyl phosphate synthetase, ornithine transcarbamylase, arginosuccinate synthetase, arginosuccinate lyase and arginase). In addition, *N*-acetylglutamate synthetase is also required for synthesis of *N*-acetylglutamate which activates carbamyl phosphate synthetase. Defects in all these enzymes have been described.

A few days after birth affected infants develop vomiting and lethargy, progressing to convulsions and coma. They are often misdiagnosed as having sepsis. Older affected children develop vomiting, ataxia and disturbed behaviour, precipitated by infection or a high protein meal.

Plasma ammonia concentration is grossly elevated. Those with carbamyl phosphate synthetase or ornithine transcarbamylase deficiency have elevated glutamine, aspartic acid and alanine secondary to hyperammonaemia. Ornithine transcarbamylase deficiency (X-linked dominant, the remainder are autosomal recessive) produces elevated urinary orotic acid. Argininosuccinic acid synthetase deficiency produces elevation of plasma citrulline; argininosuccinic acid lyase deficiency produces elevation of argininosuccinic acid, and arginase deficiency produces elevation of arginine.

Deficiency of *N-acetylglutamate* synthetase is suggested by improvement after oral administration of carbamyl glutamate; confirmation is by specific enzyme assay.

The aim of treatment is to remove the ammonia and to decrease the rate of ammonia production with calories (lipids) and essential amino acids. Other drugs which remove ammonia are sodium benzoate (combines with glycine) phenylacetate (combines with glutamine) and arginine (combines with carbamyl phosphate to form citrulline) except in arginase deficiency. The resulting compounds are readily excreted by the kidney. If these measures fail to decrease the hyperammonaemia, peritoneal dialysis is required. Long-term therapy consists of protein restriction, benzoate phenylacetate, and arginine (citrulline in ornithine transcarbamalase deficiency).

17 Nephrology and urology

Nephrology refers to the study of disorders of the kidney, and urology is the study of the urinary system. With the routine use of antenatal ultrasound, many defects of the urinary system are detected and form a considerable workload for paediatric surgeons.

Urinary tract infections

Epidemiology
At any time 2% of girls will have significant bacteriuria when a mid-stream sample of urine is cultured. Colonization is much rarer in boys. At least 5% of girls will develop a symptomatic infection in childhood.

INTRODUCTION

Urinary tract infection can be defined as the multiplication of bacteria somewhere within the urinary tract, producing inflammation.

AETIOLOGY AND PATHOGENESIS

The urinary tract apart from the lower end of the urethra should normally be sterile. The introduction of bacteria, usually from the bowel flora, may produce infection. Since the urethra is much shorter in a girl than a boy such infections are much more common in females. The exception is the neonatal period when boys have a higher incidence of infection than girls. It is likely that bacteria are introduced into the urinary tract quite commonly and in most cases do not lead to infection as they would be 'washed out' at the next micturition. Abnormalities of 'plumbing' such as vesicoureteric reflux, congenital obstructions and bladder dysfunction will predispose to infection since they allow for stasis giving the bacteria an opportunity to proliferate (Fig. 17.1). The other predisposing factor for urinary infection is a particular characteristic of the bacterium that is introduced. Certain *E. coli* possess surface proteins called fimbriae, which allow them to adhere to epithelial cells in the urinary tract and thus resist being 'washed' out. These bacteria therefore have a higher potential for causing infection, even in those with a normal urinary tract.

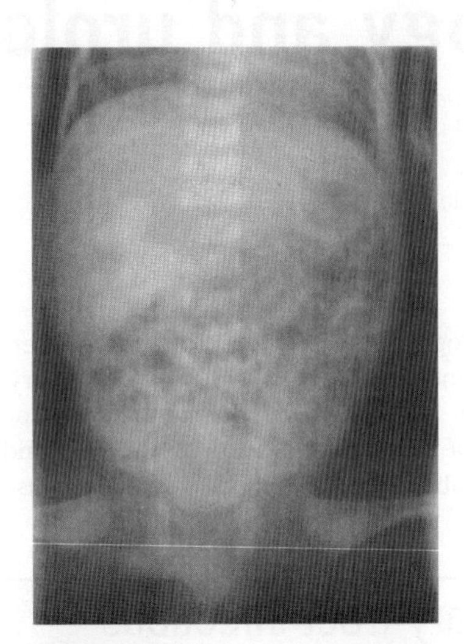

(a)

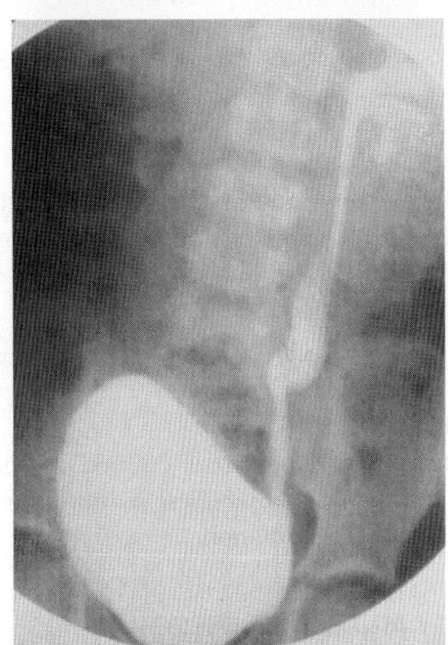

(b)

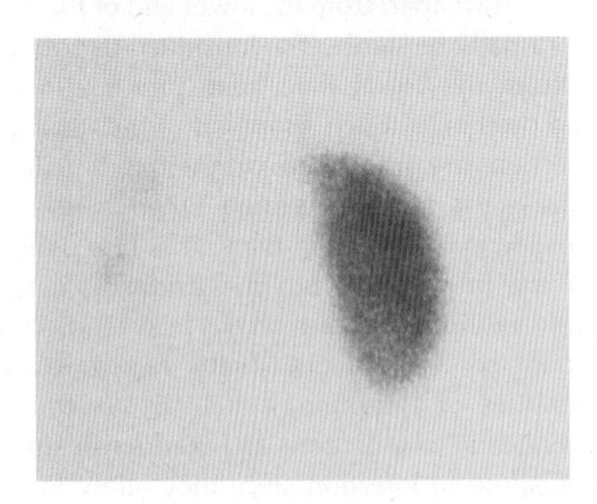

(c)

Fig 17.1
(a) Congenital abnormalities of the renal tract predispose to infection. Right hydronephrosis and nonfunctioning left kidney. (b) Micturating cystourethrography (MCU) shows ureteric reflux. (c) DMSA (dimercaptosuccinic acid)-scan confirms nonfunctioning left kidney.

CLINICAL PRESENTATION

This depends on the age of the child. In the neonatal period a nonspecific presentation may include poor feeding, vomiting, or irritability. Alternatively the child may become profoundly ill with 'sepsis' if the organism invades beyond the urinary tract to cause septicaemia or meningitis. After the neonatal period children may present with fever, irritability and diarrhoea or vomiting or both. Unlike at older ages frequency and dysuria are not reliable symptoms. Examination may or may not reveal suprapubic or loin tenderness. These children often therefore present with a clinical picture more suggestive of gastroenteritis than urinary tract infection.

In the school-age child the symptoms of urinary infection are much more similar to those in adults with frequency and dysuria, which may be associated with suprapubic or loin pain. Dysuria may result from inflammation of the vulva or foreskin and needs to be distinguished from 'genuine' urinary tract infection. Loss of bladder control may be the result of urinary tract infection. Urinary tract infection is sometimes completely asymptomatic and discovered incidentally on routine urine testing.

DIAGNOSIS

In the neonate the main differential diagnosis will be sepsis elsewhere in the body. In preschool children it will be gastroenteritis or other bacterial infection such as otitis, meningitis and pneumonia. In school-age children it is likely to be local vulval irritation and infection in girls or balanitis in boys.

The diagnosis is confirmed by obtaining a urine sample for microscopy and culture. The latest generation of reagents for 'stick testing' provides fairly reliable bedside evidence of infection, being able to detect in addition to blood and protein, white cells and nitrite (the latter being highly suggestive of bacterial infection). However in addition to carrying out the stick test it is essential to send a urine sample to the laboratory for confirmation and for identification of the organism and its antibiotic sensitivities. In the laboratory the urine is examined under the microscope and is then set up for culture and a bacterial colony count (Information box 17.1).

Collection of a clean urine specimen provides its own practical problems (see Practical box 17.1).

The most reliable urine specimen is that obtained by suprapubic urine aspiration. In this process a needle is inserted in a vertical trajectory just above the pubic symphysis and into the bladder. Urine is aspirated and should always be sterile; any growth will be significant as will be any white cells. The procedure is not nearly as nasty and invasive as it sounds and it is often easier than collecting a blood sample! Unless there is great urgency to obtain a urine sample in this way, such as suspected septicaemia in a very sick infant, it is best to

Information Box 17.1

Urinary findings in infection

- White cell count usually, but not invariably, raised (normal range is $<10^4$/mm^3
- Bacteria may also be seen on microscopy
- Normal viable count is $<10^5$/ml
- Usually single species (mixed growth in contamination)
- $>10^5$/ml

perform the procedure when the bladder is likely to be full. Ideally the fullness of the bladder should be confirmed by ultrasound before attempting to aspirate. In children beyond the age of 1 year the technique becomes much more difficult because of the impossibility of immobilizing the child, and the need to obtain a sample becomes less acute. Finally, specimens of urine obtained by catheterization have been used for diagnosing urine infection. Unless there is a need to catheterize a child for other reasons it is best avoided since there is a high risk of causing a urine infection even if there was not one before.

White cells will be present in the urine in vulvovaginitis.

The presence of white cells without a significant bacterial growth may be seen as an incidental finding in children with a high fever and sometimes in the presence of appendicitis. It is also seen in nonspecific urethritis and rarer disorders such as renal tuberculosis or glomerulonephritis.

MANAGEMENT

In young infants and neonates treatment with a broad-spectrum antibiotic needs to be started rapidly intravenously, to lessen the risk of disseminated infection. In older children there is less urgency but in the sick symptomatic child it is also best to treat as quickly as possible. This will often involve an empirical choice of antibiotics since culture results take 24–48 hours. Trimethoprim or a second-generation cephalosporin or clavulinic acid/amoxycillin are reasonable empirical choices. If the child fails to respond then modification of treatment can be made in the light of the culture result. Ideally, if samples are collected by bag, two separate specimens should be obtained before treatment is started but this is not always possible. Furthermore it is advisable to repeat testing of a specimen of urine after the antibiotic course is finished in order to confirm resolution of the infection. A 5–7 day course is sufficient for most urine infections unless they are complicated by septicaemia when a longer course is necessary. Single dose treatment has not been evaluated in this age group.

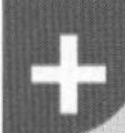

Practical Box 17.1

Collection of urine samples in children

- Midstream urine samples are not available in babies and young children
- Collection using an adhesive bag is the standard method
- More successful in boys
- The urine is not sterile as it washes the skin of the perineum, which is often colonized by enteric bacteria
- Low colony count, especially of a mixed growth, from bag urine suggests no infection
- A pure culture of $>10^5$/ml is fairly conclusive
- Intermediate results are common
- Alternatives include:
  - Suprapubic aspiration or catheter specimens
    These are invasive
    Any culture is significant
  - Clean-catch urine
    Optimal method
    Time-consuming
    Involves sitting with a sterile container, waiting for the baby to pass urine, some of which is caught in mid-air
    Easier in boys but not impossible in girls
    Results are easier to interpret than those from bag specimens

Follow-up investigation of children with urinary tract infection is usually necessary. It has been shown that a high proportion (one-third) of children with even their first urinary infection have an underlying urinary tract abnormality of which vesicoureteric reflux is the most common. Renal scarring is a common consequence of reflux and infection in young children and, if not recognised and treated, may lead to chronic renal insufficiency (if the scarring is extensive) or later hypertension. Scarring is most likely to occur in the first 5 years of life; the younger the child the greater the risk. Children over the age of 5 seldom develop new scars, but pre-existing scars can become more extensive if infection is not prevented. For this reason, there are different schemes for investigation of children of different ages and protocols may differ from centre to centre according to local experience with the various imaging modalities. Ultrasound in particular is highly operator-dependent and isotope scanning depends on good technique to acquire high quality images without movement artefact. Intravenous urography (IVU), although long-established, is less often employed nowadays as it is associated with a higher radiation dose than the alternatives. Micturating cystourethrography (MCU) is the most invasive of the investigations as it requires catheterization of the bladder, which may be difficult and traumatic, particularly in toddlers. In an attempt to avoid MCUs in older children, some centres are using indirect isotope (MAG3) cystography to detect reflux. Information box 17.2 gives one protocol of investigation.

If there is ureteric reflux the child should be put on prophylactic antibiotics which are continued for a minimum of 2 years or, in the case of renal scarring, until the reflux has resolved or has been surgically corrected. An antibiotic such as trimethoprim or nitrofurantoin is taken once a day at night. The idea is to prevent further infections which because of the reflux have a greater likelihood of causing renal scarring.

With time ureteric reflux often disappears in childhood at a rate of approximately 10% per year. In children with normal kidneys, it may not be necessary to repeat the MCU before stopping antibiotics. Since scarring has not occurred by age 5 years, it is very unlikely to occur later, even if further infections occur.

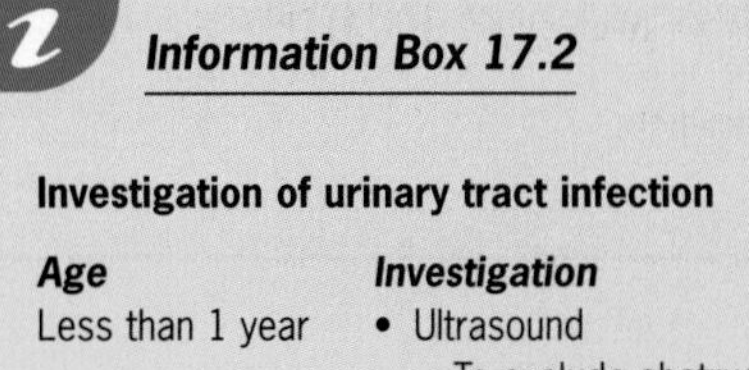

Information Box 17.2

Investigation of urinary tract infection

Age	*Investigation*
Less than 1 year	• Ultrasound – To exclude obstruction and major malformations • Micturating cystourethrography (MCU) – To detect reflux – To detect urethral obstruction in boys • DMSA (dimercaptosuccinic acid) scan – To detect renal damage – To assess renal function
1–5 years	• Ultrasound and abdominal X-ray • DMSA scan (*Note* Intravenous urography (IVU) as a single investigation can substitute for ultrasound and DMSA) • MCU or indirect isotope (MAG3) cystography – For children with abnormal first-line investigations or recurrent infections
Over 5 years	• Ultrasound and abdominal X-ray (or IVU) – Other investigations only if clinically indicated

One potential risk period for girls is that reflux and the potential for scarring may recur during pregnancy and the families should be counselled accordingly.

Some authorities would manage ureteric reflux by the surgical approach which involves reimplanting the ureters in such a way as to prevent reflux occurring. This is not without complication, and since most children do well on prophylactic antibiotics, the authors believe that this approach should be reserved for those children who get breakthrough urinary infections with resistant organisms while taking prophylaxis, or if there is poor compliance with medical treatment. If reflux persists after the age of 5 years and if the kidneys are scarred, surgery should be considered as an alternative to prophylactic antibiotics.

Students may feel that paediatricians tend to overinvestigate children with urinary tract infection. However the investigations are done because congenital abnormalities are common and, if undiagnosed, may lead to renal damage in the vulnerable kidneys of young children, which can be easily prevented. It has to be remembered that even in the most recent breakdowns of the reasons for patients to go onto chronic renal dialysis programmes, it is found that a large proportion still involve chronic pyelonephritis which almost certainly has its origins in early childhood.

Anatomical defects of the genitourinary system

Epidemiology

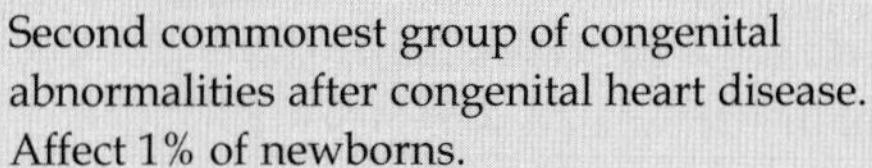

Second commonest group of congenital abnormalities after congenital heart disease.
Affect 1% of newborns.

Exostrophy of the urinary bladder (ectopia vesicae)

In this failure of development of the lower abdominal wall (Fig. 17.2), the bladder protrudes from the abdomen and the mucosal surface is exposed. The pubic rami are widely separated and the umbilicus is low. Male infants have complete epispadias; the urethra opens on the top of the penis.

Early and complex surgery is required to produce a reasonably sized bladder and repair the sphincter.

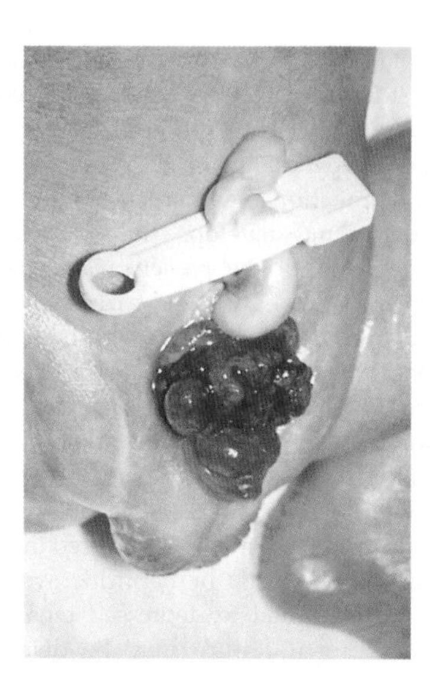

Fig 17.2
Exostrophy of the bladder.

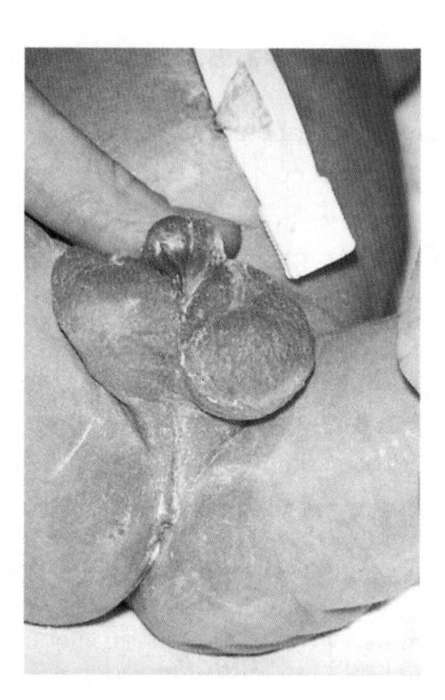

Fig 17.3
Hypospadias. Note the hooded prepuce, chordee and urethral opening at the base of the penis. The scrotum is bifid which may indicate inter sex.

Hypospadias

Definition
This Greek word means that the penis is abnormally formed with the urethral opening on the underside (Fig. 17.3).

Epidemiology
Mild degrees are relatively common (about 1 in 500), but fortunately extreme cases are rare.

Sometimes the condition is very mild with only a slight bend (or chordee) to the penis so that the boy can pass urine normally. Inguinal herniae and undecended testes are other common associations. If the opening is lower down on the shaft of the penis, or worse, at its base, it may be very difficult or impossible to pass urine standing up. Karyotyping should be performed in those with severe defects to exclude conditions resulting in masculinization of a female fetus, such as congenital adrenal hyperplasia (see p. 197).

The condition is bound to alarm parents greatly and to embarrass the boy as he grows. It is, however, nearly always possible for a skilled surgeon to do an excellent corrective operation that permits both normal urination and sexual intercourse. This is often best done before the boy starts school. Severe cases may require a series of operations. The foreskin is needed for this and circumcision must be prevented.

The condition is caused by abnormal development of the penis in the early weeks of intrauterine life. The reason for this is unknown.

Medullary sponge kidneys

This cystic dilatation of the collecting ducts in the renal papillae is of unknown cause and may be asymptomatic. It may be complicated by:

- Kidney stones (nephrolithiasis)
- Defective urine concentrating ability
- Distal renal tubular acidosis.

Pelviureteric obstruction

In this condition there is congenital obstruction of the pelviureteric junction, which is unilateral in 80% of cases. It may present as:

- Antenatal hydronephrosis
- Urinary tract infection
- Haematuria
- Pain in the flank.

In the newborn, providing one kidney is normal, follow up is justified. Many improve spontaneously. In the older child, surgical resection of the pelviureteric junction is required.

Phimosis

Surgical correction is required for this narrowing of the opening of the foreskin after 3 years of age.

Paraphimosis is a narrowing of the opening of a retractile foreskin. The constriction ring causes oedema of the glans and reduction of the retracted foreskin is difficult. Circumcision may be required, but only if there is obstruction to the urinary stream on direct observation of micturition.

Prune belly syndrome

Very occasionally infants are born with abnormally weak muscles to the abdominal wall which therefore bulges. The wrinkled abdominal skin gives the peculiar name to this condition, also known as Eagle–Barrett syndrome. The condition is often associated with severe obstruction to the renal tract. The disorder mainly affects boys. There is no clear-cut genetic pattern, and there are probably several different 'prune belly syndromes'. They are usually associated with urinary tract disorders, with dilatation of the ureters and bladder. The testes may be undescended and parts of the genital tract underdeveloped. Skeletal and cardiac abnormalities can also occur. Serious forms are often lethal in utero, and in surviving children the manifestations are very variable from mild to severe.

Reconstructive surgery to improve drainage of the kidneys or bladder is often needed.

Posterior urethral valves

These membranous structures in the posterior urethra cause dilatation of the bladder and hydronephrosis.

When these have been discovered prenatally, various methods have been tried to drain the bladder antenatally. These are at present experimental techniques.

Postnatally the child may present with a distended bladder and poor urinary stream. If the condition is missed the infant will present later with urinary tract infection or renal failure. The valves are demonstrated by cystourethrography.

Once the urethra is large enough the valves can be destroyed by the transurethral approach. Meanwhile the urinary tract is drained by vesicostomy.

Glomerular disorders

Glomerulonephritis

Cause
An important cause of glomerulonephritis is the group A β-haemolytic streptococci.

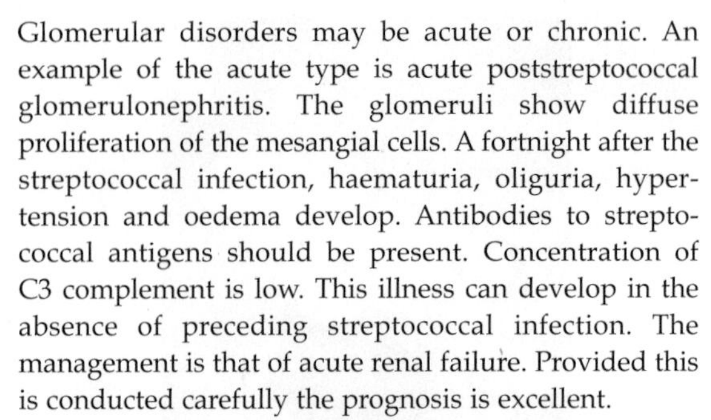

Glomerular disorders may be acute or chronic. An example of the acute type is acute poststreptococcal glomerulonephritis. The glomeruli show diffuse proliferation of the mesangial cells. A fortnight after the streptococcal infection, haematuria, oliguria, hypertension and oedema develop. Antibodies to streptococcal antigens should be present. Concentration of C3 complement is low. This illness can develop in the absence of preceding streptococcal infection. The management is that of acute renal failure. Provided this is conducted carefully the prognosis is excellent.

The commonest type of chronic glomerulonephritis is membranoproliferative. This disorder is also associated with low C3 levels. The capillary walls are thickened and C3 complement is deposited in them. The lesion produces nephrotic or nephritic syndrome or haematuria with normal to depressed renal function. Progression to renal failure may be delayed with steroids and antiplatelet drugs. The lesion can develop in transplanted kidneys.

Other disorders affecting the glomeruli, such as haemolytic uraemic and Henoch–Schönlein syndromes are dealt with elsewhere.

Haemolytic uraemic syndrome

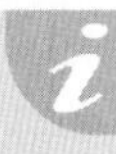

Epidemiology
The commonest cause of acute renal failure in children in developed countries.

This is commonly associated with an illness caused by a diarrhoeagenic *Escherichia coli* of serotype O157:H7 called haemorrhagic colitis, because the stools contain blood. These *E. coli* produce toxins called verocytotoxins resembling that of *Shigella dysenteriae* 1 which also causes haemolytic uraemic syndrome. The capillaries of the glomeruli and other organs become occluded with fibrin thrombi. The platelet count is low due to consumption of platelets in the thrombi. The threads of fibrin in the capillaries cleave passing red cells. This process is referred to as microangiopathic haemolytic anaemia. Dialysis may be required until urine flow returns.

Nephrotic syndrome

Epidemiology
Idiopathic nephrotic syndrome may be familial. It is twice as common in boys and is commonest in 2–6-year-olds.

Information Box 17.3

Histological types of nephrotic syndrome

	Histology of glomeruli	*Frequency in idiopathic nephrotic syndrome*	*Response to steroids*
Minimal change	Normal with retracted foot processes of the glomerular epithelial cells on electron microscopy	85%	>95%
Mesangioproliferative	Diffuse increase in mesangial cells and matrix	5%	55%
Focal glomerulosclerosis	Segmental scarring of juxtamedullary glomeruli	10%	20%

INTRODUCTION

Excessive loss of protein in the urine (generally greater than 2 g/24 hours) results in oedema. Most of the protein in the urine is albumin. Oedema usually occurs when serum albumin falls to 25 g/l.

AETIOLOGY AND PATHOGENESIS

The histological types of nephrotic syndrome are shown in Information box 17.3 together with frequency and response rate to steroids. Focal sclerosis frequently progresses to end-stage renal failure and may recur in the transplanted kidney.

The underlying cause of the glomerular capillary leakiness is unknown. The hypoalbuminaemia causes a fall in plasma osmotic pressure which allows fluid to move from the intravascular to the interstitial spaces. As the intravascular volume shrinks there is less renal perfusion, and the renin–angiotensin–aldosterone system is stimulated. The released aldosterone encourages distal tubular reabsorption of sodium. Antidiuretic hormone (ADH) is also stimulated by the low intravascular volume. ADH stimulates reabsorption of water in the collection duct. The pathophysiology of oedema in nephrotic syndrome must be more complex than this because patients have been reported with an increased intravascular volume and low plasma concentrations of aldosterone.

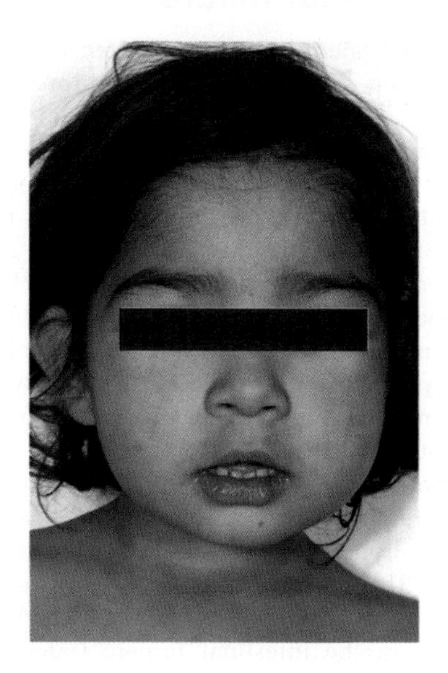

Fig 17.4
Nephrotic syndrome. Note oedema of the upper eyelids.

CLINICAL PRESENTATION

The child is not hypertensive. The oedema is initially periorbital, becoming generalized pitting oedema as urine output falls. Ascites and pleural effusions develop (Fig. 17.4). Plasma albumin is usually less than 20 g/l. C3 concentration is normal. Urinalysis shows protein without gross haematuria. Creatinine clearance is low because renal perfusion may be decreased due to low intravascular volume.

MANAGEMENT

Treatment is started with prednisolone 1 mg/kg/day up to 60 mg/day. Strict salt restriction is unnecessary. Diuresis usually occurs after 2 weeks after which the dose of prednisolone is given on alternate days for 3–6 months then withdrawn. Relapses are treated the same way. Steroid cover will be required for serious illness or surgery for up to 1 year after steroid therapy.

Those children who develop massive oedema should be hospitalized for diuretic therapy. Albumin infusions may be necessary for the diuretics to work but the effect is transient and puts the patient at risk for volume overload. The complication of spontaneous bacterial peritonitis, often due to *Streptococcus pneumoniae*, should be borne in mind. The symptoms may be masked by the steroid therapy. Pneumococcal vaccination is recommended during remission. Another complication is venous thrombosis as the condition produces a hypercoagulable state.

Many patients, termed 'steroid-dependent' will relapse. They are candidates for therapy with cyclophosphamide for 8 weeks. If proteinuria is still present after 1 month, the disease is termed 'steroid-resistant'. A renal biopsy is performed to look for mesangial proliferation, which is less likely to respond to steroids or focal glomerular sclerosis which causes progressive glomerular disease. The family should be reassured about the eventual good prognosis for steroid-sensitive nephrotic syndrome.

Renal failure

Epidemiology

The commonest cause of acute renal failure in children in Europe and North America is the haemolytic uraemic syndrome.

INTRODUCTION

Renal failure occurs if the kidneys cannot maintain homeostasis of fluid and electrolytes. In acute renal failure the urine output is usually less than 250 ml/m^2.

AETIOLOGY AND PATHOGENESIS

The causes of acute renal failure (Information box 17.4) are classified into prerenal (e.g. hypovolaemia due to haemorrhage, hypotension due to septicaemia), renal (e.g. glomerulonephritis, acute tubular necrosis due to shock) and postrenal (e.g. obstruction to both ureters due to tumour).

In prerenal causes there is defective perfusion of the kidney leading to decrease in glomerular filtration rate. If the underlying cause can be corrected in time, then renal failure will be avoided. Rapidly progressive glomerulonephritis can lead to renal failure.

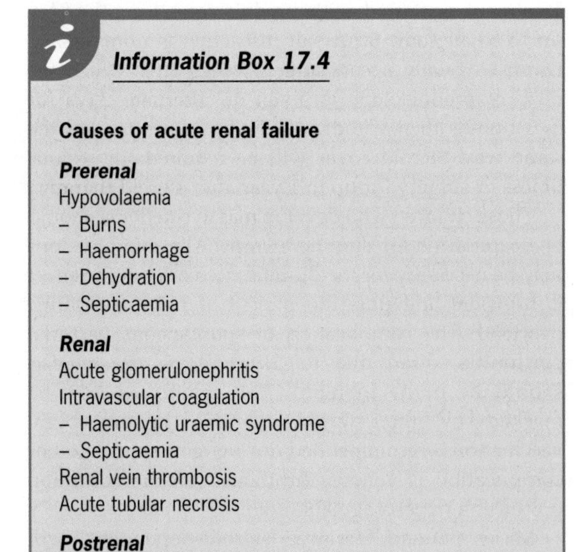

Information Box 17.4

Causes of acute renal failure

Prerenal

Hypovolaemia
- Burns
- Haemorrhage
- Dehydration
- Septicaemia

Renal

Acute glomerulonephritis
Intravascular coagulation
- Haemolytic uraemic syndrome
- Septicaemia

Renal vein thrombosis
Acute tubular necrosis

Postrenal

Acute urinary tract obstruction

CLINICAL PRESENTATION

The child becomes oedematous and hypertensive. Volume overload produces congestive cardiac failure. Serum creatinine and urea will be grossly elevated.

MANAGEMENT

Prerenal failure must be differentiated from renal failure and obstruction to the renal tract must be excluded by plain X-ray of the abdomen and ultrasound with occasional recourse to radionuclide scan and retrograde pyelography. Percutaneous nephrostomy will reverse the obstruction. Children with hypovolaemia have urine osmolalities greater than 500 mOsm/kg containing less than 20 mmol/l of sodium. In tubular necrosis, urine osmolality is less than 350 mOsm/kg and sodium concentration greater than 40 mmol/l. In hypovolaemia 20 ml/kg of isotonic saline are given, which should produce a diuresis, followed by 2 mg/kg frusemide if this fails. If urine flow is not restored, fluid restriction is required. Potassium is excluded to avoid hyperkalaemia. When potassium rises to 5.5 mmol/l, a potassium–sodium exchange resin (sodium polystyrene sulphonate) is given orally. If this fails to decrease potassium, calcium gluconate, sodium bicarbonate and glucose are given and dialysis commenced. Dialysis is also required for fluid, electrolyte and severe acidosis. The prognosis depends on the underlying cause of the acute renal failure.

Chronic renal failure

Chronic renal failure in young children is commonly due to long-standing reflux nephropathy and hypoplasia of the kidney. In older children, glomerulonephritis, polycystic disease and Alport syndrome are more likely. Children with chronic renal failure fail to grow, and poor calorie intake is partially responsible. They require carbohydrate and fat supplements. If urea is greater than 30 mmol/l, nausea occurs and dietary protein should be restricted. Most children maintain water and electrolyte homeostasis until dialysis is required. Acidosis is commonly present but sodium citrate or bicarbonate is only given if serum bicarbonate is less than 20 mmol/l.

As renal function declines serum phosphorus rises, thus depressing serum calcium and leading to secondary hyperparathyroidism and renal osteodystrophy. This can be corrected with a low phosphate diet and oral calcium carbonate which binds phosphate in the intestinal lumen. Calcium malabsorption may contribute to hypocalcaemia because of deficiency of the active form of vitamin D (1,25-

dihydroxycholecalciferol) which is normally made by the healthy kidney. Supplements can be given to maintain normal alkaline phosphatase and heal the rickets of renal osteodystrophy.

An important factor in the anaemia of chronic renal failure is deficiency of erythropoietin, which is also produced by the healthy kidney. Recombinant human erythropoietin is now available for treatment.

Hypertensive crises are treated with intravenous diazoxide. Frusemide, propranolol and hydralazine are given for sustained hypertension.

Continuous ambulatory peritoneal dialysis (CAPD) is commenced when serum creatinine reaches 900 μmol/l, or the child develops problems with fluid overload or metabolic disturbances, with a view to renal transplantation.

Metabolic disorders of the kidney

Bartter syndrome

This hyperplasia of the juxtaglomerular apparatus results in increased production of renin and aldosterone, and hypokalaemia with muscle weakness, constipation, inability to concentrate urine and stimulation of synthesis of prostaglandins. Blood pressure is normal.

Inhibition of prostaglandin synthesis with indomethacin reverses the abnormalities. The condition may be autosomal recessive.

Fanconi syndrome (de Toni–Debré–Fanconi syndrome)

Cause
Defective proximal renal tubule, leading to loss of water, amino acids, glucose, phosphate, and sometimes bicarbonate, potassium, sodium, uric acid and protein.

Some of the causes of Fanconi syndrome are shown in Information box 17.5. The resulting hypophosphataemia leads to rickets. In addition to the treatment of any underlying cause, high doses of vitamin D and phosphate, and extra water, sodium, potassium and bicarbonate (or bicarbonate precursor such as citrate) are given.

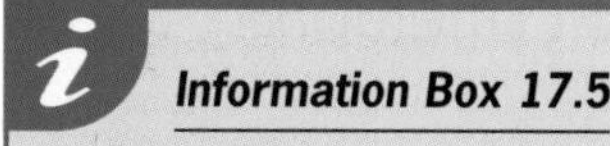

Information Box 17.5

Causes of Fanconi syndrome

Idiopathic (sporadic)

Genetic
Dominant
Recessive
X-linked recessive

Inborn errors of metabolism
Cystinosis
Fructose intolerance
Galactosaemia
Glycogenosis
Lowe syndrome
Tyrosinaemia
Wilson disease

Drugs
Azathioprine
Gentamicin
Out-of-date tetracycline

Heavy metals
Cadmium
Lead
Mercury

Lowe syndrome (oculocerebral dystrophy, oculocerebrorenal syndrome)

This X-linked recessive syndrome presents with mental retardation, hypotonia, congenital cataracts, and glaucoma, causing marked visual impairment.

Associated abnormal proximal renal tubules make this disorder one cause of Fanconi syndrome (see above); there is amino aciduria and renal rickets due to phosphaturia. Renal failure occurs in later life.

No specific treatment is available.

Nephrolithiasis (kidney stones)

Kidney stones usually result from chronic infection or excess urinary excretion of calcium, uric acid, oxalate or cystine. The presenting complaints are abdominal pain, flank pain, gross or microscopic haematuria and symptoms of urinary tract infection.

Some surgical conditions

Circumcision

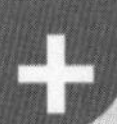

Practical Box 17.2

Circumcision

This operation is usually performed for cultural reasons. Medical reasons advanced for the procedure include prevention of:

- Balanitis (inflammation of the foreskin)
- Phimosis (narrowing of the opening in the foreskin)
- Paraphimosis (nonretractile foreskin)
- Urinary tract infection
- Cancer of the penis.

Complications include:

- Bleeding
- Sepsis
- Amputation of glans
- Removal of excessive amount of foreskin
- Urethral fistula.

Circumcision is contraindicated if there is hypospadias as the skin may be required for the repair. The operation is the cause of much controversy.

Treatment of torsion of the testes

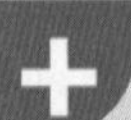

Practical Box 17.3

Torsion of the testes

A common cause of acute painful swelling of the scrotum. If the tunica vaginalis invests the testis, epididymis and end of the spermatic cord, instead of the anterior surface of the testis then the testis is free to rotate (bell clapper deformity). The scrotum becomes swollen and very tender.

Prompt surgical exploration is required to avoid ischaemic damage to the testis. Both testes should be fixed to the scrotum as the bell clapper deformity is often bilateral.

Epididymitis is the commonest cause of testicular pain in teenagers and exploration is required to exclude torsion.

18 Neurology

Neurological problems are an important part of paediatrics. Before reaching school age, 3% of children will have had a convulsion (mainly febrile). Headache is an almost universal symptom in children. Much of the developmental screening of community paediatrics is underpinned by paediatric neurology.

Anatomical defects

Agenesis of corpus callosum

Failure of development of the commissural plate that develops near the anterior neuropore may be X-linked recessive, autosomal dominant or part of a chromosomal disorder.

This may form part of the Aicardi syndrome, a neurodegenerative disorder occurring only in females with agenesis of the corpus callosum. Other features include convulsions, severe mental retardation, vertebral abnormalities and colobomata (fissures) of the optic discs.

The impact on brain function depends on whether other defects of brain structure are present. The abnormalities can be asymptomatic if it is an isolated finding.

Craniosynostosis

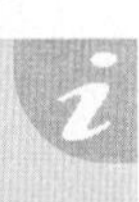

Importance
A preventable cause of mental retardation.

The skull bones are formed as separate plates held together with fibrous tissue at the growing edges. They normally fuse together once skull growth is complete. This is a gradual process, head growth being particularly rapid in the early months and being largely complete by age 6. The disappearance of the anterior fontanelle around the first birthday is an illustration of this process. Occasionally some and more rarely all the skull bones start to fuse abnormally early. The cause is unknown although genetic disorders are associated. In most infants with small heads the brain itself is not growing rather than the skull. If there is a question of poor head growth and early closure of the fontanelle, a skull X-ray will demonstrate the condition of the skull sutures and whether they have closed. Premature closure of the sagittal suture results in a long, narrow skull (scaphocephaly; Fig. 18.1). Fusion of one coronal suture results in unilateral flattening of the forehead (frontal plagiocephaly). Fusion of the frontal suture produces trigonocephaly with a narrow forehead. Fusion of multiple sutures results in a conically shaped head (acrocephaly; Fig. 18.2) or prominent temporal bones (clover-leaf-shaped skull or Kleeblatt-Schädel). It is sometimes possible to operate on the skull (craniectomy) and insert plastic substances between the skull bones in order to prevent fusion. If one suture is fused, the indication for operation is cosmetic, but fusion of several sutures can cause raised intracranial pressure and optic atrophy.

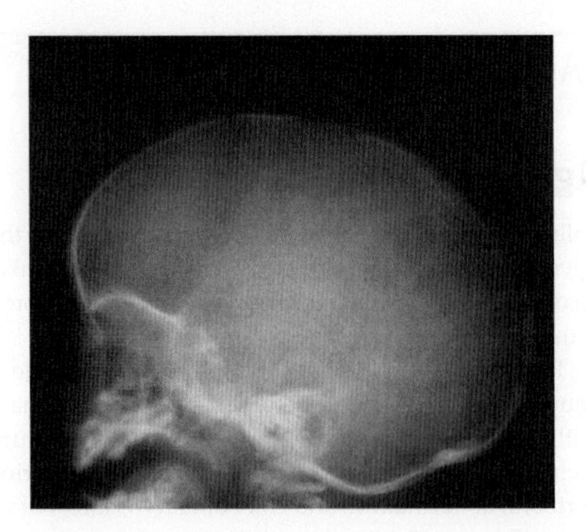

Fig 18.1
Scaphocephaly: partial fusion of the sagittal suture.

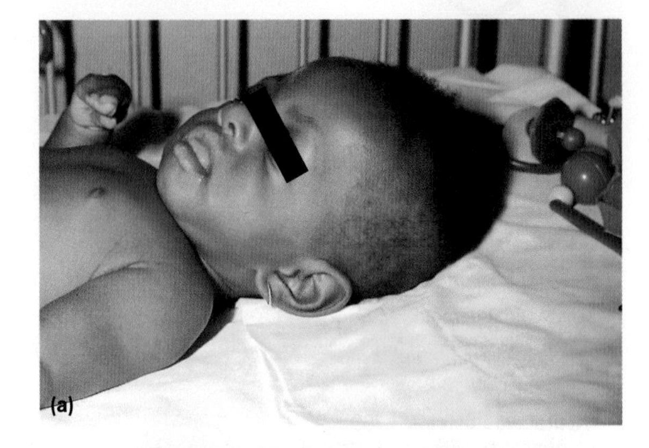

(a)

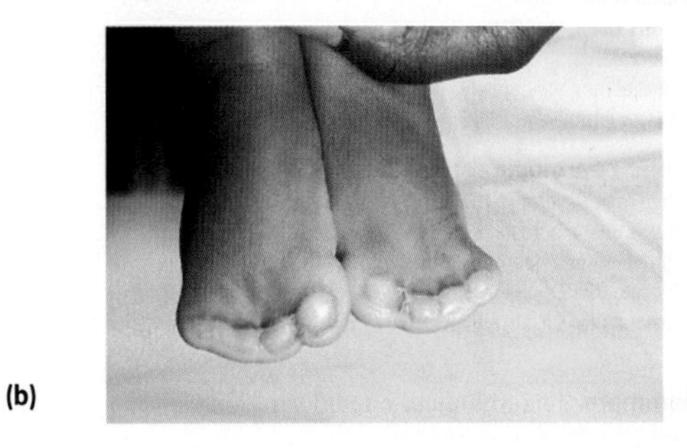

(b)

Fig 18.2
(a) and (b) Apert syndrome. This child has acrocephaly and syndactyly.

Crouzon syndrome is an example of an autosomal dominant disorder affecting the facial skeleton; unknown factors in the development of the skull bones result in a characteristic deformity which includes proptosis due to shallow orbits and dental irregularity. Some have craniosynostosis and increased intracranial pressure.

In Apert syndrome there is premature fusion of multiple cranial sutures and syndactyly of fingers and toes (Fig. 18.2). The abnormal shape of the skull is termed acrocephaly (high forehead and flat occiput). The fused sutures may have to be reopened surgically to allow the brain to grow. It is usually sporadic but may be autosomal dominantly inherited.

In recent years, the development of complex surgical techniques has brought new hope for those affected by these conditions.

Porencephaly

Definition
Fluid-filled space or cyst of very variable size within a brain hemisphere.

There are many possible reasons why a child might have a brain cyst. Often they are called porencephalic cysts (or in plain English, a hole in the brain tissue). Much will depend on their cause, position in the brain, whether there are multiple or single cysts and why they formed.

Among possible causes are: resolved blood clot due to cerebral trauma following accidental or non-accidental injuring or shaking; a cavity due to infestation by a parasite such as an amoebic or hydatid cyst, found in tropical countries; the end result of meningitis or encephalitis, or degeneration of a brain tumour. Some are never explained and are presumably developmental cerebral abnormalities caused by some intrauterine insult. A left-sided weakness suggests that the cyst is on the right side of the brain because motor messages which originate in the brain cross to the other side of the body; speech defect may be due to involvement of the centres of the brain that initiate and control speech. It is important to realize that there may be generalized brain disorder as well as the cyst.

Whatever the pathological cause, the outcome will be affected by whether the cyst enlarges, shrinks or is amenable to surgery. Seizures will need anticonvulsant treatment.

Neural tube defects

Epidemiology
Commonest congenital anomalies of the central nervous system.

Spina bifida

Anencephaly (see also Myelomeningocele)
Infants with anencephaly (Fig. 18.3) are born without a scalp, vault to the skull cerebrum and cerebellum. Only a residual brain stem is present. The embryonic basis is the same as myelomeningocele (see below), except that failure of fusion of a portion of the neural tube is responsible. The defect used to occur in 1:1000 births, but is becoming less common due to prevention by folic acid supplements in pregnancy.

Antenatal diagnosis is by ultrasound and measurement of alpha-fetoprotein in serum and amniotic fluid. The recurrence risk is 4%.

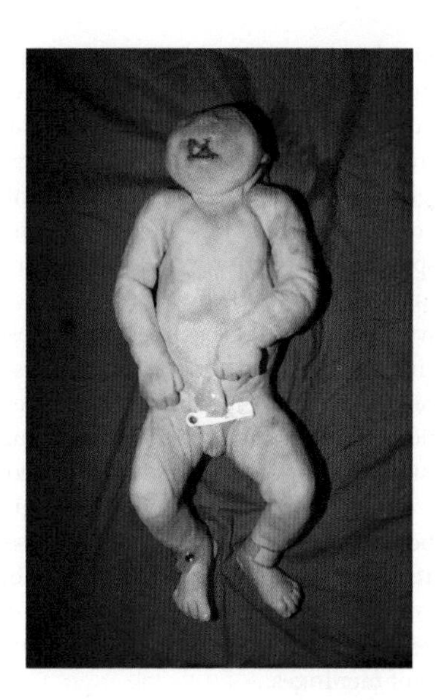

Fig 18.3
Anencephaly.

Encephalocele
This is the cranial equivalent of myelomeningocele (see below). It usually occurs beneath the occiput. If the sac contains only meninges (cranial meningocele), the prognosis is better than for encephalocele containing part of the cerebral cortex, cerebellum or brain stem.

Myelomeningocele (Fig. 18.4)
This occurs in 1:1000 live births. However, the incidence is falling because of antenatal diagnosis and prevention by supplementation with folic acid to pregnant mothers. The risk after an affected pregnancy is 4%.

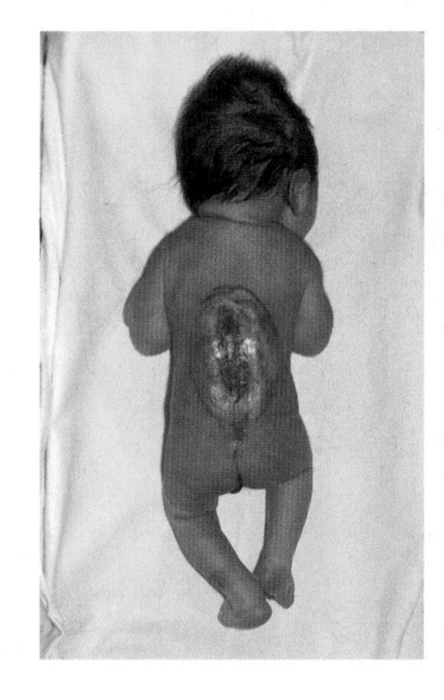

Fig 18.4
Spina bifida: myelomeningocele.

The lesion consists of a sac-like structure protruding through a defect in the vertebral column and containing rudimentary nervous tissue. Most lesions are in the lumbosacral region. A lesion in the sacral region affects only bowel and bladder function, while a lumbar lesion will also compromise walking. Cervical lesions tend not to affect spinal cord function. Most affected infants also have hydrocephalus (see below).

In active treatment, the back lesion is closed and a shunt is inserted if there is hydrocephalus. Regular bladder catheterization is required in the treatment of neurogenic bladder of myelomeningocele, and enemas may assist in the development of faecal continence. Club feet or dislocated hips may need attention; this may not be undertaken if the legs are paralysed.

Variants of this condition include spina bifida occulta, only the vertebral arches being cleft, and meningocele in which there is no nervous tissue in the herniation of meninges.

Hydrocephalus (Fig. 18.5)

Cerebrospinal fluid (CSF) is produced by the choroid plexus in the lateral ventricles. It flows via the foramina of Munro into the third ventricle and via the aqueduct of Sylvius into the fourth ventricle. The fourth ventricle is drained laterally by the foramina of Luschka and in the midline by the foramen of Magendie into the basal cisterns. The CSF then passes over the surface of the brain and is absorbed by the arachnoid villi.

Obstruction to CSF flow results in hydrocephalus. Obstruction in the ventricles is called obstructive or noncommunicating. Obstruction to the basal cisterns is referred to as nonobstructive or communicating. Skull X-rays show widening of the sutures and increased convolutional markings (beaten-silver appearance). CT or MRI scans help to identify a specific cause.

A ventriculoperitoneal shunt is usually required to prevent progression.

Microcephaly (Fig. 18.6)

The abnormally small head circumference of this condition is diagnosed by comparing the infant's head circumference to standard charts. Microcephaly may be inherited by an autosomal dominant or recessive mode and may be part of a syndrome, e.g. Down, Edward or 'cri du chat' (see p. 240). Intrauterine infection and exposure to alcohol are other causes. Microcephaly will follow any severe insult to the brain, such as hypoxic–ischaemic encephalopathy or meningitis.

Genetic counselling may be required, and associated developmental delay will require assessment and special education.

Familial megalencephaly

Familial megalencephaly is part of the differential diagnosis of macrocephaly.

The child's head is large, and as the condition is dominantly inherited, so is that of one of the parents.

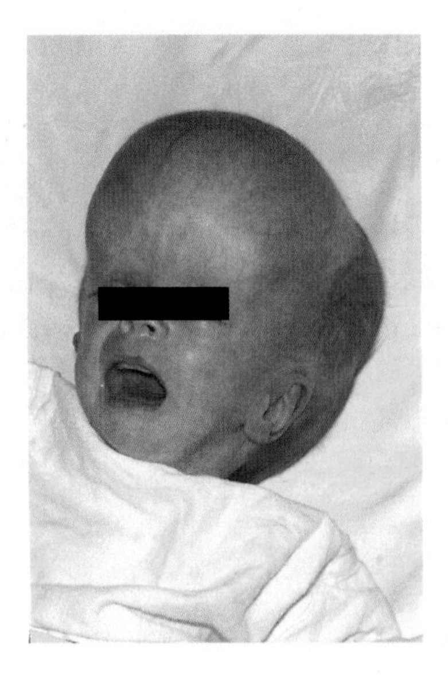

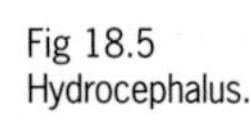

Fig 18.5
Hydrocephalus.

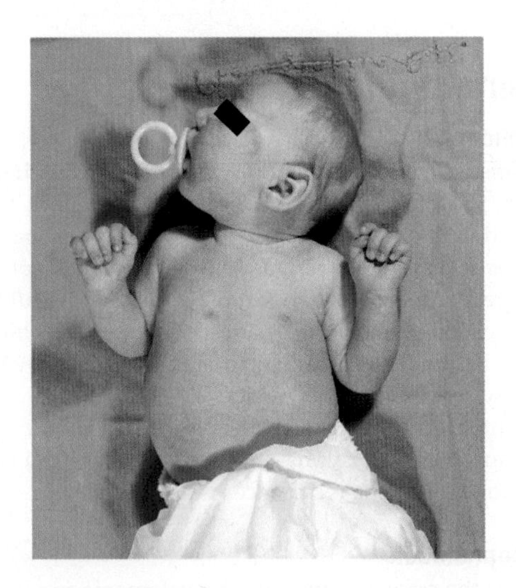

Fig 18.6
Microcephaly.

The cerebral ventricles are normal in size and the head grows at a normal rate.

Diastematomyelia

In this disorder the spinal cord is split by a bony or cartilaginous septum extending posteriorly from the vertebral body. There may be a haemangioma of the overlying skin. Traction on the cord produces talipes, which may progress to leg weakness, sensory loss and urinary incontinence. MRI scanning is required to demonstrate a cartilaginous septum.

Treatment is by excision of the septum.

Genetic neurological disorders

Angelman syndrome

This is an extremely rare condition found in a distinct group of mentally handicapped children. It is characterized by odd, jerky ataxic movements which resemble the action of a puppet. The face is remarkably similar in all affected children; the teeth may be uneven and the ears are low set. Many have epilepsy.

Typically the child never speaks at all, unlike other severely disabled children who usually make some speech sounds. From infancy, however, the child develops a loud, normal-sounding but totally inappropriate (or gelastic) laugh. Angelman syndrome is an example of disomic inheritance. The gene is inherited from the mother, in exactly the opposite situation from Prader–Willi syndrome where an identical gene is inherited from the father causing a very different disorder (see p. 244).

Ataxia telangiectasia (Louis-Bar disease)

Telangectasia are enlarged blood vessels which are seen on the skin and sclerae in this condition. The child is usually perfectly healthy at birth, but in infancy, cerebellar ataxia and occular movement abnormalities begin. There is a deficiency of IgA and IgE, and serum alpha-fetoprotein and carcinoembryonic antigens are elevated.

Impaired DNA repair predisposes to malignancy, usually a lymphoma. The long-term prospect tends to be bleak, with a gradual downhill course usually associated with mental deterioration although not in every affected child.

Inheritance is usually autosomal recessive, involving chromosome 11. The affected gene (ATM) encodes a protein controlling the cell cycle.

Batten disease (ceroid lipofuscinosis)

Ceroid lipofuscinosis should be remembered when encountering any child, especially around school starting age, who presents with gradual loss of vision, fits and developmental regression.

Deterioration is relentless and no medical treatment is helpful.

In some countries the same condition is called Spielmeyer–Vogt disorder, and if it starts in infancy the name Jansky–Bielschowsky syndrome may be used.

Batten disease is but one of a group of conditions collectively described as 'ceroid lipofuscinosis'. Within the nervous system there is degeneration of neurons. Abnormal fatty substances accumulate within the nerves. The most convenient site for the biopsy which is needed to prove the diagnosis is the rectum. The eye may show retinal degeneration, and EEG, electroretinogram (ERG) and visually evoked responses (VER) are abnormal.

These conditions are autosomal recessive disorders. Prenatal diagnosis is possible. In some affected families the abnormalities are mapped on chromosome 1.

Chorea

Chorea is usually thought of as abnormal movements occurring during rheumatic fever (see p. 180). It may rarely be dominantly inherited as familial paroxysmal choreoathetosis (where athetosis describes 'writhing' movements), or as Huntington chorea.

In the latter condition presenile dementia occurs in the third decade, and affected children have behavioural problems. There is generalized epilepsy. The disorder is linked to a gene on chromosome 4. There is no treatment, and prevention is by genetic counselling.

Spinal muscular atrophy (Werdnig–Hoffman syndrome, anterior horn cell disease)

(Fig. 18.7)

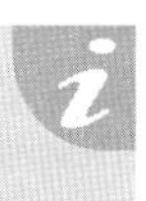

Epidemiology
About 1 in 20 000 births, or once in 5 years in a busy maternity unit

It is probable that the condition originally described by Drs Werdnig and Hoffman in the 1890s is not the same as the condition that now bears their names. This

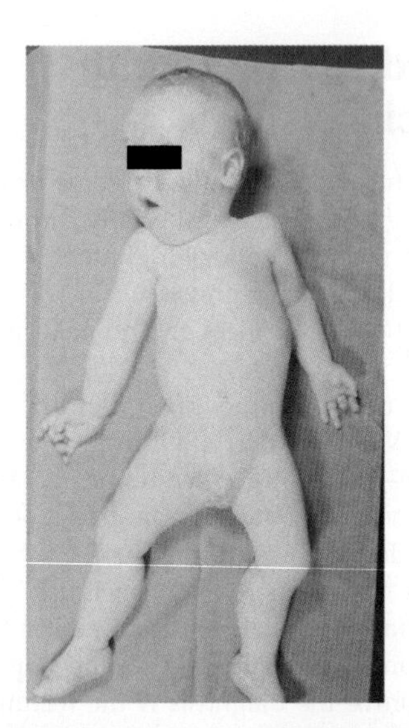
(a)

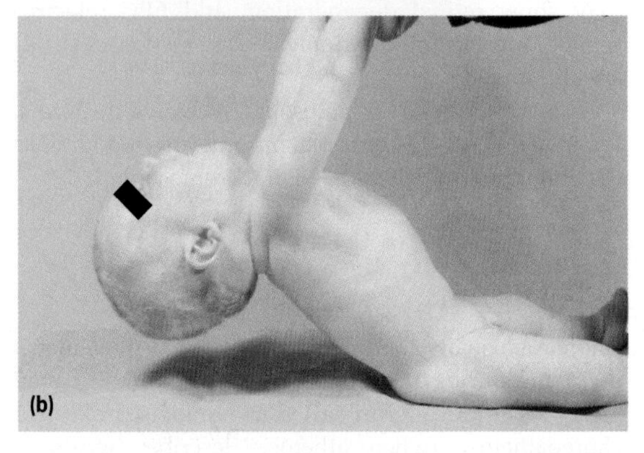
(b)

Fig 18.7
(a) and (b) Spinal muscular atrophy. Note the mask-like face; affected infants are socially aware, however.

disorder is a rare and very serious form of spinal muscular atrophy seen in infants. The child is often noted to kick poorly in utero, and to be reluctant to breathe and cry after delivery. Many have congenital orthopaedic deformities due to muscular weakness, and many have to be tube-fed because of poor sucking.

As the weeks go by, poor muscle tone prevents the infant from making normal progress. Most remain very thin and weak and cannot lift their bodies off the cot. Shivering movement of the tongue (fasciculation) is a sign that the muscles are not contracting properly. Despite the best care few infants live for more than 18 months, death usually being due to chest infection. The condition is usually autosomal recessive.

There are also less severe conditions with some similar features which present at a later age, such as Kugelberg–Welander disease, though there are other conditions with some of these features. It is important that the diagnosis is fully confirmed in every case. Spinal muscular atrophy is due to failure of normal development of motor nerve cells in the anterior half of the spinal cord; the reason remains unknown. Nothing can be done to prevent this happening in affected infants nor is there any useful drug or surgery. The defective gene lies on chromosome 5.

Inflammatory neurological conditions

Bell palsy (facial nerve paralysis)

This acute unilateral facial nerve paralysis is not caused by intracranial pathology. It is a post-infectious demyelinating condition, following infections such as mumps or glandular fever. It may also be a complication of otitis media or forceps delivery.

Early use of a short course of high-dose steroids may shorten the course. Methyl cellulose eye drops at night prevent the development of exposure keratitis as the eye cannot close completely.

The majority recover completely, but in those who do not recover, a primary or secondary tumour of the nerve should be considered.

Transverse myelitis

An acute disorder of the spinal cord may present with a profound weakness of all muscles innervated below the level of a lesion to the cord, due to temporary or permanent damage to myelin which affects the ability of nerve tissue to transmit impulses. When the condition affects an entire cross-section of the spinal cord, the results are known as transverse myelitis.

The condition may be inflammatory and linked with virus diseases, such as coxsackie, rabies, *Herpes zoster* or polio, or (in the past) smallpox vaccination, or it may be associated with a generalized infection. Transverse myelitis may also be caused by trauma, compression from a tumour, vascular abnormality or thrombosis.

Generally no specific treatment is available, but large doses of steroids may reduce the initial swelling and help recovery. Physiotherapy and occupational therapy are also employed.

Cerebral palsy

Definition
Static, nonprogressive but not unchanging disorder affecting posture and movement, caused by damage sustained by the immature and developing brain.
Beyond 6 years, similar damage causes a 'stroke' leading to a different pattern of disability.

Epidemiology
The prevalence of 2–3 : 1000 live births has increased slightly in recent years. This trend has been found in most developing countries.
The prevalence is increased by low birth-weight, multiple pregnancies and prematurity.

INTRODUCTION
Cerebral palsy has essential features which represent the attempts of the still growing brain to compensate for damage.

AETIOLOGY AND PATHOGENESIS
Potential causes of cerebral palsy are shown in Information box 18.1. In the majority of cases there is no obvious cause; hence those listed account for a minority of cases.

Prolonged perinatal hypoxia is associated with the development of an ischaemic encephalopathy. It should never be assumed, however, that just because a baby is hypoxic at birth this is the prime cause of cerebral palsy in any individual case. Recent evidence suggests that birth asphyxia can be a manifestation in some cases of antenatal disorders that lead to cerebral palsy. The clinical classification is shown in Information box 18.2.

True cerebral palsies may be spastic, due to damage in the motor brain areas and descending neural pathways. Some infants are noted to be severely brain damaged from birth. In others there may be no obvious physical signs in the early months. The infant may then be noted to be floppy and fail to sit up by 6 months; the primitive neonatal reflexes (see p. 35) may persist. Affected infants show hand preference (which is almost always abnormal in early life) and scissoring (crossing over) of the legs. Eventually the limbs start to stiffen and variable degrees of limb contracture develop; in worst cases the hips may dislocate. The child may have bulbar problems leading to feeding, breathing and speech difficulties.

Athetoid (dyskinetic) cerebral palsy, due to damage to the basal ganglia, in the past was a sequel of severe prolonged kernicterus; deafness often occurs as well. Present-day cases tend to be associated with hypoxic brain damage, usually in the term neonate. The predominant features are unsynchronized writhing movements of the limbs and head and trunk making hand control, swallowing and speech very difficult. Often the intelligence is not affected leading to an intelligent person being trapped in a poorly controllable body.

Information Box 18.1

Causes of cerebral palsy

Antenatal
Genetic abnormality
Intrauterine infection (rubella, CMV)
Intrauterine malnutrition
Cerebral malformation (cortical dysplasia)

Intranatal
Infection
Prolonged hypoxia

Postnatal
Haemorrhage (preterm neonates)
Accidents
Suffocation
Shaking injury
Intracranial infection
Hyperbilirubinaemia (kernicterus)
Hypoglycaemia

Information Box 18.2

Types of cerebral palsy

Classification by topography
Monoplegia: affecting one limb only
Hemiplegia: affecting one side of the body
Quadriplegia: affecting all four limbs
Double hemiplegia: both sides affected but to a dissimilar degree

Classification by motor symptoms
Spastic: damage to motor cortex (see below)
Athetoid (*dyskinetic*): damage to basal ganglia (see below)
Ataxic
Mixed

The film *My Left Foot* gave a dramatized but fair portrait of athetoid cerebral palsy; do try to see it. Affected children usually present because of concern about delay in passing normal developmental milestones.

MANAGEMENT

Diagnosis is clinical and made by an experienced medical specialist who works closely with appropriate therapists who have their diagnostic contribution to make.

Often no investigations are needed; in some cases brain scanning is required to evaluate intracranial pathology and blood and urine tests for progressive metabolic disorders and congenital infections.

Treatment is multidisciplinary and aims to prevent complications and maximize the child's chances to achieve his or her full potential. Early diagnosis is needed so that a therapy plan can be worked out as soon as possible – well before the child has had time to demonstrate all the potential features of the condition. Once even a tentative diagnosis has been made, parents need full counselling and to be introduced to the child development team at their local child development centre. Then a full assessment can be started. In every case this will include speech, hearing and vision as well as mapping out the affected areas. Sometimes gait analysis is needed prior to reconstructive surgery that is giving promising results in specialized centres. Much has been written about special treatment centres such as the Peto method from Hungary where multiskilled therapists or conductors are employed. This is but one of many approaches; there is no universal panacea for the amelioration of the cerebral palsies. Physiotherapy with the goal of preventing contractures and enhancing mobility is the first essential; special shoes and wheelchairs that must be properly fitted may be needed. Lioresal (baclofen) can control severe muscular spasms. Botulinum toxin injections may make physiotherapy more effective. Cerebral palsy is a multifaceted condition; good management requires professional teamwork: the team members teach the parents to become the child's personal therapists and maintain morale. At an early stage a plan for appropriate schooling is needed (see Statementing on p. 323).

Reflux oesophagitis is common and requires investigation and treatment. Dietitians play an important role as affected infants usually have feeding problems and some need gastrostomy feeding. Seizures require careful evaluation and treatment. It is also worth involving an orthopaedic surgeon at an early stage to monitor and try to prevent the development of contractures, scoliosis and dislocated hips.

The prognosis is very variable. Good compensation for the effects of mild cerebral palsy can occur; in severe cases the main aim is to get as good an outcome as possible and prevent deterioration. The prognosis for life is dependent on associated factors including nutrition, presence of seizures, risk of accident, aspiration pneumonia and psychological health.

Muscle disorders

Muscular dystrophies

Duchenne muscular dystrophy and Becker variant

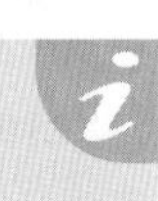

Epidemiology
About 100 affected boys are born in the UK yearly; a rate of 1 : 3000 male births.

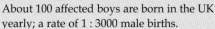

This tragic disorder is named after the French doctor who described it in 1868. It probably only affects boys because of the X-linked recessive inheritance pattern. They seem normal at birth and in their first year or two but gradually develop weakness of the muscles, firstly around the hips so that standing up and walking is affected most. Gradually the whole body becomes weak. One common early sign is difficulty in arising from the ground. The child has to pull himself up. Walking may start at the usual age or late but the gait is always waddling. At first the disease may be difficult to recognize but gradually the diagnosis becomes distressingly apparent. The creatinine phosphokinase (CPK) activity in the blood is very high. Muscle biopsy and blood for DNA studies help clinch the diagnosis; without it the disease could be mistaken for other conditions. Accurate diagnosis and then genetic counselling is vital. By 12 years most will only be able to get around in wheelchairs; electric ones are soon needed. The Becker variant is less severe with walking preserved until 16 years or later. Cardiomyopathy and conduction defects are often found. Many but not all have a lower than normal intelligence level. Some develop an odd euphoric state.

The important thing is that affected children must be cherished and allowed to live as full a life as possible, something that may cause difficulty to distraught families. Great support from families and school is essential. Most die in their twenties if not in their late teens when the disease hampers respiration. It is important that the bereavement process does not start while the boy lives. A lot of living has to be compressed into a few years. Skilled nursing advice and family support are the key. Obesity should be avoided as this makes care needlessly difficult. About two-thirds of affected boys come from families where the problem is carried via the mother. In theory half her sons would be affected and half her daughters carry the condition, to the potential detriment of half their offspring. One-third are 'new mutations' and further affected brothers are most unlikely.

Dystrophia myotonica (myotonic muscular dystrophy)

Nomenclature
Myotonia means that the muscles relax slowly after contraction.

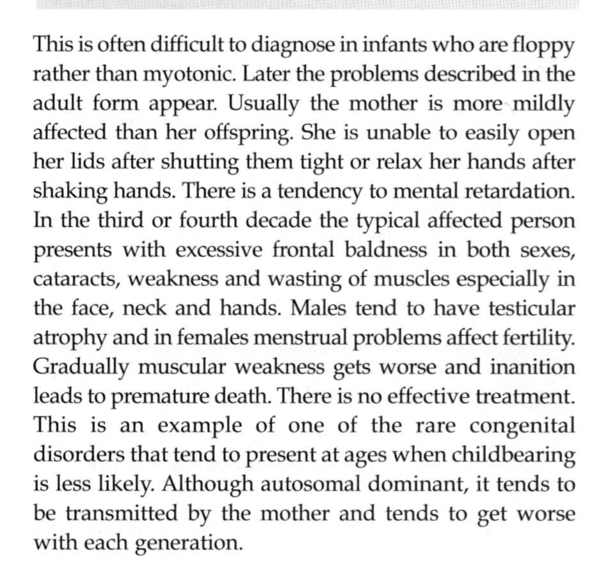

This is often difficult to diagnose in infants who are floppy rather than myotonic. Later the problems described in the adult form appear. Usually the mother is more mildly affected than her offspring. She is unable to easily open her lids after shutting them tight or relax her hands after shaking hands. There is a tendency to mental retardation. In the third or fourth decade the typical affected person presents with excessive frontal baldness in both sexes, cataracts, weakness and wasting of muscles especially in the face, neck and hands. Males tend to have testicular atrophy and in females menstrual problems affect fertility. Gradually muscular weakness gets worse and inanition leads to premature death. There is no effective treatment. This is an example of one of the rare congenital disorders that tend to present at ages when childbearing is less likely. Although autosomal dominant, it tends to be transmitted by the mother and tends to get worse with each generation.

Facioscapulohumeral muscular dystrophy

This dominantly inherited weakness of facial and shoulder girdle muscles may not present until adult life. Muscle biopsy demonstrates the condition, showing increased fibrous tissue, hypertrophic and atrophic, degenerating and regenerating muscle fibres, and sometimes a lymphocytic infiltrate.

There is no treatment. The defect has been mapped to chromosome 4.

Scapulohumeral muscular dystrophy (scapuloperoneal muscular dystrophy)

This is another X-linked muscular dystrophy, which is rarer than the Duchenne and Becker types. Weakness, wasting and contracture of muscles occur, rather than hypertrophy. The muscles most affected are highlighted in the names for this condition.

Cardiomyopathy is a common cause of death in adult life, and respiratory failure compounded by scoliosis also contributes.

Myasthenia gravis

Epidemiology
Rare.
Girls are far more likely to develop this condition.
More common in adults.

Myasthenia means 'severely weak muscles'. An infant of an affected mother may show the signs of this disorder for several weeks after birth and need temporary treatment. The typical presentation is droopiness of the eyelids and complaints of double vision. As time goes by the patient will notice that she finds muscular activity of all types becoming increasingly difficult. The explanation is that acetylcholine, the chemical substance which transmits messages from nerve to muscle can no longer act normally because of the presence of antibodies against the acetylcholine receptor, present in the neuromuscular junction. This puts myasthenia in the same family as other poorly understood disorders such as thyroiditis and disseminated lupus erythematosus. These autoimmune antibodies are influenced for the worse by the thymus gland in the neck. Many affected people are helped by a thymectomy though this is unlikely to be fully curative. Drugs that ease the passage of neurotransmitter from nerve to muscle such as physostigmine help greatly, though their use has to be strictly monitored and regulated. Some children with myasthenia gravis get better spontaneously in adult life.

Myopathies

Myotonia congenita (Thomsen)

Affected children have very large, albeit weak, muscles in this autosomal dominant or recessive disorder. Myotonia, that is the slow relaxation of muscles after contraction, is striking. The histology of muscle biopsies is virtually normal, and the condition is nonprogressive.

Myotubular myopathy

In this, X-linked recessive condition, the muscle cells resemble those of a 15-week fetus histologically.

'Myotubular' refers to the arrangement of myofibrils in a cylinder around the periphery of the muscle cell; the nuclei are positioned centrally within the cylinder.

Muscle weakness is such that most affected infants die and survivors have severe handicaps preventing mobility.

Nemaline rod disease

Nemaline rods (Greek *nema*, a thread) are abnormal structures demonstrated by special histological techniques in the muscle fibres of children with this myopathy. Inheritance is variable and may be autosomal dominant recessive or X-linked dominant; thus girls can be affected.

The prognosis is poor: death may occur in the neonatal period from generalized muscle weakness and survivors will spend life in a wheelchair.

Seizure disorders

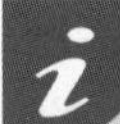

Pathogenesis

The pathogenesis of seizures and epilepsy is not fully understood. It is thought to be due to cortical neurons exhibiting abnormalities of membrane potential and firing patterns. These abnormalities may be due to imbalance between excitatory and inhibitory neurotransmitters or abnormalities of voltage-controlled membrane ion channels.

INTRODUCTION

It is wrong to think of seizures in children as a single disorder. Just as there are many types of congenital heart disease so there are many types of seizures. We can talk of seizures, fits or convulsions synonymously. They may be secondary to an intense stimulus affecting the brain such as hypoxia, hypoglycaemia or head injury. Such fits are not epileptic. An epileptic seizure is unprovoked. It is a disorder characterized by recurrent, unprovoked seizures. Most of us regard epilepsy as 'two or more episodes of altered consciousness, behaviours, emotion, sensation or movement, resulting from cerebral neuronal discharge with no obvious stimulus before the attack'. Do not call people 'epileptic' (or 'cystic' or 'diabetic'); that is unkind.

AETIOLOGY AND PATHOGENESIS

No specific cause may be found in 60–70% of cases. Some recognized causes are shown in Information box 18.3.

INCIDENCE

The lifetime cumulative incidence of epilepsy is approximately 3%. The overall incidence is 20–50 per 100 000 population per year and the prevalence is 4–10 per 1000. The frequency of seizures in the newborn period is high at 0.1%. Febrile convulsions occur in about 3% of children aged between 6 months and 6 years with a 30% chance of recurrence. Generalized tonic–clonic seizures represent 50% of true epilepsy and absence seizures approximately 2.5–5% of all epilepsies in childhood.

CLINICAL PRESENTATION

Seizure disorders are classified into three main groups: pseudoseizures, febrile convulsions and epilepsy.

Pseudoseizures (Information box 18.4)

Many fits, faints and 'funny turns' in children such as breath-holding attacks are very alarming. About 5% of children have this problem, particularly in their early years. In quite a number of children a false label of epilepsy is given. This can have a devastating effect and sometimes children are given antiepilepsy drugs quite

Information Box 18.3

Some recognized causes of seizures and epilepsy

Febrile seizures
Irreversible brain damage acting as a focus for seizures
- Brain haemorrhage
- Asphyxia

Defective cerebral development during fetal life
Infection
- Congenital infections
- Meningitis

Metabolic
- Hypocalcaemia
- Hypoglycaemia
- Hyponatraemia
- Hypomagnesaemia
- Hypoxia
- Inborn errors of metabolism

Toxic
- Alcohol
- Tricyclics

Trauma to the head
- Accidental
- Nonaccidental

Genetic
- Down syndrome
- Tuberous sclerosis

Brain tumours

Information Box 18.4

Conditions which may mimic epilepsy

Faints (vasovagal syncope)
Breath-holding
– Blue (cyanotic) due to anger or frustration
– White (reflex anoxic) due to pain
Cardiac
– Arrhythmias
– Outflow obstruction
Benign paroxysmal vertigo
Paroxysmal torticollis
Hypnogogic hallucination
– Normal myoclonic jerks on falling asleep
Narcolepsy
Night terrors
Nightmares
Masturbation
Tics
Behaviour disorders
– Temper tantrums
Munchausen by proxy

unnecessarily. It is thus very important that children are not labelled as having epilepsy unless they really do have it. Pseudoseizures need to be recognized for what they are and managed accordingly. If in doubt a second opinion should be sought rather than trying anticonvulsants just to see what happens. Occasionally childhood epilepsy is fabricated (Munchhausen syndrome).

Febrile convulsions

Typically febrile convulsions are generalized; occur between the ages of 6 months to 6 years; last less than 15 minutes, and occur when the child's temperature is rising. Usually the children are normal neurologically and developmentally, and often have a positive family history of febrile convulsions. If no fever is recorded one cannot make a diagnosis of a febrile convulsion. One must also appreciate that sometimes children who are starting a form of epilepsy that will later occur in the absence of fever ('afebrile') are perfectly entitled to have a fever at the same time as they have a fit.

The prognosis of a true febrile convulsion is good. Two-thirds of children who have a febrile convulsion never have another. They do just as well at school as children who have never had fits. The risk of subsequent epilepsy is 2–5%. This complication is more likely if the attack lasted more than 15 minutes and was repeated, was focal, occurred in the first year of life or was followed by a hemiparesis. Febrile convulsions can be extremely alarming. A lot of assurance is needed. One has to do one's best to track down the source of infection and treat the fever symptomatically. Just occasionally meningitis presents with a fever and a convulsion. That is the reason for making sure that an informed watch is kept over children who have had such a convulsion. As long as close observation is maintained it is no longer regarded as necessary to automatically carry out lumbar puncture in such children.

Epilepsy

Conventionally children who have had febrile convulsions are excluded from this diagnosis.

Classification

There are two ways of describing seizures.
The traditional nomenclature of petit and grand mal, etc. has been superseded by the international classification which divides seizures into primary (cause unknown) or secondary (cause known).
A fit can be generalized or partial; affecting all or part of the body respectively.
Partial seizures can be simple (no loss of consciousness) or complex (with loss of consciousness).
Many doctors still cannot get away from the traditional terms used in describing seizure types.

Generalized tonic–clonic seizures

- Often starts with some sensation or aura that something odd is about to happen, and the child may feel frightened
- All limbs stiffen then shake repeatedly (tonic and clonic phases) and the child goes blue
- Incontinence may occur
- This phase may last for many minutes
- Subsequently the fit stops but the child may be sleepy for at least an hour or more afterwards.

Absence seizures

- Usually overdiagnosed
- Attacks can be precipitated by hyperventilation
- In a true absence seizure the child momentarily stops what they are doing without loss of tone, their eyes may roll up and they look vacant
- Within 5–15 seconds they have returned to normal
- The EEG is a very good diagnostic help because typically it shows a 3 Hz spike and wave pattern (Fig. 5.21)

- Commoner in girls than in boys
- Generally stop after puberty.

Benign focal nocturnal seizures

- Emanate from the rolandic (centrotemporal) area of the brain
- Nearly always occur during sleep time
- Child may be noticed to be restless and twitching
- Excellent, benign prognosis
- Treatment (usually with carbamazepine) may be needed to calm the parent rather than the child.

Temporal lobe seizure (psychomotor)

- Associated with altered mood or stereotyped motor activities
- Due to areas of localized hyperactive cerebral tissue in or around the temporal lobes, or focal lesions including tumours, and vascular malformation
- Hence further investigation is required.

Drop attacks

- Cause affected children to collapse with no warning from an upright position, often hurting themselves
- Extremely intractable condition
- Sodium valproate (Epilim) may be tried but often surgery is the only effective treatment.

Photosensitive epilepsy

- Causes a proportion of children to have a seizure attack particularly when tired whilst watching flashing lights, e.g. video games, a badly tuned television or in a disco
- For photosensitive epilepsy it is best to sit as far from the television screen as possible and use a remote control. Colour television is probably better than black and white
- Computer monitors with a fast screen refresh rate (100 times a second) are less likely to trigger seizures.

Juvenile myoclonic epilepsy

- Gene found on chromosome 6
- Peak age 12–16 years
- Characterized by myoclonic jerking episodes with preservation of consciousness
- Affects upper limbs mainly ('flying cornflakes')
- Occur in runs on awakening or following sleep deprivation
- Can be associated with generalized seizures
- Excellent response to sodium valproate.

Infantile spasms

- Age 3–12 months
- Commoner in boys
- Extensor spasms involve trunk, neck and arms (so-called 'salaam' attacks)
- 75% are secondary to perinatal asphyxia, cerebral malformation (e.g. tuberose sclerosis), infections
- Prognosis is poor in this group with associated mental retardation (West syndrome) whereas the prognosis is better where there is no underlying cause
- EEG shows hypsarrhythmia (disorganized brain waves)
- Treatment is traditionally with ACTH or prednisolone; vigabatrin (Sabril) is becoming the first-line choice.

Dravet syndrome

- Otherwise known as severe myoclonic epilepsy, and one of the newly recognized epilepsy syndromes.
- A minority of children with epilepsy are very resistant to treatment.
- Dravet syndrome starts in the first year with prolonged febrile convulsions. These are followed by repeated short convulsions that are very resistant to all forms of drug therapy.
- Initially there are no abnormal physical signs on examination, and EEG and CT scan are likely to be normal. However, with the passage of time the child displays marked mental retardation, and eventually the EEG becomes abnormal with rapid bursts of spike waves.
- There is a strong family history of convulsive disorders of various types, but the cause of this disorder is unknown.
- Around 18 months the fit type changes from clonic unilateral or bilateral attacks to myoclonic (drop attacks) often unassociated with unconsciousness.
- Partial seizures with automatisms may also occur.
- The disorder should be differentiated from Lennox–Gastaut syndrome (see below); it is recognized to be a discrete entity.

Lennox–Gastaut syndrome

- Complex myoclonic and tonic epilepsy
- Slow spike waves on EEG
- Refractory to anticonvulsants
- Learning delay and behaviour disorders frequent.

DIAGNOSIS

Diagnosis is clinical, from the history, from witnesses and a full examination. One-quarter of children with epilepsy may be wrongly diagnosed.

INVESTIGATION

Estimation of serum glucose, calcium and magnesium is required. EEG is a help particularly in sorting out rare forms of epilepsy. A normal EEG does not mean that epilepsy is not present; a specialist opinion should be sought before coming to that conclusion. CAT and MRI scanning are overperformed for epilepsy. They only occasionally show an abnormality in children and there is no need to rush into performing these. They should be done in all cases with focal seizures. They are usually undertaken because the parent twists the doctor's arm. Occasionally a surprise is obtained.

MANAGEMENT

General management includes education and support of the child and family, including the provision of information leaflets and information about support groups. Parental permission should be obtained to inform the child's school. Advice is given on sports such as cycling and swimming which require close supervision and mountain climbing which should be avoided. The parents should know about managing prolonged fits lasting more than 20 minutes by placing the child in the recovery position and administering rectal diazepam (Stesolid). The side-effects of anticonvulsants should be discussed and the importance of not suddenly discontinuing treatment, and the need to continue treatment for at least 2 years.

At regular follow up, compliance with anti-convulsant therapy is checked. Advice is given on the learning and behavioural difficulties that can be associated with epilepsy.

Absence seizures generally respond well to either sodium valproate, iamotrigine or ethosuximide. Sodium valproate, lamotrigine or carbamazepine successfully suppresses partial and general fits. Sodium valproate is best not given to little children unless there is no reasonable alternative, and liver function tests should be undertaken at the onset of therapy. It appears that hepatic failure tends to occur in children who have intractable seizures, are less than 3 years old and are on multiple drugs. Every effort should be made to avoid multitherapy with antiepileptic drugs because they readily interfere with each other's metabolism.

The role of surgery for children with intractable epilepsy is being evaluated. Vagal nerve stimulation may become a useful adjunct.

Congenital neuropathies

Familial dysautonomia (Riley–Day syndrome)

The gene for this autosomal recessive condition is carried by 1 in 100 eastern European Jews, but is rare in other ethnic groups. It is a disorder of the sensory and autonomic nerves whose manifestations include:

- Feeding difficulties
- Vomiting
- Aspiration
- Excessive sweating
- Impaired thermoregulation
- Lack of tears
- Insensitivity to pain
- Corneal ulceration
- Tongue biting
- Lack of sensation from muscles
  - Clumsiness
- Developmental delay
- Convulsions.

One of the simplest diagnostic tests is to place methacholine eye drops in one eye; as a result of parasympathetic denervation the pupil constricts.

There is no specific treatment.

Congenital insensitivity to pain

The disorder is found more commonly in boys. Affected children do not seem to appreciate pain. They do not sweat (anhidrosis), and readily become pyrexial.

The peripheral nerves lack the unmyelinated nerve fibres which convey pain and autonomic functions.

Degenerative conditions

Friedreich ataxia

Ataxia means incoordination of voluntary movements; this leads to uncontrollable wobbling. The lower limbs are most affected resulting in pes cavus (high arched feet). Inheritance may be autosomal dominant or recessive.

Degeneration of the posterior columns of the spinal cord causes marked loss of vibrational and position sense. There is dysarthria and nystagmus and some develop diabetes mellitus. Intelligence is normal. Most affected individuals die of hypertrophic cardiomyopathy.

Infectious neurological conditions (see also Meningitis, p. 280)

Poliomyelitis

Polioviruses are RNA enteroviruses of the Picornaviridae family. No animal host is involved, transmission being from child to child. The viruses are ingested and travel via gastrointestinal associated lymphoid tissue to the central nervous system. The anterior horn cells of the spinal cord are infected.

Febrile illness is associated with rigidity of the spine. Paralysis involves groups of muscles, and also bladder and bowel (paralytic ileus). Respiratory muscles may be involved.

Increased use of polio vaccines has eliminated polio from developed countries. It is hoped that developing countries will soon follow suit.

Spongiform encephalopathies

> Epidemiology
> About 30 people have died so far from 'new variant' Creutzfeldt–Jakob disease which is thought to be identical to bovine spongiform encephalopathy.

Creutzfeldt–Jakob disease is one of the spongiform encephalopathies, so-called because of the vacuolation of neurons that it produces. One suggested cause is an infectious protein or 'prion', rather than a virus that also contains nucleic acid. There is also a genetic component in that the disease may be inherited with an autosomal dominant pattern. The disease has become notorious because of 'mad cow disease' (bovine spongiform encephalopathy) and scrapie (in sheep). In humans it may have been transmitted by cannibalism ('kuru' in Papua New Guinea) and in growth hormone and gonadotrophins derived by extraction from human pituitary obtained at postmortem. The risk from hormone therapy is no longer present, now that these are made by molecular biological techniques, but corneal grafts and neurosurgical instruments are potential sources of infection. Progressive dementia and death within a year or two are the usual results.

Guillain–Barré syndrome

This ascending paralysis is due to demyelination of motor nerves following infections with viruses, *Mycoplasma pneumoniae* or *Campylobacter*. Sensory and autonomic nerves may be affected and respiratory muscles may be involved.

Recovery begins a few weeks after onset, as a rule, but relapse can occur. Treatment includes high dose intravenous immunoglobulin and steroids.

Traumatic conditions

Horner syndrome (oculosympathetic paralysis)

Constriction (miosis) of the pupil, ptosis of the eyelid with enophthalmos (recession) of the eyeball, and heterochromia iridis (hypopigmentation of the iris) are associated with Horner syndrome.

There is also lack of facial sweating due to damage of the sympathetic nerves supplying the eye.

The condition is usually due to damage to the sympathetic nerve trunk as it leaves the spinal cord in the lower neck region to entwine around the carotid artery. Injury causing Horner syndrome can also occur in the midbrain, brain stem, neck, middle cranial fossa or orbit or during thoracic surgery. It can also occur as a complication of haemangiomas, vertebral anomalies, Klumpke paralysis or tumours.

Intracranial haemorrhage

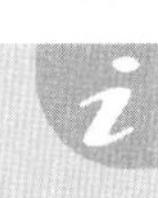

> Aetiology
> Taken up by the mass media as the notorious 'shaken child' syndrome.

Subdural haematoma (Fig. 18.8)

This is a collection of blood between the dura and the brain due to rupture of the venous drainage of the cerebral cortex.

Extradural haematomata

The bleeding is from meningeal arteries of dural veins resulting in a collection of blood between the dura and the skull. Both subdural and extradural haematomata follow head trauma; forceful shaking of children can lead to formation of subdural collections. As the red cells in the haematoma lyse, the volume of the collection increases by osmotic pressure and intracranial

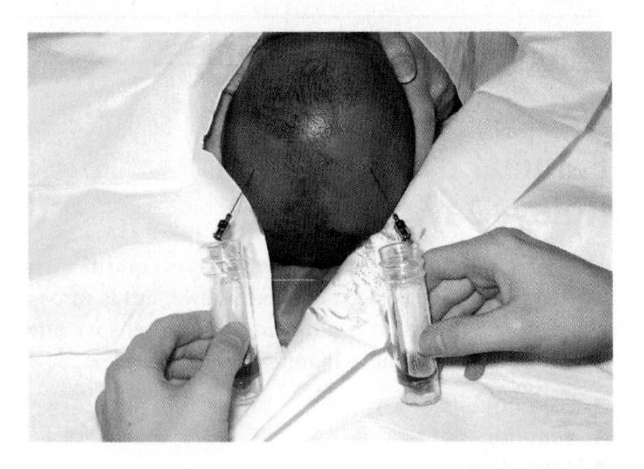

Fig 18.8
Tapping subdural haematomas.

pressure increases. The haematomata can be demonstrated by CT scan. The prognosis is good if the diagnosis is made before cerebral compression occurs, surgical drainage is performed promptly, and the underlying brain has not been directly injured by the trauma.

Subarachnoid haemorrhage

This is a complication of cephalopelvic disproportion at birth. The prognosis is good in an otherwise well baby.

Intraventricular haemorrhage

(Fig. 18.9)

This is very common in extremely low birthweight neonates (<750 g birthweight). Such infants should be routinely examined in the first week of life by cerebral ultrasonography for the development of intraventricular haemorrhage. This begins in the brain tissue surrounding the cerebral ventricles (subependymal germinal matrix). The immature blood vessels in this region are prone to leak in response to hypoxia, changes in cerebral blood flow and blood pressure, pneumothorax and abnormal haemostasis. The resulting haemorrhagic infarction termed 'periventricular leukomalacia' (softening of the white matter around the ventricles) later becomes cystic (porencephaly). The corticospinal tract may also be damaged in the internal capsule. The infant becomes unresponsive and often develops shock, increased frequency of apnoeic attacks and convulsions. Complications include posthaemorrhagic hydrocephalus and cerebral palsy. Therapy includes anticonvulsants, transfusion and correction of disordered bleeding and clotting.

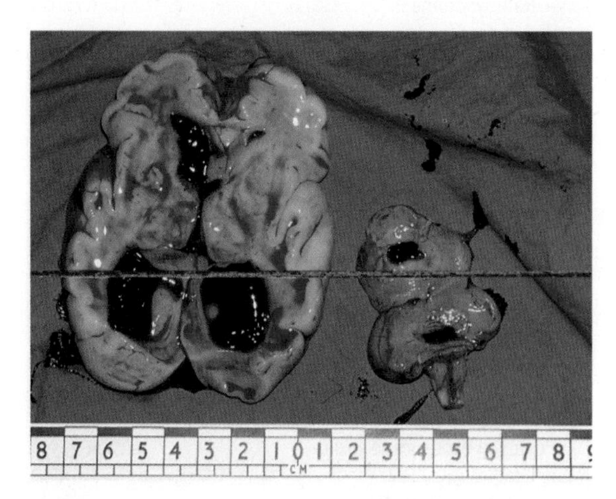

Fig 18.9
Intraventricular haemorrhage.

Leukodystrophies

Krabbe disease (globoid cell leukodystrophy)

Globoid cell leukodystrophy is an autosomal recessive condition, in which there is progressive degeneration of cerebral white matter due to storage of the glycolipid galactose ceramide in the lysosomes. The enzyme galactosylceramide-β-galactosidase is found to be deficient when measured in white cells and cultured skin fibroblasts. Antenatal diagnosis is possible by measuring the enzyme in amniocytes.

Metachromatic leukodystrophy

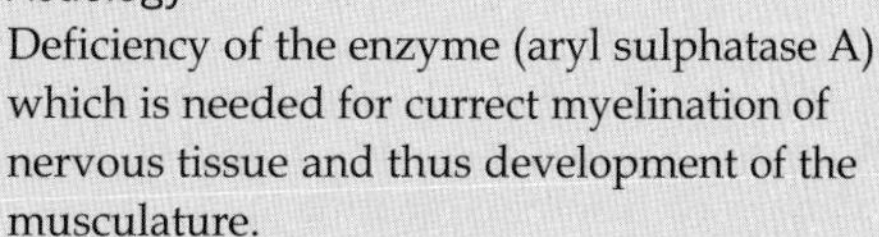
Aetiology
Deficiency of the enzyme (aryl sulphatase A) which is needed for currect myelination of nervous tissue and thus development of the musculature.

This is a rare but very serious congenital disorder. Both sexes are affected; the condition is recessive. The condition gets its name from the appearance of stained preparations of brain or nerves viewed under a microscope. The problems are due to the abnormal formation of myelin, the fatty sheath that develops around nerve tissue in the first year of life. It is needed for conduction and full neurological function. The diagnosis is made by enzyme assay in blood and muscle biopsy. A high protein concentration in the CSF suggests the possibility of the disorder. MRI studies on the brain show the extent of the neurological abnormality.

There is no specific treatment; genetic advice is essential as it may be possible to diagnose a future fully affected infant by amniocentesis. Children with this disorder may be mentally well preserved until late in the final stage but some are mentally retarded. Typically, the child is well at birth. The first signs usually occur late in the first year with difficulty in standing and starting to walk. The tendon jerks are brisk. Gradually the limb muscles become very weak with the development of a peripheral neuropathy and the child runs a downhill course with problems with swallowing and feeding. At the same time intellectual development is lost and the child becomes mentally retarded. This is a very bleak and ultimately lethal condition. There is no drug treatment. Think about metachromatic leukodystrophy in a child with initially mild cerebral palsy that gets worse.

Learning disorders

Definition
IQ less than 70.

Epidemiology
Fewer than 1% of school age children have learning difficulties.
10% of school children can be regarded as needing extra help in order to make their maximum progress at school.
About 3% can be regarded as unable to cope academically in normal school classes and will require some form of special education.
About 0.5% are severely educationally disabled and will need intensive special educational care.

Learning disorder is not a specific disease, disorder, syndrome or specific disability. It is a blanket term for a wide variety of disorders sharing one feature: an abnormally low IQ. In mild mental retardation the IQ is between 50 and 70. In severe retardation the IQ is less than 50. The majority of instances of mental disability are relatively mild and represent the left hand end of the Gaussian distribution of the intelligence scale.

AETIOLOGY AND PATHOGENESIS

Some causes of learning disorders are listed in Information box 18.5.

SOCIOLOGY

The more severe the educational disability the greater the likelihood of a diagnosable syndrome. Repeated surveys show that mildly mentally disabled individuals tend to come from the poorer end of the social stratum; their problems tend to be a compound of adverse environment, both intrauterine and postnatal. They are more at risk of accident, substitute care is poorer, they are more likely to have unsupported single parents. There is little hard evidence that mild mental disability is genetic.

A large study of adopted children showed that such children tend to take on the ability level at school of their adoptive rather than birth parents. In societies where standards of living rise, overall educational achievement levels rise and vice versa.

Understanding of the medical factors in severe disability is improving and children who were investigated some years ago should be re-studied; for example, fragile X syndrome was not routinely sought until recently.

Medical as distinct from societal problems are thus mainly found among the severely mentally disabled.

CLINICAL PRESENTATION

There is no clinical picture common to all affected individuals because it varies enormously depending on the aetiology. The child may present with:

- Learning disability
- Behaviour problems
- Fits
- Dysmorphism
- Developmental delay with visual and hearing impairment
- CNS and systemic signs.

There is a reliable rule: disabling problems rarely come singly – the deaf child often has a heart problem, and so on. This is why multiple assessment by child development teams is so important.

DIAGNOSIS

Assessment should include enquiring about familial/hereditary and psychosocial circumstances, pregnancy, delivery, developmental progress, and past medical history. Examination includes plotting growth and head

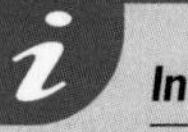

Information Box 18.5

Some causes of learning disorders

Genetic disorders
- Down syndrome
- Fragile X syndrome
- Rett syndrome

Part of specific syndromes of multiple congenital abnormalities
Intrauterine infections
- CMV
- Rubella

CNS
- Infections
- Trauma
- Haemorrhage
- Dyspraxia
- Dyslexia

Exposure of fetus to drugs
- Alcohol
- Cocaine

Perinatal factors
- Hypoxic–ischaemic encephalopathy

Postnatal exposure to toxins
- Lead

Inborn errors of metabolism
Other metabolic disorders

circumference, neuromotor assessment, careful inspection of the skin, and testing of hearing and vision including fundoscopy. Any dysmorphic features are recorded.

Investigations usually include full blood count, glucose, urea and electrolytes, liver function tests, calcium, phosphate, CPK, thyroid function tests, chromosome studies (especially for fragile X syndrome), plasma and urine amino acids, urinary organic acids and mucopolysaccharidosis screen.

One of the aims of the infant screening programme is to detect such children at the earliest possible stage in order to get compensatory education, diagnosis and treatment started as early as possible.

MANAGEMENT

Specific approaches are available for a minority of causes of mental retardation, examples being replacement therapy for hypothyroidism, dietary therapy in phenylketonuria and prevention of rubella embryopathy by immunization.

Early diagnosis, education of the family and special education measures are crucial. Multidisciplinary team assessment and management are vital: genetic advice, physiotherapy, occupational therapy, speech therapy, dietetics, neurology, orthopaedics, general practice, health visiting and social work all play a role in the management of such children.

STATEMENTING

For a child to receive special educational help in the UK and for extra resources to be given to the school, a 'statement of special educational need' has to be drawn up. This can be initiated by parents or involved professionals. Each writes a description of the child's needs as seen from their standpoint. This process is coordinated by the local educational authority who in the light of the written evidence has to make a suitable educational placement. This can be challenged by the parents. There is much argument over whether disabled children should be educated in mainstream schools or separately in special schools.

Dyspraxia

Dyspraxia is the inability to make fine and accurate voluntary movements presumably because of problems in the cerebral cortex. These can affect control of speech muscles (oromotor dyspraxia). Speech is distorted because of great difficulty in making the more complex speech sounds, and the child may tend to use gestures in order to be understood. Dyspraxias can also affect the use of other muscles such as those needed for writing: the child may know what to do, but cannot manage to produce the fine hand control needed to write normally.

Skilled multidisciplinary assessment and treatment are needed to help the child make the most of their abilities. Word processors can help these children communicate.

Dyslexia

The specific reading disability of dyslexia is a developmental defect of symbol recognition. It must be differentiated from delayed reading due to learning difficulties, social deprivation, defects in vision or word blindness (alexia) from a cerebral lesion. Abnormalities in writing are associated, with mirror writing and letter reversal.

Vision should be checked and corrected, and remedial teaching requested (see p. 137).

Rett syndrome

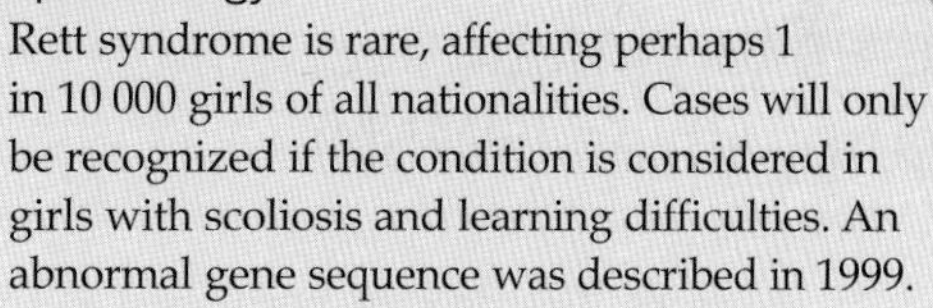

Epidemiology

Rett syndrome is rare, affecting perhaps 1 in 10 000 girls of all nationalities. Cases will only be recognized if the condition is considered in girls with scoliosis and learning difficulties. An abnormal gene sequence was described in 1999.

This cause of serious mental retardation, seen only in girls was first described in 1962 by Dr Rett in Austria. Rett syndrome is thought to be a dominant condition. Presumably the condition in a male fetus is lethal, so only affected females are born. The girls are normal at birth, but at some time between 9 and 24 months they begin to deteriorate for no explicable reason, losing skills they had acquired earlier. Many lose the ability to walk and develop fits that are difficult to control with antiepilepsy drugs. One characteristic feature is a tendency to make spontaneous hand-wringing movements. This characteristic hand-wringing forms the emblem of the Rett Syndrome Association. The head size is normal at birth but grows inadequately later. There is poor circulation to the hands and feet and breathing abnormalities (apnoea and hyperventilation). Behaviour has an autistic element. The limbs become stiff and may be regarded as showing spastic quadriplegia, though the mechanism is clearly different from that of classic cerebral palsy. Other problems include severe scoliosis.

DIAGNOSTIC REVIEW

Several other serious neurological diseases such as metachromatic leukodystrophy and Leigh disease (see p. 292) present at around the same age. Understanding Rett syndrome could help research into autism and scoliosis as well as into some types of epilepsy and other conditions associated with retardation.

It is in the best interests of all disabled children to

have their diagnoses reviewed from time to time. 'New' conditions are continually being described, and as children get older new signs present. Accurate genetic guidance can only be given when a diagnosis is made. This is needed even where parents have decided not to have more children for the sake of their relatives and descendants.

Autism

The child with autism has severe developmental delay in communication skills. They have a strong preference for routine; any change can provoke rages. Imaginative play is lacking – ritualistic spinning of objects such as wheels on toys is characteristic. Siblings may be affected. Therapy is based on special education. The prognosis is guarded. Less severely affected children are classified as Asperger's syndrome. The cause is unknown.

Hereditary motor–sensory neuropathies (HMSN)

This is a group of disorders of peripheral nerves, examples of which are peroneal muscular atrophy (HMSN type I and II) and Refsum disease.

Peroneal muscular atrophy (Charcot–Marie–Tooth disease, HMSN type I)

HMSN type I is an autosomal dominant condition with a prevalence of 4 : 100 000. In this progressive demyelinating peripheral neuropathy, denervation of the muscles of the anterior compartment of the lower leg and the feet, which begins in the second year of life, results in development of foot drop and pes cavus. Hands and forearms are involved later. Sensory nerve involvement causes paraesthesiae ('pins and needles'). No treatment is available.

Peroneal muscular atrophy (HMSN type II)

HMSN type II has a slower progression rate compared with type I, and causes axonal degeneration rather than demyelination.

Refsum disease

Refsum disease, an autosomal recessive condition, is most common in Scandinavia, and is named after the Norwegian doctor who described it. It is very rare but not unknown in the UK.

Neurological problems tend to start after the age of 20, with unsteady gait, weakness of limbs and impaired vision (especially in the dark, due to retinitis pigmentosa), hearing and smell. The skin can become abnormally scaly and dry and peripheral neuropathy also occurs. The diagnosis is suggested by a combination of these problems that may present at almost any age.

The disorder is caused by an inherited inability to break down and use phytanic acid. The latter is produced in the body from substances found in the pigment chlorophyll which is present in green leaves and finds its way into milk. Eliminating these substances from the diet helps to slow the serious effects of this disorder.

It is most important that an accurate diagnosis is made. The child should remain under the supervision of a specialist familiar with the condition, who must liaise closely with the dietician and other supportive therapists.

Neurocutaneous syndromes

Definition
A group of neurological problems which can be recognized by characteristic skin or retinal lesions.

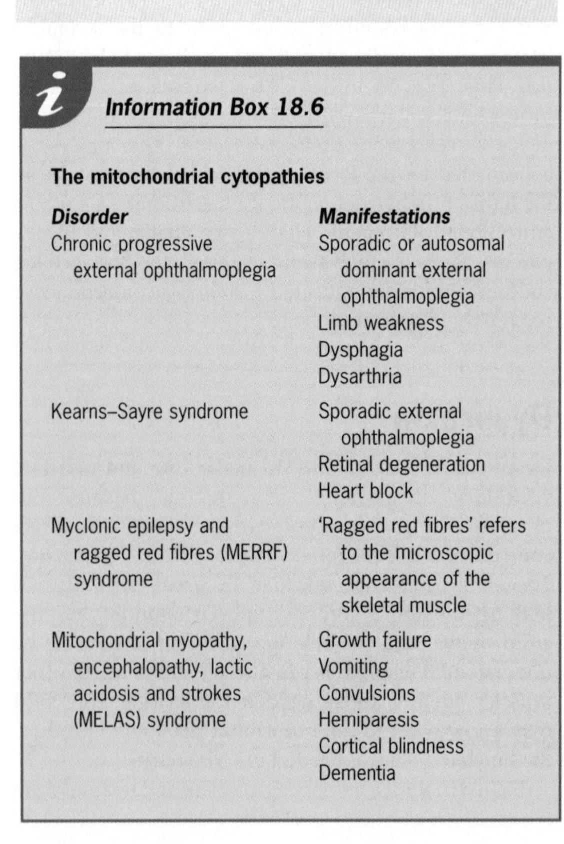

Information Box 18.6

The mitochondrial cytopathies

Disorder	***Manifestations***
Chronic progressive external ophthalmoplegia	Sporadic or autosomal dominant external ophthalmoplegia Limb weakness Dysphagia Dysarthria
Kearns–Sayre syndrome	Sporadic external ophthalmoplegia Retinal degeneration Heart block
Myclonic epilepsy and ragged red fibres (MERRF) syndrome	'Ragged red fibres' refers to the microscopic appearance of the skeletal muscle
Mitochondrial myopathy, encephalopathy, lactic acidosis and strokes (MELAS) syndrome	Growth failure Vomiting Convulsions Hemiparesis Cortical blindness Dementia

Neurofibromatosis (von Recklinghausen disease)

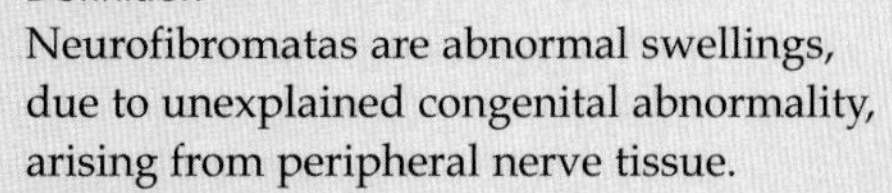

Definition
Neurofibromatas are abnormal swellings, due to unexplained congenital abnormality, arising from peripheral nerve tissue.

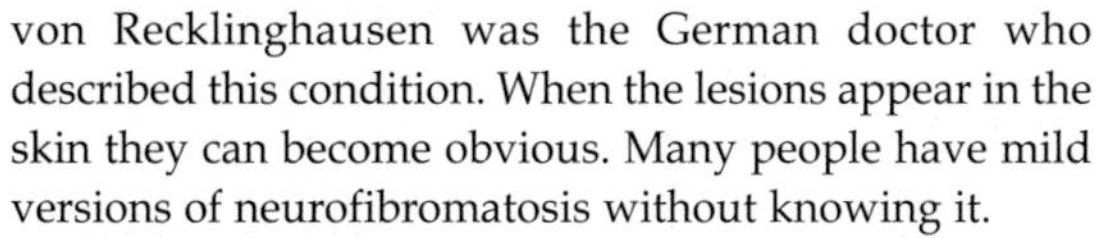

von Recklinghausen was the German doctor who described this condition. When the lesions appear in the skin they can become obvious. Many people have mild versions of neurofibromatosis without knowing it.

The typical diagnostic sign is permanent pale coffee (café-au-lait) coloured spots. It is important to appreciate that most children with café-au-lait patches are not affected. For a diagnosis of neurofibromatosis more than six patches larger than a 10p coin must be present. Some other conditions such as tuberose sclerosis and McCune–Albright syndrome (where there are bone and endocrine abnormalities) have this skin sign as well. There may be marked freckling, especially around the armpits, and excess pigmentation, especially around the groin and shoulders. Sometimes the skin spots grow to form spongy raised growths of very variable size. They are disfiguring and surgical removal may help, though there are often too many to eradicate.

More fundamental problems are caused by unseen internal lesions that spring from cranial nerves; these can cause deafness and other neurological problems including epilepsy and blindness due to optic glioma. Pressure on bones can lead to their distortion, the skull can become misshapen and a large variety of neurological problems occur that can impair development and lead to seizures.

Hypertension occurs secondarily to phaeochromocytoma or renal artery stenosis. This type of neurofibromatosis is called NF-1. The characteristic feature of NF-2 is bilateral acoustic neuromata and absence of cutaneous lesions.

There is no suppressive treatment. Although some affected people deteriorate, only those who are severely affected tend to be seen in hospital. Intelligence and lifespan are often unimpaired, though there is a risk of neurofibromata becoming malignant. It is important to find whether the condition occurred in a totally unaffected family, where the condition can be regarded as a fresh mutation or whether a parent is affected, even if mildly. Once known, genetic guidance can be given. Usually the condition is transmitted as dominant inheritance, and 50% of children of an affected individual are at risk of developing the condition. NF-1 is inherited on chromosome 17 and NF-2 on chromosome 22.

von Hippel–Lindau disease

In this autosomal dominant disorder, cerebral haemangioblastomas, which produce raised intracranial pressure, are associated with retinal angiomata. The cerebral haemangiomata are removed surgically, and retinal angiomata are treated with a laser. The commonest cause of death is renal carcinoma.

Sturge–Weber syndrome

This presents at birth with a unilateral vascular naevus (port wine stain) of the upper half of the face (Fig. 9.5). CT scanning shows calcification and atrophy of the cerebral cortex on the same side. Cerebral abnormality predisposes to focal tonic–clonic seizures, and removal of the abnormal hemisphere may be required if the convulsions are resistant to treatment. The port wine stain may be improved by laser therapy.

Glaucoma and hemiplegia are further complications.

Tuberose sclerosis

Tuberose (or 'tuberous' in the USA) sclerosis gets its name from potato-shaped degenerative swellings in the brain. These are but one manifestation of a condition that causes the deposition of abnormal tissue in many parts of the body including the eyes, kidneys and bones.

When this affects the skin, many different manifestations may be found. These include patches of milky coffee coloured staining. (Many unaffected people also get this; usually at least five patches are seen in tuberose sclerosis.) The patches are referred to as 'shagreen' because of a resemblance to shark skin, and as ash leaf skin lesions (Fig. 18.10) because of their shape. Patches of reddened thick acne like tissues over the cheeks led to the old alternative name, adenoma sebaceum, a misleading name as the sweat glands are not involved. This 'hamartoma' tissue can become malignant.

The condition can present in widely differing degrees. Most cases, however, are due to new mutations and the parents are unaffected, but the disease can be dominant. Many people with it are minimally affected. In some it is only diagnosed after an affected child is born and the parents are carefully examined. The main problems are epilepsy and mental retardation. Remember that mildly affected patients get neither and do not let them become needlessly anxious.

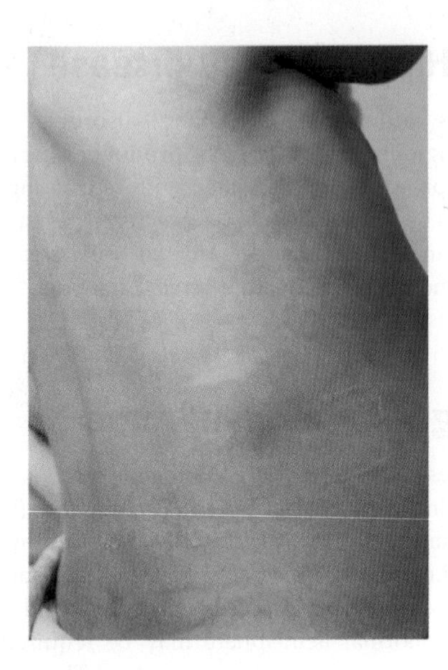

Fig 18.10
Ash leaf patch.

Other neurological disorders

Ondine curse

Epidemiology
Very rare.

Although 'Ondine's curse' is well described in standard medical textbooks, the history of Ondine whose name is given to this condition is not. Ondine is the French name for Undine, a female water sprite from German legend, who had no soul but was told that she would obtain one if she married a mortal and bore a child. The conventional teaching on Ondine is that the curse applied to a mythical character who could only breathe if she was awake and thus was fated to die if she slept. In contemporary medical practice the term, 'Ondine curse' is given to a condition in which the sufferer 'forgets' to breathe especially when asleep. This is a potentially life-threatening state and a tracheotomy and artificial ventilation may be needed.

In some sufferers the basis of the problem is a lesion in the midbrain or the connecting nerve pathways and the condition may be associated with intracerebral pathology. In most patients no anatomical abnormality can be found. The patient is then said to have primary alveolar dysfunction. The normal reflexes are under-responsive to CO_2 in the blood which normally stimulates respiration. Although this mechanism has been suggested as an explanation for cot death there is little hard evidence that this actually occurs.

Opitz syndromes

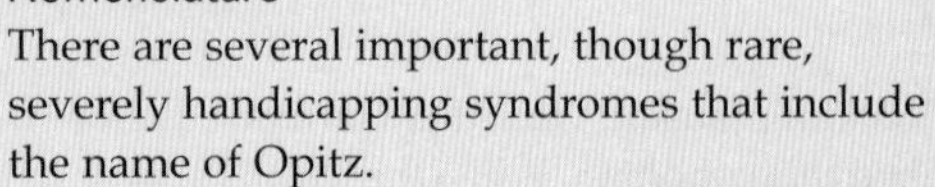

Nomenclature
There are several important, though rare, severely handicapping syndromes that include the name of Opitz.

The Opitz trigonocephaly syndrome is otherwise known as C syndrome after the first patient recognized. The head is microcephalic with a triangular shape narrowing on top. The forehead has a bulge down the middle. There is severe mental retardation, often a severe squint, downward sloping eyelids and a very narrow palate. The skin hangs loosely, limbs are very limp and joints may dislocate; hands and fingers are very short and digits may be joined together (syndactyly). It will be obvious that the infant is abnormal at birth and may die. The blood cholesterol is low. One has to know this syndrome to be able to recognize it among many other causes of microcephaly. It is an autosomal recessive condition.

A different Opitz syndrome had been described earlier. Here, affected infants have wide apart eyes and males have hypospadias. A wide variety of other abnormalities may also be found including variable degrees of mental retardation, heart abnormality, cleft palate, squint and imperforate anus. Inheritance is dominant.

The third Opitz syndrome is the Smith– Lemli–Opitz syndrome found in low birthweight infants who fail to thrive. They have microcephaly, droopy eyelids, low set or otherwise odd ears, squints, and upward slants to the end of the nose. Boys often have undescended testes and hypospadias. The infants are difficult to feed, and readily get infections. The brain is severely and patchily underdeveloped. Many die early. The inheritance pattern is autosomal recessive.

Septo-optic dysplasia

In this developmental anomaly involving midline structures in the brain, the optic nerves are hypoplastic as are the optic chiasm and tracts. There is agenesis of the corpus callosum and septum pellucidum. Involvement of the hypothalamus can lead to panhypopituitarism (see p. 204) and diabetes insipidus (p. 198). Neonatal hypoglycaemia is an important presenting symptom. The condition has occurred in siblings, and the genetics are emerging.

19 Nutritional disorders

Nutritional disorders are frequent but their nature is polarized according to whether children are from rich or poor countries. Malnutrition makes an enormous contribution to mortality from infection in developing countries because of adverse effects on immune function. Malnutrition adversely affects gastrointestinal function, so that attacks of diarrhoea last longer. By contrast a large proportion of children in developed countries are obese, with the likelihood of morbidity and premature mortality in adult life.

Malnutrition

Marasmus (Fig. 19.1)

Epidemiology

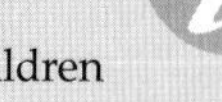

In developing countries 100 million children are probably affected.
In developed countries about 30% of children in children's hospitals are malnourished.

Marasmus is severe loss of weight due to inadequate intake of food, persistent diarrhoea or systemic illness. In developed countries it is seen in association with disorders such as Crohn disease and anorexia nervosa. In contrast to another clinical form of malnutrition, kwashiorkor, there is no oedema. The name comes from the Greek for wasting. The child appears wizened and wasted and may be hypothermic. The abdomen may be scaphoid or distended. The weight is less than 60% of the mean weight for age. Skinfold thickness is decreased. Without treatment, growth velocity and then

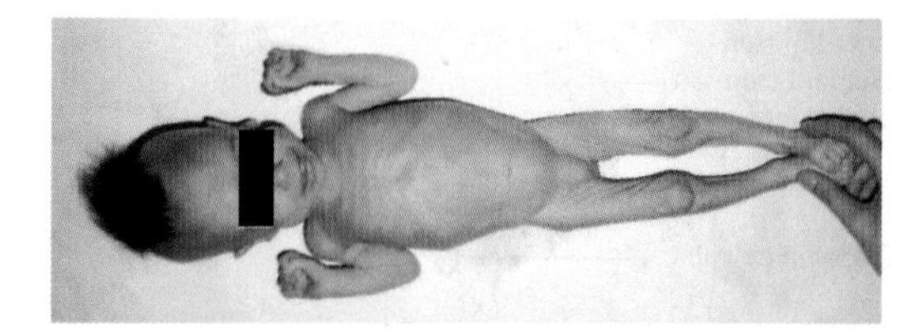

Fig 19.1
Marasmus.

head growth decrease. If the child has persistent diarrhoea, milk may not be tolerated because of secondary lactose intolerance. Elemental formulae may be required which are lactose-free and the protein is hydrolysed to peptides. Alternatively a special diet may be formulated using comminuted (finely ground) chicken and rice.

Kwashiorkor (protein-calorie malnutrition) (Fig. 19.2)

Epidemiology
Seen mainly in Africa, West Indies and parts of India.

Kwashiorkor is a type of malnutrition characterized by generalized oedema, skin lesions, fatty infiltration of the liver, and hair and skin depigmentation. It means 'deposed child', drawing attention to the onset of the condition with weaning when a new baby arrives. The condition is corrected by expert nutritional support, although the child's growth and development may be permanently impaired.

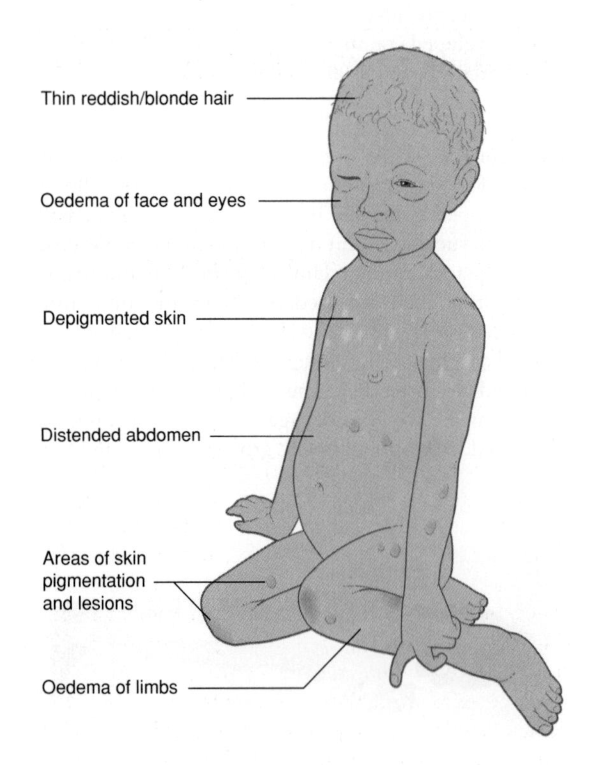

Fig 19.2
Typical clinical presentation in kwashiorkor.

Obesity

Epidemiology
Commonest nutritional problem in the developed world.

About one-third of English children are overweight. One-half of schoolgirls diet. The hazards of obesity are well known (premature vascular and joint disease and diabetes), but management is usually unsuccessful. Much teasing results from obesity. Affected children find physical activity difficult and the resulting decrease in activity compounds the problem without excessive eating. Their families are often obese. Breastfeeding protects.

One way of measuring obesity is to compare the weight of the child with the 50th percentile weight for the child's age from a growth chart. If the child's weight is greater than 120% of the 50th percentile weight for age then the child is obese. This method does not take into account the child who is heavy because of well developed musculature and skeleton. A better method is to measure the thickness of the skinfold over the triceps using a special calliper.

Affected children are best managed in special clinics by paediatricians, dietitians and psychologists. Energy intake restriction, exercise and behaviour modification are emphasized. Relapse is frequent.

An extreme form of obesity includes alveolar hypoventilation, polycythaemia, cyanosis, cardiac failure and somnolence (sleepiness). This is termed 'Pickwickian syndrome' after Dickens's character, the Fat Boy.

Water-soluble vitamin deficiencies

Beri-beri

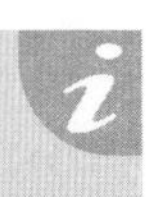

Prevention
Diversification of the diet and enrichment of rice with thiamine are preventative.

Deficiency of vitamin B1 (thiamine), which is a coenzyme in the tricarboxylic acid cycle and hexose monophosphate pathway, causes beri-beri. Nuts, peas, beans, pulses and brewer's yeast are the richest sources. The name for the deficiency state is derived from the Malay word beri, meaning weak. It can occur when the intake falls bellow 0.4 mg thiamine per 1000 calories.

Infantile beri-beri can occur in infants breastfed by mothers eating a diet of polished rice, which contains less than 0.15 mg/1000 cal of vitamin B1. It can produce acute high output cardiac failure (wet beri-beri) which can lead to sudden death. There is an aphonic (absent voice) type where there is laryngeal oedema. The pseudomeningeal type produces drowsiness and meningism. Older children develop the sensory and motor neuropathy of so-called dry beri-beri. The diagnosis is made by measuring red cell transketolase activity in the presence and absence of thiamine. If thiamine increases activity by 25%, this indicates deficiency. Thiamine hydrochloride 50–100 mg i.v. should be given immediately the diagnosis is suspected, followed by 5–10 mg/day for 1 week. If the infant is breastfed, the mother should also be treated.

Pellagra

Prevention
The diet may be fortified with niacin to prevent pellagra.
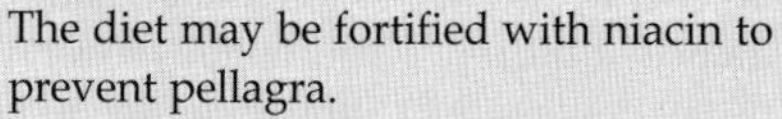
A high tryptophan strain of maize (opaque-2) may be planted.

Pellagra (*Pelle*, skin, *agra*, rough) is a dietary deficiency of niacin which can occur in a number of ways. Niacin may be synthesized from the amino acid tryptophan using vitamin B6 (pyridoxine) as a cofactor. Hence deficiencies of niacin, tryptophan and pyridoxine may all be responsible. It is endemic in South Africa, where the maize diet, in which niacin has a poor bioavailability, is also low in tryptophan. In the body, niacin is incorporated in nicotinamide, a constituent of NAD^+ and $NADP^+$ (nicotine adenine dinucleotide and the phosphate derivative) which are coenzymes in many redox reactions. Pellagra causes a light-sensitive dermatitis, diarrhoea, deafness and dementia (and death if untreated). The treatment is oral nicotinamide 100 mg 4-hourly.

Scurvy

Prevention
The provision of fresh citrus fruit is preventative.
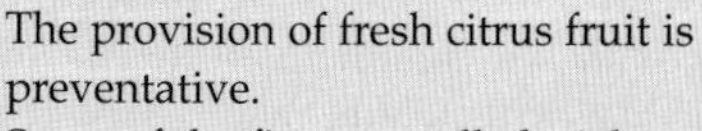
Some of the first controlled trials ever conducted were on seamen with scurvy, by James Lind in the 18th century.

Scurvy is caused by deficiency of vitamin C (L-ascorbic acid) which is a biological reducing agent and a cofactor for hydroxylation of proline and lysine (important in collagen synthesis). Vitamin C is also important in assisting the absorption of iron from the diet. The daily requirement of 20–30 mg is obtained from citrus fruit and green vegetables. Deficiency is rare because ascorbic acid is found in most fresh foods.

Clinical features include swollen bleeding gums and bleeding around hair follicles. 'Pseudoparalysis' occurs because of painful limbs. X-rays show subperiosteal haematomata with calcification. The metaphyses have a 'ground glass' appearance due to atrophy of the bony trabeculae. Epiphyses are surrounded by a dense rim of cortical bone: the so-called 'smoke-ring' epiphyses. The clinical features can be explained by defective synthesis of the collagen matrix of bone, dentine and cartilage. The capillary haemorrhages are due to defective basement membrane lining the capillaries and intercellular substance joining the endothelial cells together.

Plasma concentrations below 1 mg/l (5.7 μmol/l) or white blood cell concentrations below 70 mg/l (400 μmol/l) indicate risk of scurvy. Oral ascorbic acid 500 mg daily for 1 week should be given urgently with correction of dietary practices. The clinical features respond rapidly, except for the skeletal changes which may take months to resolve.

Fat-soluble vitamin deficiencies

Rickets (Fig. 19.3)

Epidemiology
Can be seen mainly in Asian, African and Caribbean children in cities in the UK. Children with malabsorption are also prone to develop rickets.

Rickets is caused by failure of mineralization of growing bone because of vitamin D deficiency, which is usually due to inadequate exposure to sunlight or inadequate dietary intake. After puberty rickets is called osteomalacia. The provitamin 7-dehydrocholesterol is present in the skin. Ultraviolet light catalyses the conversion of 7-dehydrocholesterol to cholecalciferol. Calciferol is hydroxylated in the liver to 25-OH-cholecalciferol then in the kidney to 1,25-OH-cholecalciferol, the active form of vitamin D. The chief dietary sources are oily fish and fortified margarine. Dairy products and breast milk are relatively poor sources. The principal effect of vitamin D is to facilitate calcium absorption from the intestine.

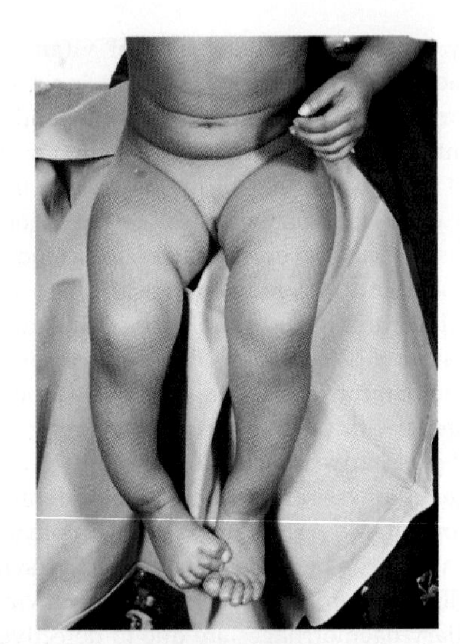

(a)

(b)

Fig 19.3
Rickets. (a) Note the swollen ankles and bowed legs; (b) X-rays show widening of the metaphyseal plate and concavity of the diaphysis.

Rickets (Anglo-Saxon *wrikken*, a twist) causes defective calcification of metaphyseal cartilage in growing children. Serum calcium is low only in severe cases, as intestinal absorption decreases. Parathormone production increases causing hypophosphataemia because of increased urinary phosphate excretion. Alkaline phosphatase activity is elevated from osteoblasts in metaphyseal uncalcified ('osteoid') tissue.

Skeletal lesions include craniotabes (softened areas of skull bones, which can be indented), 'bossing' of the frontal and parietal bones and delayed closure of the fontanelle. The epiphyses, most noticeably the distal radii, are swollen. The costochondral junctions are enlarged (rickety rosary) with pectus carinatum (pigeon chest) and Harrison sulci (depression of the ribcage at the site of insertion of the diaphragm). The tibiae become bowed (genu valgum) and eventually growth is retarded. Other features include irritability, hypotonia, tetany, laryngospasm, convulsions and aminoaciduria.

The diagnosis is made on the basis of raised alkaline phosphatase for age, low phosphate and/or calcium. X-rays show widening of the metaphyseal plate, and concavity of the ends of the diaphysis (shafts of the bone).

Treatment is with vitamin D 25–125 μg/day (1000–5000 IU/day). If compliance is a problem a single dose of 7.5 mg (300 000 IU) can be given by injection. Treatment is continued until alkaline phosphatase is normal, then a prophylactic dose (10 μg/day) is given. Calcium requirements can be supplied by 500 ml/day of milk. Greater exposure to sunlight should be encouraged. Extensive remodelling of deformed bones occurs, but orthopaedic surgery may be required for the severest deformities.

Unless a child is receiving a vitamin D-fortified milk, they should receive 10 μg/day for the first year. Preterm babies are especially at risk because of lack of stores in the liver and their rapid growth. Antiepilepsy drugs induce liver enzymes which accelerate vitamin D breakdown; hence children with epilepsy require prophylaxis. Excess vitamin D intake causes hypercalcaemia, which leads to vomiting, constipation, polyuria, irritability, drowsiness, and metastatic calcification of blood vessels and kidneys.

Xerophthalmia

> **Prevention**
> Some studies have shown that mass vitamin A supplementation for children in developing countries resulted in striking decreases in childhood mortality from diarrhoeal and respiratory diseases.

'Dry eye' is caused by vitamin A deficiency. Vitamin A is an essential component of retinal pigment rhodopsin (visual purple). Deficiency leads to squamous metaplasia of epithelial surfaces. Important animal sources of vitamin A include liver, milk, butter, cheese and eggs. An important vegetable source is the pigment carotene, which is a dimer of vitamin A.

Deficiency may occur when the diet lacks dairy produce, fresh vegetables and fruit, or when there is malabsorption. Night blindness is an early symptom. Xerophthalmia comprises conjunctival xerosis (dry, wrinkled conjunctiva) with white, foamy spot (Bitot spot). Corneal xerosis then develops with clouding of the cornea due to keratinization. Eventually keratomalacia (softening of the cornea) leads to necrosis of the cornea and loss of eyesight. Serum vitamin A is less than

200 μg/l. Treatment is with 300 mg retinol for 3 days then 9 mg/day for 2 weeks. Prevention involves encouraging the intake of green, leafy vegetables and yellow or orange fruit.

Trace element deficiency

Iron

See Iron deficiency anaemia, page 250.

Copper

See Wilson disease, Menkes kinky hair syndrome, page 292/293.

Zinc

See acrodermatitis enteropathica, page 292.

Food allergy

See Chapter 11, page 227

Parenteral nutrition

Historical
First applied successfully to beagle puppies in 1968 and soon after to infants. Parenteral nutrition is now a routine therapy in neonatal and paediatric intensive care units.

Parenteral nutrition is a lifesaving therapy in intestinal failure. The indications are shown in Information box 19.1.

Nitrogen is administered as a mixture of crystalline, essential and non-essential L-amino acids. Carbohydrate is given as D-glucose. The solutions are hypertonic and of low pH, and hence are irritant to peripheral veins. Lipid is given as an emulsion of soy bean oil in egg phospholipid. Electrolytes, vitamins and trace elements are also added. The solutions are compounded in the pharmacy, in a laminar flow cabinet to prevent contamination. The mixture is usually given via a catheter into the superior vena cava. This route improves the quality of life for the child by avoiding extravasation of the solutions from peripheral veins and frequent re-siting of drips. Quality of life can be further enhanced in children requiring long-term parenteral nutrition if this is undertaken at home. However central venous feeding predisposes to infection of the catheter, leading to septicaemia. Thombosis of the central veins and pulmonary emboli can also occur.

While the child is receiving parenteral nutrition, every effort is made to give as much nutrition as possible into the gut. This means that the child can be weaned off parenteral nutrition as soon as possible. Every aspect of gastrointestinal function is affected adversely when the supply of enteral nutrient is stopped.

Information Box 19.1

Indications for parenteral nutrition in paediatric practice

- Protracted diarrhoea of infancy
- Gut dysmotility in preterm infants
- Major gut surgery in newborns
- Necrotizing enterocolitis
- Intensive care of low birthweight infants
- Severe inflammatory bowel disease
- Severe trauma
- Extensive burns
- Acute renal failure

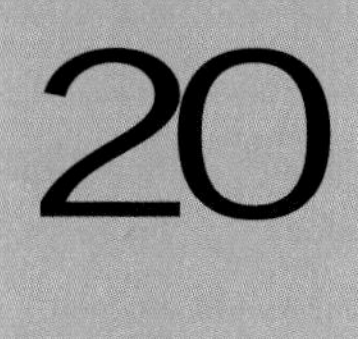

20 Oncology

Malignant disease is the second commonest cause of death (after accidents) in childhood. Remarkable progress has been made in the treatment of childhood cancer through the development of highly effective but potentially toxic drugs. This has sometimes been at the expense of long-term problems, particularly with growth and endocrine function and the development of a second tumour.

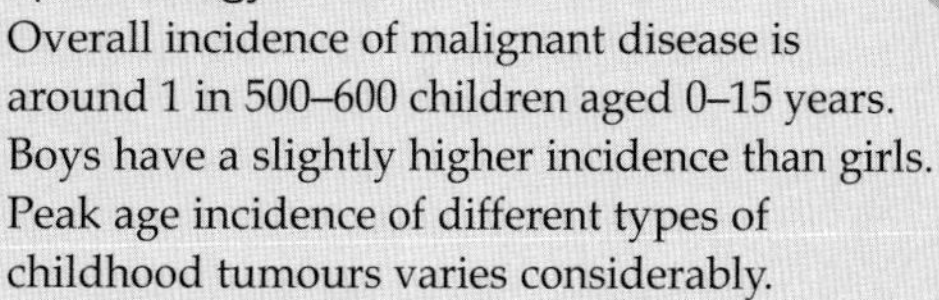

Childhood cancer – general principles

> **Epidemiology**
> Overall incidence of malignant disease is around 1 in 500–600 children aged 0–15 years.
> Boys have a slightly higher incidence than girls.
> Peak age incidence of different types of childhood tumours varies considerably.

INTRODUCTION

Cancer in childhood differs from that in adults in that carcinomas are very rare while many of the paediatric tumours arise from primitive embryonal cells.

INCIDENCE

The important childhood cancers are listed in Table 20.1, with their cell or tissue of origin, relative incidences, peak age incidence in childhood and common presenting features.

Leukaemia is the most common form of malignancy with tumours of the central nervous system second. There is evidence that both of these show an increasing incidence in recent years. Though there is speculation on environmental causes for this increase, as yet, proof is lacking.

AETIOLOGY AND PATHOGENESIS

A number of predisposing conditions can be identified. These are listed in Information box 20.1.

There are many other conditions predisposing to carcinoma development in adulthood but which may be diagnosed in childhood (e.g. familial polyposis coli).

CLINICAL PRESENTATION

This is described in Table 20.1.

Table 20.1
Important childhood cancers

Cancer	Cell/tissue of origin	Relative incidence, %*	Peak age of incidence in childhood years	Common presenting features	Tumour markers useful for diagnosis and monitoring
Leukaemia	Bone marrow progenitor cell	33.6	Lymphoid 2–5 Myeloid 0–15	Pallor, bruising, tiredness, bone pain, infection	Gene rearrangements Cytogenetic abnormalities
Lymphoma (non-Hodgkin)	Lymph node	6.1	0–15	Localized lymph node swelling, symptoms like leukaemia, central nervous system features, fevers	Some specific gene rearrangements
Lymphoma (Hodgkin)	Lymph node	4.3	10–15	Localized lymph node swelling, fevers	None
Central nervous system†	Glial cells (glioma, astrocytoma) Primitive neuroectodermal cells (medulloblastoma) Pineal (pineal tumours) Craniopharyngioma	23.5	3–8 depending on type	Headache, vomiting, visual disturbance, squint, unsteady gait, convulsions, behavioural change Hypopituitarism and optic chiasm compression (craniopharyngioma) Wasting (tumours of hypothalamus – diencephalic syndrome)	None
Neuroblastoma and other sympathetic nervous system tumours	Neural crest cells (sympathetic chain)	6.8	0–3	Local swelling, bone pain (secondaries), fevers	Urinary catecholamines (HVA and VMA)• elevated in 85–90%
Nephroblastoma (Wilms) and other renal tumours	Renal cells	5.2	2–5	Abdominal mass, haematuria, loin pain, fevers (Fig. 20.1)	None
Ewing sarcoma	Primitive neural cells in bone or occasionally soft tissues	1.9	10–15	Local pain and swelling	Elevated lactate dehydrogenase (LDH) in some
Osteosarcoma and other bone tumours	Osteoblasts	3.2	13–18	Local pain and swelling	None
Rhabdomyosarcoma and other soft tissue sarcomas	Primitive mesenchymal cells in striated muscle (rhabdomyo) or other soft tissues	5.5	0–5	Local pain and swelling, interference with adjacent structures, e.g. nerves	None
Germ cell tumours	Primordial germ cells in gonads or other sites (commonly sacrococcygeal area)	2.4	15–19	Local mass Sacrococcygeal in the neonatal period Gonadal at puberty	α-fetoprotein in most; β-human chorionic gonadotrophin in some; elevated LDH in yolk sac tumours
Retinoblastoma	Embryonal cells in retina	2.7	0–2	Opaque mass visible through iris, squint, absent red reflex. Routine examination if family history	None
Hepatoblastoma, hepatocellular carcinoma	Liver cells	0.9	Hepatoblastoma 0.3. Hepatocellular carcinoma 0–4 or 12–15	Abdominal distension, vomiting, malaise, anorexia, pain	Hepatoblastoma: α-fetoprotein in 67%; β-human chorionic gonadotrophin in a few Hepatocellular carcinoma: α-fetoprotein in 50%

* From Parker et al (1988) International Childhood Cancer Incidence. IARC Scientific Publications No 87. International Agency for Research in Cancer, Lyon.
† The distinction between benign and malignant tumours of the CNS is not clear-cut or, in most cases, useful.
• HVA = homovanillic acid, VMA = vanillyl mandelic acid. Both are end-products of catecholamine metabolism.

DIAGNOSIS

Presenting features depend largely on the site of the primary tumour. There are some tumours which produce specific biochemical markers which can be useful in diagnosis and in monitoring response to therapy.

MANAGEMENT

Since most of the childhood tumours have the potential to metastasize, it is important to stage the tumour before treatment starts (to assess the extent of the primary tumour and the presence or absence of metastases). This may involve radiological assessment including CT or MRI scans, isotope scans and often bone marrow examination. Neuroblastoma staging can be facilitated by administering a radiolabelled precursor for catecholamine-producing cells followed by gamma camera scans. This technique also has therapeutic potential using higher doses of radioisotope.

A detailed account of the individual treatment protocols for childhood tumours is beyond the scope of this book. However the student should be familiar with some general principles.

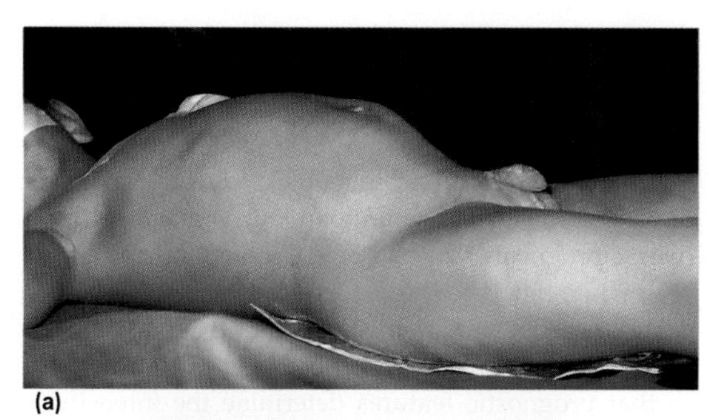

(a)

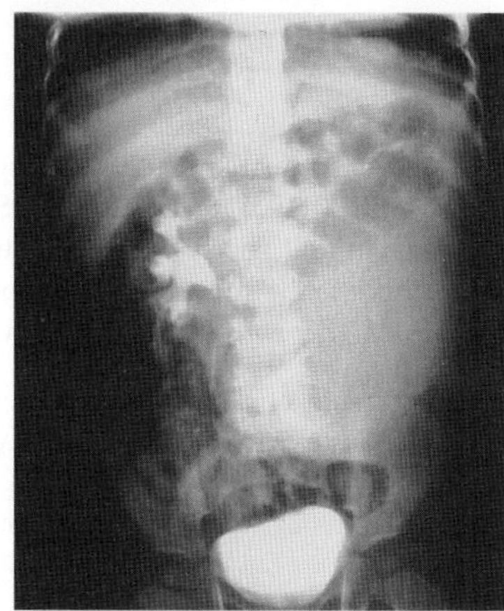

(b)

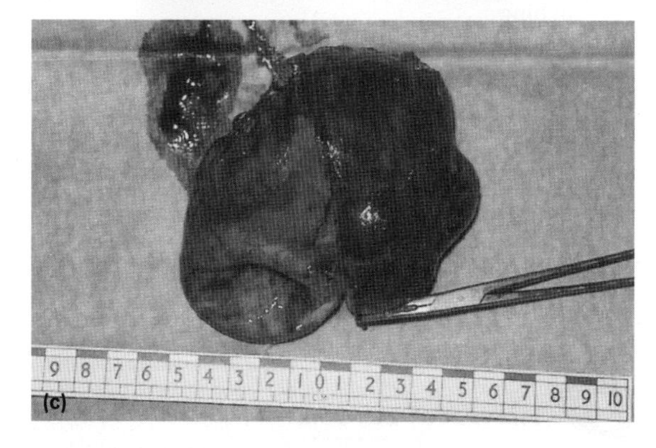

(c)

Fig 20.1
Nephroblastoma. (a) Abdominal swelling; (b) distortion of left kidney seen in intravenous urogram; (c) operative specimen.

In general, children tolerate oncological therapy better than adults, both physically and psychologically. It is very important to involve those children who are old enough in discussions and explanations and always to be truthful with them and their families. Since most treatments involve repeated injections and venesections, it is standard practice where tumours require intensive treatments to insert central venous catheters to minimize injections. Though these catheters pose an increased risk of infection, this is outweighed by the benefits. Drug-induced nausea and vomiting

Information Box 20.1

Conditions leading to increased susceptibility to malignancy in childhood

Condition	***Malignancy***
Chromosomal disorders	
Down syndrome	Leukaemia
Klinefelter syndrome (47, XXY)	Breast cancer
Gonadal dysgenesis (XO/XY)	Gonadal tumours
Aniridia (with 11p-deletion*)	Nephroblastoma
13q-deletion†	Retinoblastoma
Chromosomal breakage disorders	
Fanconi anaemia	Leukaemia
Bloom syndrome	Leukaemia/lymphoma
Ataxia telangiectasia	Leukaemia/lymphoma
Xeroderma pigmentosum	Skin cancer
Immunodeficiency (genetic)	
Wiskott–Aldrich syndrome	Mostly lymphoma
Ataxia telangiectasia	Mostly lymphoma
Immunodeficiency (acquired)	
HIV/AIDS	Mostly lymphoma
Immune suppression after organ transplantation	Mostly lymphoma
Miscellaneous	
Neurofibromatosis	Gliomas, astrocytoma
Hemihypertrophy	Nephroblastoma
Beckwith–Weidemann syndrome (p. 245)	Hepatoblastoma
Tyrosinaemia (p. 259)	Hepatocellular carcinoma
Coeliac disease (p. 224)	Small bowel tumours

* Deletion involving the short arm of chromosome 11
† Deletion involving the long arm of chromosome 13

should be prevented by prophylactic use of the modern, powerful antiemetics. Pain should also be treated aggressively. Painful procedures such as lumbar puncture and bone marrow sampling should be performed under general anaesthesia.

The range of therapies for childhood tumours involve combinations of the following.

Surgery confirms diagnosis and allows histological grading (which is becoming increasingly important in planning treatment). It may also be used for removal of localized disease (before or after other treatments).

Radiotherapy is most important in treating tumours of the central nervous system. It is also used for some other tumours and as a part of 'mega' therapy.

Conventional chemotherapy, usually with combinations of drugs, is becoming increasingly sophisticated.

'Mega' therapy is used for cases with poor prognosis. It allows very large doses of chemotherapy and/or

radiotherapy with restoration of bone marrow function by allogeneic or autologous bone marrow transplant. A variation on the latter is autologous stem cell transplantation in which stem cells are harvested from the blood before therapy and used to reconstitute bone marrow function afterwards.

Side-effects during treatment include the following.

Tumour lysis syndrome is characterized by massive release of breakdown products including uric acid, causing renal impairment and metabolic upset.

Gastrointestinal upset including vomiting, diarrhoea and mucositis.

Hair loss. This is reversible.

Haematological toxicity leads to thrombocytopenia (bleeding), anaemia and neutropenia (infection). The occurrence of a significant fever in a neutropenic individual (febrile neutropenia) should be urgently investigated and treated. If the neutrophil count is less than 500 x 10^9/l, there is a high likelihood that the fever is due to bacteraemia or septicaemia and this may progress to septic shock and death in a matter of hours. This is particularly likely if the organism is a gram negative enteric bacillus such as *Pseudomonas aeruginosa*. After collection of appropriate cultures including blood cultures, an empirical broad-spectrum combination of antibiotics should be commenced immediately.

Immunosuppression increases susceptibility to opportunistic infection (e.g. *Pneumocystis carinii*), and severe viral infections (e.g. chickenpox).

Late sequelae to treatment for childhood cancers include:

- Endocrine dysfunction, particularly affecting growth and puberty, but also other functions (e.g. thyroid)
- Reduced fertility
- Localized growth abnormalities after local radiotherapy
- Psychological/emotional problems
- Subtle learning difficulties after cranial irradiation
- Second neoplasms, which occur in up to 5% of cases. The occurrence is highest after radiotherapy but may be an increasing problem as chemotherapeutic regimens intensify.

In addition to the above listed general side-effects of treatment, specific chemotherapeutic agents have their own particular side-effects. Examples are given in Information box 20.2.

PROGNOSIS

The prognosis is generally better for childhood tumours than for carcinomas in adults. However there is great variability with type of tumour, stage of disease at diagnosis, histological grade of the tumour and age of the child. The age may act in either way; for example neuroblastoma has a much better prognosis in infancy than in older children, while some leukaemias have a worse prognosis in infancy.

The overall 5-year disease-free survival rate for children with the common form of acute lymphoblastic leukaemia (CALL) is around 75%. Adverse prognostic factors in this form of childhood leukaemia include age (worse prognosis <2 years or >12 years), having a very high white blood cell count at presentation and having central nervous system involvement.

Increasingly, treatment protocols are being adapted so that prognostic features determine the intensity of the treatment.

PALLIATIVE AND TERMINAL CARE

Despite the advances in treating childhood malignancy many children still die of their disease. Sensitive handling of the child and family during this time is of immense importance to the subsequent emotional well-being of that family. There are a number of key areas:

- To give full and truthful explanations to the child and family and to support them in dealing with this information
- To relieve symptoms by whatever means possible
  - Pain
  - Nausea/vomiting
  - Itching
  - Bowel/bladder dysfunction
- To support the family in the environment best suited to them. This is likely to be their home in most cases, but some families prefer to be in either a hospital or a hospice.

Information Box 20.2

Side-effects of some chemotherapeutic agents

Agent	Side-effect
Vincristine/vinblastine	Reversible peripheral neuropathy (including autonomic)
Methotrexate	Hepatotoxic
Platinum-based drugs (cisplatin, carboplatin)	Renal Auditory
Anthracyclines (Adriamycin, daunorubicin)	Cardiotoxicity (nonreversible)
Cyclophosphamide	Haemorrhagic cystitis (in high doses)
Bleomycin	Pneumonitis

Langerhans cell histiocytosis (histiocytosis X)

The rare histiocytosis syndromes were known as Hand–Schüller–Christian and Letterer–Siwe diseases, and eosinophilic granuloma, previously classified as 'histiocytosis X'. These are now called Langerhans cell histiocytoses.

This condition is not a true malignancy. There is an abnormal proliferation of Langerhams cells with an associated pleomorphic cellular reaction. This can produce lytic lesions of the skeleton, especially in the skull, and may be painful. Infiltration of the skull produces exophthalmos and anterior and posterior pituitary insufficiency including diabetes insipidus. Pathological fractures can occur. A skin rash resembling seborrhoeic dermatitis is common. Pulmonary infiltration (Fig. 20.2), hepatosplenomegaly and lymphadenopathy may occur. The diagnosis is made by biopsy of an infiltrate.

Anticancer drugs such as steroids, vinblastine and etoposide are used. The prognosis varies from 50% to 90% for 5-year survival. Children under 2 years with organ involvement have the worst prognosis.

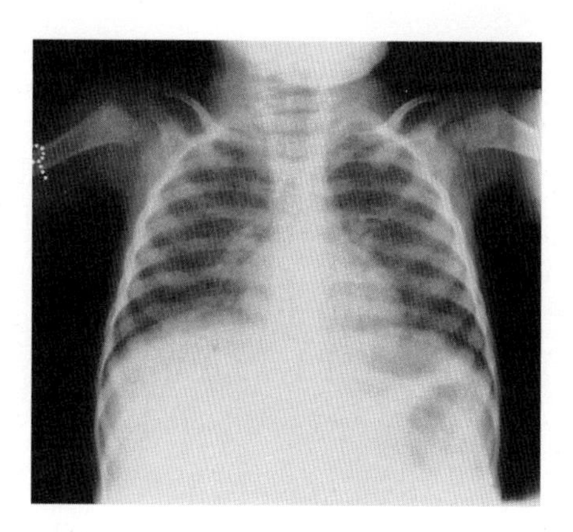

Fig 20.2
Pulmonary infiltration in Langerhans cell histiocytosis.

Xeroderma pigmentosum

The name means 'dry pigmented skin'. This rare and very serious disorder presents in infancy or early childhood with any one of a number of possible skin signs, including severe reddening, scaling and crusting of sunlight-exposed areas. The eyes can also be affected, with intense soreness and eventual blindness. Affected children lack the normal mechanism for DNA repair whereby the skin naturally heals itself when exposed to ultraviolet light from the sun. They must be very carefully protected from direct sunlight, with appropriate clothes and sun creams. Unfortunately the skin changes tend to become malignant.

The condition is autosomal recessive. Antenatal diagnosis is possible.

21 Ophthalmology

Expert assessment of squints is required at any age, to avoid blindness in the squinting eye. Ophthalmologists are also required to advise on relatively common, and potentially life-threatening, infections around the eye.

Glaucoma

Increased intraocular pressure causes:

- Increased tear production
- Photophobia
- Blepharospasm (spasm of eyelids)
- Cloudy corneas (due to oedema)
- Buphthalmos (enlarged eye)
- Optic atrophy with loss of visual acuity.

Most glaucomas are caused by persistence of embryonic tissue in the outer rim of the iris, which prevents drainage of the aqueous humour. Glaucoma may complicate retinopathy of prematurity. It also occurs in Sturge–Weber syndrome, neurofibromatosis, Lowe syndrome, Marfan syndrome (due to dislocation of the lens), and congenital rubella, which are dealt with elsewhere. Inheritance is multifactorial.

Surgery is directed to improving drainage of aqueous humour to prevent optic nerve damage.

Cataracts

Cataracts may occur:

- Transiently in preterm babies
- Following antenatal infections
- In galactosaemia and galactokinase deficiency
- In hypoparathyroidism
- As a result of chromosome defects
- With steroid therapy
- As a result of trauma.

Dominant inheritance occurs.

If vision is affected the lens is removed. Vision is corrected by lens implant, contact lenses or spectacles.

Defects of the iris

Aniridia

The iris fails to develop properly in aniridia ('without iris'). The pupils always look exceptionally large. Vision is poor, and bright light can be painful. Other eye problems are associated including glaucoma and cataract.

Type I is caused by an autosomal dominant mutation on chromosome 2. Type II is associated with a deletion on the short arm of chromosome 11; there are also abnormalities of the urinary tract, including Wilms tumour (nephroblastoma).

Coloboma

In this deformity of the iris, and sometimes the eyelid as well, the large gap will result in damage to the cornea from exposure. Dermoid cyst of the eye globe can be associated, and coloboma of the iris can occur with a cleft of the retina and optic nerve.

Simple colobomata are often autosomal dominant and may occur in syndromes such as CHARGE (**C**oloboma, **H**eart disease, choanal **A**tresia, **R**etardation and **G**enital and **G**enetic abnormalities, **E**ar defects). They represent defective closure of the embryonic fissure.

Waardenburg syndrome

This syndrome has an autosomal dominant inheritance. It is one cause of having irises of different colours (heterochromia iridis). The eyes are widely set, and there is depigmentation of the forelock hair, and hearing impairment. The gene responsible has been identified.

Defects of the pupil

Anisocoria (unequal pupils)

Anisocoria can occur in healthy individuals, but it may be an indication of neurological problems (e.g. Horner syndrome, see below), congenital defects of the iris (aniridia, colobomata), or local iris disorders (adhesions to the lens or synechiae).

Horner syndrome

See Chapter 18, page 320.

Inflammatory ophthalmic conditions

Dacryocystitis

The lacrimal duct may be incompletely canalized at birth (dacryostenosis). Dacryocystitis presents with overflow of tears (epiphora) and chronic, mucopurulent discharge from the affected eye.

With simple cleansing of the lids with warm water, the condition usually resolves by the age of 1 year. If not, the duct should be probed under anaesthesia.

Infection may involve the nasolacrimal sac, producing local swelling and reddening of the overlying skin. Antibiotics and early surgery to relieve the obstruction are required.

Iridocyclitis

Acute iridocyclitis causes lacrimation, pain and photophobia. Chronic iridocyclitis produces much less marked symptoms. Affected eyes have hyperaemic conjunctivae, most marked around the limbus, which overlies the ciliary body. Slit lamp examination will show inflammatory deposits (keratic precipitates) on the posterior surface of the cornea, and inflammatory exudate ('flare') in the aqueous humour. Chronic iridocyclitis causes corneal and lens opacities.

Conditions associated with iridocyclitis, such as juvenile chronic arthritis, inflammatory bowel disease and Kawasaki disease, are discussed elsewhere.

Iridocyclitis can also follow eye infections. Other causes include corneal abrasions, corneal ulcers, *Herpes simplex*, bacterial and fungal infections, and intraocular foreign bodies.

Iridocyclitis associated with infection is treated with antibiotics, and the noninfective type with topical or systemic steroids. Atropine is used to prevent adhesion of the iris to the lens.

Periorbital cellulitis (Fig. 21.1)

The tissue of the orbit can be infected by direct extension from ethmoid sinusitis, a penetrating injury, nasolacrimal sac, lacrimal glands or by extension from cellulitis. The infection can lead to proptosis, limitation of eye movement, chemosis (oedema of the conjunctiva) and eyelid swelling. Conjunctivitis can spread to the eyelids resulting in pre-septal orbital cellulitis, in which case there is no proptosis. Systemic antibiotics effective against *Haemophilus influenzae*, staphylococci, streptococci and pneumococci are required to prevent

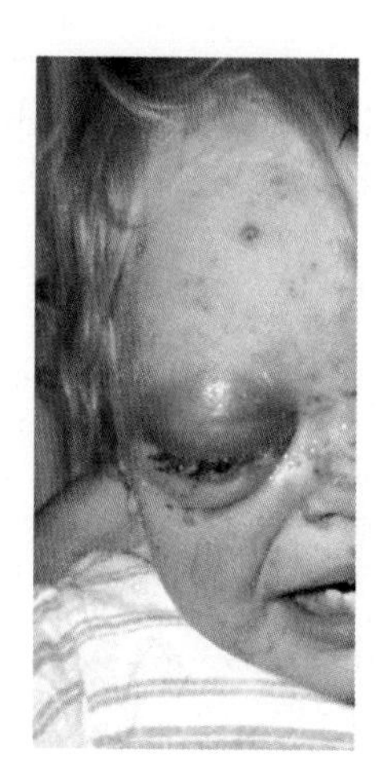

Fig 21.1
Pre-septal orbital cellulitis (complicating chickenpox).

damage to the eye or extension of the infection into the cranium. Thrombosis of the sagittal sinus is a rare complication. Hence affected children should be promptly hospitalized and given systemic antibiotics. Surgical drainage of the ethmoid sinuses may be required.

22 Orthopaedics

Congenital conditions and deformities

Talipes (club foot) (Fig. 22.1)

The usual deformity is for the foot to be turned down (equinus) and inwards (varus), probably because of intrauterine posture. The range of movement of a normal neonatal foot is that the little toe can be touched against the anterior surface of the tibia; this is impossible in talipes equinovarus.

Provided the diagnosis is made at birth, before the soft tissues become fixed, most talipes will resolve by being splinted in the correct position.

Talipes can also occur as a part of neurological disorders, such as post-traumatic cerebral palsy and polio.

Developmental dysplasia of the hip (congenital dislocation)

The hip joint may be dislocatable, in which case the femoral head is in the acetabulum at rest but can be removed by manipulation. In developmental dysplasia (dislocation) of the hip (DDH) the femoral head is outside the acetabulum at rest but is reducible by manipulation.

The incidence of DDH is about 1% of neonates. There may be a family history. It is more common in female infants and multiple births and breech presentations predispose. After birth, cerebral palsy predisposes. Some resolve spontaneously as the ligaments tighten.

The diagnosis is made clinically by abducting the hip while holding the knee flexed with the infant supine. If there is DDH, re-entry of the femoral head into the acetabulum is felt as the hip is abducted. If the hip is already dislocated, abduction is restricted. Not all are detected clinically and screening by ultrasound is being introduced. X-ray examination is unreliable to confirm the diagnosis before 3 months of age, because of lack of ossification of the femoral head.

The relocated hip is maintained in position with a special harness for at least 3 weeks. Open reduction is required for failures of conservative management or delayed diagnosis. This avoids later complications of

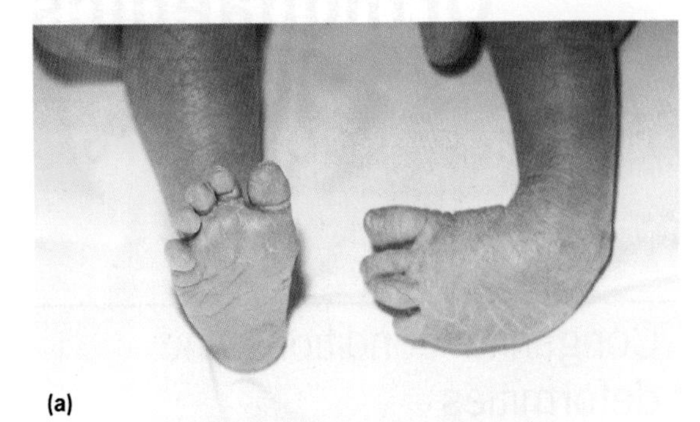

(a)

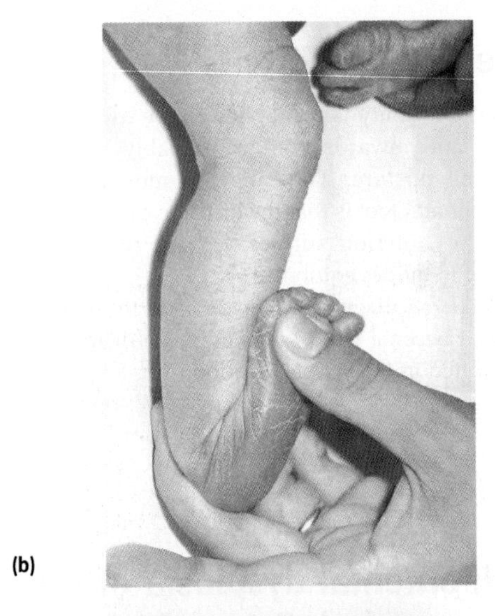

(b)

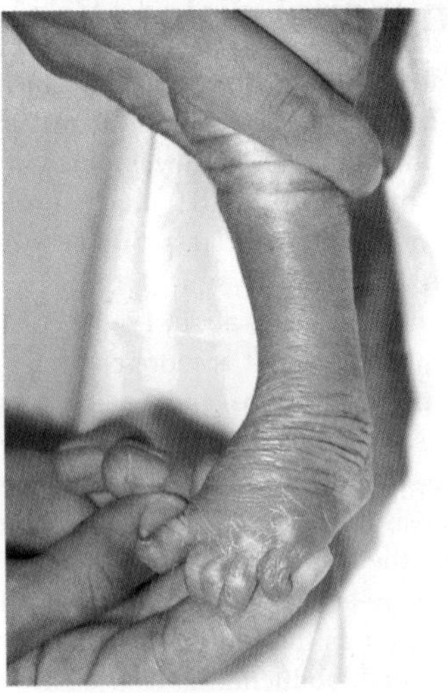

(c)

Fig 22.1
(a) Left talipes equinovarus; (b) normal range of movement in the right ankle; (c) restricted range of movement in the left ankle.

waddling gait (bilateral) or limp (unilateral) and later degenerative hip arthritis when the child tries to walk.

Absence of the radius

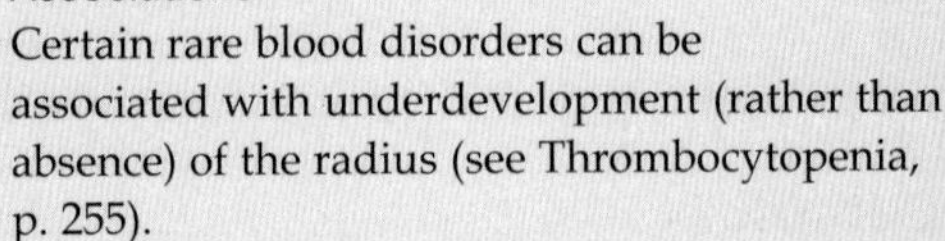

Associations
Certain rare blood disorders can be associated with underdevelopment (rather than absence) of the radius (see Thrombocytopenia, p. 255).

Several rare congenital conditions involve abnormality of the radius. In one group the only abnormality is that the radius (and occasionally the ulna instead) is missing. This results in an abnormal forearm in which the wrist is only supported by the ulna; as a result the hand bends in a radial (or thumb side) direction causing a 'clubbed hand'. This must be prevented by splinting and very skilled surgery. Short stature, small thumbs, browning of the skin, genital abnormalities and retardation comprise the Fanconi anaemia. Rather worse disorders including absence of radius as well as blood disorder and congenital cardiac defect are seen in a variant of this condition known as radial aplasia–thrombocytopenia (thrombocytopenia–absent radius; TAR) syndrome. It can be part of trisomy 18.

Why abnormality of the radius should be associated with other conditions remains a mystery. It suggests that the radius is laid down in intrauterine life at the same time as some elements needed in blood formation. There is much need for more research here.

Atlantoaxial instability (atlanto-occipital dislocation)

This may occur because of hypoplasia of the odontoid process, trauma or inflammation (e.g. rheumatoid arthritis). In Down syndrome the transverse ligaments are lax. There may be pain, limited movement or quadriplegia.

Posterior fusion of the upper cervical spine may be required.

Cleidocranial dysplasia

This is one manifestation of a group of congenital conditions known as the genetic skeletal dysplasias, caused by abnormal formation of bone in a specific pattern. Cleidocranial dysplasias principally affect the anterior end of the clavicle (Greek *cleido*), making the shoulders droop, as well as the anterior part of the sacrum. The cranium is also affected with late closure of the fontanelles and frontal bossing. The teeth are often irregular. Affected children tend to be short. Intelligence is normal.

There is no specific treatment. Good orthodontic care should be given and physiotherapy to help posture.

These disorders are autosomally inherited.

Klippel–Feil syndrome (brevicollis) (Fig. 22.2)

This rare congenital malformation is caused by fusion of two or more cervical vertebrae. It is associated with skeletal, cardiac, neurological and renal malformations.

Kyphoscoliosis

> **Definition**
> A spinal deformity resulting from an accentuation of the normal curvatures of the spine.
> Kyphosis refers to deformities in the sagittal plane; there is an exaggeration of the normal dorsal curve of the spine. Scoliosis occurs in the coronal plane; it is a lateral curvature of the spine associated with a rotational deformity.

The deformity may be congenital in association with abnormalities of the vertebral bodies (Fig. 22.3) or other disorders such as chondrodysplasia punctata (p. 294), mucopolysaccharidoses (p. 289), Noonan, (p. 241), Marfan (p. 245), and Rett (p. 323) syndromes. It can also be part of neuromuscular disorders. Both kyphoscoliosis and the range of movement of the spine are best demonstrated by asking the child to bend forwards (the forward bend test).

Idiopathic kyphosis (Scheuermann juvenile kyphosis) begins in adolescence with the development of a wedge-shaped deformity of one or more vertebrae. Idiopathic scoliosis is familial and the more severe deformities are commoner in girls. Minor deformities do not require treatment; as many as one in 20 children are affected. The commonest age of onset is adolescence. Severe untreated scoliosis impairs cardiorespiratory function because of the associated chest deformity. Severe kyphosis may cause damage to the spinal cord. Spinal X-rays are required to determine the nature and direction of the curvature.

Congenital kyphosis requires surgery. Scoliosis of greater than 30° in childhood usually progresses and requires treatment. Idiopathic kyphosis and scoliosis are treated with an external brace which is worn continuously until growth has ceased, with surgery reserved for treatment failures.

(a)

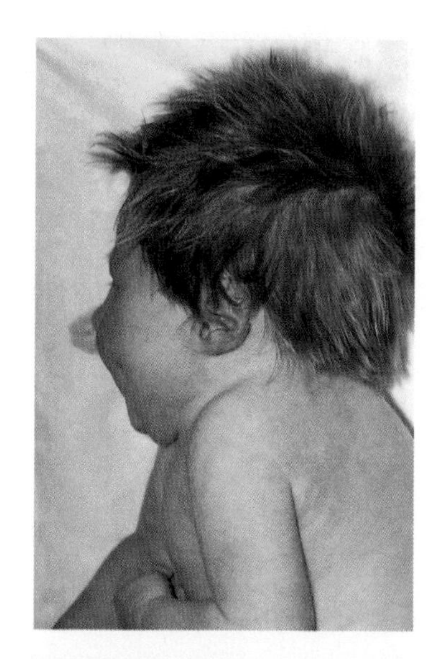

(b)

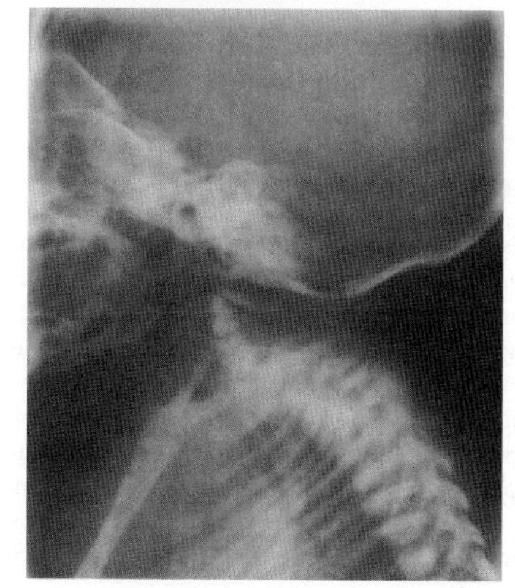

Fig 22.2
(a) Klippel–Feil syndrome. (b) Cervical spine X-ray in Klippel–Feil syndrome.

Metaphyseal dysplasia

This group of disorders affecting the long bones may be autosomal dominant or recessive. Affected individuals are of short stature due to shortening and bowing of the legs. Joints are swollen, and superficially resemble the bony changes of rickets. One recessively inherited type (McKusick), called 'cartilage-hair hypoplasia', is associated with ectodermal dysplasia (see p. 189) and immunodeficiency.

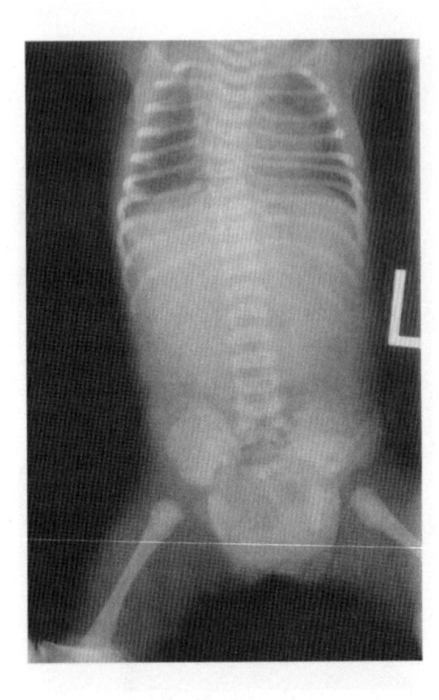

Fig 22.3
Scoliosis due to fusion of two vertebral bodies.

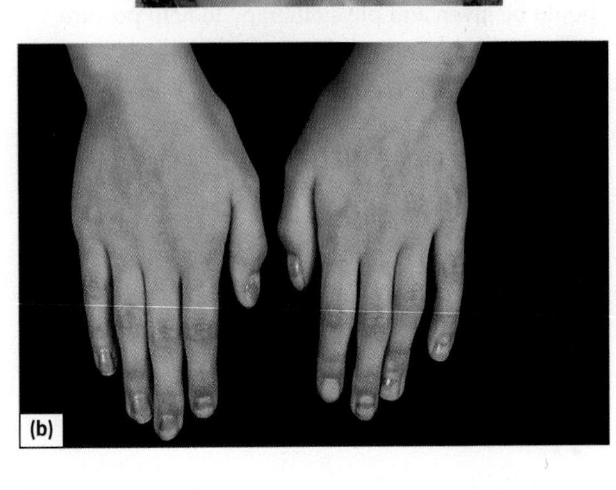

Fig 22.4
Osteogenesis imperfecta. (a) Note blue sclerae. (b) Arachnodactyly.

Osteogenesis imperfecta (Fig. 22.4)

Type I is the commonest (1 : 30 000) and is dominantly inherited. It is characterized by deep blue sclerae, fragile bones and severe osteoporosis, with reduced synthesis of collagen type I. Some infants have fractures present at birth. Fractures are not an inevitable consequence of trauma. Skeletal deformities such as kyphoscoliosis develop later in life but fractures become less frequent. Some families have discoloured fragile teeth (dentinogenesis imperfecta). X-rays confirm the osteoporosis, showing evidence of previous fractures and normal callus formation.

In type II there are multiple intrauterine fractures and an abnormally shaped thoracic cage, which are incompatible with life.

Type III is of intermediate severity, with an autosomal recessive inheritance.

Type IV has bone fragility as the sole manifestation.

The mainstays of treatment are expert orthopaedic care and genetic counselling.

Osteopetrosis (marble bone disease)

Overgrowth of bone into the marrow cavity results in bone marrow failure. It may present with anaemia, thrombocytopenia and serious infection. The foramina in the skull, through which the optic nerves run, are narrowed. The liver and spleen enlarge as sites of extramedullary haemopoiesis, and X-rays show increased bone density with loss of medullary cavity. Death from bone marrow failure is usual.

Bone marrow transplantation can be a successful therapy. The optic nerve foramina may require surgical decompression.

A milder variant, osteopetrosis tarda, is also known as Albers–Schönberg disease.

Inflammatory orthopaedic conditions

Osteomyelitis (see also p. 283)

> Epidemiology
> Osteomyelitis occurs at any age but most commonly in boys under 1 year of age and in mid-childhood.

INTRODUCTION

Osteomyelitis is the infection of bones by bacteria. The diagnosis should be considered in any child with fever or limp. The child should be examined for skeletal tenderness, swelling, reddening of the skin and limitation of movement (pseudoparalysis) (Fig. 22.5).

AETIOLOGY AND PATHOGENESIS

Local bone injury seems to predispose to infection. *Staphylococcus aureus* is the commonest cause, with

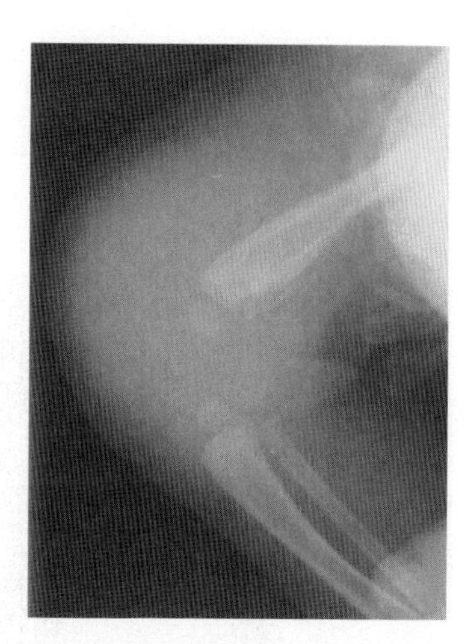

Fig 22.5
Neonatal osteomyelitis of lower femoral metaphysis. Note soft tissue swelling, bone destruction and subperiosteal new bone formation.

Escherichia coli and group B streptococci occurring in young infants, and *Streptococcus pneumoniae* in older infants. Salmonellae osteomyelitis is seen in those with sickle cell anaemia (see p. 252) and anaerobic organisms, if the infection spreads from the skull (originating from sinuses). The infection arrives in the blood stream, often from a nonapparent source, to form an abscess at the metaphysis (between the shaft of the bone or diaphysis and the growth plate or epiphysis), an area of stasis where phagocytic cells are not numerous. In young infants the infection tends to spread to an adjacent joint. Lateral spread through cortical bone results in a subcutaneous abscess.

CLINICAL PRESENTATION

Three clinical types are recognized. Acute haematogenous osteomyelitis presents with fever and bone pain of less than 1 week's duration. Subacute osteomyelitis evolves over 1–4 weeks, and has less systemic manifestations. Bone pain is the most striking finding. Chronic osteomyelitis lasts longer than 1–2 months.

Clinical manifestations vary with more systemic upset tending to occur in young infants. In older children, one-third may be afebrile and manifest only local bone pain. Blood culture and needle aspiration of the bone are required to isolate the infecting organism. X-ray changes are absent for the first 2 weeks of infection but bone scans are positive much earlier.

Treatment is with intravenous antibiotic (flucloxacillin and fusidic acid, intravenously). Infants require initial cover against *E. coli* (ceftriaxone or cefataxime) until the correct organism is identified. Clindamycin or metronidazole are required for skull infections. If the child is improving after 1–2 weeks, oral antibiotics may be introduced. If the infection does not improve, surgical exploration is required.

Complications include recurrence if therapy is stopped too soon, septic arthritis and disturbances in bone growth.

Septic arthritis (Fig. 22.6)

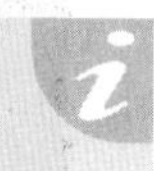

Epidemiology
Commonest in the under 3-year-olds.

Staphylococcus aureus is the commonest agent in neonates together with group b streptococci, *Escherichia coli* and *Candida albicans*. *Haemophilus influenzae* and *S. aureus* predominate in childhood, with *S. aureus* becoming the commonest organisms in children over 5 years old. The infection is due to haematogenous spread or contiguous spread from an osteomyelitis.

In the neonate, signs can vary from unwillingness to move a limb (pseudoparalysis) to septicaemia. Older children show pseudoparalysis and joint swelling. ESR and white cell count are high. X-rays show soft tissue and joint swelling. The diagnosis is established by arthrocentesis, which guides the choice of antibiotics.

Flucloxacillin is given for staphylococcal infection; ceftriaxone for *H. influenzae* and coliforms, and amphotericin for candida, for 4–6 weeks (2 weeks i.v.). Repeated joint aspiration or open surgical drainage may be required.

The outcome is poorer in infancy, in hip infections, in the presence of osteomyelitis, and following delayed treatment.

Discitis (Fig. 22.7)

Discitis is inflammation of the intervertebral disc due to infection with bacteria, most commonly *Staphylococcus aureus*, viruses or unknown causes. The infection results in low grade fever and back pain. A bone scan will be

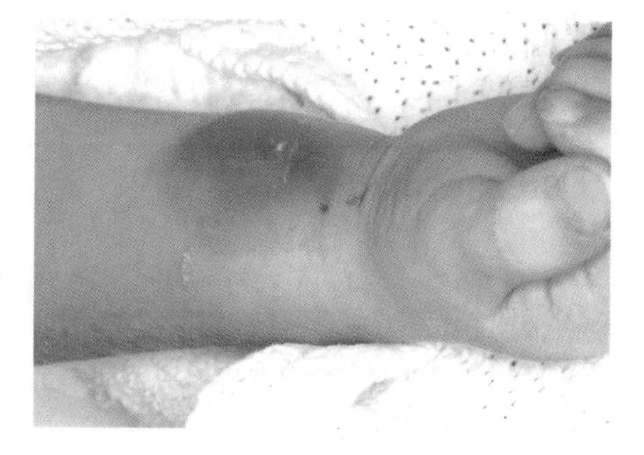

Fig 22.6
Septic arthritis of the wrist. The portal of entry of infection was an intravenous cannula.

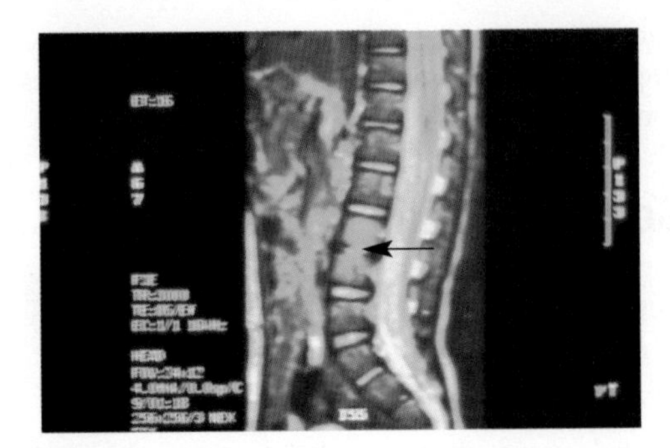

Fig 22.7
Discitis: MR imaging.

positive before X-ray changes of a narrowed disc space are found after 2 weeks. If there is high fever, neutrophil leukocytosis or positive blood or disc aspirate culture, antistaphylococcal antibiotics are given for 6 weeks. Other measures include anti-inflammatory drugs and immobilization.

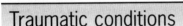

Traumatic conditions

Dislocation (subluxation) of the head of the radius (pulled elbow)

This dislocation is caused by sudden traction on the outstretched arm of young children. Supination is limited. The pain is relieved immediately by careful supination of the forearm with the elbow held at 90°.

Chondromalacia patellae

This produces anterior knee pain, a grating sensation on knee flexion and tenderness of the undersurface of the medial side of the patella in susceptible adolescents.

It is associated with recurrent dislocation of the patella. Quadriceps-strengthening exercises, with analgesia and rest for acute pain, are required.

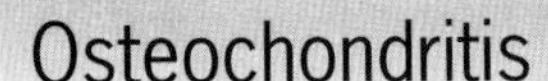

Osteochondritis

Epidemiology

Perthes disease occurs in 1 in 2000 children.
Boys outnumber girls by five to one.
The epidemiology of the other osteochondritides is less well studied.
Osgood–Schlatter disease (Fig. 22.8) is quite common.

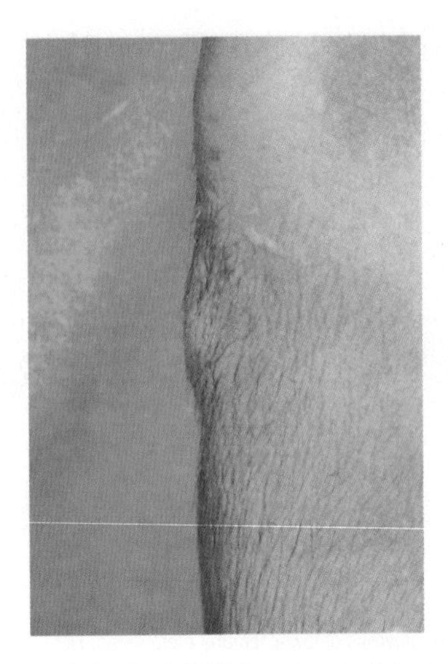

Fig 22.8
Osgood–Schlatter disease.

Osteochondritis is thought to be due to avascular necrosis of individual bones (see Information box 22.1).

Treatment consists of rest and prevention of strain.

The most significant of the osteochondritides is Perthes disease (Fig. 22.9) which involves the hip. It results from recurrent loss of blood supply to the head of the femur (both femora in 10% of cases) causing avascular necrosis. The underlying cause is unknown although one in five cases is familial, especially affecting deprived families.

The child usually presents with slow onset of groin pain, limp and stiffness of the hip. At the onset, the hip X-ray is normal although a bone scan will show increased uptake of isotope and an MRI scan will confirm avascular necrosis. Later the femoral head will be radiodense and become fragmented.

Treatment is based around rest, bracing or surgery to maintain the femoral head within the normal aceta-

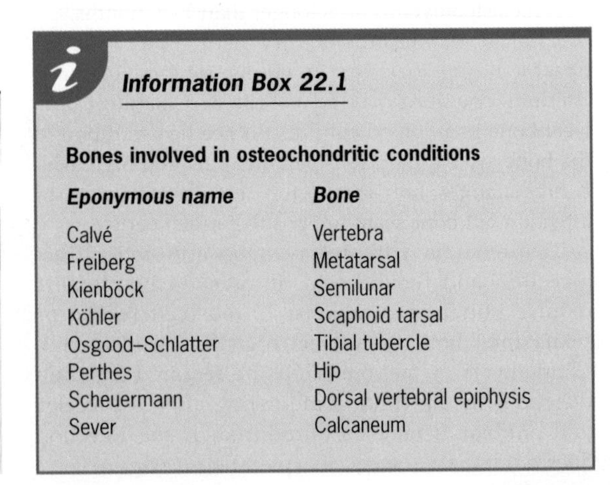

Information Box 22.1

Bones involved in osteochondritic conditions

Eponymous name	***Bone***
Calvé	Vertebra
Freiberg	Metatarsal
Kienböck	Semilunar
Köhler	Scaphoid tarsal
Osgood–Schlatter	Tibial tubercle
Perthes	Hip
Scheuermann	Dorsal vertebral epiphysis
Sever	Calcaneum

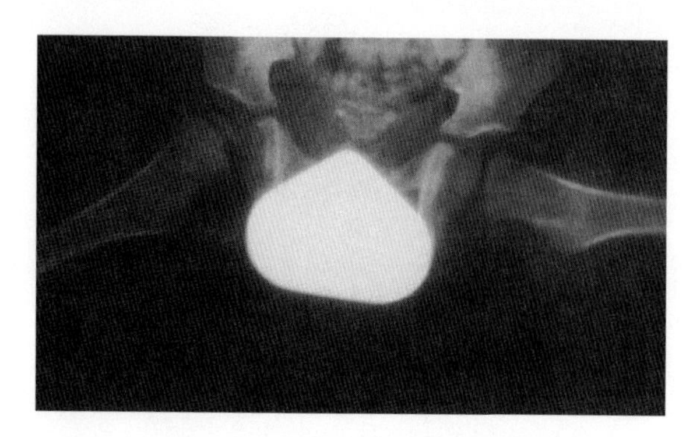

Fig 22.9
Perthes disease. Note abnormal right femoral epiphysis.

bulum. The aim is to maintain the spherical shape of the head to prevent later degenerative arthritis. As always there is a compromise between overenthusiastic treatment and the normal psychological development of the affected child. Surgery has the advantage of earlier mobilization. Problems arise later in middle age, especially if treatment in childhood was suboptimal. The femoral head may need replacing.

23 Respirology

Respiratory conditions are amongst the most frequently occurring and important in childhood. Worldwide, respiratory infections are now the commonest cause of death. The survival of low birthweight babies is dependent on the successful management of their immature lungs. Respiratory tract infections occur on average every 6 weeks in toddlers. Asthma affects up to 30% of children and seems to be increasing. Thus respiratory disorders cause enormous morbidity and mortality in childhood.

Congenital disorders

Asphyxiating thoracic dystrophy

The ribcage fails to develop as the child grows, leaving insufficient room for lung and heart to expand. Many affected children die in infancy of respiratory insufficiency, often with associated lung infection. There is a wide variety of associated features, including shortness of stature and limbs, because of the failure to form cartilage properly; the kidneys may be abnormal and fail.

This is a bleak diagnosis: there is no known cure, only symptomatic relief.

Inheritance is autosomal recessive. Some affected children have survived; individual advice is needed in any particular case.

Primary ciliary dyskinesia

Each cell lining the respiratory tract bears approximately 300 cilia beating at 1 kHz. These transport mucus backwards in the nose and upward in the lower respiratory tract to the pharynx where it is swallowed. Defective motility may be secondary to respiratory infections and cystic fibrosis. Primary ciliary dyskinesia causes chronic sinusitis, otitis media and bronchiectasis. Association with dextrocardia and abnormal sperm motility is called Kartagener syndrome. The dextrocardia, and sometimes situs inversus indicate that functional cilia are important for normal development of the embryo.

Cilia from the respiratory tract are examined by electron microscopy and primary organ culture derived from nasal brushing. The beating pattern is examined by phase contrast microscopy. Repeated examination may be required as abnormal cilia can be found during infections. Normal lifespans have been reported if early, effective antibiotic treatment and physiotherapy are given.

The condition is autosomal recessive. Defects in many different genes responsible for ciliary structure can result in this syndrome.

Cystic fibrosis

> **Epidemiology**
> In Europid races the cystic fibrosis carrier frequency is about 1 in 25.
> The disease affects about 1 in 2500 live births.
> Only common in Europids.

INTRODUCTION

Cystic fibrosis (CF) is an autosomal recessive disorder. It is manifested in homozygotes chiefly by pancreatic insufficiency and chronic suppurative lung disease.

AETIOLOGY AND PATHOGENESIS

The abnormal gene is located on the long arm of chromosome 7. It codes for a membrane protein in epithelial cells which regulates chloride transport, the cystic fibrosis transmembrane regulator (CFTR) protein. In up to 70% of affected children the mutation is one known as the Δ508 mutation. Over 300 other mutations have been identified.

Water follows the movement of chloride ions across epithelia and defective transport of chloride leads to dehydrated secretions. The pancreatic ducts become blocked by inspissated mucus secretions preventing enzyme production and leading to malabsorption. The pancreas eventually fibroses. In the lungs, dehydrated viscous mucus causes defective mucociliary clearance which predisposes to chronic infection and eventually bronchiectasis. Dehydrated intestinal secretion can lead to intestinal obstruction (DIOS) in older children. Later complications include diabetes mellitus, biliary cirrhosis and male infertility.

CLINICAL PRESENTATION

Neonates may present with meconium ileus (10–20%) due to inspissated meconium (Fig. 23.1) or persistent jaundice. Older children present with frequent chest infections (Fig. 23.2), persistent wheeze or cough, failure to gain weight and offensive, fatty stools. They can lose sodium excessively in their sweat (and taste salty when kissed!) and become hyponatraemic in hot weather. CF must be excluded in any child presenting with nasal polyps or rectal prolapse.

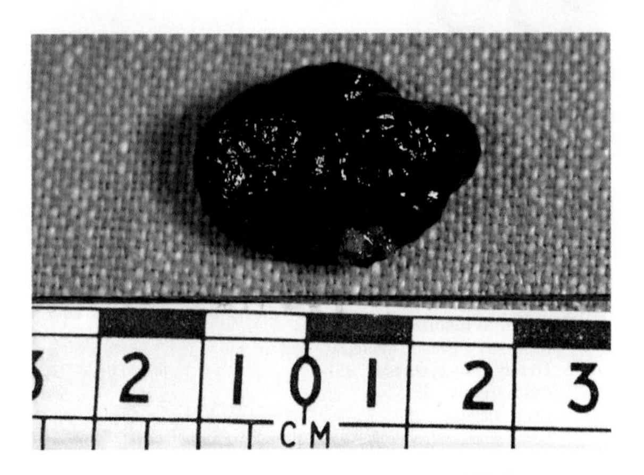

Fig 23.1
Meconium plug.

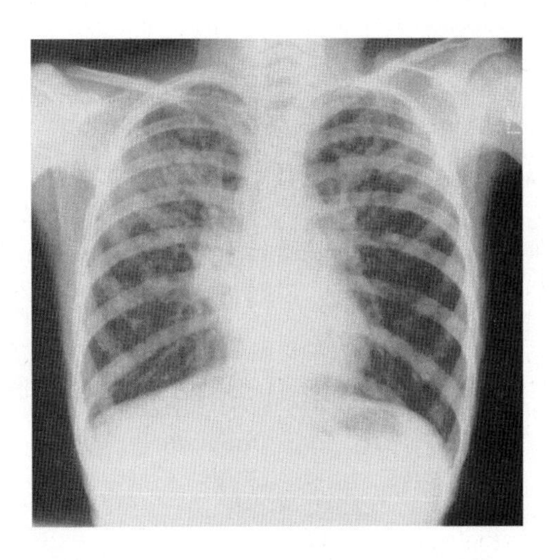

Fig 23.2
Chest X-ray in cystic fibrosis.

DIAGNOSIS

Neonatal screening can be performed by testing for elevated serum immunoreactive trypsin on blood spots. Prenatal diagnosis is available for couples who have had an affected child in whom the mutation has been identified.

After the neonatal stage sweat output increases making it possible to collect enough sweat for electrolyte estimation (see Practical box 23.1).

A sweat sodium or chloride in excess of 70 mmol/l is diagnostic of cystic fibrosis. Demonstrating cystic fibrosis mutations from both parents would also be diagnostic but both mutations cannot always be identified.

MANAGEMENT

Regular chest physiotherapy is given to shift mucus. Various techniques may be employed with differing

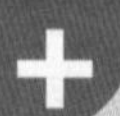

Practical Box 23.1

Performing a sweat test

- Clean and dry an area of skin on the back.
- Induce sweating by forcing pilocarpine into the skin by iontopheresis using a battery and wire circuit.
- Excess sweating is induced locally.
- This is collected onto dry filter paper, the electrolytes eluted and levels of Na^+ and Cl^- determined.
- At least 100 mg sweat is required for a reliable result.

degrees of parental participation depending on the child's age.

Intensive control of chest infection using appropriate antibiotics guided by sputum culture and sensitivities is needed. The common organisms are *Staphylococcus aureus, Haemophilus influenzae* and *Pseudomonas aeruginosa* including mucoid species. Nebulized antibiotic may be helpful for those with chronic respiratory colonization with *Pseudomonas aeruginosa.*

Nutrition is optimized by giving pancreatic enzyme supplementation with every meal and snack, encouraging a high calorie (not low fat) diet, supplemented if necessary with high calorie drinks or even continuous overnight feeding via nasogastric tube or gastrostomy, and giving vitamin (particularly fat-soluble) supplements.

Complications such as salt depletion, DIOS, diabetes, etc., are treated or prevented.

Psychological problems are common in coming to terms with a chronic illness and should not be overlooked. Lifespan has greatly increased however in the last decade with many surviving to their thirties and beyond. Of males, 98% are sterile due to blockage of the vas deferens, though women can give birth.

Death is usually due to cor pulmonale. Lung or heart lung transplantation is an option for some. Gene therapy (local incorporation of normal genetic material) offers one hope for the future.

Choanal atresia

In this condition there is a unilateral or bilateral bony or membranous partition between the pharynx and the nose. When it is bilateral, cyanosis relieved by crying occurs from birth, or during the first feed, depending on how successful are the infant's attempts at mouth breathing. Unilateral atresia presents with a unilateral discharge. The diagnosis is confirmed when a catheter cannot be passed via the nostril, or by fibreoptic rhinoscopy.

An oral airway is inserted if necessary and the obstruction is relieved by elective surgery.

Choanal atresia can be part of the CHARGE syndrome (see Coloboma, p. 340).

Laryngomalacia (congenital laryngeal stridor, tracheomalacia)

Stridor is present from birth due to floppiness of the supraglottic folds and walls of the upper airway in this disorder. Symptoms vary in severity and may be relieved in the prone position. Diagnosis is by direct laryngoscopy which excludes other malformations of the larynx.

The condition usually resolves spontaneously. Very occasionally, tracheostomy is required.

Inflammatory conditions

Allergic rhinitis (hay fever)

Allergic rhinitis may occur in spring (seasonal) or all year round (perennial). Inhaled antigens provoke production of IgE antibodies in atopic individuals. When antigens bind to IgE, release of vasoactive substances such as histamine from mast cells produces the symptoms of sneezing, watery rhinorrhoea, mouth breathing and itching of the nose, ears and eyes. The nasal mucosa looks swollen and lilac-coloured.

Treatment includes avoidance of dust, and use of oral antihistamines and nasal sprays such as sodium cromoglycate and beclomethasone.

Anaphylaxis

Anaphylaxis is a severe, systemic (type I hypersensitivity) allergic reaction. It may lead to respiratory distress due to laryngeal oedema and/or bronchospasm, or to circulatory failure (shock) or, most commonly, to a combination of both.

Without treatment, death may occur within 15–20 minutes: *anaphylaxis can be a medical emergency.*

The reaction is caused by massive histamine release from mast cells through antigen interaction with specific IgE. Most affected children have a background of atopic disease.

In recent years the frequency of these reactions seems to have increased, and they are a source of considerable anxiety to parents and healthcare workers involved with atopic children. In practice given the high prevalence of allergy and atopy in the paediatric age group, the incidence is low.

The antigens most commonly causing anaphylaxis in children are:

- Foods: peanuts, tree nuts, fish, shellfish, egg, milk
- Bee or wasp stings
- Drugs, e.g. penicillin, anaesthetic agents.

In adults latex sensitivity is a relatively common cause (especially in healthcare workers).

Treatment is described in Emergency box 23.1.

Families of children considered at risk should be equipped with preloaded adrenalin syringes and instructed in their use and in basic resuscitation. Children at risk or with a history of anaphylaxis need referral to a specialist with expertise in allergic disorders, for identification of the causative antigen and advice on its avoidance. Desensitization can be undertaken for bee/wasp stings but is not generally used for other allergies.

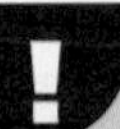

Emergency Box 23.1

Treatment of anaphylaxis

- Urgent administration of adrenalin, 1 in 1000 pre-loaded syringe (e.g. Epipen®), by the intramuscular or subcutaneous route. This should never be given intravenously – fatal arrhythmias are likely to ensue.
- This is followed by intravenous antihistamine and hydrocortisone.
- Urgent transfer to hospital is needed.
- A second dose of adrenalin may be needed after 10 minutes if there is no improvement.

Asthma

Epidemiology
Prevalence figures vary widely between countries: the disorder affects 1–25% of children, but depends on the epidemiological definition of 'asthma'.
In a recent English study, 16% of children aged 8–10 years had a history of wheezing in the last year.

INTRODUCTION

Asthma is probably the most common chronic illness of children in developed countries. Despite advances in the understanding of the condition and in its treatment, management is still frequently suboptimal.

DEFINITION

Asthma is a disorder of airway inflammation. It is characterized by an increased responsiveness of the airways to various stimuli, and manifested by airways obstruction that varies spontaneously or as a result of therapy.

PATHOGENESIS AND AETIOLOGY

Most asthmatic children are atopic, i.e. they have an inherited propensity for type I (IgE mediated) hypersensitivity. Lung inflammation is probably initiated by an allergic reaction to inhaled allergens such as house dust mite, cat fur, grass pollen, etc. In response to allergens, IgE is produced, which activates mast cells and eosinophils. This process sets up a vicious cycle of ongoing inflammation from the release of numerous mediators that cause hyper-responsive epithelial damage and shedding. Airways obstruction is generated by bronchospasm, mucosal swelling and plugging of airways. It should be understood that once airway inflammation has ensued, contact with the original allergen is not required to cause an asthma attack; indeed the commonest trigger is a viral respiratory infection.

PREVALENCE

In countries where comparable serial estimates have been made, the prevalence of asthma has undoubtedly been rising. The reasons are still not clear. Currently, there is no evidence for, and some evidence against air pollution being a major factor. Acute rises in atmospheric pollution may be associated with an increase in asthma exacerbations, but overall, the levels of, for example, sulphur dioxide have decreased in recent years. Enhanced exposure to allergens during infancy would seem to be a more likely factor. Asthma prevalence in places with very clean air, such as the islands in the North Sea, is just as high as in the more polluted parts of the mainland UK.

CLINICAL PRESENTATION

The cardinal sign of asthma is wheezing, which is defined as a continuous respiratory noise with a musical pitch heard mainly in expiration. It is caused by turbulent air flow in the large airways (trachea and major bronchi). In asthma turbulent air flow is caused by distortion (dynamic compression) of the large airways due to the increased expiratory force required to push air through obstructed smaller airways. Anything that causes turbulent air flow in the large airways may also cause wheezing (e.g. an inhaled foreign body). Wheeze can be heard by the unaided ear or with a stethoscope. Wheeze however is not always present and this is particularly so in young children in whom there may be a history of chronic asthma with persistent cough worse at night or brought on by exercise or exposure to irritants such as cold air. At times, the cough may be almost paroxysmal and followed by vomiting of mucus.

Usually, the child presents to the GP or hospital clinic with a history of wheezing but little may be found on examination. The chest may be overinflated. Signs of chest deformity (Harrison sulci; pectus carinatum) indicate more severe persistent disease. Asthma does not cause finger clubbing. There may be symptoms or signs of other atopic diseases (eczema, p. 192; rhinitis, p. 353). A family history of asthma supports the diagnosis.

DIAGNOSIS

Asthma is probably the commonest cause of wheezing. Diagnosis in infancy is difficult because many infants wheeze during viral respiratory infection but do not go on to have atopic asthma. Differential diagnosis is shown in Information box 23.1.

However, there may not be wheezing or chronic signs at presentation. Diagnosis is then dependent on history but may be confirmed by response to anti-asthma treatment. Lung function measurement showing airway obstruction that improves after inhaling a bronchodilator, is useful in older children who can perform the tests reliably (usually older than 5–7 years). In the child with persistent cough without wheezing, the diagnosis is more difficult to make. If the cough shows some of the typical features (e.g. nocturnal or worse on exercise) then often a trial of anti-asthma medication may need to be given. A favourable response confirms the diagnosis.

MANAGEMENT

The problem should be explained to the parents and to the child. Precipitating factors may be identified from the history and (where possible) the family counselled on how to avoid these. Drastic avoidance measures are rarely necessary. The acquisition of pets should be discouraged. The parents should be dissuaded from smoking. Common trigger factors for childhood asthma are listed in Information box 23.2.

Asthma is treated with bronchodilators and/or anti-inflammatory agents. Drugs for asthma are best thought of as *relievers* (bronchodilators) and *preventers* (inhaled corticosteroids, long acting β_2 agonists, sodium cromoglycate and theophylline). The use of drugs is dictated by the pattern and severity of asthma. There are three patterns: infrequent episodic, frequent episodic, and persistent. Prophylactic treatment is indicated in persistent, often in frequent episodic and not in infrequent episodic. Most children with persistent asthma should receive an inhaled corticosteroid as should all children with chronic chest deformity due to asthma. Long acting β_2 agonists are used as an adjunct to inhaled corticosteroids, and not on their own. Theophylline has become an alternative or adjunct to long acting β_2 agonists and is hardly ever used as primary prophylaxis because of its behavioural and gastro-intestinal side-effects. β_2 agonists are available as oral preparations but are best given by inhalation. The method of administration will vary with the age of the child. Table 23.1 lists some of the commonly used inhalation devices and the ages at which their use may be attempted.

Administration of oral β_2 agonists such as salbutamol (Ventolin®) or terbutaline (Bricanyl®) are less effective than inhaled treatment and more likely to cause side-effects. The appropriate inhaler device

Information Box 23.1

Differential diagnosis of wheezing

Small airways obstruction
Bronchiolitis
Other viral respiratory tract infections
Cystic fibrosis
Recurrrent inhalation bronchitis

Large airways obstruction
TB (hilar) nodes
Foreign body

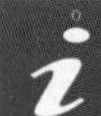

Information Box 23.2

Trigger factors for childhood asthma

Viral respiratory infections

Exposure to airway irritants
Sudden air temperature changes (especially to cold)
Cigarette (or other) smoke
Chemical irritants
Environmental pollutants

Exercise

Allergen exposure
House dust mite
Animal dander
Pollens
Foods

Emotional upset

Gastrooesophageal reflux

Drugs
Aspirin (in certain children only)
Beta blockers

Table 23.1
Earliest ages at which various inhalation devices may be used to administer drugs to treat asthma.

Device	Age
Metered dose inhaler + spacer* with mask	Any age
Nebulizer	Any age
Metered dose inhaler + spacer alone**	2½–3 years
Dry powder device***	4 years
Metered dose inhaler†	Greater than 12 years†

* e.g. Nebuhaler®, Volumatic®, Babyhaler®, Aerochamber®.
** e.g. Nebuhaler®, Volumatic®.
*** e.g Turbohaler®, Acuhaler®, Diskhaler®.
† Metered dose inhalers require considerable skill and should not be used to deliver inhaled corticosteroids.

should always be prescribed. A nebulizer should never be the first choice. Care should be taken to ensure that if nebulizers are used they do not delay the seeking of medical advice during a severe attack. Bronchodilators are best used on an intermittent basis rather than continuously.

For children with persistent symptoms, or with intermittent episodes that occur with high frequency, long-term prophylactic anti-inflammatory treatment should be used. For example if the child uses an inhaled β_2 agonist more than three times a week, then prophylaxis should be considered. This is best given by inhalation and there are two main classes of drug used. Mast cell stabilizers such as disodium cromoglycate (Intal®) are exclusively used for long-term prophylaxis and have no place in the treatment of an acute attack. Inhaled corticosteroids such as beclomethasone (Becotide®), budesonide (Pulmicort®) and fluticasone (Flixotide®) act directly to reduce airways inflammation. Many studies have now shown that in standard doses these drugs, even when used on a long-term basis, do not produce significant adverse effects. Acute systemic effects can be demonstrated with standard doses but do not appear to be adverse in the long term. As a result, these agents are being increasingly used. Preparations are available for use with all of the inhalation devices listed. Systemic corticosteroid therapy is rarely needed in long-term management but it is required for treating acute attacks. Regimes vary but generally a high oral dose is employed for between 3 and 5 days.

Continuous daily monitoring with symptom diaries and recording peak expiratory flow rate (PEFR) is an added burden on the child and should be reserved for only the most severely affected children who are likely to benefit. It is helpful to record the child's best PEFR when well to compare with readings obtained when unwell. There will be times when monitoring PEFR for short periods may give helpful information (for example when trying a new treatment).

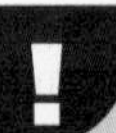

Emergency Box 23.2

Management of severe acute asthma

A child admitted severely ill with asthma should be treated as a medical emergency. Supplemental oxygen and nebulized β_2 agonists (2–4-hourly depending on response) should be given immediately while an assessment is being performed. This assessment should include:

- Whether or not the child can talk
- Presence or absence of pulsus paradoxus
- Central cyanosis
- Usage of accessory muscles (subcostal, intercostal and supraclavicular)
- Hyperinflation of the chest with air trapping
- The wheeze may decrease as the amount of air moving through the airways decreases ('silent chest' is a particularly grave sign)
- Peak flow decreases markedly.

A chest radiograph is only required for first attacks or if a complication such as an air leak, chest infection or inhaled foreign body is suspected. Corticosteroid therapy takes 5 or 6 hours to give relief in acute asthma and should be given at the earliest opportunity. Prednisolone is given initially.

Assessment of response to initial treatment will determine:

- The frequency of subsequent nebulizer therapy
- Whether to use ipratropium
- Need for: i.v. hydrocortisone, i.v. aminophylline (omit loading dose if child has had theophylline recently), i.v. salbutamol, or mechanical ventilation.

Salbutamol and steroids can cause a fall in serum potassium but this is rarely a major problem.

Bronchiectasis

The tubular dilatation of bronchi (Fig. 23.3) may rarely be congenital. However it usually results from chronic infection or one of the following:

- After measles
- Whooping cough
- Cystic fibrosis
- Aspiration of foreign body
- Compression of bronchi by mediastinal nodes
- Primary ciliary dyskinesia (see p. 351)
- Immunodeficiencies.

Copious mucopurulent sputum results with haemoptysis and clubbing.

Bronchoscopy is used for assessment of severity and obtaining sputum samples.

Treatment is by postural drainage and antibiotics. Resection is required for localized disease.

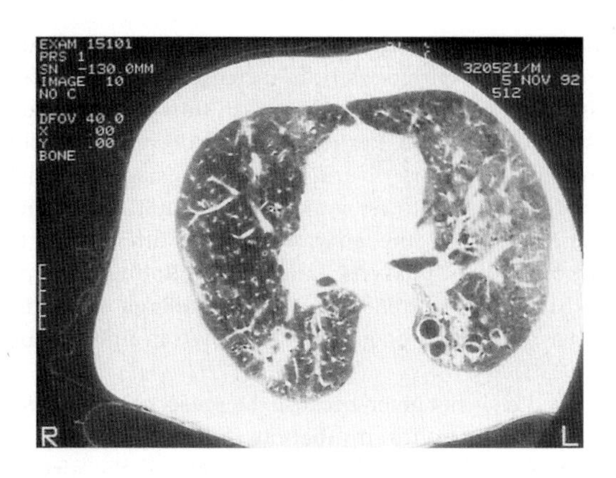

Fig 23.3
Bronchiectasis. Note the tubular dilations of bronchi at the lower right.

Bronchiolitis

> Epidemiology
> Infection with respiratory syncytial virus (RSV) is one of the most common viral infections in young children.
> About 10–15% of infants develop some degree of bronchiolitis.

INTRODUCTION

Bronchiolitis is an acute infective illness of infants in which inflammation of the very small airways (bronchioles) occurs.

AETIOLOGY AND PATHOGENESIS

Infection with the respiratory syncytial virus (RSV) causes 80% of cases of bronchiolitis. The others are caused by a variety of other respiratory viruses including influenza, parainfluenza and adenovirus. Occasionally rhinoviruses and *Mycoplasma pneumoniae* can also produce this clinical picture. These agents all cause respiratory illness in all age groups but only in infancy does the clinical picture of bronchiolitis seem to develop. There is evidence that the pathological process causing inflammation of the airways is a type 3 hypersensitivity reaction in the lung, possibly associated with circulating antibody levels that are insufficient to clear the virus but sufficient to cause inflammation. This may be one explanation for the age incidence since most cases occur after the age of 3 months, at a time when maternally derived antibody levels are in decline.

INCIDENCE

Serological surveys suggest that 50% of children have encountered this virus by their first birthday and 85% by their second birthday. In the vast majority, bronchiolitis is a self-limiting disease. In children with preexisting heart or lung conditions however, infection with this virus may produce a severe disease with a high mortality rate. In the United Kingdom RSV bronchiolitis occurs in the community every year through the winter months. Cases usually start appearing in November and the virus persists in the community until the early spring.

CLINICAL PRESENTATION

Initial symptoms are of upper respiratory coryzal illness, which over a few days progresses to give lower respiratory symptoms including tachypnoea, cough and wheezing. The tachypnoea may be so severe as to produce feeding difficulties. Systemic upset and fever are usual but not invariable.

Examination will reveal an ill child with coryzal symptoms and marked tachypnoea with wheeze. There will often be recession and dramatic usage of accessory muscles. Central cyanosis may be present in the more severely infected infants. Auscultation usually reveals wheeze and extensive areas of fine crackles throughout both lung fields. The clinical picture may however be variable and wheeze and crackles may come and go. Chest radiography typically shows hyperinflation with patchy, often streaky atelectasis.

DIAGNOSIS

In the young infant with the typical clinical presentation the diagnosis is usually straightforward. If the infant presents during the winter epidemic of RSV a confident diagnosis can be made. The main differential diagnosis is of a widespread broncho-pneumonia. The chest X-ray showing increased shadowing of the lung fields will be helpful in distinguishing bronchopneumonia from bronchiolitis.

In older infants, in addition to pneumonia, the possibility of asthma with associated upper respiratory viral infection has to be considered. This is particularly so if the clinical signs reveal wheeze without crackles and if there is a positive family history of atopy and asthma. Chest radiography is not helpful in differentiating these two. The demonstration of RSV by immunofluorescence on nasopharyngeal aspirate is not necessarily helpful, since during the RSV season many upper respiratory infections that trigger asthma are caused by this virus.

MANAGEMENT

Mildly affected children are normally managed by their parents and the general practitioner at home. Parents will need to watch for signs of deterioration that include poor feeding, irritability, increasing respiratory rate and cyanosis. For infants who are hospitalized, supportive measures including attention to fluid intake, supplemental oxygen where necessary and antipyretics are all that is required. In the deteriorating child or the child with preexisting heart or lung disease the broad-spectrum inhaled antiviral agent ribavirin is sometimes used, but its efficacy is at best marginal.

The child who goes into respiratory failure needs mechanical ventilation which is often technically extremely difficult because of the tendency of air to be trapped in the distal airways and atelectasis.

There is no evidence that antia-sthma drugs help in bronchiolitis, though often they will be given, particularly ipratropium, if there is the possibility of asthma. Systemic corticosteroids have been shown to have an adverse effect in bronchiolitis and are therefore contraindicated.

Children who have suffered a severe attack of bronchiolitis in infancy have a tendency to recurrent wheezing episodes which may persist for many years. The mechanism is unclear and seems to be unrelated to the atopic state.

The consequences of this virus infection are quite considerable in the childhood population. Unfortunately there is no immediate prospect of a vaccine although there is ongoing work in this field. Earlier attempts at vaccination proved disastrous in that immunized children developed a tendency to more severe illness, presumably because of enhancement of the immunopathological process which occurs in this disease. A monoclonal anti-RSV antibody has been developed for passive protection of high risk infants (e.g. preterm babies with bronchopulmonary dysplasia) and is under evaluation.

Bronchiolitis obliterans

In this condition progressive fibrosis of the bronchioles with obliteration of the lumen by granulation tissue causes cough, wheezing, increasing dyspnoea and cyanosis. It usually follows lower respiratory infection or lung transplantation.

The condition may be fatal.

Laryngotracheobronchitis (croup)

Definition

'Croup' refers to the characteristic cough which occurs in association with partial obstruction of the larynx.

It has been described as 'the worst sound a parent can ever hear' because it is potentially life-threatening.

The commonest cause is parainfluenza virus. Group A streptococcus, pneumococcus and staphylococcus are some of the bacteria which cause croup. As croup progresses, respiratory stridor increases and respiratory distress begins (nasal flaring and indrawing of the soft tissues of the neck). Restlessness and decreased stridor precede respiratory obstruction. At this stage the child must be moved to an intensive care unit for further management of the airway, without attempting to examine the pharynx and precipitating airway obstruction. Recurrent croup may be allergic in origin. Other differential diagnoses are shown in Information box 23.3.

Oxygen is not given because the presence of cyanosis is an indicator for intubation. Recently, nebulized budesonide has been shown to decrease the airway swelling. If the airway obstruction is properly managed the prognosis is excellent.

Epiglottitis

Epiglottitis is caused by *Haemophilus influenzae* type b. Immunization has greatly reduced the incidence of this condition.

There is a dramatic course, with sudden respiratory obstruction and drooling as the pharynx is too sore to allow swallowing of saliva. The child sits and leans forward with open mouth. The child should be intubated by an expert. Laryngoscopy shows the enlarged, cherry red epiglottis. This should only be performed during intubation, to avoid total obstruction, by the swollen epiglottis, of the larynx. Ceftriaxone is administered.

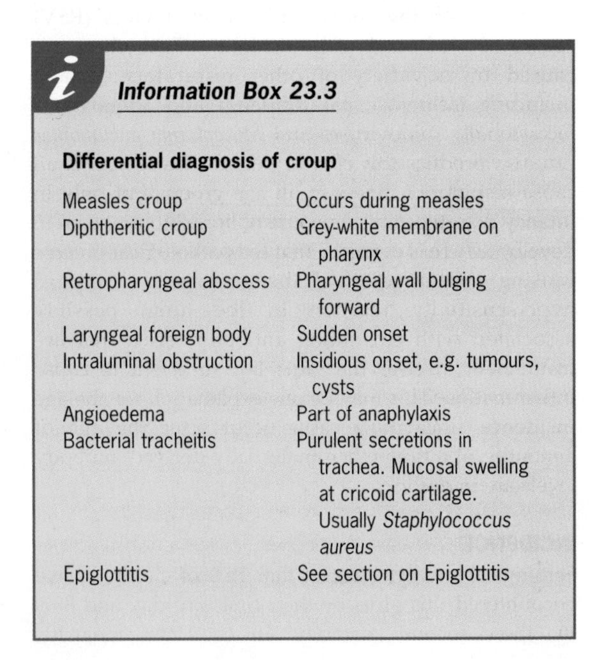

Information Box 23.3

Differential diagnosis of croup

Measles croup	Occurs during measles
Diphtheritic croup	Grey-white membrane on pharynx
Retropharyngeal abscess	Pharyngeal wall bulging forward
Laryngeal foreign body	Sudden onset
Intraluminal obstruction	Insidious onset, e.g. tumours, cysts
Angioedema	Part of anaphylaxis
Bacterial tracheitis	Purulent secretions in trachea. Mucosal swelling at cricoid cartilage. Usually *Staphylococcus aureus*
Epiglottitis	See section on Epiglottitis

Loeffler syndrome (eosinophilic pneumonitis)

In Loeffler syndrome there is a high eosinophil count with abnormal chest X-ray. The lungs are infiltrated with eosinophils and the child wheezes. Triggers include parasitic infections from larvae of the worm *Toxocara canis* from dogs and *Toxocara cati* from cats. Many other worms cause the syndrome in children in tropical countries. Drug reactions have also been implicated.

Pneumonia

Clinical significance
Pneumonia has displaced diarrhoea as the commonest cause of death in developing countries.
It remains a frequent cause for hospital admission in developed countries.

Pneumonia is an infection of the lung (see Information box 23.4).

Information Box 23.4

Infective causes of pneumonia

Bacterial
Streptococcus pneumoniae
Haemophilus pneumoniae
Staphylococcus aureus
Klebsiella pneumoniae
Pseudomonas aeruginosa
Legionella pneumophilia

Mycoplasmal
Mycoplasma pneumoniae

Viral
Respiratory syncytial
Parainfluenza
Adenovirus
Enterovirus
Rhinovirus
Influenza
Herpes simplex

Fungal
Pneumocystis carinii
Histoplasma sp.
Aspergillus sp.

Streptococcus pneumoniae (pneumococcus) is the commonest cause of bacterial pneumonia. The disease tends to be lobar in children, with bronchopneumonia in infants. Older children have an upper respiratory tract infection followed by a sudden onset of rigors, high fever, tachypnoea, unproductive cough and drowsiness alternating with restlessness. Signs of consolidation are present from the second day of the illness and the appearance of crackles (indicating return of aeration) is a sign of resolution. Infants have respiratory distress with cyanosis, less cough, abdominal distension (ileus and swallowed air) and meningism (especially from right upper lobe infections). Lung signs are less apparent than in older children. Pneumococci may be isolated from tracheal aspirate, blood, pleural fluid, and urine. Consolidation may be seen on X-ray before signs are present and after clinical recovery (Fig. 23.4).

Treatment is with penicillin G and oxygen. Resistant strains are occurring, particularly in Spain. The onset of *H. influenzae* pneumonia is slower than that of *S. pneumoniae*. The infection may spread to blood, pericardium, meninges and joints. There is no typical chest X-ray. Ceftriaxone is usually given as ampicillin resistance is increasing. *S. aureus* bronchopneumonia occurs mainly in infancy and may result in multiple lung abscesses. Onset of fever, cough and respiratory distress is sudden. The illness may be accompanied by shock, vomiting and diarrhoea. X-ray changes may involve an entire lung.

Pneumatoceles (acquired lung cysts) are characteristic of staphylococcal pneumonia but may occur in bacterial pneumonia of other causes. Treatment is with flucloxacillin or cephtriaxone.

K. pneumoniae tends to infect the immunocompromised or those with previously damaged lungs. The disease may begin with diarrhoea and vomiting with rapid formation of pulmonary abscesses and

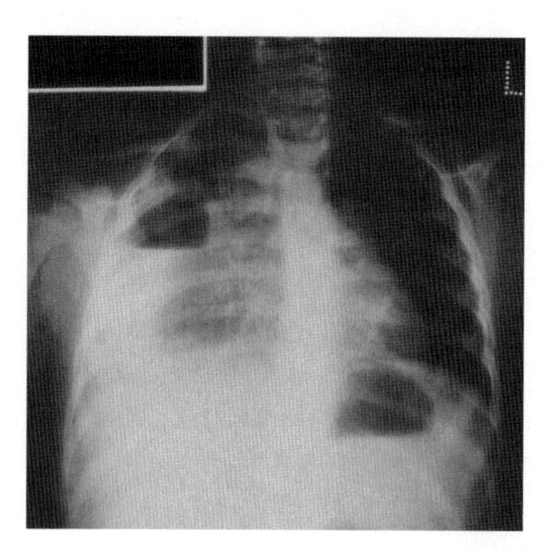

Fig 23.4
Staphylococcal pneumonia.

empyema. Ceftriaxone with gentamicin may need to be combined with drainage of abscesses and empyema.

P. aeruginosa produces a necrotizing bronchopneumonia in previously damaged lungs. Ceftazidine with an aminoglycoside is the best treatment.

M. pneumoniae causes tracheobronchitis and bronchopneumonia in school-age children and may precipitate an 'acute chest syndrome' in sickle cell anaemia. The signs and symptoms may resemble asthma or bronchiolitis. X-rays show unilateral opacities and hilar lymphadenopathy. Numerous possible complications may occur including Coombs positive haemolytic anaemia (due to production of cold haemagglutinins), Stevens–Johnson syndrome, Guillain–Barré syndrome and transverse myelitis. Culture of sputum may isolate *M. pneumoniae* but only after the first week of illness. Detection of cold haemagglutinins supports the diagnosis. Mycoplasma are sensitive to erythromycin.

Viral pneumonia may be difficult to distinguish from bacterial or mycoplasmal pneumonia, particularly as they may coexist. Wheezing is characteristic of RSV pneumonia. The chest X-ray may show a diffuse perihilar infiltrate. Ribavirin may be given to infants with RSV pneumonia who also have cystic fibrosis, other chronic lung disease or congenital heart disease.

P. carinii affects immunosuppressed children. The presentation is striking with insidious onset of increasing tachypnoea and cyanosis over 1–4 weeks. There are no added sounds. The X-ray shows a diffuse, granular appearance. Sputum obtained by bronchoalveolar lavage should be examined first for the parasite; bronchial washings or lung biopsies are often required to make the diagnosis. High dose cotrimazole and pentamidine are required. Pneumonia also follows aspiration of vomitus, baby powder and hydrocarbons.

Adenoidectomy and tonsillectomy

Adenoidectomy

Recurrent infections of the adenoids result in hypertrophy, and the enlarged adenoids obstruct the choanae and eustachian tube. Symptoms of adenoidal hypertrophy include:

- Mouth breathing
- Snoring
- Sleep apnoea
- Pulmonary hypertension
- 'Nasal' speech
- Otitis media.

Enlarged adenoids can be visualized by a bronchoscope or lateral X-ray of the postnasal space.

Adenoidectomy is performed for severe symptoms.

Tonsillectomy

Many symptoms are attributed to chronically infected tonsils, such as anorexia, poor weight gain and respiratory infections. The tonsils normally enlarge in childhood. Extremely enlarged tonsils can contribute to airway obstruction.

Throat infections decrease after tonsillectomy but also decrease without surgery. Severe haemorrhage can occur after tonsillectomy.

24 Rheumatology

Rheumatic disorders are relatively uncommon in children, and hence it is necessary to establish paediatric rheumatology services which assess children from a wide geographical area. This will optimize management of conditions such as juvenile chronic arthritis.

Inflammatory conditions

Juvenile idiopathic arthritis

Epidemiology
The incidence is 1 : 10 000 children; the prevalence is 1 : 1000.

INTRODUCTION

Juvenile idiopathic arthritis is a collection of diseases in which the joint lining (synovium) is chronically inflamed. It has been variously termed juvenile rheumatoid arthritis, juvenile chronic arthritis, Still disease, juvenile chronic polyarthritis and chronic childhood arthritis.

AETIOLOGY AND PATHOGENESIS

One possible aetiology is that the arthritis is the result of an undetected infection. For example salmonella, shigella, *Yersinia enterocolitica*, and campylobacter cause a reactive arthritis especially in patients with tissue type HLA-B27. *Borrelia burgdorferi*, the agent of Lyme disease, and mycoplasma also cause recurrent arthritis. Another possibility is that the disease is autoimmune. The rheumatoid factor of adult-onset rheumatoid arthritis is an autoantibody against IgG. In children, however, more than 90% are rheumatoid factor-negative.

The synovium is inflamed with an infiltration of lymphocytes and plasma cells. The synovial membranes extend into the joints as villi which adhere to the articular cartilage and eventually destroy it. Secretion of excess synovial fluid causes effusions.

CLINICAL PRESENTATION

Chronic juvenile arthritis is classified clinically into polyarticular (more than four joints involved; 30% of cases), pauciarticular (fewer than four joints; 50%), and systemic (20%).

Polyarticular

This is divided into two groups, rheumatoid factor-positive or -negative. The positive group has a worse prognosis. Many joints become stiff and swollen, often symmetrically. Pain is variable and may be absent. This type is much commoner in girls, usually in the adolescent age group.

Pauciarticular (Fig. 24.1)

The disease remains confined to four or fewer (usually large) joints for at least 6 months from onset. Type I is more common in girls and is associated with iridocyclitis. Type II usually occurs in boys and is associated with ankylosing spondylitis in association with tissue type HLA-B27. Ankylosing spondylitis causes back pain and stiffness and eventual loss of mobility of the spine.

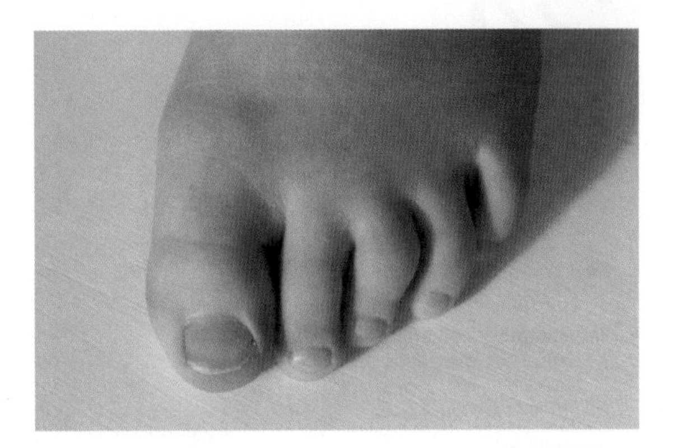

Fig 24.1
Juvenile idiopathic arthritis: pauciarticular. Knee and ankle also involved.

Systemic (Fig. 24.2)

This form is associated with high fever (often >40 °C), neutrophilia, hepatosplenomegaly, lymphadenopathy, pleuropericarditis, and multiple, small, pink macules on the trunk and proximal extremities that appear during febrile periods and rapidly fade. Arthritis is present but often not a constant feature at the onset. Later, in a proportion of patients, a destructive arthritis occurs.

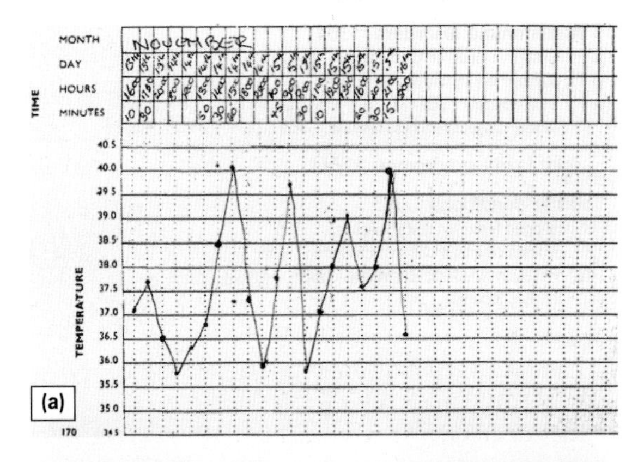

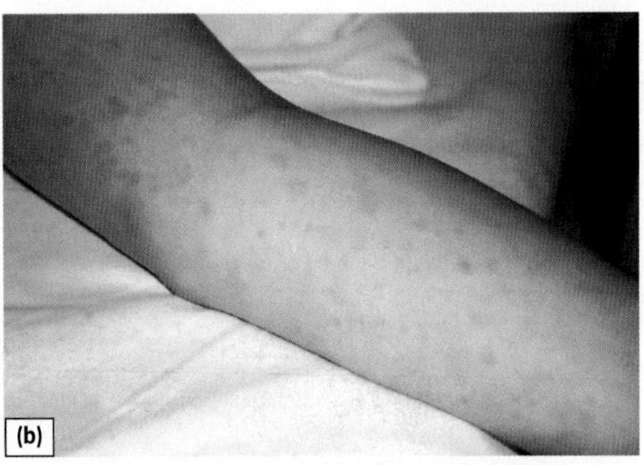

Fig 24.2
(a) Fever, and (b) rash, in systemic juvenile idiopathic arthritis.

DIAGNOSIS

The diagnosis is primarily clinical and requires that arthritis or other systemic symptoms have been present for a minimum of 3 months. The erythrocyte sedimentation rate (ESR), C-reactive protein and white cell count may be elevated and haemoglobin depressed, but not invariably. Any or all immunoglobulin classes may be elevated. The presence of antinuclear antibodies correlates with the presence of iritis. Rheumatoid factor is found in only 5% of children with juvenile chronic arthritis and carries a bad prognosis. The synovial fluid contains elevated numbers of neutrophils with low glucose and high protein. X-rays show narrowing of the joint space. Lyme disease should be considered, especially if the arthritis is pauciarticular, as well as viral arthritis, chronic inflammatory bowel disease and malignancy and leukaemia. The differential diagnosis of a monoarticular (single joint) arthritis is infection (especially tuberculosis) and malignancy.

MANAGEMENT

At least 75% of children with juvenile rheumatoid arthritis escape severe joint damage and hence the prognosis is good for most patients.

Systemic. Aspirin in doses sufficient to maintain blood levels of 200–300 mg/l is the mainstay of treatment. Intoxication is suggested by tachypnoea but not tinnitus, which is a rare side-effect in children. The aspirin should be withdrawn during chickenpox or influenza to avoid Reye syndrome. Steroids are best avoided, except for uncontrolled systemic disease and iridocyclitis unresponsive to topical steroids, as bone and cartilage destruction may be hastened.

Polyarticular and pauciarticular. Other non-steroidal anti-inflammatory agents such as ibuprofen are used, rather than aspirin. Methotrexate may be used to modify disease activity if there is no response to nonsteroidals, but little is known about possible long-term side-effects such as decreased fertility or induction of malignancy. Sulfasalazine, gold, D-penicillamine, hydroxychloroquine, and immunoglobulin may be tried; few of these agents have been tested by controlled trial in children and they are rarely used.

Iridocyclitis (Fig. 24.3). Treatment (in consultation with an ophthalmologist) is with topical steroids and mydriatics; systemic steroids are used if this fails. Parents should be encouraged to urgently report eye symptoms in their child.

In pauciarticular disease, iridocyclitis is often asymptomatic but permanent eye damage can still occur. Regular slit lamp screening is therefore essential.

Physical therapy. Exercise, and night splints are very important. Synovectomy and joint replacement may be required at a later stage.

General. A positive attitude is required, with encouragement to lead as normal a life as feasible.

Irritable hip

This inflammatory arthritis of unknown cause occurs unilaterally in children of less than 10 years old. It is self-limited except in 2–3% who develop Perthes disease.

There is pain, limited hip movement and low grade fever. Hip aspirate is normal.

The condition resolves with bed rest and analgesia.

Rheumatic fever

See Chapter 7, Cardiology, page 180.

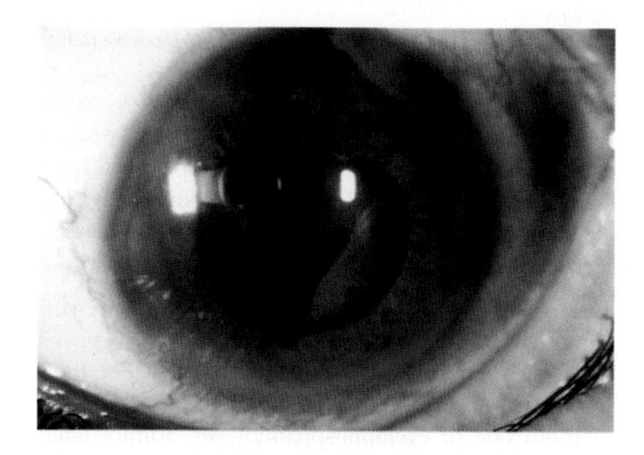

Fig 24.3
Juvenile idiopathic arthritis: chronic iridocyclitis. Note hypopyon (white cells at lower margin of cornea) and irregular pupil.

Vasculitides

Henoch–Schönlein syndrome

See Chapter 11, Gastroenterology, page 209.

Kawasaki syndrome

See Chapter 15, Immunology and infectious diseases, page 285.

Polyarteritis nodosa

This inflammatory condition of small and medium-sized arteries, of unknown cause, is rare in childhood.

An affected child is generally unwell, with fever, anorexia and weight loss. The arterial lesions can produce arthritis, myositis and skin lesions in the form of petechiae and ulcers. Interruption of the blood supply to nerves produces peripheral neuropathy, which may be of the mononeuritis multiplex type. The arterial involvement produces gastrointestinal bleeding, renal failure, cough, stroke and myocardial infarction.

High dose steroids and cytotoxic drugs are used to try to prolong survival.

Takayasu arteritis (pulseless disease)

This inflammatory process of the aorta and great vessels, of unknown cause, is associated with arthritis, pleurisy, pericarditis, fever and rashes.

It may cause ischaemia of kidneys and brain. Treatment is with steroids and arterial surgery.

Wegener granulomatosis (lethal midline granuloma)

This is a rare syndrome of chronic inflammation of the upper respiratory tract, of unknown cause. There is progressive destruction of the nasal septum and sinuses, and ulceration of the palate, pharynx, larynx and trachea. There is vasculitis of lungs and kidneys. The disease is treated with steroids and cyclophosphamide.

Autoimmune disorders

Systemic lupus erythematosus

Systemic lupus erythematosus occurs mainly in females, and is more severe in children than adults. The aetiology is unknown but it is associated with a variety of immune reactions. Antibodies are found against nuclei (antinuclear antibody), DNA, red cells, white cells and platelets. Immune complexes containing anti-DNA are deposited in glomeruli. Lupus-like illnesses can be triggered by exposure to drugs such as antiepilepsy drugs.

The rash is described as a 'butterfly', with the wings on the cheeks and the body over the nose (Fig. 24.4). Other manifestations are listed in Information box 24.1.

Non-steroidal anti-inflammatory drugs are used for arthritis. Most patients require systemic steroids and cytotoxic drugs. Cyclophosphamide has improved the prognosis; the 5-year survival is 90%.

Juvenile dermatomyositis

Dermatomyositis is a systemic disease of unknown cause associated with tissue type HLA-B8/DR3. It is less common than lupus erythematosus. In adults, but not in children, it is associated with malignancy. It is an inflammatory vasculitis of striated muscle, skin and gastrointestinal tract.

Clinical manifestations include:

- Stiffness, soreness and weakness, initially in the trunk and proximal muscles
- Nonpitting oedema of skin, progressing to atrophy, calcification and pigmentary changes

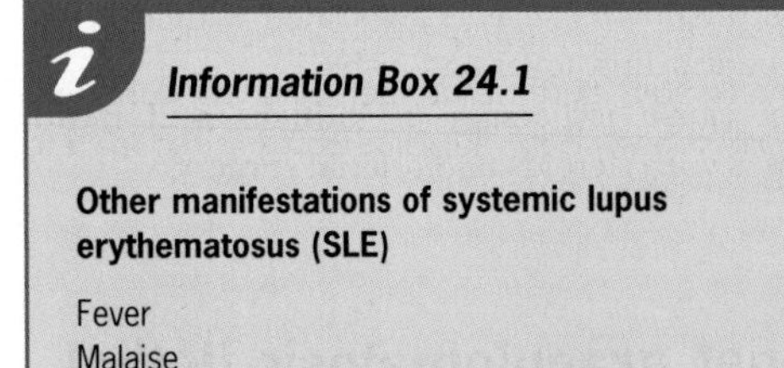

Information Box 24.1

Other manifestations of systemic lupus erythematosus (SLE)

Fever
Malaise
Arthritis
Purpura
Haemolytic anaemia
Pleurisy
Pericarditis
Peritonitis
Renal involvement
CNS involvement
Diarrhoea and vomiting

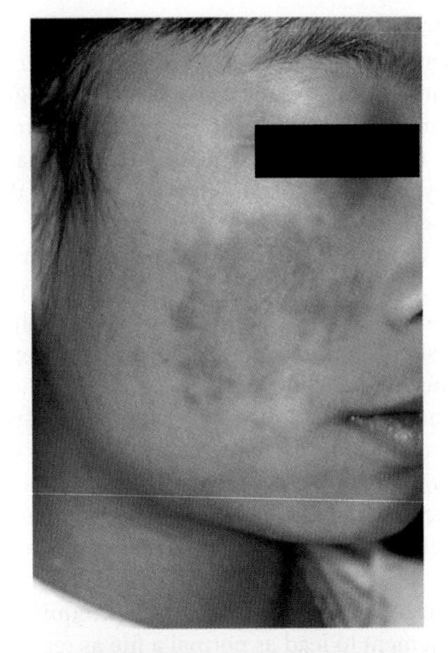

(a)

(b)

Fig 24.4
(a) 'Butterfly' rash in systemic lupus erythematosus. (b) Lupus-like rash induced by phenytoin.

- Violet (heliotrope) discoloration of upper eyelids and 'butterfly' rash (like lupus erythematosus)
- Abdominal pain, gastrointestinal bleeding, constipation.

Treatment is with prednisolone 1–2 mg/kg/day, with slow withdrawal as muscle strength improves. Salicylates are given as adjunctive therapy. For those who fail to respond to steroids, azathioprine, methotrexate or cyclophosphamide are administered. Physiotherapy is also used. Respiratory function and swallowing are monitored (for respiratory and pharyngeal muscle involvement). Death may follow pharyngeal or respiratory involvement and gastrointestinal haemorrhage.

The disease usually becomes inactive after several years; there may be residual contractures.

Scleroderma

In this chronic fibrosis of connective tissue of unknown aetiology, there may be localized skin involvement (morphoea, the commonest form in childhood), or generalized involvement including internal organs (systemic sclerosis). Morphoea consists of areas of shiny, atrophic skin which become fixed to underlying structures. In systemic sclerosis, the skin involvement is principally of face, hands, feet, and trunk. Raynaud phenomenon and ulceration of finger tips are associated. Oesophageal involvement causes dysphagia and aspiration.

Treatment includes:

- Physiotherapy to prevent contracture
- Avoidance of cold to prevent Raynaud phenomenon
- Corticosteroids, salicylates, cytotoxics, chloroquine and penicillamine, which have been tried without convincing effectiveness.

The involvement of heart, lungs or kidneys may be fatal.

Mixed connective tissue disease

The occurrence of a condition with features of systemic lupus, rheumatoid arthritis, scleroderma and dermatomyositis is know as mixed connective tissue disease. Symptoms are treated with corticosteroids, and physiotherapy is required for musculoskeletal involvement.

Joint laxity syndromes

Ligamentous laxity is common in children, and causes joint pain and sometimes swelling after exercise. The condition tends to improve with age. Management involves physical treatment to build up muscle strength, and reassurance that the condition is not a true arthritis.

(See also: Marfan syndrome, p. 245; Ehrlers–Danlos syndrome, p. 189; achondroplasia, p. 244, and Morquio syndrome, p. 289.)

Other conditions

Slipped femoral capital epiphysis

This is a stress fracture through the femoral capital epiphyseal growth plate, usually during the pubertal growth spurt before fusion. It occurs much more commonly in males, with an incidence of 1–4:100 000.

It is usually unilateral, and can follow trauma but the epiphysis may displace slowly in obese or rapidly growing individuals. Pain and limitation of movement are caused, and the X-rays show medial displacement of the epiphysis. The latter must be fixed, using pins, to prevent further slipping.

Nonspecific limb pains of childhood

This describes symmetrical pain in the lower legs, often coming on at night, and often referred to as 'growing pains'. Heat and massage may be effective. Limb X-rays may be required to exclude osteoma and reassure parents. There is no specific treatment but reassurance can help.

Reflex sympathetic dystrophy

In this condition a limb is immobilized by severe pain, caused by autonomic nervous dysfunction. Osteoporosis is associated. Physiotherapy is required to remobilize the affected part.

Osteochondritis

See Chapter 22, Orthopaedics, page 348.

Appendix 1: Therapeutics

At any one time around 20% of children are taking a prescribed medication. Most of these medications are used for respiratory conditions such as asthma.

Prescription and administration of drugs

General rules for prescribing

The same general principles of prescribing apply for children as for any groups of patients. These include:

- Use generic drug names.
- For most common purposes use a relatively small 'pool' of drugs with which you are familiar.
- Prescribe only when necessary. (Some groups of agents, including antitussives, should rarely, if ever, be used. It is better to treat the underlying cause.)
- Avoid, where possible, large numbers of drugs in the same patient (polypharmacy).
- Always check that the dosage is correct.
- Beware of drug interactions.

Paediatric prescribing: special points

1. Dosage

Children vary greatly in size. All drug doses administered systemically should be calculated according to size (not age).

- For children of less than 1 year, prescribe on a per kg basis.
- For children of more than 1 year, surface area (m^2) is the best measure (used for chemotherapy and some other drugs). Otherwise, prescribe on a per kg basis.

Information about dosage should be available in a paediatric prescribing manual of which there are many to choose from, for example Medicines for Children (1999) *Royal College of Paediatrics and Child Health*, London or under 'Child' in a standard National Formulary.

It is important to distinguish between total daily (24-hour) dose and individual dose (given more than once a day).

2. Prescribing in newborns

Particular care is needed because of:

- Immaturities in renal/hepatic function necessitating dose reduction and/or reduction in dose frequency
- Specific adverse reactions in neonates, for example chloramphenicol and the grey baby syndrome.

3. Unusual adverse drug reactions in young children

Children's responses to drugs are occasionally unexpected and at variance with the response of adults. Examples include:

• Chloramphenicol	Grey baby syndrome
• Aspirin	Reye syndrome
• Phenobarbitone	Stimulant (exaggerates hyperkinetic syndrome)
• Amphetamine family	Sedative

4. Drugs not licensed for paediatric usage

Drugs commonly used in adults may not be licensed for children. There are two possible reasons:

1. The drug has particular adverse affects or lack of efficacy in children.
2. There are not sufficient data on paediatric usage to merit a licence application for children.

In most circumstances the latter applies. It is sometimes necessary to use such agents when no alternative exists. In considering this it is important to ensure that there are no real contraindications, to obtain the best possible advice on dosage and to be certain that the parents and (if of a sufficient age) the child are aware of the situation (see Informed consent, p. 383).

Drug administration in children

Children may be resistant to the idea of being treated. Some are good medicine takers, others poor, and their general behaviour does not necessarily predict which will be the case.

Paediatric prescriptions should always specify the route of administration. This should be done after discussion with the parents and, for hospitalized patients, with experienced paediatric nursing staff.

There are a few general points:

1. The oral route is usually preferred. Reasons for not using this are:

- Drugs poorly absorbed
- Intestinal problems
  - Vomiting
  - Ileus
  - Obstruction
  - Diarrhoea/malabsorption
- Neurological problems
  - Coma
- The need to get rapid high blood levels of drug
  - Emergency treatment
  - Treatment of meningitis (high peak blood levels facilitate transfer across the blood–brain barrier).

2. Intramuscular injections are rarely used in paediatric practice. The intravenous route is preferred when possible.

3. A well-sited indwelling cannula is used for administering drugs intravenously. For longer-term treatments a central venous catheter is often employed. Great care should always be taken. Possible problems include:

- Extravasation of drug into the tissues which, depending on the drug in question and the pH of the solution, may cause severe tissue injury e.g. vincristine (used in lymphatic leukaemia). This may occur as a result of the child wriggling if the cannula is not securely placed. Strategies for treating such injuries may involve injection of saline with or without hyaluronidase to dilute and disperse the drug, or the injection of an anti-inflammatory agent such as hydrocortisone. Urgent expert advice from plastic surgeons and from a drug information department should be sought.
- Excessively rapid injection of a number of drugs may produce unexpected (usually cardiovascular) potentially serious side-effects. The manufacturers' guidelines on rates of infusion should always be followed.
- If the child is hypersensitive to the drug the intravenous route is likely to produce a more dramatic (possibly fatal) reaction than the oral route.

4. Other routes used in children include the rectal, sublingual and subcutaneous routes. The intrathecal route is used for the administration of chemotherapeutic agents in some childhood malignancies such as acute lymphoblastic leukaemia. Disasters have occurred as a result of the incorrect drug being administered by this route.

Fluid therapy

Approximate daily fluid requirements at different ages are given in Table A1.1. These will vary, depending on route of administration (generally less given intravenously than orally), environmental conditions, and the presence of a fever or other condition which increases insensible fluid loss.

Fluid therapy is needed:

- To maintain normal fluid requirements
- To replace deficits caused by
  - Inadequate intake
  - Excessive losses
- To support the circulation in shock states.

Oral rehydration therapy

This is discussed under acute diarrhoea in Chapter 11.

Intravenous fluid therapy

It should be remembered that the body is not designed to receive fluids by this route. Intravenous (i.v.) fluid therapy should therefore be regarded as being on a par with pharmacological therapy, and treated with respect. This is particularly relevant in young children who may become fluid overloaded very quickly.

Table A1.2 presents the types of intravenous fluid.

Treatment of dehydration

Most dehydration involves losses of both water and sodium. Therefore at least part of the rehydration should involve fluid from category 2 in Table A1.2. Colloids are used for resuscitation if the dehydration is severe enough to cause circulatory failure. Exceptionally, dehydration involves water only (diabetes insipidus, lack of fluid intake in preterm infants)

Table A1.1
Fluid requirements

Age range	Approximate daily requirement ml/kg bodyweight
0–6 months	150
6–12 months	120
1–3 years	100
3–7 years	90
7–12 years	70
Adult	50

This varies between individuals and with other factors such as environmental conditions and presence of fever.

Table A1.2
Types of intravenous fluid

Category	Constituents	Application
1. Colloid (Distribution restricted to vascular space, at least initially)	Albumin solutions Synthetic macromolecular preparations (encompassing polymers of glucose or amino acids) Blood products	Used for rapid expansion of the intravascular compartment (in shock due to hypovolaemia or sepsis); not in cardiogenic shock
2. Predominantly sodium-containing solutions (distributed predominantly throughout the extracellular fluid compartment)	Normal saline (154 mmol Na/l) 0.5 N saline (70 mmol Na/l) Hartmann solution (120 mmol Na/l)	Used for dehydration to replace extracellular fluid and sodium losses Used in shocked states if colloid is not available
3. Predominantly glucose-containing solutions (distributed throughout total body water)	5% or 10% dextrose 4% dextrose with 0.18 N saline (30 mmol Na/l) dextrose saline	Used for 'maintenance' i.v. fluid Dextrose saline normally used Replacement fluid in mild dehydration

leading to hypernatraemia. Although it might be considered that category 3 fluids are needed for this, in fact category 2 fluids should be used as they are safer and lessen the risk of 'rebound' swelling of the dehydrated intracellular fluid compartment causing, for example, cerebral oedema. Occasionally hypernatraemic dehydration also occurs in gastroenteritis in infants.

Calculating the degree of dehydration and therefore volume of rehydration fluid

This can be done in a number of ways:

1. Assessing the lost fluid by comparative weights – most accurate, but usually not available
2. Estimating percentage fluid loss (5, 10, 15%) dehydration from clinical signs.
   5% = mild dehydration
   5–10% = florid signs of dehydration
   10–15% = severe dehydration with circulatory compromise
   >15% = hypovolaemic shock
3. Estimating the response to fluid challenge: a good diuresis with dilute urine suggests absence of severe dehydration (assuming normal renal function)
4. Measurement of circulatory status
   - Peripheral–central temperature gap
   - Central venous pressure.

Times for correction of dehydration

Normo- or hyponatraemic dehydration (give normal maintenance fluid plus the deficit over 24 hours)	24 hours
Hypernatraemic dehydration (use solutions with relatively high sodium to prevent too rapid a drop in plasma sodium which could cause cerebral oedema) (give normal maintenance plus the deficit over 48 hours). Once circulation is restored, oral rehydration may be safer.	48 hours

General points about fluid therapy

- Always use a pump (never free flow) – overload happens quickly in children.
- Check drip site regularly.
- Ensure good splinting and bandaging to prolong life of cannula.

Appendix 2: Practical procedures in children

The term 'invasive procedure' is used in medicine to describe treatments, or more commonly, investigations which involve physically breaching the body's integrity, for example, to obtain biopsy materials. Sometimes there is a degree of risk attached. Generally speaking simple procedures such as venous blood sampling in adults are not considered invasive, but this may not be the case in a young child where even the simplest of procedures handled badly may be exceedingly traumatic for all concerned. There are a number of guiding principles in performing such procedures:

1. Consider whether the test is really necessary.
2. Offer a full explanation of the procedure to parents and child.
3. Ensure that samples to be collected are clearly listed beforehand so that there are no omissions necessitating a repeat procedure.
4. Decide on sedation/local anaesthesia beforehand with the parents and child.
   (a) For minor local procedures such as venesection, topical local anaesthetic creams are excellent, provided sufficient time is allowed for absorption into the skin.
   (b) For procedures which are not painful but require the child to remain still for prolonged periods (e.g. some forms of radioisotope scanning), a simple sedative will usually suffice (e.g. chloral hydrate, sedative antihistamines, or both).
   (c) For painful (or uncomfortable) procedures, a much more potent sedative and an analgesic are required. Some of those involving opiates are potentially dangerous and require medical supervision of the child. A short general anaesthetic administered by an experienced anaesthetist may be safer and guaranteed is to work.
5. Decide beforehand with the parents whether or not they will remain present throughout. They should be warned precisely what will happen. Preferably they should be seated. (Even the most outwardly stoical have been known to faint!)
6. Make sure all lighting and equipment is set up beforehand.
7. Maintain a confident approach with the child.

The particular techniques involved are mostly similar to those used in adults but with smaller equipment. Two common procedures which differ significantly in children are described here.

Lumbar puncture

- Fine disposable needles are used.
- Local anaesthetic injection (which would use a needle of similar size) is usually unnecessary.
- Routine lumbar punctures, e.g. for administering chemotherapy in leukaemia, are usually performed under a general anaesthetic.
- The test is always performed with the child lying on his/her side on a firm surface, to avoid any lateral flexion of the spine.
- The assistant holds the child in a flexed 'knee to chin' position to open up the interspinous spaces.
- Post-lumbar puncture headache, not infrequent in adults, is relatively rare in children.

Urine collection

Obtaining a clean uncontaminated urine specimen may be difficult in young children and newborn infants. A number of techniques are used.

Bag collection

- This is used mainly in very young children in nappies, who cannot urinate on request.
- The perineum and genitalia are carefully washed to reduce colonizing bacteria.
- A specially designed polythene bag with an adhesive top is applied over the perineum. The bag has upper and lower chambers connected by a small hole, so that ideally when urine is passed it can reach the lower chamber where it is not in contact with the perineum; in practice this does not always happen.
- The bag is checked frequently, and removed as soon as possible after urination to lessen bacterial contamination and multiplication in the warm nappy environment.
- A small removable tab at the bottom of the bag allows the urine to be transferred to a pot.

'Clean catch' method

- This is the nearest thing to a midstream specimen in young children.
- It is used in young children who are potty trained.
- It can also be used in 'nappy age' children; a wide necked pot is kept ready when the nappy is being changed.
- Contact of receptacle with perineal skin is avoided.
- Successful collection is easier in boys, but can be achieved in girls.

Suprapubic aspirate (SPA)

- This is used in newborns and infants up to 6 months of age, but should not be attempted in older children.
- It is performed when the bladder is full (determined by percussion of the abdomen and/or the presence of a dry nappy).
- The infant is held supine on the couch with legs extended.
- A standard 5-ml syringe with a standard hubbed needle is used.
- The needle is inserted vertically in the midline just above the pubic symphysis to a depth of 2–3 cm. It is then aspirated and withdrawn at the same time until urine appears.
- Passes of the needle should always be in the vertical plane only. No more than two passes should be made at any one time.

The problems with interpreting the results of urine samples obtained by these various methods are discussed in the section on urinary tract infections (see Chapter 17, Nephrology and urology, p. 297).

Appendix 3: Screening for disorders of growth

Normal growth is a sensitive index of wellbeing in every child and it is, therefore, essential to identify abnormal patterns of growth at an early stage.

Suboptimal growth may be an indicator of endocrine dysfunction, such as growth hormone deficiency or Cushing syndrome, or it may be an early sign of an intracranial tumour or systemic disease, such as Crohn or coeliac disease.

Early fall-off in growth may be picked up by careful community screening, and it is currently recommended that every child has a measurement of weight, supine length and head circumference at birth and 3, 6, 12 and 18 months.

Standing height should be measured at 2, 3 and 5 years, and most growth specialists would in addition suggest further measurements of height at 7, 9, 11 and 13 years, although this is not currently routine practice. It is essential to interpret any measurement of height with parental height, and if possible measured or reported heights of parents should be plotted on the child's growth chart.

United Kingdom Child Growth Standards were published in 1994, to replace the charts first compiled by Tanner & Whitehouse in 1965. The new charts are significantly different and take into account an average 1.5-cm increase in the height of children throughout the UK since the data for the original charts was collected. In addition, puberty appears to occur earlier. The significance of this upshift should not be lost, since several thousand children who have been regarded as 'normal' for at least the last 10 years may now be presenting with concerns about their growth. It must be stressed that these standards are based on the indigenous British population and do not, therefore, include centiles for ethnic communities. Non-caucasian children continue to be assessed under the generalization that Asians are smaller and lighter and Afro-Caribbeans are taller and heavier than the British caucasian.

Any child whose height falls below the 0.4th centile or above the 99.6th centile should be referred to a paediatrician, as should any child who is inappropriately tall or short with regard to his parents. A child whose growth curve crosses one centile line between two measurements should be reviewed, and referred at the next measurement if the trend continues. If two centile lines are crossed between one pair of measurements then referral should be made. When a growth problem is suspected, parameters such as height, parental heights, weight and birthweight, help trace the reasons behind any shortfall in growth. A child with a height less than 3 standard deviations below the mean has a 50% chance of having an organic cause for their short stature. The new charts advising the 0.4th centile as a cut-off should help in the detection of children with underlying pathology, while at the same time ensuring children are not referred unnecessarily for specialist investigation.

It is clearly important in older children to take into account pubertal status, as constitutional delay in growth and puberty will often present at around 11 or 12 when the children become conspicuously shorter than their peers who are in true puberty at an average time.

Screening investigations include an assessment of skeletal maturation, that is to say bone age, karyotype (particularly in any short, slowly growing girls who may have Turner syndrome), blood count, biochemistry and thyroid function. Any child who suddenly stops growing should have MRI or CT to exclude an intracranial tumour. More sophisticated assessment of underlying dysfunction of the hypothalamo–pituitary axis should be undertaken only in a specialist centre.

In any child who appears to be growing slowly for no obvious reason, one must always consider the possibility of emotional or physical abuse. In severe abuse, children may have symptoms of hypothalamic dysfunction, such as polydipsia, polyuria and hyperphagia, all of which resolve when the child is removed from the adverse environment.

With any child who is tall or growing abnormally quickly one must consider the possibility of premature sexual maturation, and at every assessment the child's secondary sexual characteristics must be assessed; central precocious puberty can present as early as 18 months.

Growth disorders – some possible diagnoses	
Small for chronological age	growth delay
Chronic diseases	for example, renal failure, coeliac disease, Crohn disease, cystic fibrosis
Abnormal karyotype	chromosome abnormalities, e.g. Turner or Down syndrome
Russell–Silver syndrome	low birthweight, asymmetry and dysmorphism
Abnormal hypothalamo-pituitary function	endocrine disorders, i.e. growth hormone insufficiency, hypothyroidism, Cushing syndrome, premature sexual maturation, emotional/physical/sexual abuse
Bony dysplasia	for example, achrondoplasia, hypochrondoplasia
Inappropriately tall stature	constitutional tall stature, Marfan, Klinefelter or Sotos syndromes
Precocious puberty	

Girls' growth chart 0–1 yr © Child Growth Foundation

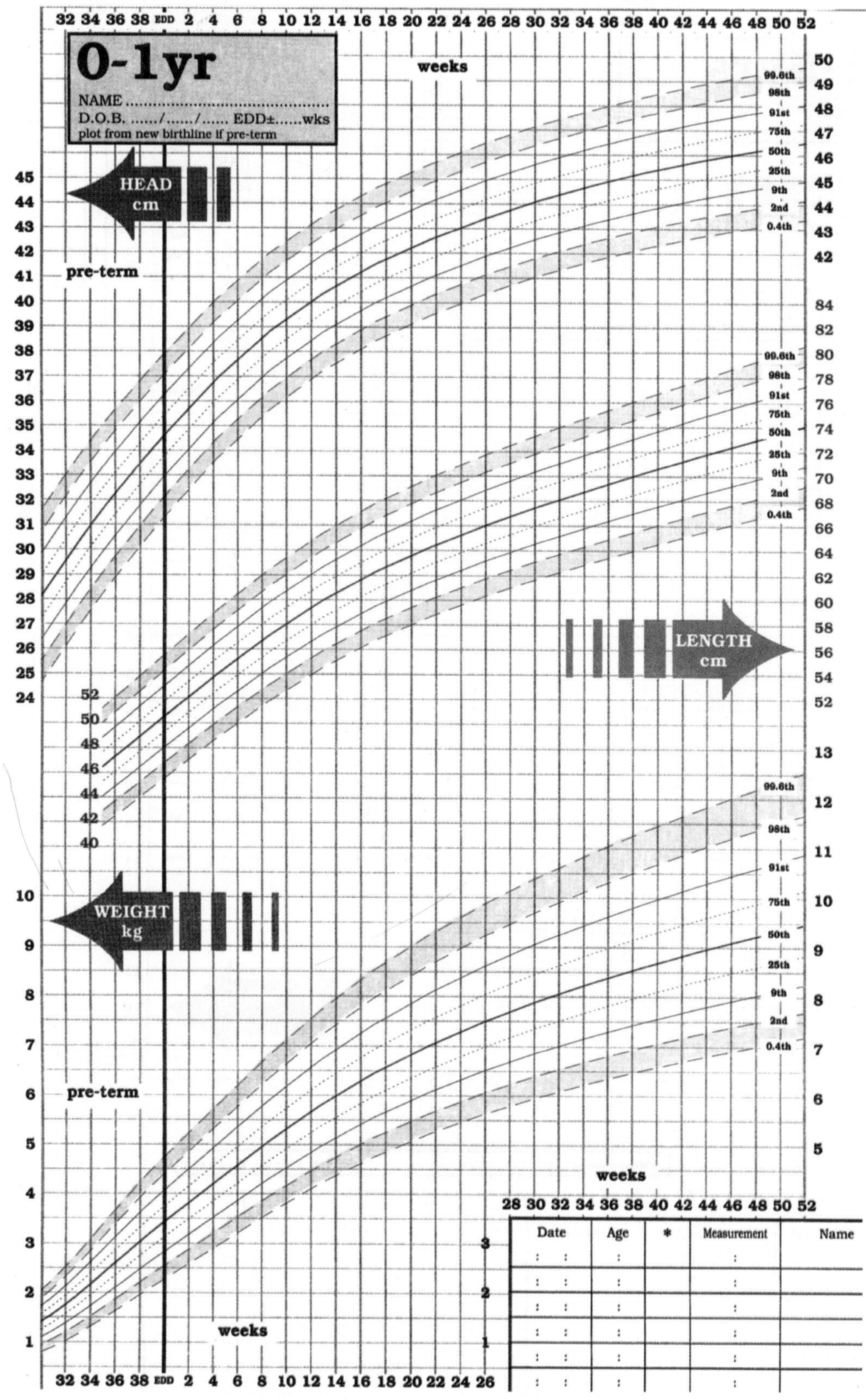

Date	Age	*	Measurement	Name
: :	:		:	
: :	:		:	
: :	:		:	
: :	:		:	
: :	:		:	
: :	:		:	

Girls' growth chart 1–5 yr © Child Growth Foundation

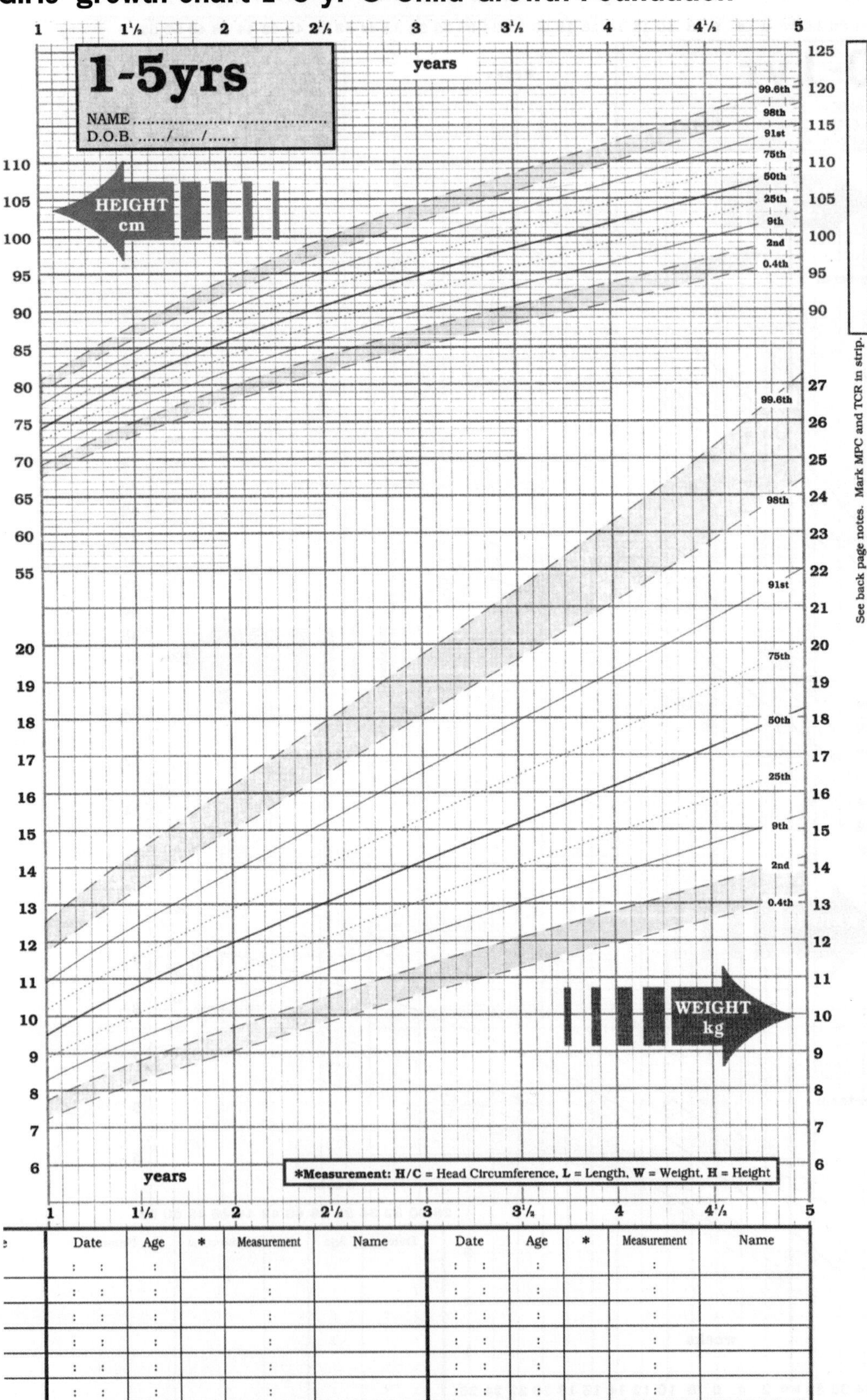

Date	Age	*	Measurement	Name	Date	Age	*	Measurement	Name
: :	:		:		: :	:		:	
: :	:		:		: :	:		:	
: :	:		:		: :	:		:	
: :	:		:		: :	:		:	
: :	:		:		: :	:		:	
: :	:		:		: :	:		:	

Girls' growth chart 5–18 yr © Child Growth Foundation

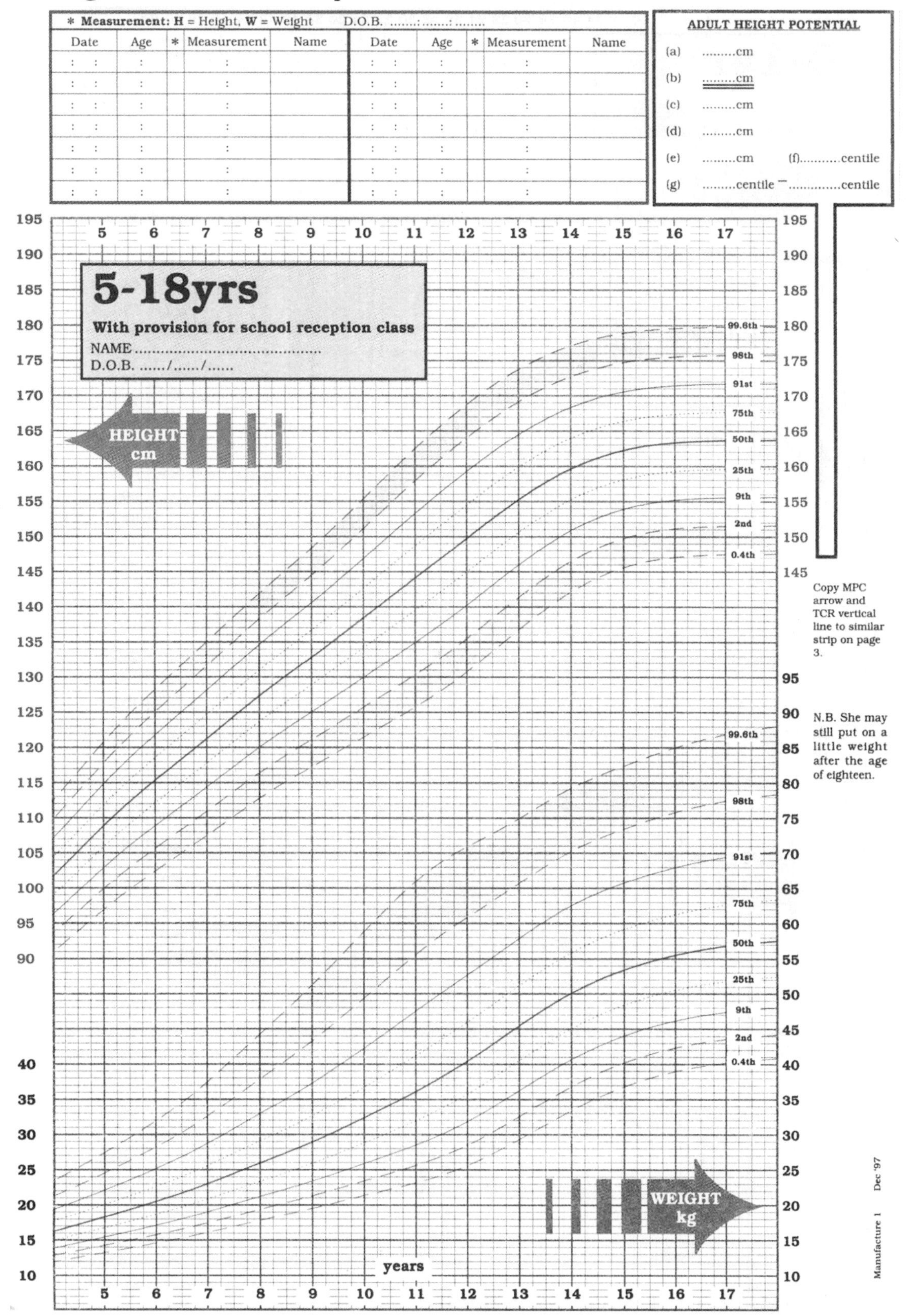

Boys' growth chart 0–1 yr © Child Growth Foundation

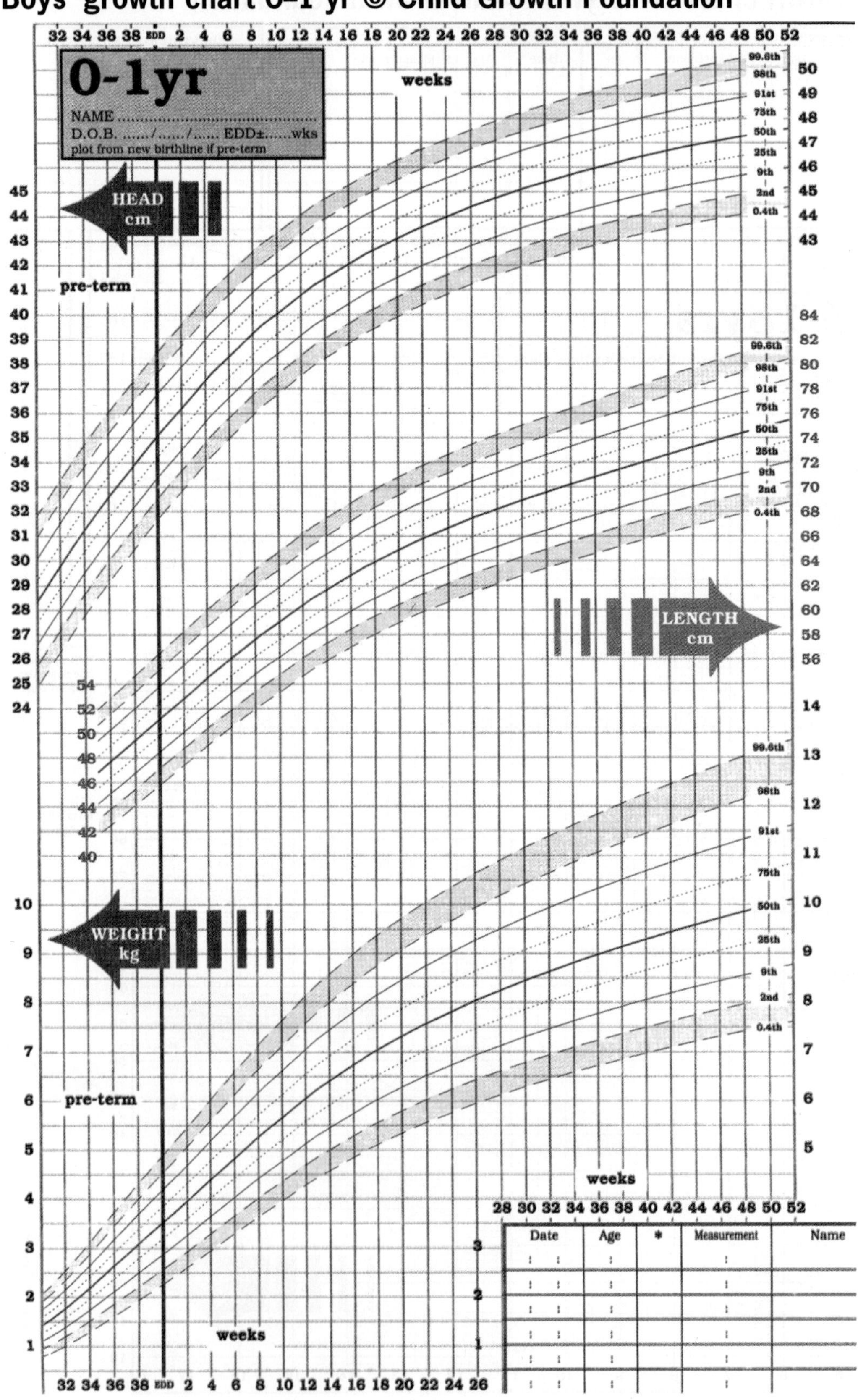

Boys' growth chart 1–5 yr © Child Growth Foundation

1 1½ 2 2½ 3 3½ 4 4½ 5

years

1-5yrs

NAME ....

D.O.B. ....../....../......

HEIGHT cm

130 125 120 115 110 105 100 95 90 85 80 75 70 65 60

99.6th 98th 91st 75th 50th 25th 9th 2nd 0.4th

See back page notes. Mark MPC and TCR in strip.

WEIGHT kg

27 26 25 24 23 22 21 20 19 18 17 16 15 14 13 12 11 10 9 8 7 6

99.6th 98th 91st 75th 50th 25th 9th 2nd 0.4th

years

*Measurement: H/C = Head Circumference, L = Length, W = Weight, H = Height

1 1½ 2 2½ 3 3½ 4 4½ 5

Date	Age	*	Measurement	Name	Date	Age	*	Measurement	Name
: :	:		:		: :	:		:	
: :	:		:		: :	:		:	
: :	:		:		: :	:		:	
: :	:		:		: :	:		:	
: :	:		:		: :	:		:	
: :	:		:		: :	:		:	

Boys' growth chart 5–18 yr © Child Growth Foundation

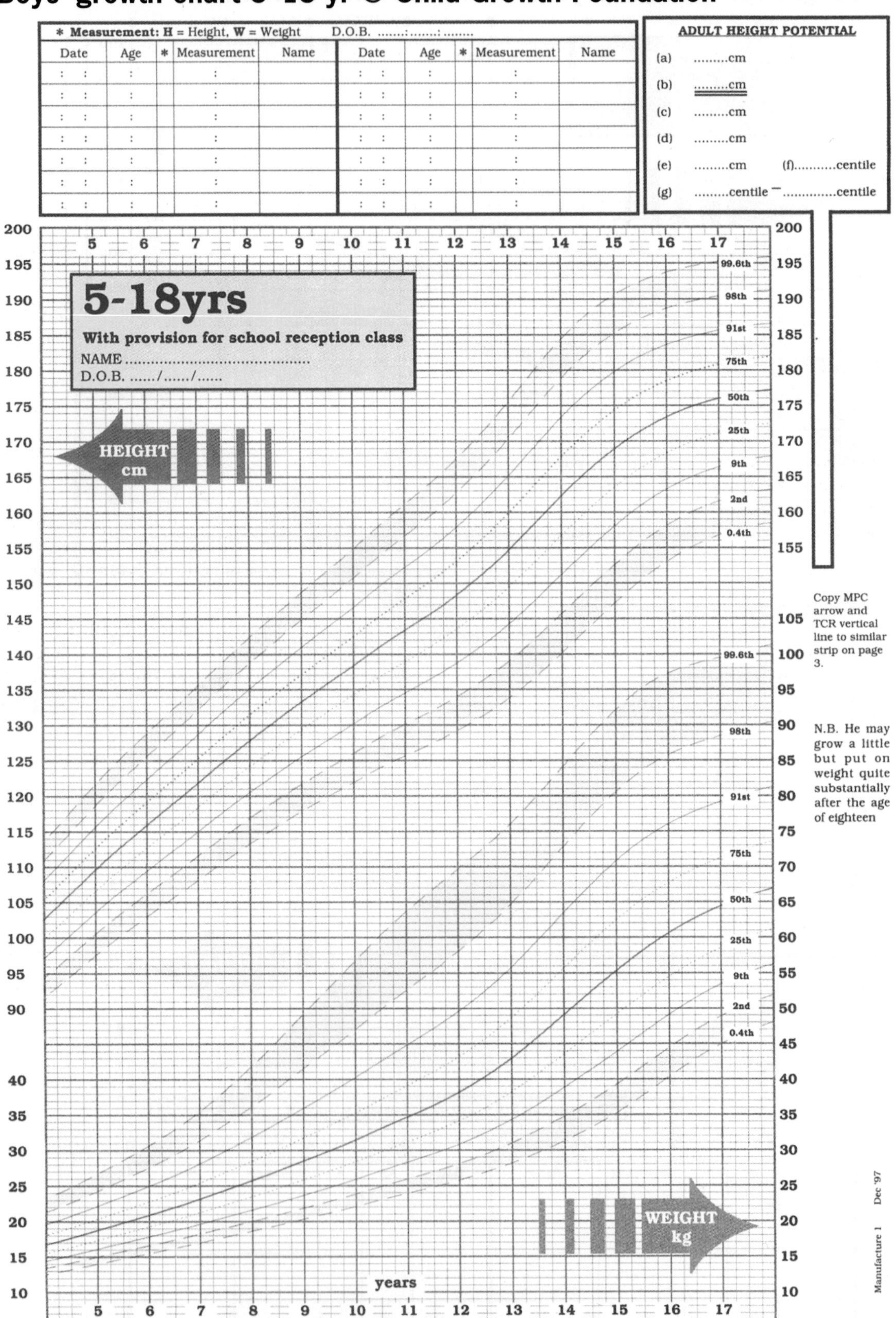

Appendix 4: Informed consent

This issue was addressed in the Children Act (1991). This states that children who are considered old enough to understand the issues, should be involved in the process of giving consent for medical procedures, trials, etc. This age will vary from child to child and from issue to issue. The age question is potentially one which would be the subject of legal debate in litigation cases.

In the USA an age limit of 9 years is defined for consent (for any procedure). In practice, involving children means that they give their assent rather than consent and it is not common practice (nor good practice) to insist that minors sign consent forms, this should remain the prerogative of the parents/guardians.

It is the responsibility of paediatric doctors and nurses to ensure that the child is given every opportunity to understand and assent to the issues involved.

Clinical trials on children

Traditionally new modalities of treatment are tried out initially on adult patients. While this is understandable, it does mean that children who might benefit from such treatments are deprived of them for long periods of time or sometimes altogether. Many paediatricians believe that this should not be the case and children should be involved in such trials from an early stage. To ensure that children are not misused in the name of medical research there are a number of guiding principles:

- There must be a clinically important question which needs to be answered and is of major importance to children.
- The trial should be conducted by personnel trained specifically in the care of children (doctors and nurses).
- Sample collection and other painful/uncomfortable procedures should be kept to a minimum that answers the research questions.
- As well as parental informed consent the informed assent of the child should be sought (when the child is of sufficient age to understand the issues – see above).

Local Research Ethics Committees should take particular care in assessing projects especially with regard to the above points and a national Multicentre Research Ethics Committee (MREC) has been set up to consider multicentre research studies.

Index

Page numbers in **bold** refer to main discussions, and in medical conditions include aspects such as epidemiology, aetiology and pathogenesis, clinical presentation, diagnosis and treatment

A

B

D

H

I

J

K

L

M

N

Q

R

S

T

U

V

W

X

Z